THE
PATELLOFEMORAL
JOINT

NOTICE

THE
PATELLOFEMORAL
JOINT

Edited by

James M. Fox, M.D.
Wilson Del Pizzo, M.D.

Southern California Orthopedic Institute
Van Nuys, California

McGraw-Hill, Inc.
Health Professions Division

New York   St. Louis   San Francisco   Auckland   Bogotá   Caracas
Lisbon   London   Madrid   Mexico   Milan   Montreal   New Delhi
Paris   San Juan   Singapore   Sydney   Tokyo   Toronto

THE PATELLOFEMORAL JOINT

1 2 3 4 5 6 7 8 9 0 KGPKGP 9 8 7 6 5 4 3 2

ISBN 0-07-021753-X

This book was set in Melior by Monotype Composition, Inc. The editors were
Jane E. Pennington and Peter McCurdy. The production supervisor was
Clare Stanley. The text and cover were designed by Marsha Cohen/Parallelogram
and the index was prepared by Elizabeth Babcock-Atkinson.

Library of Congress Cataloging-in-Publication Data

The Patellofemoral joint / edited by James M. Fox, Wilson Del Pizzo.
    p.   cm.
  Includes bibliographical references and index.
  ISBN 0-07-021753-X
  1. Patellofemoral joint—Wounds and injuries.   2. Patellofemoral
joint—Diseases.   3. Patellofemoral joint—Surgery.   I. Fox, James
M.   II. Del Pizzo, Wilson.
  [DNLM: 1. Joint Diseases.   2. Knee Joint.   3. Patella.
4. Patella—injuries.,   WE 870 P295]
RD561.P38 1993
617.5′82—dc20
DNLM/DLC
for Library of Congress   92-48244
                                                     CIP

CONTENTS

v

SECTION III

Malalignment / 123

SECTION IV

Non-Osseous Lesions / 177

SECTION VIII

Rehabilitation / 279

SECTION IX

Surgical Technique / 305

SECTION X

Case Presentations / 351

CONTRIBUTORS

NOTE: The numbers in brackets refer to the chapters written or co-written by the contributor

Richard A. Berger, M.D.   *[3]*
Orthopaedic Surgery Resident
Department of Orthopaedic Surgery
University of Pittsburgh

Philippe Cartier, M.D.   *[20]*
Director of Orthopaedic Surgery,
Clinique des Lilas
Paris, France

Richard A. Cautilli, M.D.   *[8]*
Clinical Instructor
  of Orthopaedic Surgery
Thomas Jefferson University

G. Cerullo, M.D.   *[12]*
Radiology Department
Ospedale S. Maria di Collemagio
L'Aquila, Italy

M. Cipolla, M.D.   *[12]*
Clinica Valle Givlia
Rome, Italy

Marlene De Maio, M.D.   *[21]*
Former Fellow, Louisiana State University

F. De Paulis, M.D.   *[12]*
Radiology Department
Ospedale S. Maria di Collemagio
L'Aquila, Italy

Wilson Del Pizzo, M.D.   *[18]*
Southern California Orthopedic Institute
Van Nuys, California

Andrew L. Deutsch, M.D.   *[5]*
Attending Radiologist, Cedars-Sinai Medical Center
Associate Clinical Professor of Radiology
University of California, San Diego
San Diego, California

David J. Drez, Jr., M.D.   *[21]*
Clinical Professor and Head
Louisiana State University Knee and Sports
  Medicine Fellowship Program
Lake Charles, Louisiana

Mary Dutka, RN, MS   *[13]*
Massachusetts General Hospital
Surgical Day Care Unit

Scott F. Dye, M.D.   *[1]*
Assistant Clinical Professor of Orthopaedic Surgery
University of California, San Francisco
San Francisco, California

Robert A. Eppley, M.D.   *[9]*
Berkeley Orthopaedic Medical Group
Consultant, University of California, Berkeley
Berkeley, California

J. Whit Ewing, M.D.   *[25]*
Crystal Clinic, Akron, Ohio
Professor of Orthopaedics
Northeastern Ohio Universities College of Medicine

Richard D. Ferkel, M.D.   *[26]*
Clinical Instructor of Orthopedic Surgery
UCLA School of Medicine
Chief of Arthroscopy Section
Wadsworth VA Hospital, Los Angeles
Attending Physician
Southern California Orthopedic Institute
Van Nuys, California

Marc J. Friedman, M.D.   *[27]*
Attending Physician
Southern California Orthopedic Institute
Van Nuys, California
Assistant Clinical Professor of Orthopedic Surgery
UCLA School of Medicine

Freddie H. Fu, M.D.   *[3]*
Blue Cross of Western Pennsylvania Professor of
  Orthopedic Surgery
Vice Chairman/Clinical
Department of Orthopedic Surgery
Chief, Division of Sports Medicine
University of Pittsburgh

John P. Fulkerson, M.D. *[8]*
Professor of Orthopaedic Surgery
University of Connecticut School of Medicine
Medical Director, Sport Rehabilitation Center
University of Connecticut Health Center
Head Team Physician, Hartford Whalers
(National Hockey League)

Ronald P. Grelsamer, M.D. *[20]*
Assistant Professor of Orthopaedic Surgery,
Columbia University
Clinical Director—Knee Division
Orthopaedic Research Laboratory
Columbia-Presbyterian Medical Center

Letha Y. Griffin, M.D., Ph.D. *[23]*
Staff Physician, Peachtree Orthopaedic Clinic
Clinical Instructor, Emory University School of
Medicine

Jeffrey L. Halbrecht, M.D. *[7]*
Private Practice
California Orthopedic
and Sports Medical Group
San Francisco, California

Thomas Helpenstell, M.D. *[19,28]*
Fellow, Orthopedic Surgery
Orthopedic and Fracture Clinic
Eugene, Oregon

Jack C. Hughston, M.D. *[4]*
Clinical Professor
Tulane University School of Medicine
Department of Orthopaedics
Chairman, Hughston Sports Medicine
Foundation, Inc.
Columbus, Georgia

Mary Isham, M.D. *[19,28]*
Orthopedic Surgeon,
Kaiser Permanente Hospital
Santa Clara, California

Douglas W. Jackson, M.D. *[7]*
Medical Director
Southern California Center for Sports Medicine

Robert W. Jackson, M.D. *[22]*
Chief, Department of Orthopaedics
Baylor University Medical Center
Dallas, Texas
Clinical Professor of Orthopaedics, University of
Texas
Southwestern Medical Center

Lanny Johnson, M.D. *[29]*
Clinical Professor of Surgery
Mississippi State University

Ronald P. Karzel, M.D. *[18]*
Attending Physician
Southern California Orthopedic Institute
Van Nuys, California

Gregory C. R. Keene, MBBS *[11]*
Director, Sportsmed SA (Orthopaedic Division)
Adelaide, Australia

L. Andrew Koman, M.D. *[17]*
Professor, Department of Orthopaedic Surgery
The Bowman Gray School of Medicine of Wake
Forest University

Cato T. Laurencin, M.D., Ph.D. *[13,14]*
Clinical Fellow in Orthopaedic Surgery
Massachusetts General Hospital, Harvard Medical
School
Boston, Massachusetts
Instructor of Biochemical Engineering
Division of Health Sciences and Technology
Massachusetts Institute of Technology
Cambridge, Massachusetts

Henry J. Mankin, M.D. *[2]*
Chief of Orthopaedic Service
Massachusetts General Hospital

Howard J. Marans, M.D., M.Sc. *[11]*
Staff Orthopaedic Surgeon
Fountain Valley Regional Hospital
Irvine Medical Center
Hoag Memorial Hospital

Alan C. Merchant, M.D. *[10]*
Clinical Professor of Surgery, Orthopaedic Division
Stanford University School of Medicine
Stanford, California
Active Staff Surgeon
Department of Orthopaedic Surgery
El Camino Hospital
Mountain View, California

Lyle J. Micheli, M.D. *[6]*
Director, Division of Sports Medicine, Children's
  Hospital
Boston, Massachusetts
Past President of the American College of Sports
  Medicine

Jerrold H. Mink, M.D. *[5]*
Director, Magnetic Resonance Imaging Services,
  Cedars-Sinai Medical Center
Medical Director, Tower Musculoskeletal Imaging
  Center

Todd J. Molnar, M.D. *[24]*
Attending Physician
Southern California Orthopedic Institute
Van Nuys, California

Dinesh Patel, M.D. *[13,14]*
Assistant Clinical Professor of Orthopaedic Surgery
Associate Orthopaedic Surgeon
Chief of Arthroscopic Surgery Unit
Massachusetts General Hospital, Harvard Medical
  School

Lonnie E. Paulos, M.D. *[15]*
The Orthopedic Specialty Hospital
Co-Director, Orthopedic Biomechanics Institute
Associate Clinical Professor
University of Utah School of Medicine

John L. Pinkowski, M.D. *[15]*
Northeast Ohio Orthopaedic Associates
Northeast Ohio Sports Medicine Institute
Instructor in Orthopaedic Surgery
Northeast Ohio Universities College of Medicine
Akron General Medical Center Campus

Gary G. Poehling, M.D. *[17]*
Department of Orthopaedic Surgery
The Bowman Gray School of Medicine of Wake
  Forest University

F. Edward Pollock, Jr., M.D. *[17]*
Resident, Department of Orthopaedic Surgery
The Bowman Gray School of Medicine of Wake
  Forest University

Giancarlo Puddu, M.D. *[12]*
Sports Orthopaedic Surgeon
Professor of Biomechanics at I.S.E.F.
Rome, Italy

Michael J. Seel, M.D. *[3]*
MD/PhD Candidate
Department of Orthopaedic Surgery
University of Pittsburgh

Frank G. Shellock, Ph.D. *[5]*
Department of Radiology
Cedars Sinai Medical Center
Tower Musculoskeletal Imaging Center
Assistant Professor of Radiological Sciences
UCLA School of Medicine

Kenneth M. Singer, M.D. *[19,28]*
Clinical Assistant Professor Surgery
Orthopaedic/Rehabilitation
Oregon Health Sciences University
Eugene, Oregon

Neal L. Thomson, MBBS *[16]*
Consultant Orthopaedic Surgeon
Mater Misericordiae Hospital
Longueville Private Hospital
Sydney, Australia

Akihiro Tsuchiya, M.D. *[13,14]*
Research Fellow in Orthopaedic Surgery
Massachusetts General Hospital
Harvard Medical School

FOREWORD

Almost 45 years ago, when I was an instructor in anatomy at Duke University Medical School, the renowned Professor Joseph Markee (honorary member AAOS) assigned to me the patellofemoral joint as one of my projects for instructing the freshman class. It is amazing that since that time the complexities of this joint have continuously and progressively become recognized, so that we now, here, have an entire book dedicated solely to the patellofemoral joint.

The patellofemoral joint is center stage for the extensor mechanism. It is free floating with an automatic transmission. It is our greatest weight-bearing joint, serving as the decelerator (brake) for the weight and velocity of the entire body. The complexity of the extensor mechanism lies in its dynamic interaction with the entire lower extremity. One must see the big picture. The big picture reaches from the hip to the foot. A mildly weak hip abductor results in an almost imperceptible Trendelenburg gait requiring slight internal rotation and adduction of the thigh to place the knee and foot under the more central point of weight load of the pelvis. The stress at the knee results in anteromedial patellofemoral pain. Or, in the athlete, it may result in overcompensation by the iliotibial apparatus, resulting in anterolateral knee pain that can be confused with the so-called lateral patellar compression syndrome. Remember, the active iliopatellar ligament attaches to the lateral aspect of the patella.

A tight hamstring, nothing more, requires increased compensatory extensor mechanism forces which result in anterior patellofemoral pain. Tight heel cords induce a slightly flexed-knee gait with increased strain and painful malfunction of the patellofemoral complex.

Malalignment of the lower limbs becomes simple to recognize compared to the dynamic dysfunctions.

Then we look with more focus on the knee itself and see all sorts of disability (patellar tendinitis, quadriceps tendinitis, Osgood-Schlatter disease, patellofemoral malacia, synovial plica irritation, etc.) resulting from patella alta, which produces an inadequate braking surface for repetitious, forceful deceleration.

A careful history and physical are paramount. Fortunately, treatment decisions infrequently need to be hurried and a majority of malfunctions respond to rehabilitation. Incorrect rehabilitation is recognized by resultant increased pain and disability. The rehabilitation can be easily changed and corrected, whereas a hurried and misapplied surgical intervention adds greatly to the complexity of an already complex system and often is very difficult to correct.

The orthopaedic clinician is presently suffering through the proliferation and confusion of instrumentation, mechanization, and all sorts of moving radiographics. If he chooses to use these for supportive and scientific purposes, all well and good. However, these exciting technological advances should hardly ever supercede a smart clinical evaluation.

Clinical practices of orthopaedics vary; however, in my practice I have shown that patellofemoral problems characterize a little more than 50 percent of the knee problems we see in our clinic. The incidence is obviously high.

The text of this book is comprehensive and covers examination, physiology, anatomy, radiography, rehabilitation, and surgery (the last resort). Each chapter is authored by a recognized expert with a history of long, sustained worry and experience with the patellofemoral joint.

This text will be a timely and valuable contribution to the literature. I can't say much more in this foreword for fear that my generalities will get me into trouble with the learned authorities and their specific contributions herein.

Remember, this is a complex joint. Its complexity is in its dynamics.

Jack C. Hughston, M.D.

PREFACE

Problems of the patellofemoral joint have been the most difficult area in the care of the knee joint. This subject is frustrating, not only for the orthopaedic surgeon but for the patient who suffers as well.

In this text, authorities in many areas of orthopaedics shed light on the many and diverse problems of the patella and extensor mechanism of the knee. The text has been divided into various sections as a matter of organization and for rapid referencing by the reader.

Many operations have been developed for extensor mechanism problems. Dr. Jack Hughston has stated for many years, "There is no problem that cannot be made worse by surgery." Among problems with the knee, this dictum is never more relevant than when approaching difficulties with the extensor mechanism. Thus, we discuss not only the various surgical techniques but also emphasize the importance of diagnosis and nonoperative care.

This text can truly be dedicated to those patients and orthopaedic surgeons who have suffered with the patellofemoral joint and in so doing blazed new trails of knowledge. It is on that experience which we try today to continue forward.

ACKNOWLEDGEMENTS

Appreciation to Ms. Eleanor O'Brien, Research and Publications Coordinator at Southern California Orthopedic Research and Education (S.C.O.R.E.), for her tireless efforts in collating the vast amount of verbiage submitted to her and trying to maintain all of us on the appropriate time schedule; Mr. Christopher Richter, in the Audiovisual Department of S.C.O.R.E., for his diligent efforts in the chapters requiring audiovisual aids; Dr. Jane Pennington, Senior Medical Editor of the Health Professions Division of McGraw-Hill, for her patience and understanding in dealing with physicians, whose deadline priorities often are not the same as publishers'; the physicians and staff of the Southern California Orthopedic Institute, where professionalism, dedication, and caring have made it an honor to be a partner; and lastly, to our families, the Del Pizzos—Sharon, Andrea, Kristin, Diana, and Wilson—and the Foxes—Ellen, David, Josh, and Lisa—for their patience, understanding, love and support.

CHAPTER 1

Patellofemoral Anatomy

Scott F. Dye

INTRODUCTION

The human knee, one of the most complex systems in the biologic realm, functions in concert as a type of biologic transmission or torque converter. In this mechanical analogy, the ligaments act as linkages within the transmission, meniscal and articular cartilage surfaces as bearings, and the muscles function as living engines and brakes. This system is designed to accept and redirect high loads—on the order of magnitude of multiples of body weight.[1,2,3] That the highest compressive and tensile loads of the knee are withstood by the patellofemoral components is reflected in its design. The patellofemoral system (as well as the whole knee comprised of approximately 100 billion vertebrate cells) has an asymmetrical structural form with, for example, typically greater surface area of the lateral facet and femoral trochlea (L., "pulley") (Fig. 1-1) and greater bulk and distal insertion of the medial musculature (Fig. 1-2). This chapter presents the functional anatomy of the patellofemoral joint, detailing appropriate facts of the evolution and embryological development of the patellofemoral system and a layer-by-layer anatomical description of the multiple structural constituents.

EVOLUTION

The overall asymmetrical design of the knee is extremely ancient in origin. The major components of this system, with the exception of the patella, were probably well established more than 300 million years ago.[4] According to the fossil evidence so far discovered, the patella evolved as an independently derived characteristic in many mammalian, avian, and reptilian knees (some lizards) about the end of the Cretaceous period, 65 million years ago. The pa-

tella must be considered, therefore, a rather late evolutionary addition to the tetrapod knee compared to the cruciate ligaments or menisci. However, the current importance of the patellofemoral system to knee function is significant because of its continued pres-

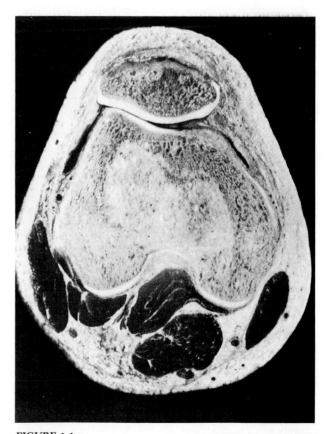

FIGURE 1-1
A coronal section of the knee through the midpatella, revealing an asymmetrically longer lateral patellar facet and femoral trochlea. [From W. Müller, 1983, (Ref. 19), with permission.]

ence across a broad spectrum of tetrapod orders. Even in some mammalian species where an osseous patella is absent, such as the red kangaroo (*Macropus rufus*), a fibrocartilage pad with the form of a bony patella is present.[5] The tetrapod knee evolved in flexion, and the patella of most species functionally remains well within the confines of an often symmetrical femoral trochlea. In humans, who are bipedal and plantigrade, however, the knee is frequently loaded in or near full extension. Thus, the patella is often positioned *superior* to the trochlear cartilage resting on a fibrofatty pad with synovial lining over the distal nonarticular femur.

The patella can be considered the largest of all sesamoid (Gr., "sesame-shaped") bones.[6] It is not uncommon for soft tissues, such as tendons, placed in a biomechanical environment of frequent compression, tension, and friction, to become thickened with ossification taking place, resulting in sesamoid structures. These systems are thus able to withstand high repetitive loading by providing a larger bearing surface as well as protecting the tendon from possible structural failure due to abrasion. In addition, the patella acts as a type of biomechanical lever arm increasing the effective extension capacity of the quadriceps musculature, particularly in the midrange of knee flexion.

EMBRYOLOGY

In the human knee the patella and trochlea form by enchondral ossification (Figs. 1-3 and 1-4).[7–9] The anlage of the patellofemoral components can be traced to the pelvic limb buds. The joint space of the patellofemoral component is the first to form. The patella typically lies more proximal initially in the region of the future suprapatellar pouch and later descends to its eventual position.[8] Cihak and Puzanova[10] noted that the tendon of the rectus femoris forms *anterior* to the patella and continues distally, connecting with the patellar tendon from the inferior pole. They also commented that the vastus medialis and vastus lateralis connect to the patella through tissue "disks" with only the vastus intermedius inserting directly into the patella along its proximal border. As Doskocil[8] has observed, even in these initial stages of development, the patella (and corre-

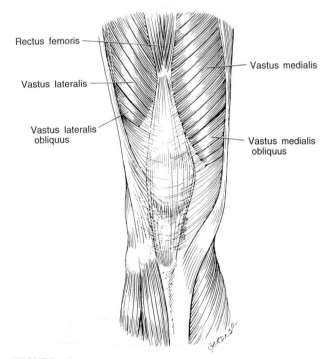

FIGURE 1-2
Anterior rendering of the right knee, manifesting a more distal insertion for the vastus medialis compared to that of the vastus lateralis.

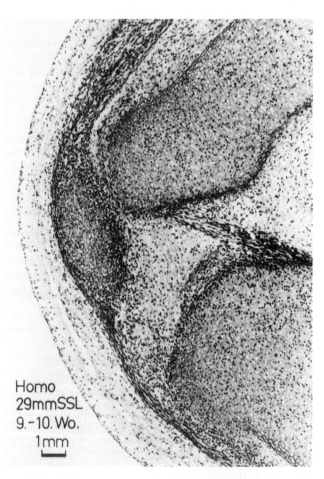

Homo
29mmSSL
9.–10. Wo.
1mm

FIGURE 1-3
Sagittal section of a 9- to 10-week-old embryo at the proximal part of the patellofemoral joint. [From W. Müller, 1983, (Ref. 19), with permission.]

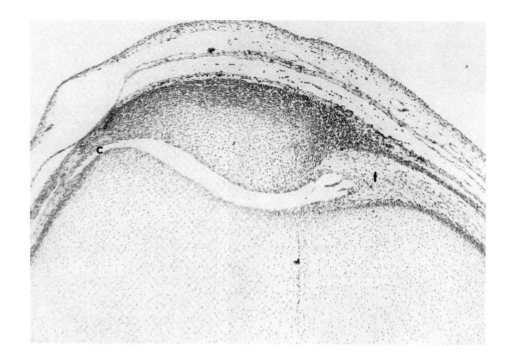

FIGURE 1-4
Coronal section of a 9- to 10-week-old embryo showing the cartilaginous patella in relationship to the distal femur. Mesenchymal tissue (t) is located medially whereas cavitation (c) is noted more laterally. *[From Ogata, 1990, (Ref. 9), with permission.]*

sponding articular surfaces of the femur) is already markedly asymmetrical. Maldevelopment of the patellofemoral components during these early stages could result in conditions such as patella alta (failure of the normal patellar descent), patella hypoplasia, and congenital dislocation of the patella leading to later ambulatory dysfunction.

The knee of a 24-week fetus prepared with an enzyme clearing technique[11] is shown in Figs. 1-5*A* and 1-5*B*. The distal femur, proximal tibia, and patella are seen as translucent blue cartilage, and the bone of the femur and tibia diaphysis is seen as red.

The patella typically begins to ossify from a single center by age three, with completion of ossification in females by age ten and males by age thirteen to sixteen.[12] Multiple centers of secondary ossification can occur laterally, which may become clinically manifest in adulthood as symptomatic bipartite patellae.

The tibial tubercle develops as an outgrowth of hyaline cartilage that in the fetal period grows progressively more distal to become positioned anterior to the metaphysis. At about the sixth postnatal month, a growth plate develops by invasion of fibrovascular tissue forming the tibial tuberosity.[13] Eventual fusion of the tuberosity to the proximal tibia does not usually occur until the sixteenth to eighteenth year. The tibial tubercle is a complex structure under tremendous tensile loading during activities of daily life. Physiologic or structural failure of this system, particularly during adolescence (e.g., Osgood-Schlatter), is a common occurrence.

PATELLOFEMORAL ANATOMY

Despite its seemingly simple construction, the anatomy of the patellofemoral joint is, in fact, one of the more highly complex regions of the knee that has defied accurate description to date. Much controversy exists in the literature regarding the anatomy of the patellofemoral system, especially the fascial, tendon, and ligamentous components. Not only is there disagreement in the terminology of these soft tissue structures, but there is also disagreement regarding their shape, origin, insertion, and even existence.[3,14–20] An attempt will be made in this chapter to provide an accurate depiction of these complexities based on a synthesis of the available literature and on dissections of multiple fresh adult cadaver knees.

Dissection of Soft Tissue Layers

One of the problems with describing the soft tissue anatomy of the anterior knee is that often the layer of one component is connected through dense fibrous tissue to the next layer (in essence, "spot welded"), making dissection of the two nearly impossible. With the caveats stated above, this depiction of the patellofemoral anatomy will proceed layer by layer from superficial to deeper structures as one might encounter them in a fresh cadaver dissection.

Subcutaneous Layer

Little subcutaneous fat or few fascial cutaneous ligaments are usually found directly over the patella and

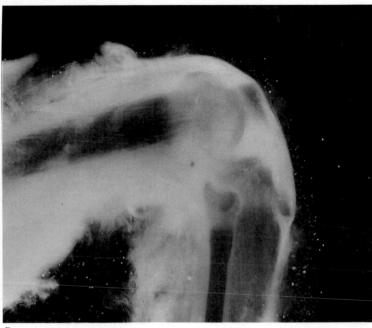

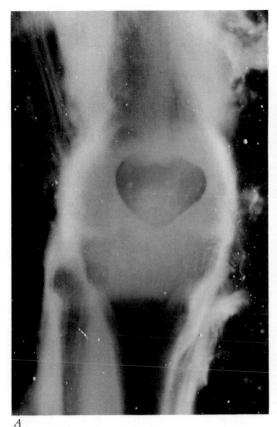

A   B

FIGURE 1-5
A. The anterior view of a 24-week-old human fetus with the cartilage stained with halcyon blue and the bone with alizarine red. (Prepared by the method of Dingerkus). *B.* The lateral view of a 24-week-old human fetus with stained cartilage and bone. Note the distal extension of the tibial tubercle cartilaginous anlage. (The white dots are bubble artefacts within the glycerine suspension solution.)

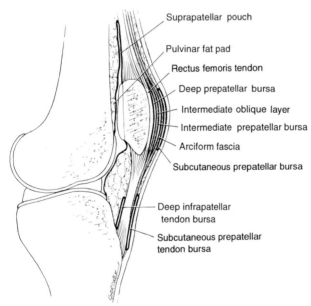

Suprapatellar pouch

Pulvinar fat pad

Rectus femoris tendon

Deep prepatellar bursa

Intermediate oblique layer

Intermediate prepatellar bursa

Arciform fascia

Subcutaneous prepatellar bursa

Deep infrapatellar tendon bursa

Subcutaneous prepatellar tendon bursa

FIGURE 1-6
Schematic representation of bursae about the anterior knee, including the subcutaneous prepatellar bursa, intermediate prepatellar bursa, deep prepatellar bursa, subcutaneous prepatellar tendon bursa, and deep infrapatellar tendon bursa. The tissues over the anterior patella have been enlarged to show detail.

in the patellar tendon region. Typically this area is composed mostly of loose areolar tissue. The skin is thus highly mobile over the deeper structures, allowing for a tremendous range of movement without restriction. The number of the small perpendicular fascial cutaneous ligamentous connections increases further medially and laterally from the patella. (This is easily distinguishable clinically by comparing the skin differential movement.) The region anterior to the patella between the skin and superficial fascia is a zone of potential fluid collection and volume expansion and constitutes the subcutaneous prepatellar bursa (L., "wineskin"), one of at least four bursae about the patellofemoral system (Fig. 1-6). These bursae are notoriously variable both anatomically and clinically. A separate subcutaneous prepatellar tendon bursa can exist that may or may not communicate with that over the patella.

Superficial Fascia—The Arciform Layer

The most superficial fascia over the anterior patella has been termed an extension of the fascia lata[21] and has been described as the arciform layer by Kaplan[22] and others[15,18] because the fiber orientation is mostly transverse "arcing" over the anterior knee. (I prefer the term *arciform layer*.) This most superficial fascial layer of transverse fibers covers the iliotibial band, the distal muscles of the quadriceps and the patellar tendon, becoming less dense and ending at about the level of the tibial tubercle (Fig. 1-7*A*). These are the fibers transected in harvesting the patellar tendon for an anterior cruciate ligament reconstruction. One can also find at this level, proximal to the patella, multiple circumferential fibers I call "hoop" fibers.

Intermediate Oblique Layer

In my experience there frequently exists a fascial layer anterior to the patella that is called the *intermediate oblique layer*. It can easily be found in fresh dissections or at surgery in many knees by carefully incising and reflecting the arciform layer proximal to the inferior pole of the patella. This layer is somewhat thicker than the arciform layer and is composed of fibers contributed by the anterior-most rectus femoris, vastus medialis, and vastus lateralis. The fibers blend into the deeper layers just medial and lateral to the patellar margins. The intermediate oblique layer typically ends distally at the level of the inferior pole of the patella and, unlike the next deepest layer, seemingly does not contribute fibers to

the patellar tendon (Fig. 1-7*B*). This layer is often the same as the patellotibial ligaments connecting the patella both medially and laterally to the anterior tibia. The potential space between the arciform layer and this intermediate layer constitutes an intermediate prepatellar bursa. The intermediate layer can be completely absent in some individuals.

Deep Longitudinal Layer

The next deepest layer is primarily composed of the longitudinal and distal expansion over the anterior patella of the rectus femoris tendinous fibers (Fig. 1-7*C*). This layer is extremely adherent, with multiple fibrous connections into the bone of the anterior patella such that it cannot be peeled off easily, even with a scalpel. The fibers of this layer are contiguous with the patellar tendon from the inferior pole and continue distally to insert over the broad area of the tibial tubercle. Some fibers in this layer are also contributed by the vastus medialis and vastus lateralis. The space between this layer and the next superficial layer constitutes the deep prepatellar bursa.

Deep Transverse Layer

Part of the important *static* guidance and limiting components of the patellofemoral system, i.e., the

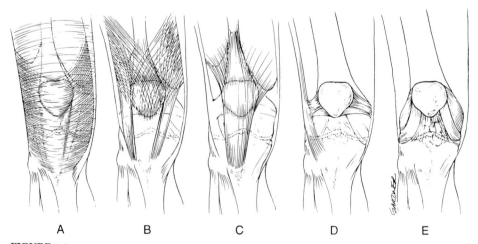

A B C D E

FIGURE 1-7
A. A line drawing of the superficial arciform layer with mostly transverse orientation of fibers over the patella and patellar tendon. *B.* A line drawing representation of the intermediate oblique layer with chevron-oriented fibers from the rectus femoris, vastus medialis, and vastus lateralis covering the patella and ending at the level of the inferior pole. This is at the same layer as the medial and lateral patellotibial ligaments. *C.* A deep longitudinal layer comprised primarily of the continuation of the longitudinal rectus femoral fibers, which are extremely adherent to the anterior surface of the patella and continuing distally to blend in with the fibers of the patellar tendon. *D.* A deep transverse layer comprised of the lateral transverse retinaculum, which blends in with the deep fibers of the iliotibial band and the medial transverse retinaculum that inserts in the region of the medial femoral epicondyle. *E.* A deep capsular layer revealing condensations termed the *medial* and *lateral patellomeniscal ligaments*. This is the deepest layer of the transverse bracing system.

deep transverse structures, forms the medial and lateral *retinacular* system (L., "rope" or "cable," from L. *retinere*, "to restrain"). The depiction of the anatomy of this layer is quite controversial. I believe that the descriptions of Blauth and Tillmann[20] are most accurate. The lateral transverse ("horizontal" in their terminology) retinaculum passes deep to the iliotibial tract to blend with this structure without necessarily inserting directly into the femur (Fig. 1-7*D*). The medial transverse retinaculum, although more variable in consistency does insert into the region of the medial femoral epicondyle.

Deep Capsular Layer

Condensations of the medial and lateral capsule from the patella to the medial meniscus and lateral meniscus constitute supportive ligaments that form the deepest layer of the transverse bracing system (Fig. 1-7*E*). The insertion of these structures to the middle region of meniscus is consistent, while anterior meniscal insertions are less common.

Quadriceps Muscle Group

The quadriceps muscle group is a complex asymmetrical system composed of the rectus femoris, rectus intermedius, vastus medialis, and vastus lateralis that functions most often, according to Hughston et al.,[23] in normal ambulation as a decelerator through eccentric contraction. The rectus femoris component has insertions to the superior border of the patella and continues distally over the anterior surface, becoming contiguous with the fibers of the patellar tendon. Deep to the rectus femoris is the rectus intermedius, whose muscle fibers surround the anterior distal femur (Fig. 1-8). The tendinous insertion of the rectus intermedius is to the greatest surface area of the superior border of the patella. These fibers do not insert directly into the patellar bone but through a zone of uncalcified and calcified fibrocartilage (Fig. 1-9). This cartilage transition zone is felt to diffuse forces over the entire attachment site, thus minimizing local stress concentrations.[24] A similar fibrocartilage transition zone is found at the distal patellar pole and tibial tubercle. The broad undersurface of the quadriceps tendon has been shown by Goodfellow et al.,[1] to contact the femoral trochlea and condyles and thus share in the transmission of load beyond 90 degrees of flexion.

The vastus medialis usually has greater bulk and inserts more distally than the vastus lateralis. Typically, it inserts at the superior medial patellar border with occasional insertion to the level of mid-patella. The most distal fibers of the vastus medialis are now well recognized as a separate grouping of muscle cells with a more semitransverse orientation of fibers (averaging approximately 65 degrees to the long axis of the femur).[23] These fibers clearly function as dynamic medial stabilizers of the patella when the knee is close to full extension (Fig. 1-10).

Weinstabl et al.,[17] have demonstrated that nerve fibers to the vastus medialis obliquus (VMO) are distinct and separate from the vastus medialis. They also describe an areolar fascial plane separating the VMO from the vastus medialis.

The vastus lateralis orients more longitudinally and has a long tendinous insertion to the superior lateral patellar border. As Hallisey et al.,[14] and Weinstabl et al.,[17] have described, a similar separate vastus lateralis obliquus also commonly exists for this muscle (Fig. 1-10). The *articularis genu* muscle, deep to the vastus intermedialis, originates on the distal anterior femoral diaphysis and inserts into the superior capsule of the suprapatellar pouch. This muscle is thus believed to retract the suprapatellar pouch with active contraction of the quadriceps (Fig. 1-11).

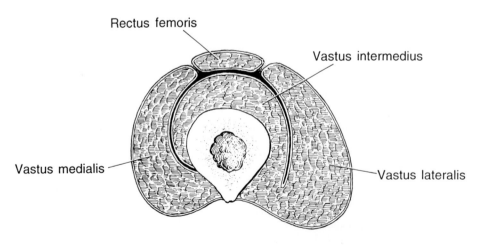

FIGURE 1-8
Schematic representation of the anatomical relationship of the quadriceps muscles at the level of the distal femur.

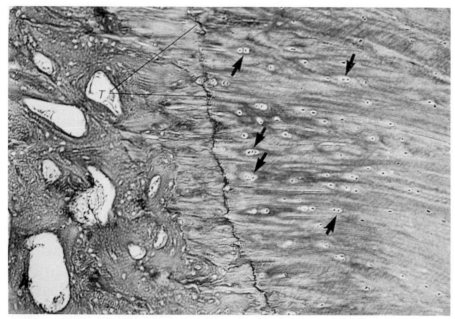

FIGURE 1-9
Section of the attachment to the proximal patella of the quadriceps tendon. Arrows indicate numerous cartilage cells in the zone of uncalcified fibrocartilage, T indicates the tidemark. Masson's trichrome, ×80. [From Evans et al, 1990, (Ref. 24), with permission.]

Patellar Tendon Anatomy

The patellar tendon, one of the largest collagenous structures of the body, is designed for the transmission of high tensile loads. The fibers originate from a broad area of the inferior pole, including the posterior surface of the patella, and blend with the anterior rectus fibers described previously. There is an equally broad region of insertion of the patellar tendon fibers to the tibial tubercle. Deep to the patellar

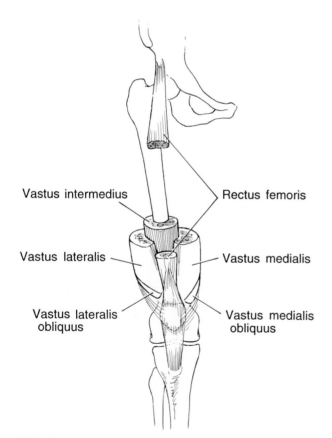

FIGURE 1-10
Representation of the separate muscle groups of the vastus medialis obliquus and vastus lateralis obliquus of the distal quadriceps muscle group.

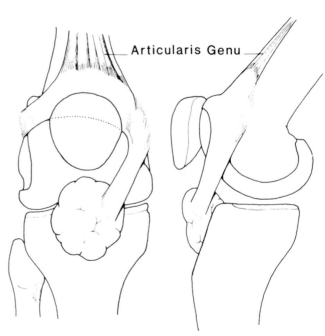

FIGURE 1-11
Schematic drawing of medial parapatellar and suprapatellar plica as well as articularis genu. [From Hughston, Walsh, and Puddu, 1984, (Ref. 23), with permission.]

tendon at the level of the anterior tibia proximal to the tibial tubercle exists the deep infrapatellar bursa. Arthrofibrosis of this zone can be a significant factor in limitation in range of motion after surgery.

Patellar Anatomy

The complex osseous and cartilaginous design of the patella reflects its function as the mobile central point of application of multiple forces. The slightly convex anterior surface has perforations for vascular structures and fibrous insertions of the rectus femoris. The superior pole is relatively flat and sloped posteriorly, accepting the fibers of the rectus and intermedius. The *nonarticular* inferior pole comprises a full one-quarter of the length of the patella. The gentile chevron configuration serves as a region of progressive transition of load via the patellar tendon fibers. The posterior cartilaginous surface is divided into asymmetrical zones with the lateral facet longer and separated from the medial facet by the rounded central ridge. A more vertical "odd" facet is adjacent to the medial facet, which articulates with the medial femoral condyle only in extreme flexion (Fig. 1-12).

Anatomists often describe the patellar articular cartilage as the thickest of the body, commonly extending 5 mm or more from the subchondral bone.[25,26]

It usually becomes thinner with age.[27] The articular cartilage attaches to the subchondral bone through the tidemark zone and a deeper calcified cartilage layer (Fig. 1-13). These layered transition regions are thought to be important in the transmission and dampening of high compressive loads withstood by the patella during normal activities.

The internal osseous design of the patella is not homogeneous.[28–31] The trabecular architecture is described by Townsend and others[28,30] as anisotropic with a design of sheets and struts (Fig. 1-14). The local stiffness of the bone varies throughout the patella with the more proximal region exhibiting greater stiffness than the mid and distal regions.

Intracapsular Synovium and Patellar Plicae

Synovial cells line the intracapsular region of the knee joint. Under normal circumstances, these cells produce a minimal amount of synovial fluid. The suprapatellar pouch extends far proximal to the superior pole of the patella. This zone can be partially or completely separated from the rest of the knee by a suprapatellar plica (L., "fold" or "pleat"). The medial parapatellar plica typically extends proximally from the fat pad and may be contiguous proximally with the suprapatellar plica (Fig. 1-11). These plicae can become enlarged, inflamed, and fibrotic; thus they can be a source of clinically significant symptoms following trauma.[23,32,33] In full extension the patella rests on a fibrous fatty pad lined with synovium that is called the *pulvinar* fat pad.

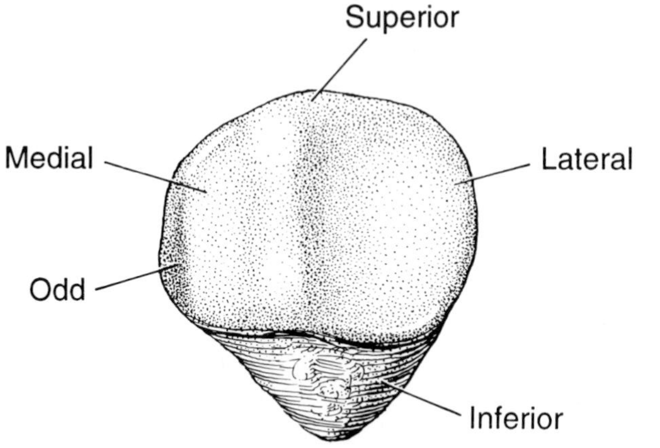

FIGURE 1-12
Representation of the articular cartilage facets including the large lateral, medial, and odd facets.

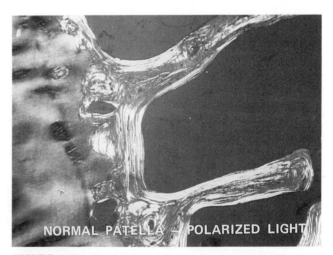

FIGURE 1-13
Microscopic section of the transition of articular cartilage to subchondral bone demonstrating articular cartilage tidemark zone, deeper calcified cartilage and subchondral bone H&E, ×125 (polarized light).

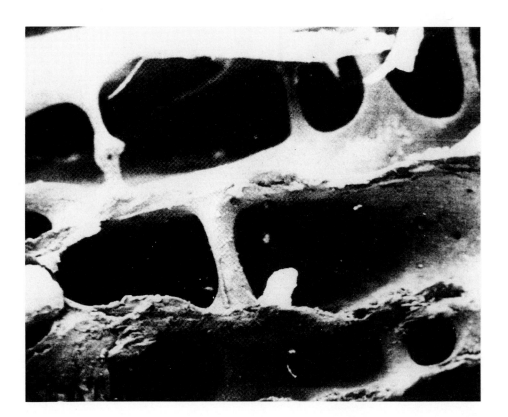

FIGURE 1-14
Scanning electron micrograph of the cancellous bone of the patella demonstrating horizontal sheets and vertical strut architecture. *[From Townsend, Miegel and Rose, (Ref. 30), 1976 with permission.]*

Patellar Blood Supply

A vascular anastomotic ring lying just anterior to the rectus fibers over the anterior patella represents the major blood supply of the patella (Fig. 1-15).[34-37] This anastomotic ring is supplied by the superior genicula, medial superior genicula, lateral superior genicula, lateral inferior genicula, and medial inferior genicula arteries (Fig. 1-16). The anterior vessels enter through fenestrations in the anterior patellar bone. The intraosseous blood supply is also supplemented by vessels from the infrapatellar anastomosis that enter the inferior pole posteriorly (Fig. 1-17). Because of this asymmetry of blood supply, the proximal pole of the patella is at risk of avascular necrosis in transverse fractures, isolating it from the main vascular supply to the mid and inferior patella.

Patellar Nerve Supply

Branches of the saphenous, anterior femoral cutaneous and lateral sural cutaneous nerves innervate the patella. The infrapatellar branch of the saphenous nerve is at risk with medial surgical exposures of the knee. Damage can lead to numbness not only medially but also lateral to the midline by virtue of its asymmetrical lateral extent, as represented in Fig. 1-18.

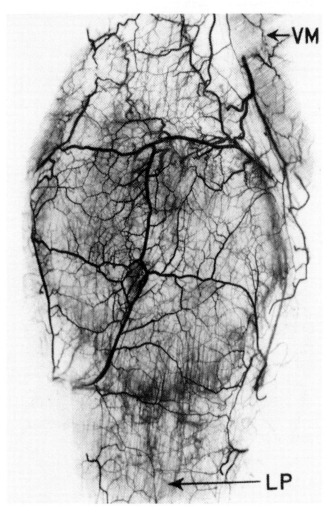

FIGURE 1-15
Vascular anastomotic ring supplying anterior patella. VM = vastus medialis, LP = ligamentum patellae. *[From Scapinelli, 1967, (Ref. 34), with permission.]*

9

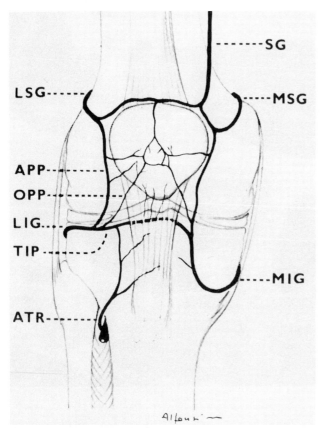

FIGURE 1-16
Schematic of peripatellar vascular supply. SG = supreme genicular artery, MSG = medial superior genicular artery, MIG = medial inferior genicular artery, LSG = lateral superior genicular artery, APP = ascending parapatellar artery, OPP = oblique prepatellar artery, LIG = lateral-inferior genicular artery, TIP = transverse infrapatellar artery, ATR = anterior tibial recurrent artery. *[From Scapinelli, 1967, (Ref. 34), with permission.]*

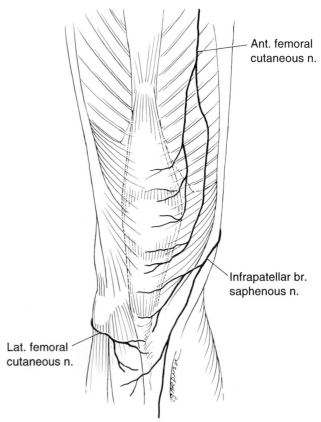

FIGURE 1-18
Nerve innervation of the patella (drawing by Gil Gardner) demonstrating region supplied by anterior femoral cutaneous, lateral sural cutaneous, and the saphenous nerves. Note that the saphenous nerve supply extends lateral to the midline. *(Adapted from W. Muller's The Knee, 1983).*

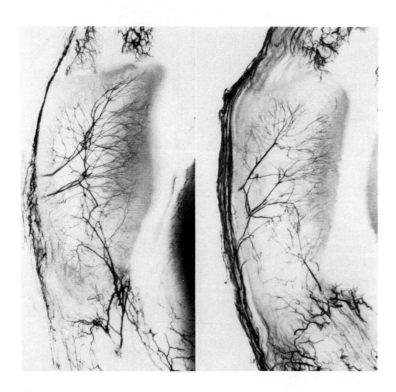

FIGURE 1-17
Two patellae in sagittal section demonstrating the vessels which enter through the foramina situated in the middle third of the patella of the anterior surface and in the lower pole behind the patellar tendon. *[From Scapinelli, 1967, (Ref. 34), with permission.]*

SUMMARY

The patellofemoral system is one of the most clinically important components of the human knee. The surprisingly complex anatomy of this region reflects the high functional requirements of compression, tension, and force transmission that often occur near the limits of biologic tissue capacity. Knowledge of some of the basic anatomic principles will assist the reader in understanding the functional biomechanics and subsequent clinical chapters.

REFERENCES

1. Goodfellow J, Hungerford DS, Zindel M: Patellofemoral joint mechanics and pathology. 1. Functional anatomy of the patellofemoral joint. *J Bone Joint Surg* 58B:287, 1976.
2. Huberti HH, Hayes, WC, et al: Force ratios in the quadriceps tendon and ligamentum patellae. *J Orthop Res* 2:49, 1984.
3. Fulkerson JP, Hungerford DS: *Disorders of the Patellofemoral Joint*, 2d ed. Baltimore, Williams & Wilkins, 1990.
4. Dye SF: An evolutionary perspective of the knee. *J Bone Joint Surg* 69A:976, 1987.
5. Holladay SD, Smith BJ, Smallwood JE, et al: Absence of an osseous patella and other observations in *Macropodidae stifle. Anat Rec* 225:112, 1990.
6. Hollingshead HW: *Anatomy for Surgeons, vol. 3: The Back and Limbs*, 2d ed. New York, Harper & Row, 1969.
7. Gardner E, O'Rahlilly R: The early development of the knee joint in staged human embryos. *J Anat* 102:289, 1968.
8. Doskocil M: Formation of the femoropatellar part of the human knee joint. *Folia Morphol* 33:38, 1985.
9. Ogata S, Uhthoff HK: The development of synovial plicae in human knee joints: An embryologic study. *J Arthroscopy* 6:315, 1990.
10. Cihak R, Puzanova L: The shape and position of the patella and the configuration of the insertions of the m. quadriceps femoris in the foetal period. *Cs Morfol* 8:15, 1960.
11. Dingerkus G, Uhler LD: Enzyme clearing of Alcian blue stained whole small vertebrates for demonstration of cartilage. *Stain Technol* 52:229, 1971.
12. Warwick R, Williams P (eds): *Gray's Anatomy*, 35th Br ed. Philadelphia, Saunders, 1973.
13. Ogden JA, Hempton RJ, Southwick WO: Development of the tibial tuberosity. *Anat Record* 182:431, 1975.
14. Hallisey MJ, Doherty N, Bennett WF, et al: Anatomy of the junction of the vastus lateralis tendon and the patella. *J Bone Joint Surg* 69A:545, 1987.
15. Terry JC: The anatomy of the extensor mechanism. *Clin Sports Med* 8:163, 1989.
16. Fulkerson JP, Gossling HR: Anatomy of the knee joint lateral retinaculum. *Clin Orthop* 153:183, 1980.
17. Weinstabl R, Scharf W, Firbas W: The extensor apparatus of the knee joint and its peripheral vasti: Anatomic investigation and clinical relevance. *Surg Radiol Anat* 11:17, 1989.
18. Terry GC, Hughston JC, Norwood LA: The anatomy of the iliopatellar band and iliotibial tract. *Am J Sports Med* 14:39, 1986.
19. Müller W: *The Knee: Form, Function, and Ligament Construction*. New York, Springer-Verlag, 1983.
20. Blauth M, Tillmann B: Stressing on the human femoro-patellar joint. I. Components of a vertical and horizontal tensile bracing system. *Anat Embryol* 168:117, 1983.
21. Reider B, Marshall JL, Costlin B, et al: The anterior aspect of the knee joint. *J Bone Joint Surg* 63A:351, 1981.
22. Kaplan EB: Surgical approaches to the lateral (peroneal) side of the knee joint. *Surg Gynecol Obstet* 104:346, 1957.
23. Hughston JC, Walsh WM, Puddu G: Patellar subluxation and dislocation. *Vol 5, Saunders Monographs in Clinical Orthopedics*. Philadelphia, Saunders, 1984.
24. Evans ES, Benjamin M, Pemberton DJ: Fibrocartilage in the attachment zones of the quadriceps tendon and patellar ligament of man. *J Anat* 171:155, 1990.
25. Ewing JW (ed): *Articular Cartilage and Knee Joint Function*. New York, Raven, 1990.
26. Meachim G: Cartilage lesions of the patella, in: Pickett JC, Radin EL (eds): *Chondromalacia of the Patella*. Baltimore, Williams & Wilkins, 1983.
27. Meachim G, Bentley G, Baker R: Affective age on thickness of adult patellar articular cartilage. *Ann Rheum Dis* 36:563, 1977.
28. Townsend PR, Raux P, Rose RM: The distribution and anisotropy of the stiffness of cancellous bone in the human patella. *J Biomech* 8:363, 1975.
29. Takechi H: Trabecular architecture of the knee joint. *Acta Orthop Scand* 48:673, 1977.

30. Townsend PR, Miegel RE, Rose RM: Structure and function of the human patella: The role of cancellous bone. *J Biomed Mater Res Symp No. 7*, 605–611, 1976.

31. Bjorkstrom S, Goldie I: Hardness of the subchondral bone of the patella in a normal state, in chondromalacia, and in osteoarthrosis. *Acta Orthop Scand* 53:451, 1982.

32. Patel D: Plica as a cause of anterior knee pain. *Orthop Clin North Am* 17:273, 1986.

33. Dandy DJ: Anatomy of the medial suprapatellar plica and medial synovial shelf. *Arthroscopy* 6:79, 1990.

34. Scapinelli R: Blood supply of the human patella. Its relation to ischemic necrosis after fracture. *J Bone Joint Surg* 49B:563, 1967.

35. Shim S, Leung G: Blood supply of the knee joint. *Clin Orthop* 208:119, 1986.

36. Brick GW, Scott RD: Blood supply to the patella. Significant in total knee arthroplasty. *J Arthroplasty* (suppl) 75, 1989.

37. Slater RN, Spencer JD, Churchill MA, et al: Observations on the intrinsic blood supply to the human patella: Disruption correlated with articular surface degeneration. *J R Soc Med* 84:606, 1991.

CHAPTER 2

Articular Cartilage, Cartilage Injury, and Osteoarthritis*

Henry J. Mankin

INTRODUCTION

The articular cartilages of any joint, such as the patellofemoral, are central to discussion of that joint, be it biologic, mechanical, or pathologic. For the most part, the health and function of the joint reside in its articular cartilages and no external system has ever been able to compensate for malfunction or damage to these structures. Even prosthetic systems are poor substitutes for the "real thing" and at least at the time of this writing are limited in their capacity to replace the normal articular surface in terms of functional capacity, resistance to wear, or duration of service.

The cartilages of the body are unique structures remarkably designed and ordered to provide a lifetime of competent function. They are almost frictionless (a coefficient of friction roughly equivalent to one-eighth that of ice gliding on ice), self-renewing, and self-lubricating; they work better under load. Although aging changes occur in the cartilage and, indeed, osteoarthritis is a disease of the elderly, age alone does not preclude good function of the cartilage and many old people have normal joints both anatomically and functionally. The cartilages are built to function for a lifetime and do so effectively unless damaged in some way or when some form of osteoarthritis supervenes.

The articular cartilages are unique in several important ways. They live in "isolation" from the rest of the body, having no blood, nerve, or lymph supply. Because nutrition depends on a double-diffusion system from the joint (nutrients must diffuse across the synovial barrier and then across the matrix of the cartilage to reach the cell), the cartilages probably receive few humoral signals from the bloodstream and are probably isolated from the body fluids. The matrix of cartilage is uniquely constituted to maintain a significant stiffness and resiliency despite a high water content; and the combination of type II collagen fibers and several families of proteoglycans (PGs), which are in large measure responsible for the physical properties of the cartilage, are unique in the body's tissues. Finally, despite sparse numbers and an effete appearance of the chondrocytes, ample evidence indicates that they are actively involved in maintaining the matrix. Despite the uniquely hypoxic circumstances of the chondrocyte's milieu, the cells enjoy an active metabolic life with some of the components of the matrix being turned over at a very rapid rate.

In this chapter we shall explore some of the biologic characteristics of the articular cartilages with special reference to the knee and patellofemoral joint and define the response of the cartilages to some of the more well-known treatment modalities. We shall discuss at some length the healing of cartilage (or lack of it) and the nature and effect of the principal failure mode for the cartilage—the osteoarthritic process.

THE STRUCTURE, BIOCHEMISTRY, AND METABOLISM OF ADULT ARTICULAR CARTILAGE

The articular cartilages vary rather widely in structure, chemistry, and metabolism from species to species, joint to joint, site to site in any joint, and with depth in the cartilage at any site. This makes any description of the cartilage somewhat likely to be an average or summary value rather than a truly valid statement. It is important to note, however, that the patellar cartilage is for the most part the thickest cartilage in the joints of the human being (or other mammalian species).[1,2] The adult human patellar cartilage may be as thick as 5 mm, which far exceeds the values for other sites, such as the hip joint or distal femur.[3] The cartilage in children and young adults is dense blue-white in color. With advancing age a yellowish hue appears, which presumably is related to staining with foreign materials, but the nature of these is not clear.[4] No evidence supports the concept that the color of the cartilage has any effect on function.[5,6] Although the surface of cartilage seems smooth and "mirror-like" (the word *hyaline* is from the Greek word for mirror) on careful examination by incident light microscopy, transmission microscopy, and scanning electron microscopy (SEM), it is evident that the cartilages are not at all smooth but have undulations and irregularities of the surface, probably reflecting the position of the cells of the gliding

*Supported in part by grant R01-16265 from NIAMS.

layer below.[7-10] The SEM picture of the cartilage clearly shows the presence of a fine filamentous fibrous layer, which presumably is part of the augmented boundary lubrication mechanism.[11]

Although examination of the cut surface of the hyaline articular cartilage from an adult joint suggests a sparsely cellular homogeneous structure with random distribution of the cells, careful study discloses that the structure is not uniform, but heterogeneous and that the cells are distributed in a distinct zonal pattern.[12-14] The most superficial zone is the *gliding layer* in which elongated cells are seen tangentially arranged parallel to the surface; deep to that is the *transitional zone,* consisting of more rounded, randomly distributed chondrocytes; next is the *radial zone,* in which the cells are in short columns; and deepest is the *calcified zone,* in which small pyknotic (and seemingly dead) cells are distributed in a cartilaginous matrix heavily encrusted with apatitic salts. On hematoxylin and eosin staining, a wavy bluish line appears, called by Collins the *tidemark,* which separates the radial zone from the calcified zone (Fig. 2-1).[14] Original description of the tidemark suggested that it is an artifact on hematoxylin and eosin-stained sections, which is associated with the margin of the calcification front. Most investigators now believe the finding is related to a "twist" in the collagen bundles as they descend to enter the calcified zone and the bone.[15,16] Furthermore, the tidemark may disappear with osteoarthritis or change its appearance with either aging or cartilage injury, suggesting that it may serve an important role in adjusting to abnormal states and protecting the cartilage from osteoarthritis.[12]

The Nutrition of Articular Cartilage

As indicated above, articular cartilage from mature animals is totally avascular, aneural, and alymphatic. The surface is not covered by either a perichondrium or a synovial layer or reflection. Electron microscopic studies have failed to show any form of limiting membrane other than the "skin," (the dense collagenous bundles running parallel to the surface of the cartilage in the superficial zone[11,17]) (Fig. 2-2) and a "lamina splendens," which conforms well to a 10-nm fine-fibered filamentous layer considered important in lubrication.[11,17]

The source of nutrition for the cartilaginous surfaces is an ancient puzzle. Because the tissue is avascular in adult life, most investigators believe that the nutritive materials diffuse through the matrix either from the synovial fluid that bathes the surface of the cartilage or from the underlying bone.[18-22] In recent years, experimental evidence has suggested that in

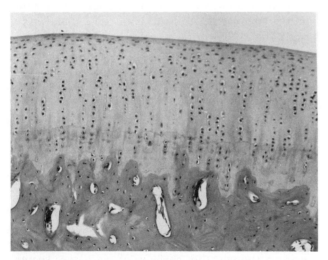

FIGURE 2-1
Photomicrograph of adult articular cartilage shows the zonal characteristics of the tissue. The cells at the surface are elongated and resemble fibroblasts. Those in the layer below (transitional zone) are rounded and seem randomly distributed. In the radial zone, the cells appear to line up in short irregular columns. Just below the radial zone is a bluish wavy line (on a hematoxylin-stained section) called the tidemark. The cells in the calcified zone are probably nonviable and the matrix is heavily encrusted with apatitic salts. H&E, ×80.

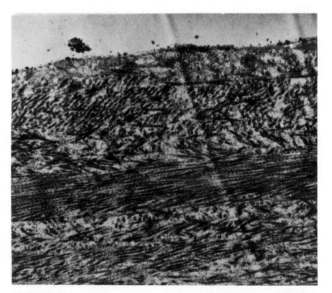

FIGURE 2-2
Electron micrograph of the most superficial portion of adult articular cartilage shows the fibrous bundles running tangential to the surface and forming the "skin" of the articular cartilage. A fine filamentous fibrous and proteinaceous layer adheres to the surface and constitutes the "lamina splendens." Courtesy of Charles Weiss, MD, ×28,000. (Reprinted with permission of the publisher from Mankin HJ: The articular cartilages, cartilage healing and osteoarthritis, in *Adult Orthopaedics,* edited by RL Cruess, WRJ Rennie. New York, Churchill Livingstone, 1984, 163–270.)

immature animals at least a portion of the substrates entering the articular cartilage do so by diffusion from the underlying bony end plate; but in the adult, with the appearance of the tidemark and a heavy deposition of apatite in the calcified zone, this type of diffusion disappears or becomes severely limited.[19,20]

Synovial fluid, then, appears to be the primary source of nutrition for the articular chondrocyte. The fluid itself arises by diffusion from the synovial vascular network and represents a diffusate of plasma (without fibrinogen and with somewhat diminished levels of urea, glucose, and plasma protein) to which the synoviocytes have added hyaluronate and some additional proteins.[23,24] The synovial fluid is sparse in quantity in normal joints, but sufficient quantities of nutrients and oxygen reach the chondrocytes, presumably by diffusion through the cartilage matrix.[25–27] Extensive studies have shown that the diffusion of nutrients through the matrix of the cartilage is not restricted and is limited by the size and charge of the molecule, and perhaps also by steric configuration.[26,27] Synovial cytokines, namely interleukin-1 (IL-1), some of the prostaglandins, and some of the growth factors, appear to traverse the matrix readily to gain access to the cell. These materials have been shown to act on the cartilage and lead us to the conclusion that regardless of prior considerations, synovial inflammation may play a critical role in the pathogenesis of osteoarthritis and other disorders of cartilage.

It is intriguing to speculate on the significance of the statement made in the Introduction that normal articular cartilage "lives in isolation." Humoral messages, such as are given to other organs by rapid transit of information peptides and proteins, may not be received by the chondrocytes because of a diffusion barrier (particularly for charged particles or for larger proteins or hormones); or, if transport of such messengers does occur, it may be considerably slower than in more vascular tissue. Furthermore, neural impulses, which regulate many of the body processes, cannot provide information to cartilage because it has no nerve supply; and cellular and humoral immune responses are not likely to have much effect in intact tissue chiefly because the size and configuration of both the monocytes and immunoglobulins tend to exclude them from the tissue. In theory at least, the chondrocytes can receive only limited information regarding the rest of the body state by the standard neural, lymphatic, or humoral pathways. On the other hand, if the cell is pressure sensitive, it may derive considerable information by alteration in the forces acting on the membrane as a result of alteration in the physical state of the tissue.

Such acts as loading, unloading, or movement of the joint may be the principal stimuli to biochemical alterations in the cartilage.[28]

The Chemistry of Articular Cartilage

Table 2-1 shows the approximate chemical composition of cartilage matrix based on current knowledge. Considering the sparse cellularity of articular cartilage, it is apparent that the chemistry reflects the composition of the matrix. Cartilage is hyperhydrated with values for water ranging from 60 percent to almost 80 percent of the total net weight. The remaining 20 percent to 30 percent is accounted for by two macromolecular materials, namely, type II collagen, which comprises up to 60 percent of the dry weight, and the various PGs, which account for a large part of the remainder. The inorganic ash content is approximately 6 percent, and the residue is composed of trace amounts of lipid, phospholipid, and an as yet poorly defined or fully characterized "matrix protein" with a molecular weight of 200,000 to 300,000 d.

WATER

The water content of articular cartilage is extraordinarily important in maintaining the resiliency of tissue, as well as contributing to the almost frictionless movement associated with a boundary lubrication system.[29,30] The content is highest at birth, with only a modest decrease recorded in adult tissues and a further slight diminution with advanced age.[31,32] An increase in total water content has been noted with immobilization,[33] denervation,[53] and joint motion

TABLE 2-1
Approximate Biochemical Composition of Adult Articular Cartilage

Material	%
Water	65–80
Solids	
Inorganic (ash)	5–6
Organic	
Collagen	48–62
Proteogylcan	30–38
Hyaluronate	1–2
Lipid	1–2
Chondronectin	<1
Anchorin	<1
Minor collagens	2–3
Matrix protein	?15

without weight bearing.[35] Water content varies from site to site in the cartilage and at the various levels from the surface.[36] The mechanism of water binding within cartilage is not entirely understood. Because most of the extracellular matrix consists of collagen and PG and because gel formation occurs when water is in contact with either of these macromolecules, this process is considered to be the major mechanism by which the tissue holds water. The water of the gel, although unable to "flow," is believed to be freely exchangeable with that of fluids on the other side of the membrane and is subjected to all of the physico-chemical laws that govern osmotic solutions or membrane theory.[29,38] Less than 5 percent of the water remains tightly bound, and it cannot be removed by heating or desiccation.[30,37,38]

PROTEOGLYCANS

The PGs are complex macromolecules that consist of a linear protein core to which are linked long-chain polysaccharide moieties (glycosaminoglycans ... GAGs; Fig. 2-3). The GAGs are polyanionic in charge, owing to the regular occurrence of carboxyl and sulfate groups along the macromolecules. The principle

form of PG (which has recently been given the name *aggrecan*) contains a large protein core (245 kd) to which numerous chains of chondroitin 4-sulfate, chondroitin 6-sulfate and keratan sulfate are covalently bound (Fig. 2-4).[39–41] The protein core consists of three distinct zones: G1 at the N-terminal portion that contains a binding site for hyaluronic acid and is involved in the aggregation process (see below); G2, a long linear segment (260 nm) to which are asymmetrically covalently bound numerous GAG chains; and G3, a globular C-terminal domain that exhibits some homology with a liver lectin.[42,43] The aggrecan PG molecules are not homogenous and at least two populations have been described—a "small" and a "large."[44,45]

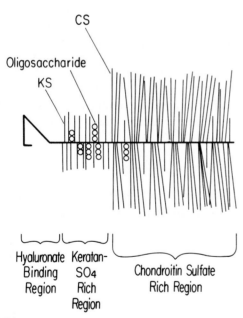

FIGURE 2-3
Drawing of a glycosaminoglycan (GAG) subunit. The core protein has three zones: a G1 *N*-terminal that is the binding site to hyaluronate, which is protein rich and has no GAG chains; G2 in which short-chain keratan sulfate, oligosaccharide, and long-chain chondroitin sulfate (GAGs) are covalently bound at special binding sites; and a terminal G3 portion that represent the C-terminal portion of the molecule. (Reprinted with permission of the publisher from Mankin HJ: The articular cartilages, cartilage healing and osteoarthritis, in *Adult Orthopaedics,* edited by RL Cruess, WRJ Rennie. New York, Churchill-Livingstone, 1984, 163–270).

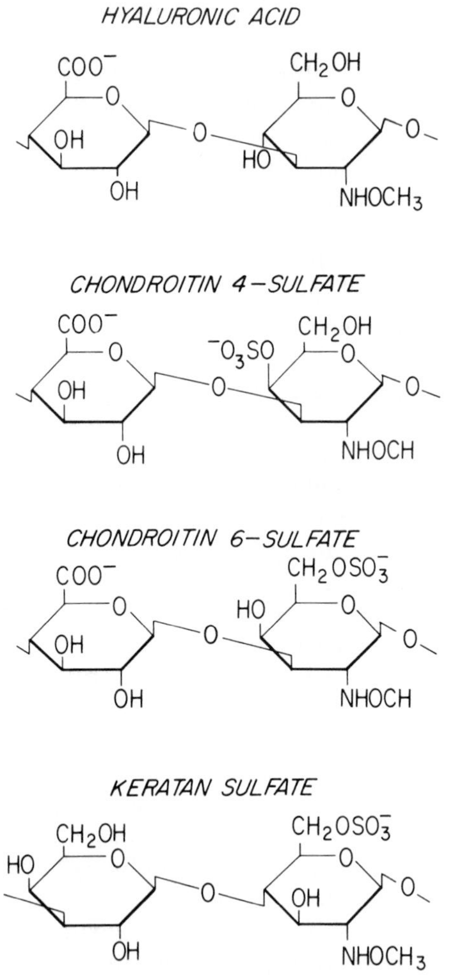

FIGURE 2-4
Chemical formulae for the repeating dimeric units of the four major glycosaminoglycan chains of articular cartilage. The key to the "stiffness" of the molecule is the repulsive force generated by the proximity of the negative charges on the keratan and chondroitin sulfates. (Reprinted with permission of the publisher from Mankin HJ: The articular cartilages, cartilage healing and osteoarthritis, in *Adult Orthopaedics,* edited by RL Cruess, WRJ Rennie. New York, Churchill-Livingstone, 1984, 163–270.)

The GAG molecules, which are covalently linked principally to G2, consist of long-chain, unbranched repeating polydimeric saccharides, and only four of these have been found in the PG subunit: chondroitin 4-sulfate; its stereoisomer, chondroitin 6-sulfate; keratan sulfate; and some short-chain oligosaccharides. The chondroitin sulfates are the most prevalent GAGs in cartilage and account for 55 percent to over 90 percent of the total GAGs depending principally on the age of the subject or the presence of osteoarthritis[48] (see below). The average chain weight for chondroitin sulfate in articular cartilage is about 15,000 to 20,000 d, so that 25 to 30 repeating disaccharide units comprise each chain.[49–51] The linkage region to the G2 portion of the protein consists of a galactosyl-galactosyl-xylosyl bridge to a serine on the protein core.[52,53]

The keratan sulfate constituents of articular cartilage are not as well defined as the chondroitin sulfates. A number of species of keratan sulfate occur in various body sites, and the composition and degree of sulfation of keratan sulfate are variable and may be considerably altered with the age of the individual.[54,55] Keratan sulfate chains of PGs from human articular cartilage are believed to be shorter than those of chondroitin sulfates, consisting of only five to six repeating dimeric units, so that the molecular weight of the entire chain is between 2300 and 2600 d.[54,55] The linkage region is believed to consist of a neuraminyl-galactosyl-disaccharide bonded to threonine or glutamic acid.[54,56]

From data reported by several research groups, it is evident that only a small fraction of the PG exists as the free subunit in articular cartilage.[55–57] The majority of the macromolecular material forms high-order aggregates, which contain many subunits and have molecular weights of 60 to 150 × 10⁶ d (Fig. 2-5).[49,56] These complex materials, together with their gel-trapped water, occupy enormous domains that, because of the polyanionic nature of the GAGs, are strongly electronegative and evoke a resistance to compressive force, which contributes materially to the resiliency of the tissue.[29,58] Studies have now established that the more aggregating factor is hyaluronic acid synthesized by the chondrocyte, which forms a filamentous backbone for the aggregate.[56,59–61] The hyaluronic acid in the aggregate is a long unbranched chainlike molecule that is able to bind several hundred PGs via interaction with the G1 regions of individual aggrecan molecules.[59–61] The average interval between PG subunits on the filamentous hyaluronate backbone has been calculated to be 2400 to 2600 nm.[62] Although hyaluronate is clearly the major factor in the aggregation of PG subunits, specific pro-

tein constituents, known as *link proteins* appear to stabilize the linkage and have been found as components of the PG aggregates from every cartilage thus far examined.[63–65] Chemical studies of the link proteins have shown them to be glycoprotein in nature and to consist of a family of two or three members varying principally in their degree of glycoslylation.[66–69]

The aggrecan PGs have a number of physical and chemical properties including viscosity, water binding, and polyelectrolytic character, all of which are important to the resiliency of articular cartilage and probably materially in providing water for surface lubrication. The PGs are closely associated with the collagen and may direct or maintain the spatial position of the fibrous protein, influence fibril formation, and possibly prevent calcification.[29,49,70,71] The aggrecans are not homogeneously distributed throughout the depth of the tissue. The surface zone is rich in collagen and relatively poor in PG.[11,75] In the transitional zone, the concentration of PGs increases, and they are more homogeneously distributed.[76,77] In the radial zone, the distribution is more variable, with some increase in the chondrocyte territorial areas as compared with the interterritorial areas.[72,73] Of considerable importance in the study of PG distribution is the affinity of these materials for certain basic dyes, especially safranin-O, which appears as a brilliant red coloration in regions of high concentration in a slide stained with the dye and fast green as a counterstain.[74]

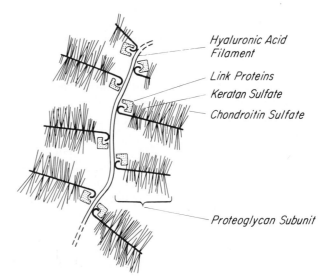

FIGURE 2-5
Diagram of the structure of the proteoglycan aggregate shows the proteoglycan subunits distributed along a long filament of hyaluronic acid. The aggrecan units are linked covalently and have as a cofactor in that linkage a glycoprotein molecule known as link protein (see text).

In addition to aggrecan, two dermatan sulfate PGs, DSPG I (biglycan) and DSPG II (decorin), are present in normal articular cartilage.[78] Biglycan contains two chains of dermatan sulfate; decorin contains one and the molecules have molecular weights of 63,000 and 100,000, respectively.[78,79] The core protein differs for the two molecules and both are distinctly different from aggrecan.[78]

The DSPGs are multifunctional, bind to various other connective tissue macromolecules, and appear to modulate their biologic functions.[80–83] The binding to fibronectin inhibits cell migration and adhesion; binding to heparin inhibits fibrillogenesis; and binding to transforming growth factor, type beta (TGF-β) probably interferes with the mitogenic effect that may be a necessary step in the healing of wounds in the cartilage (see below).

COLLAGEN

Well over 50 percent of the dry weight of adult articular cartilage consists of collagen.[12,48] For many years, the collagen of cartilage was considered to be similar and perhaps identical to that isolated from skin, bone, and other body tissues, but it is now accepted that the major collagen of cartilage, known as type II, is a distinct genetic species.[85–87] In addition, ample evidence supports the fact that type II collagen is not the only collagen found in cartilage and that types V, VI, IX, and X are present in many cartilages in varying concentrations.[85–91]

The type II collagen fibers that comprise the bulk of cartilage collagen are thinner than those seen in tendon or bone and are distinctly less soluble.[86,87] They have a macro-organization and structure thought initially to be in the form of tension-resisting arcades but have recently been shown to be more a random distribution, at least in the middle zones of the cartilage (Fig. 2-6).

Collagen is the most prevalent protein in the human body and, by definition, is the major organic component of the structural and support systems of the body. The simplest unit or extracellular collagen is the tropocollagen molecule, which measures approximately 1.5 nm in diameter and 300 nm in length. Each of these molecules consists of three polypeptide chains coiled in a rigid, left-handed, helical structure (Fig. 2-7). Tropocollagen molecules are ordered to form fibrils, and the fibrils are then ordered to form fibers that are stabilized by interfibrillar cross-links. The fibers in articular cartilage, as seen with the electron microscope, may vary in width from 10 to 100 nm and this value may be exceeded in aging or osteoarthritis.[11,92]

Although similar in appearance to other collagens, the collagen of cartilage is considerably less soluble than most others and is clearly a different

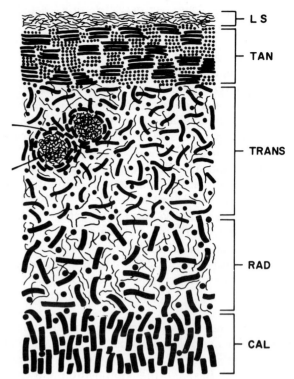

FIGURE 2-6
Diagram shows the distribution and structure of the collagen in articular cartilage. Noteworthy is the fine filamentous structure of the lamina splendens (LS); the parallel bundles tangential to the surface which serve as a "skin" (TAN); the random arrangement of the fibrillar structure in the transitional and radial zones (TRANS, RAD); and the fibers lying perpendicular to the surface in the calcified zone (CAL). Courtesy of Charles Weiss, MD. Original appeared in article by Lane and Weiss.[17] (Reprinted with permission of the publisher from Mankin HJ: The articular cartilages, cartilage healing and osteoarthritis, in *Adult Orthopaedics,* edited by RL Cruess, WRJ Rennie. New York, Churchill-Livingstone, 1984, 163–270.)

genetic species, consisting of three almost identical α 1 chains.[87,93–95] The biochemical composition is considerably different from that of collagen from other sites. Type II collagen shows a major alteration in the extent of hydroxylation of the lysyl residues and a ninefold increase in the content of hydroxylysine-linked carbohydrate, both of which increase the number of cross-links. The increased intermolecular and intramolecular cross-linkages probably account for the greater structural stability, lesser susceptibility to calcification, greater availability for PG linkage, and increased gel formation seen in cartilage.[93–95]

Over the past decade numerous studies have shown that a portion of type I (mostly in the surface layers), type V, type VI, type IX, and type X collagens are present in some cartilages in varying concentrations.[86–91] Although these collagens are grouped under the heading of "minor collagens," it is likely that they play a major role in the structure of the tissue. Type V appears to be similar in structure and perhaps a subtype of type IX and consists of either

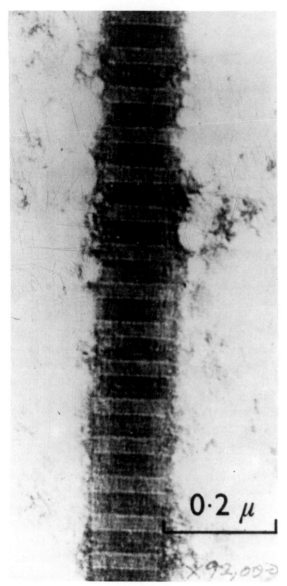

FIGURE 2-7
Electron micrograph of a collagen fiber from adult articular cartilage shows the structure. Note the banding and periodicity, which resemble collagen from other structures.

two or three helical chains of uncertain composition. Triple helical type VI collagen is present in all connective tissue usually in proximity to cells, large collagen fibers, and basement membranes, suggesting that it may be an anchoring material for these structures.[89] The type IX collagen is a major connective component of all cartilaginous structures. Although its function in cartilage is not clearly known, it is found principally around the chondrons and thought to regulate the bundle shape and structure.[88,91] Type X collagen is present in cartilage undergoing endochondral ossification and is less frequently associated with articular cartilage than with epiphyseal cartilage.[90] This form of collagen has been found in the calcified zone of articular cartilage and is believed to facilitate calcification.[86,90]

OTHER MATERIALS

An "adhesive" protein, chondronectin, has been found in articular cartilage and is presumed to be responsible for establishing a relationship between the collagen fibrils and the chondrocytes.[96,97] In addition, two other materials may play a similar role: fibronectin, which has been found in low concentration in normal but markedly increased concentrations in osteoarthritic cartilage,[98–100] and anchorin, another similar material but differing in molecular structure.[101]

Of some recent interest is the further purification and elucidation of a series of the matrix proteins of varying sizes.[102,103] These globular and probably glycoproteinaceous materials, which may account for as much as 15 percent of the total weight of the cartilage, represent a family of components whose function remains obscure but may play some role in the aggregation process.[102,105]

Lipids, which form 1 percent or less of the wet weight of human adult articular cartilage, are found both in the cells and in the matrix; their function is currently unknown but may vary with age and with the presence of osteoarthritis.[105–108] In the last several years interest has been generated in phospholipase A_2, which is synthesized by the chondrocytes and present in articular cartilage.[109–111] This enzyme may be important both in arachidonic acid metabolism and in the degradative pathway (see below).[110,111]

Pericellular osmiophilic matrix vesicles measuring 50 to 250 nm in size and containing apatitic calcific modules have been found principally in the radial zone and with increased frequency in osteoarthritic cartilage.[112,113] These membrane-bound calcific matrix vesicles appear to be increased with aging and with osteoarthritis and are thought by some to play a role in the pathogenesis of osteoarthritis.[113]

Metabolism of Articular Cartilage

Over the past 30 years, there has been ample demonstration of a surprisingly active rate of metabolism in articular cartilage. Despite inactive appearance on histologic examination, adult articular chondrocytes, synthesize, assemble, maintain, and remodel the matrix components and direct their distribution within the tissue. The synthetic apparatus is complex, because not only are proteins (core protein of the PG, collagen, glycoproteins, enzymes, etc.) synthesized by standard genetic pathways, but also sugars are assembled into GAGs, linked to the protein, and sulfated. By definition, all these actions take place under avascular and hypoxic conditions and must use an-

19

aerobic glycolysis for energy. Furthermore, considerable variation in local pressure and the physicochemical state occurs with normal activities, which must have some effect on the metabolic processes.

GLYCOLYSIS AND ENERGY PRODUCTION

One of the factors that led to the general impression that articular cartilage was inert was the early demonstration that although articular cartilage had a well-defined glycolytic system, oxygen utilization was considerably lower than that in other tissues.[114] This concept was subsequently established to be related to the sparse cell population rather than to a lack of metabolic activity but despite that there may be an excessive energy need for the actively synthesizing cell, articular cartilage uses principally the anaerobic pathway.[114–116]

PROTEOGLYCAN SYNTHESIS

Many investigators have clearly demonstrated that the chondrocyte is responsible for the synthesis, assembly, and sulfation of the PG molecule.[117,118] At the molecular level, this activity begins with the synthesis of a protein at the ribosome as dictated by messenger RNA. The sugars are then added to the molecule at the appropriate amino acid binding sites and the molecule extruded. Synthesis of some of the PG by the chondrocyte appears to occur at a rapid rate and is affected by numerous endogenous and exogenous environmental alterations. Studies have shown that such diverse physical and pathologic states as lacerative injury,[118] osteoarthritis,[118] altered hydrostatic pressure,[28] varied oxygen tension,[114,123] pH alterations,[121] calcium concentration,[122] substrate or serum concentration,[124] growth hormone,[125] cytokine mediators,[126] ascorbate,[127] vitamin E,[128] prostaglandins,[129] salicylates[130] and several other nonsteroidal anti-inflammatory drugs,[131–134] uridine diphosphate,[135] and a variety of other factors have significant effects on the PG synthesis rate. These data suggest that the control mechanisms for PG synthesis are extraordinarily sensitive to stimuli of a biochemical, mechanical, and physical nature.

One of the more extraordinary features of this tissue is the finding of a remarkably rapid rate of turnover of a small fraction of the PG.[136] The rate reported far exceeds that required to compensate for normal attrition (which cannot be very much in an almost frictionless system!). These data strongly suggest the presence of an enzymatic internal remodeling system that has the PGs as its substrate and presumably is dictated by and responsive to conditions other than attritional loss (see below). It should be emphasized, however, that the turnover rates for some of the PGs (and indeed the bulk of them) and many of the other proteins may be much slower than the small rapid fraction defined above.

COLLAGEN SYNTHESIS

The collagen of articular cartilage is much more stable than the PG, and until recently, there was little evidence for metabolic activity. It is now evident that a collagenase exists in normal cartilage and that some turnover occurs under normal conditions. This process is markedly enhanced in osteoarthritis or in those joints in which the cartilage surfaces have undergone lacerative injury.[137,138]

The synthesis of collagen in cartilage is believed to be similar to that in other connective tissues. However, in contradistinction to the collagen of skin and bone, in which two different chains are synthesized presumably under the control of two separate genes, only one gene is responsible for the synthesis of the type II collagen of cartilage.[85,87] The primary collagen product at the ribosome levels is called *procollagen,* which, in cartilage, consists of three α_1 (II) chains. These are larger than the α_1 chains of the final exported product and demonstrate some variation in the proline–hydroxyproline ratio. Enzymatic activity is necessary to convert procollagen to collagen during or after export and some of the procollagen (or fragments of it) remains intracellular and is subsequently degraded (Fig. 2-8). Two processes occur during the intracellular synthesis of procollagen, during or just after its assembly on the ribosomes. The first of these

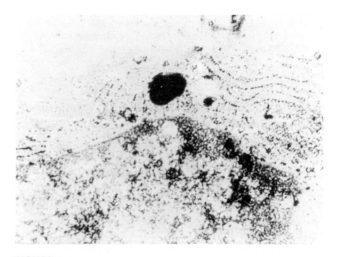

FIGURE 2-8
Electron micrograph of a lysosomal body of a chondrocyte. This serves as the source of many of the acidic destructive enzymes of cartilage including acid cathepsins, keratanase, hexosidase, and hexosaminidase.

is hydroxylation of proline and lysine to produce the amino acids hydroxyproline and hydroxylysine, which are almost unique to collagen.[139] The second process, the synthesis of hydroxylysyl glycosides, depends on the presence of galactose and glucose in the form of uridine diphosphate derivatives and two specific transfer enzymes.[87,140] Once assembled, the procollagen molecule undergoes enzymatic conversion to native collagen during or following export but to date the exact site and nature of both this conversion and the method by which the molecule is extruded from the cell are not clearly understood. The remaining processes affecting collagen occur in the matrix and consist of cross-link formation, which provides intramolecular links between the chains of the tropocollagen molecule; intrafilament bonds between the tropocollagen and molecules composing the primary unit; and interfilament cross-links between the primary filaments that make up the fibril.[87,141]

Growth Factors

Only recently have cartilage chemists begun to define the response of articular cartilage to polypeptide growth factors. It is apparent even at this early phase that these agents play a major role in the regulation of the synthetic processes of normal cartilage and perhaps an even greater role in the osteoarthritic process. The methods by which these agents act on the chondrocyte have not been fully elucidated but appear to be principally related to interaction with cell surface receptor sites on responsive cells. In the case of at least two of these, insulin-like growth factor I (IGF I) and insulin, competitive binding is present, which may alter the end result. For most of the factors, however, the cell receptor is highly specific, and the response is dictated by the concentration of the growth factor and the number of receptors on the cell.

The various growth factors include:

1.   Platelet-derived growth factor (PDGF). This factor is a major growth material for connective tissue cells and consists of a dimer of disulfide-bonded A and B polypeptide chains. Various isoforms have been identified and seem to have different activities. Although several studies have suggested that PDGF has a mitogenic effect on chondrocytes, the method of action is not clear nor does it seem likely that this material is active in the joint under normal conditions. In osteoarthritis and especially lacerative injury a greater likelihood exists for the role of these peptides in healing.[142,143]

2.   Fibroblast growth factor (basic) (b-FGF). This material, like many of the other factors, comes from multiple sources.[126,144] In the past the peptide coming from the pituitary had been described as "cartilage growth factor," whereas that generated by the cartilage was designated as "cartilage-derived growth factor." It is now evident that these are identical to b-FGF, which acts in connective tissues principally as a powerful mitogen. Studies by Osborn and colleagues[126] have shown that b-FGF alone acts as a powerful stimulator of DNA synthesis in adult articular chondrocytes in culture. Although it is contributory to matrix production, the material seems less active unless introduced with other materials such as insulin. Recent studies by Cuevas and colleagues have shown that b-FGF markedly stimulates repair of cartilage slices in an in vivo lapine model.[144]

3.   Insulin and the insulin-like growth factors I and II (IGF I and IGF II). Perhaps the best studied of the growth factors, insulin, IGF I, and IGF II are three homologous peptides that bind with varying affinity to three distinct receptors on the cells.[126,145,146] IGF I and IGF II are structurally homologous to proinsulin, almost the same size (70 and 67 amino acids) and share about 65 percent homology.[145] IGF I, formerly known as somatomedin-C, stimulates DNA and matrix synthesis in growth plate and immature and adult articular cartilage.[146] According to the studies of Osborn and colleagues, the material is more effective with coadministration with other factors including epidermal growth factor (EGF) and b-FGF but not with insulin.[126] Recent evidence suggests that the material maintains a steady state for PG synthesis in adult tissue.[146]

4.   Transforming growth factor-beta (TGF-β). TGF-β has at least five isoforms all of which are 25-kd proteins composed of two identical polypeptides linked by disulfide bonds.[148,149] The material has at least three separate receptors on the cell, which it shares with no other factors.[147] Numerous cellular activities have been attributed to this material in relation to bone and more recently cartilage and not all of these are up-regulatory.[147,148] The material seems to potentiate the stimulation of DNA synthesis by b-FGF, EGF and IGF I rather than initiating it de novo.[126] Investigative studies have shown that TGF-β is locally synthesized by the chondrocytes and appears to stimulate PG synthesis and at the same time down-regulate type II collagen synthesis.[126] In addition to its other functions, evidence suggests that TGF-β is responsible for stimulating the formation of tissue inhibitor of metalloprotease (TIMP) and plasminogen activator inhibitor-1 (PAI-1), two materials which are

believed to prevent the degradative action of stromelysin and plasmin (see section below).

   5. Epidermal growth factor (EGF). This potent mitogen for keratinocytes and other epithelial elements[150] appears to play a lesser role in cartilage metabolism, except perhaps as a cofactor with some of the others listed above.

The Degradative Enzymes of Articular Cartilage

It has been known for years that certain degradative enzymes act on articular cartilage to destroy the matrix. Papain, a crude degradative enzyme preparation extracted from the papaya plant, was noted to cause a loss of basophilia and metachromasia on histologic study and a profound depletion of the GAGs on biochemical analysis, presumably by cleavage of the core protein of the PG.[151] These same chondrolytic changes could be observed with administration of vitamin A that appeared to act by release of potent autolytic enzymes contained within the lysosomal bodies of the chondrocytes in an "inactive" form.[151,152] Lysosomal bodies have been observed on electron microscopic studies of articular cartilage (see Fig. 2-8), and analysis of cartilage for "lysosomal marker enzymes," such as acid phosphatase or B-glucuronidase, have shown them to be present in low concentration in normal tissue.[153]

   If one considers the classes of lysosomal enzymes, in theory, only two could act to degrade the intact PG. The first is a hyaluronidase, which could lyse the hyaluronate "backbone" of the PG aggregate and also the chondroitin sulfate chains (keratan sulfate is resistant to most hyaluronidases).[154] Although studies have failed to demonstrate evidence for a "true" hyaluronidase in normal articular cartilage, more recent efforts have identified a heat-stable enzyme that exhibits hyaluronidase activity in normal articular cartilage, which appears to be related to the concentration of cyclic adenosine monophosphate in the cartilage.[155]

   A second and more likely proteoglycanolytic enzyme is a cathepsin, which would attack the core protein. Investigators have demonstrated that PG could be enzymatically degraded by lysosomal acid proteases, and these have been identified as cathepsins D and B, both of which are known to occur in articular cartilage.[153,154,156] Of considerable concern, however, has been the low pH optima at which acid cathepsins act. It seems unlikely that pH values of 5.5 or less occur extracellularly in normal cartilage, except perhaps in the immediate pericellular zone, suggesting the possibility that another enzyme, a neutral proteoglycanase, operates in the tissues.[157–159]

Several groups have now identified a metal-dependent enzyme that degrades PG subunits at a neutral pH. It seems likely that this material is at least analogous to stromelysin, a metallodependent enzyme activated by IL-1, with the capacity to not only destroy the PG but under certain circumstances, activate collagenase (see below). This latter material, which has been partially purified, is maintained in an inactive state by the presence of TIMP and is believed to require plasmin for activation.[160]

   Numerous body tissues contain collagenase active at neutral pH, and the pattern of degradation of the collagen molecule is well established.[161,162] Most mammalian collagenases act on the substrate to cleave it into two fragments, which represent approximately three-fourths and one-fourth, respectively, of the length of the intact molecule. The degraded material is soluble and can be further degraded by the action of other proteases. Although an endogenous collagenase in osteoarthritic human articular cartilage has been demonstrated, to date limited evidence exists for the presence of an active collagenase in normal joint cartilage.[163] The turnover rate for collagen is sufficient, however, to require some form of enzymatic degradative system for this otherwise insoluble material, and recent observations suggest the presence of a small amount of collagenolytic activity in normal tissues. It is thought that collagenase present in the tissue is maintained in the latent form by inhibitors and requires at least two additional enzymes, stromelysin and plasmin, to activate it to a more potent destructive enzyme.

   Despite prior suggestions to the contrary, ample evidence now exists to demonstrate that plasmin is one of the principle players in the degradative cascade[164] and is probably responsible for both the activation of stromelysin and acting with that material, the activation of collagenase.[165] Tissue plasminogen activator (TPA) appears necessary to activate plasminogen to plasmin and the material which appears to prevent such activation PAI-1.

   If one now considers the degradative cascade in its current proposed form, IL-1 or perhaps to a lesser extent tumor necrosis factor (TNF) derived from synovium or other tissues stimulates a paracrine production of IL-1 by chondrocytes, which induces the synthesis of latent collagenase, latent stromelysin, and other neutral and acid proteases, latent gelatinase, and TPA (Fig. 2-9). Plasminogen is for the most part contributed by synovial cell transudation but may also be synthesized by the chondrocytes[164,168] and enters the matrix. These potentially destructive chondrolytic materials are believed to be held in the latent form by two inhibitors, TIMP and PAI-1.[166,167,169]

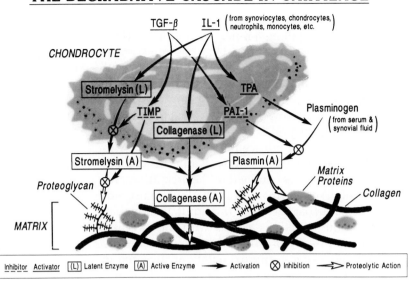

FIGURE 2-9
Drawing shows the current concept of the degradative cascade for articular cartilage. IL-1 stimulates release of the active degradative substances, plasmin and stromelysin, which in turn together activate collagenase. TGF-β appears to stabilize the situation by increasing the production of TIMP and PAI, which prevent the release of the two active enzymes.

The synthesis of both is stimulated and enhanced by the action of paracrine and autocrine TGF-β.[170] If the inhibitors are destroyed, stromelysin and plasmin are released. The stromelysin act in two ways—first as a cathepsin to destroy the protein core of the proteoglycan and second, as one "hit" in the "two-hit" system of activation of the latent collagenase. The other "hit" is supplied by plasmin, which is activated by the plasminogen activator, and the collagenase is now free to destroy the tissue.

Considerable attention has been paid to the prostaglandins, prostacyclines, etc., which initially appeared to not only cause synovial inflammation but to play some role in the degradation of cartilage. The nature of the action was not well understood but is believed to be due to an activation of lysosomal enzymes and possibly some additional effects on other parts of the degradative cascade as a result of a stimulation of synovial IL-1.[109] At least one mediator for this system may be an intracellular material, phospholipase A_2, whose synthesis is markedly increased by the chondrocyte by the action of synovial or chondrocytic IL-1.[109–111,171] The phospholipase A_2 appears to exert an effect on the synthesis of arachidonic acid and subsequent production of prostaglandins and other lipid mediators, which may in turn materially alter synthesis and degradation of the cartilage.[171]

IMMATURE ARTICULAR CARTILAGE AND THE EFFECTS OF AGING

Unlike many other body tissues, immature articular cartilage differs rather markedly from adult articular cartilage. On gross inspection, the cartilage from an immature animal appears blue-white in color (pre-sumably because of the reflection of the vascular structures in the underlying immature bone) and is considerably thicker on cut section.[172] The thickness appears to be primarily a function of the dual nature of the cartilage mass; it serves not only as a cartilaginous articular surface for the joint but also as a microepiphyseal plate for endochondral ossification of the underlying bony nucleus of the epiphysis.[173]

On histologic examination, immature articular cartilage appears considerably more cellular than the adult tissue, and numerous studies have corroborated the increased number of cells per unit volume or mass (Fig. 2-10).[174–176] The hypercellularity appears fairly uniform throughout the cartilage, with little variation noted in cell density. The structural organization of the tissue also differs from that of adult cartilage in that the zonal characteristics show major variation, particularly in the lower zones. The gliding or tangential layer remains evident in immature cartilage, although the surface cells are somewhat larger and less discoid than those seen in adult cartilage. The midzone is wider and contains a larger number of randomly arranged cells. In the lower zones, however, the orientation differs markedly; at about the halfway mark in the distance from the surface to the underlying bone, the chondrocytes are arranged in irregular columns and at further depth the short irregular columns of the micro-growth plate become evident. The cells in these columns show characteristics consistent with those of chondrocytes of the epiphyseal plate and include all the features albeit somewhat distorted in histologic appearance.[173,174]

When immature articular cartilage is examined by light microscopy, mitotic figures are readily noted and all stages of mitosis can be seen. Cell replication is not uniformly present throughout the tissue, however. In the very young animal, the mitotic activity occurs in two distinct zones. One lies subjacent to the surface and presumably accounts for the growth of the cellular complement of the articular portion of the cartilage mass; the second lies below this region and consists of a narrow band of cells that morphologically resemble the proliferative zone of the microepiphyseal plate for the subjacent bony nucleus.[174] With advancing age, the mitotic index is diminished and replicative activity is confined to the area just above the zone of vascular invasion in the lowermost portion of the cartilage.[173,174] In the adult mammalian cartilage, mitotic activity ceases with the development of a well-defined calcified zone and tidemark and in some species, approximately at the time of epiphyseal plate closure.[174,177] Careful search of nor-

mal articular cartilage from adult animals of numerous species has failed to demonstrate mitotic figures, and ^{3}H-thymidine studies have not demonstrated grains over the nucleus, indicating the absence of DNA replication.[174,177] Although it has been suggested that the chondrocyte may divide by amitotic division, only limited evidence supports such an activity, and cytophotometry and cytofluorometry have failed to demonstrate evidence of nuclear polyploidy in the adult tissue. These data support the concept that adult articular chondrocytes lose their power to replicate during health. The question remains, however, do they "break the switch" for DNA synthesis or merely "turn it off"? The answer will be forthcoming in the sections on lacerative injury and osteoarthritis (see below).

In recent years, investigations have demonstrated significant variation in the chemistry of articular cartilage with advancing age. Water content appears to be increased in immature animals and slowly diminishes to a standard figure that remains constant throughout most of adulthood. The collagen content of fetal articular cartilage is considerably lower than that of mature animals. Once the value climbs to the adult values (shortly after birth), the concentration is maintained throughout the life of the animal.

The principal chemical changes in articular cartilage matrix with advancing age appear to be in the PG molecule. The concentration of PG in articular cartilage is highest at birth and diminishes slowly through the period of immaturity.[51,178–180] The lengths of the protein core and the GAGs chains are increased in immature animals and polymerization of the GAG is greater.[180–182] As the animal approaches adolescence and maturity, the PG core becomes shorter and the GAG chain lengths, particularly those of chondroitin sulfate, diminish. Although the concentration of chondroitin 4-sulfate has been noted to be extraordinarily high in immature animals, a fairly rapid diminution in this value is noted with aging.[178,180,181] Furthermore, with advancing age, the total chondroitin sulfate concentration falls and that of keratan sulfate increases until at approximately age 30 in human beings, keratan sulfate represents 25 percent to 50 percent of the total GAG, a value that then remains constant through old age.[75,183,184] Aggregation appears to diminish with advancing age possibly on the basis of an alteration in the core protein or link protein but not reflected in the concentration of hyaluronate.[185]

In vitro synthesis of PGs is diminished for lapine and bovine articular chondrocytes from animals of advanced age, suggesting that the alteration in synthetic activity is related to a structural change in the cell associated with the senescent process.[186] The rate

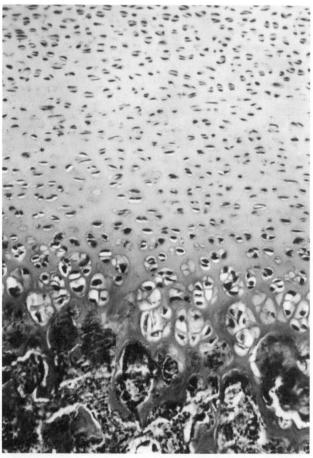

FIGURE 2-10
Histologic picture of immature articular cartilage from a 2-month old rabbit's distal femur. Note the differences between this section and that shown in Fig. 2-1. The cartilage shows increased cellularity and variation in the size and distribution of the cells. The calcified zone and tidemark are absent. H&E, ×80. (Reprinted with permission of the publisher from Mankin HJ: The articular cartilages, cartilage healing and osteoarthritis, in *Adult Orthopaedics,* edited by RL Cruess, WRJ Rennie. New York, Churchill Livingstone, 1984, 163–270.)

of such decline is not great, however, and suggests that in health articular chondrocytes from even the elderly are competent in maintaining the matrix structure and composition.[187]

CARTILAGE HEALING

Although articular cartilage is a hardy tissue and appears generally to carry out its tasks with little problem over a lifetime, in a world of high velocity trauma the cartilages are frequently mechanically injured and undergo some significant functional loss. Furthermore, any individual who has had repeated minor trauma to the knees or hips or some significant malalignment is clearly at risk for the slow process of "degeneration" (a misnomer . . . see below), believed to lead to the almost universal disease of the elderly, osteoarthritis. Although the two symptoms are considerably different in terms of histology and biologic response, it is clear that for both the major and central changes occur in the hyaline articular cartilage. Findings in the underlying bone, synovium, and capsule may be present and participatory in the pathogenesis of the process, but most investigators believe cartilage injury and osteoarthritis are "true" cartilage diseases.

The general response of vascular mammalian tissues to injury is a phasic one so similar for most organs and structures as to be almost stereotypical. The response may be divided into four rather distinct phases: necrosis, inflammation, repair, and scar remodeling. The phase of necrosis begins immediately and is characterized by tissue death, which varies in extent depending on the type of injury and the richness of the tissue blood supply. Inflammation follows shortly thereafter and is similar to that seen in infectious challenge in that it is almost entirely mediated by the vascular system. It is characterized by vascular dilatation, increased blood flow, transudation, hematoma formation, exudation, and ultimately development of a fibrin clot in which are entrapped inflammatory cells. The phase of repair supervenes when the fibrin clot is invaded by blood vessels and fibroblasts begin to produce first granulation tissue and subsequently a fibrous repair tissue that welds the wound edges together. In the final phase of scar remodeling, the fibrous repair tissue organizes and matures into scar and then over a variable period of time becomes less vascular and more heavily cross-linked to bring the wound edges into closest relationship. It should be evident to anyone interested in connective tissues that there are at least two exceptions to the rule—bone, which normally heals with bone rather than fibrous tissue, and cartilage, which if it heals, does so with a mixture of hyaline and fibrocartilage.

Superficial Injuries

In considering the application of this schema to injuries confined to the substance of the hyaline articular cartilage, cartilage can and does undergo necrosis with injury during phase one. Cells die and the matrix is disrupted at the site of the trauma. Because there are no blood vessels in cartilage (articular cartilage is avascular), the phase of inflammation is absent. No blood escapes from ruptured vessels and no clot is produced. No hyperemia, transudation, or exudation occurs and thus no plasma or cells are available to provide either the fibrin framework, the pleuripotential stems cells, or the high concentration of the numerous growth factors necessary for stimulation of wound healing (PDGF), b-FGB, IGF I, and TGF-β. All repair must be carried out by the cartilage itself, which surprisingly even in adult tissues is stimulated to carry on active DNA and matrix synthesis far in excess of the normal. The repair process is disappointingly short-lived and limited in scope and under ordinary circumstances in adult cartilage is incapable of producing other than a few cells to fill the necrotic zone adjacent to the margin of the injury.

Thus, despite recent reports to the contrary (mostly from arthroscopic observations), lacerative injuries to mature articular cartilage that do not violate the tidemark (and hence are confined to the matrix of the cartilage) show an initial necrotic phase the extent of which depends on the type and character of the injury. Although the synovial fluid and sometimes blood from the joint provide some cells and a wispy fibrinous material in the wound site, the inflammatory phase is lacking and the growth factors provided by the chondrocytes are usually only sufficient to compensate for some part of the wound edge necrosis. The repair phase both for cells and matrix components, although initially brisk, is not only limited in scope but in duration and disappears in the adult cartilage in a matter of weeks.[188,189] No repair supervenes and the cartilage wound edges remain unhealed.[188-195] Of considerable importance is the obvious fact that despite no healing, there is limited evidence for the development of osteoarthritis unless joint incongruity supervenes (see below) and the slices, whether perpendicular, oblique, or tangential to the surface, remain identifiably as such, presumably for the life of the joint (Fig. 2-11). It should be evident that the lacerative injury of adult cartilage is an old experiment (the earliest reported study dates back to John Hunter in the mid-18th century[196]) and

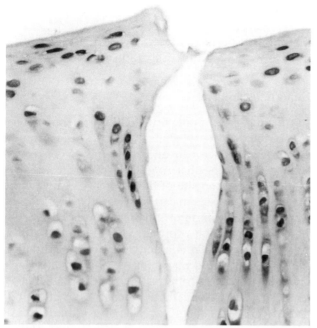

FIGURE 2-11
Photomicrograph of a histologic section taken through adult rabbit articular cartilage 1 y after a slice was made in the surface using a blade. Note that the injury was "superficial," i.e., did not penetrate the tidemark. Although some of the cells show evidence of having filled in the necrotic zone adjacent to the slice margin, there is no evidence of healing. H&E, ×150.

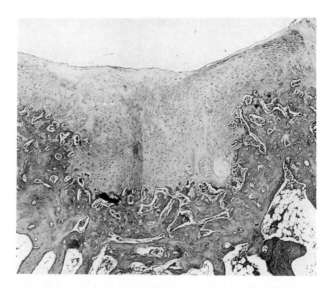

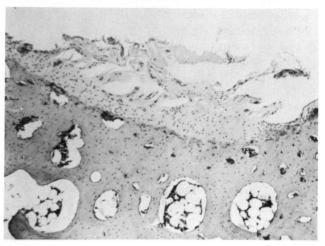

B

FIGURE 2-12
Photomicrographs of a deep coring defect in adult rabbit articular cartilage at an early phase in the repair process (*A*) and later (*B*). Note in the early phase that the defect is filled with what appears to be excellent cartilage with good restoration of the surface architecture. Later (at approximately 1 y) the cartilage shows changes of advanced osteoarthritis. (Courtesy of Dr. Lawrence C. Rosenberg. Fig. 2-12*A*.) (Reprinted with permission of the publisher from Mankin HJ: The articular cartilages, cartilage healing and osteoarthritis, in *Adult Orthopaedics,* edited by RL Cruess, WRJ Rennie. New York, Churchill-Livingstone 1984, 163–270.)

the results for mature cartilage not only do not vary but appear to be independent of species, site, and method of producing the injury. Despite suggestions to the contrary, performing intracartilaginous lacerative surgery through the arthroscope does not stimulate cartilage healing any more than if done as an open procedure; and using a shaver, laser, or cautery does not change the results from all of the hundreds of studies described for similar injuries created with a knife. If the injury is superficial—it does not heal!

Deep Injuries to Cartilage

The response of articular cartilage to injuries that are full thickness and thus penetrating to or through the underlying bone is considerably different from response to superficial injuries. In deep injury, the necrosis is usually more extensive because the penetration into the bone requires more violence. The presence of a vascular bed in the bone provides not only a source of the low molecular weight mediators and cytokines, but also supports a brisk inflammatory response, thus allowing the tissue to recapitulate all the phases of the healing seen in other soft tissues and in theory at least, since the bone is involved, that for fracture healing of osseous tissue as well.

The lesional area immediately fills with blood and the hematoma becomes organized into a fibrin clot in which are trapped cellular elements from the blood and bone marrow. Pluripotential precursor cells mobilized by the injury and the inflammatory response lay down a bed of vascular and other connective tissue elements, which initially becomes a granulation tissue and with maturation becomes more fibroblastic (Fig. 2-12). One might anticipate the repair tissue remaining fibrous in nature (early scar) as ordinarily occurs with injuries to skin, soft tissues, and most organs; or becoming osseous as one might expect in an injury to bone for which the pattern of fracture healing is well defined. Instead, the tissue almost miraculously undergoes "chondrification," becoming at first a fibrocartilage and then a histologically typical hyaline cartilage. The cartilaginous material produced has a high concentration of PG (with an appropriate distribution of GAGs for cartilage) and contains principally type II collagen although early in the repair process the collagen type more closely resembles that seen in fibrous tissue or fibrocartilage. The healing cartilaginous tissue fills the wound, joins the slice margins together (which have in the interim responded just as with superficial laceration by a meager and short-lived repair phase) and at least for a period of time appears to be an excellent substitute for the lost cartilaginous material.[190–192,197–201] Studies of the biochemistry of the cartilaginous surfaces shows that the repair tissue, although at least in part hyaline, has neither a sufficient concentration of PG nor a high enough content of type II collagen to perform as well as the normal hyaline material[192,197] and over time the tissue deteriorates. Localized osteoarthritis occurs at a rate and to an extent which depend on the size of the defect, the site, and the stresses acting on the tissue.

The ultimate fate of this mixture of hyaline and fibrocartilage is crucial to consideration of clinical management of joint disease and once again the reader should not be confused by promises of restoration following one or another form of therapy. Numerous studies have demonstrated that regardless of management system the cartilaginous tissue does not appear to "hold up" and over time a localized osteoarthritis develops at the site. Immobilization, electrical stimulation, administration of drugs either systemically or locally, active movement, and continuous passive motion have all been advocated as helping to improve the state of the cartilage.[202–208] To date, no single system or combination appears to be successful in either altering the mix of fibrocartilage and hyaline cartilage or in protecting the cartilage from localized osteoarthritic failure.

Drilling or shaving an adult cartilage defect down to or through the underlying bone regardless of how performed or how treated subsequently causes new cartilage to appear and in comparison with superficial injuries, at a brisk rate. It has been suggested that the rate and initial quality of the cartilage may be altered by continuous passive motion, but the cartilage is unfortunately not normal and does not "bear up," eventually showing all the findings consistent with the biologic process defined by the term osteoarthritis (see below). If the defect is small, the osteoarthritic focus appears to be localized to the site of the deep defect and does not progress rapidly to extensive disease in the remainder of the joint.

Response of Articular Cartilage to Blunt Trauma

Mammalian articular cartilages by their nature and in response to functional demands can accommodate to single or multiple moderate- and high-impact loads. A number of studies have sought to define the effect of either a single "excessive" high impact, which causes injury to the cartilage without causing a break in the surface, or repetitive "below-threshold" traumas, which cause damage to the cartilage as a cumulative effect.[209,210] Using the single weight "drop tower" technique, either on the exposed or the closed skin over an animal's patella or condyle or multiple repetitive injuries to a cartilaginous surface, it is evident that cartilage can be damaged by the process of impact and that the damage may be significant.[209–212] Chondrocyte death, matrix damage, fissuring of the surface, injury to the underlying bone, and thickening of the tidemark region occur after trauma caused by the impact of either a single heavy load or repetitive below-threshold blows.

Perhaps the most provocative aspect of these studies is the suggestion by several investigators that impact, perhaps a single one or more likely repetitive multiple injuries, leads to thickening of the tidemark, increases in the thickness of the calcified zone, and ultimately stiffens the cartilage–bone junction. The alterations in these parameters are alleged by proponents of this theory to increase the stresses acting on the cartilage with normal function and presumably can lead to an osteoarthritic focus. Certainly this is one of the theories suggested as causative in osteoarthritis and although perhaps less likely than some of the others, it has its attractive features for proponents.

OSTEOARTHRITIS

General Considerations

Osteoarthritis is by far the most prevalent of the clinical entities within the domain of the orthopaedist, and the clinical picture is exceedingly well documented.[213] Occasionally a patient is encountered with another disorder that can be confused with osteoarthritis but such cases are rarely difficult to solve. In general, osteoarthritis is suspected on the basis of history and epidemiologic considerations, presumptively diagnosed on physical examination, positively identified by radiographic imaging, and "confirmed" by arthroscopy.[214]

With a disorder such as osteoarthritis for which the cause remains entirely unknown, the disease is best described by an analysis of its clinical, pathologic, and biologic characteristics. One such definition (as modified to emphasize clinical presentation from a more global one proposed during a workshop on Etiopathogenesis of Osteoarthritis[215] is as follows:

Osteoarthritis is a slowly progressive monoarticular (or less commonly polyarticular) disorder of unknown cause and obscure pathogenesis. The condition occurs late in life, principally affecting the hands and large weight bearing joints and is characterized clinically by pain, deformity, enlargement of the joints and limitation of motion. Pathologically the disease is characterized by focal erosive lesions, cartilage destruction, subchondral sclerosis, cyst formation and large osteophytes at the margins of the joint. The disease appears to originate in the cartilage, and the changes in that tissue, virtually pathognomonic, are progressively more severe with advancing disease; while structural aberrations in the underlying bone and when present, inflammatory alterations in the synovium are usually milder and thought to be secondary. Systemic abnormalities have not been detected. Therapeutically, the disorder is characterized by lack of a specific healing agent.

Before considering the gross, histologic, biochemical, and metabolic alterations in articular cartilage from mechanically injured or osteoarthritic human joints or from animal models, several important qualifying remarks must be introduced to explain divergent views that have appeared in the literature in recent years. If one seeks to determine an abnormality in the appearance or biology of a segment of articular cartilage, it is logical to have as a comparison normal tissue that comes from a corresponding site of the corresponding joint from an individual of the same age, sex, body habitus, and so on. Although this is a reasonable application of the scientific method, it is frequently difficult or impossible to achieve in studies of osteoarthritis. As noted previously, the appearance and biochemical composition of articular cartilage may vary considerably from species to species, individual to individual, joint to joint, and site to site within a joint and with the depth of the cartilage from surface to calcified zone. Diffusion of materials through the cartilage may vary, depending on the thickness of the tissue studied and the integrity of the collagenous "skin"; cell density may vary widely in small segments of cartilage adjacent to one another. Furthermore, there is ample reason to believe that significant differences may exist between the biochemical abnormalities seen in osteoarthritic

cartilage recovered at autopsy from individuals who were asymptomatic during life and cartilage involved with "end-stage disease" obtained at the time of surgical extirpation of the joint. Drawing conclusions regarding the nature of a process on the basis of the latter specimens (which are readily obtainable in current orthopaedic practice) may lead to erroneous conclusions (and frequently has).

Current animal models of both lacerative injury and osteoarthritis, although accepted as demonstrating facets of the disease, may differ considerably from the human or naturally occurring mammalian condition, depending on the nature of the insult used to cause the disease, the species and age of the animal, and so on. Lacerative injury in the mouse differs from that in the horse, and that in the proximal tibia may differ from that in the distal tibia. Similarly, immobilization osteoarthritis differs in its gross and microscopic characteristics from that seen in the partial meniscectomy model or from the dog model in which the anterior cruciate has been severed. Furthermore, in models of osteoarthritis that depend on mechanical instability, the degree of usage of the unstable joint will affect development of the disease.

Lesions resulting from chemical insults may vary widely from those occurring as a result of mechanical conditions. Even the naturally occurring models (hip dysplasia in the dog and naturally occurring osteoarthritis in rodents) may be questioned because of differences in age of the animals and biologic differences in the animals.

Pathology of Osteoarthritis

On gross examination of a knee joint affected by osteoarthritis, it is clearly evident that all of the joint structures are affected.[14,216–218] The capsule of the joint is usually quite thickened and at times adherent to the deformed underlying bone, a condition that may figure rather prominently in the causation of the limitation of movement.[219,220] The synovial lining in osteoarthritic joints often shows a moderate to marked degree of inflammatory change.[221,222] The surface of the synovium is often hypervascular and hemorrhagic, the lining is thickened and nodular and at times demonstrates hypertrophic villous folds.[218,219,222]

Consistent with the terminology which introduces the Latin root *osteo-* into the name of the disease, the bones even somewhat remote from the subchondral region in osteoarthritic joints often show remarkable changes.[14,216–218] Considerable remodeling of the underlying bone is evident on the basis of alterations in gross structure, thickening of the cortices, and change in trabecular stress lines (Fig. 2-13) Patellar enlargement, bowing, or knock-knee deformities originally related to intra-articular pathology seem over many years to result in marked alterations in the bony architecture with considerable cortical and medullary remodeling.

The bone of the joint itself shows the most striking changes. Osteophytes, a cardinal feature of the disease and particularly prominent in the patella, arise from the bony margins of the osseous components of the joint, surround it and grossly alter the bony contours[14,217–219,223,224] (Fig. 2-14). The size, shape, and extent of these bony excrescences vary considerably from patient to patient and from joint to joint.[14,224,225] The majority of the articular osteophytes are covered with hyaline cartilage but occasionally display only fibrous tissue or bare bone at the surface.[216,218]

Gross examination of the split surface of the bone almost invariably shows sclerosis of the subchondral bony end plate immediately subjacent to the diseased cartilage.[218] The change is most severe at the point of maximum pressure against the opposing cartilage surface. The subchondral bony shell is enlarged and very dense and displays extensions of sclerotic trabecular descending into the old epiphyseal region.[226–228] The sclerotic change may extend to the osteophytes.[226]

Osteoarthritic cysts, another cardinal feature of the disease, are frequently noted lying close to the subchondral region of the knee joint, but occasionally appear at a considerable distance, even at times extending into the metaphyseal areas.[216–219,224,225] The margins of the cysts are often sclerotic, which helps to distinguish them from the cysts seen in patients with rheumatoid arthritis in whom the bones themselves are far less dense and the cyst margins usually are poorly marginated. When cysts are transsected they contain not a true fluid but a glairy, homogenous clear or cloudy gelatinous material with a consistency resembling that found within ganglions adjacent to tendon sheaths.[218,219,224]

The gross appearance of the hyaline articular cartilage in the osteoarthritic joint shows a highly variable pattern and is markedly focal in the alterations observed.[14,218,224,228,229] In some areas the cartilage shows "softening" and a yellowish or brownish discoloration, whereas in others the normally smooth glistening surface appears as a soft velvety feltwork (Fig. 2-15). Remnants of old irregularity scarred or ulcerated cartilage may lie adjacent to a pebble-grained newly formed material, which is dull white in color and lacks the smoothness of surface ordi-

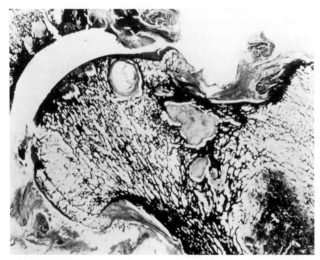

FIGURE 2-13
Histologic section of the upper end of the femur shows all the cardinal features of osteoarthritis. The joint space is narrow and sclerosis of the bony end plates is clearly evident. Cysts are present on both sides of the joint, and osteophytes are present medially and laterally on both femoral and acetabular sides of the joint. The architectural changes in the bone are displayed. H&E × 2. Courtesy of Clement B. Sledge, MD.

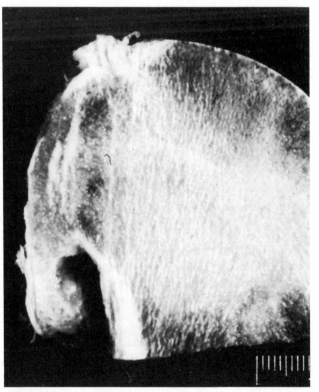

FIGURE 2-14
Classical appearance of an osteophyte on an arthritic femoral head. Note the extent of the excess bone and the "double line" of cartilage. (Reprinted with permission of the publisher from Mankin HJ: The articular cartilages, cartilage healing and osteoarthritis, in *Adult Orthopaedics,* edited by RL Cruess, WRJ Rennie. New York, Churchill-Livingstone, 1984, 163–270.)

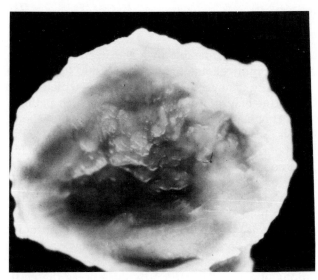

FIGURE 2-15
Photograph of the patella of a 38-year-old woman with severe chondromalacia shows extensive ulceration and alteration of contour. The margins of the patella are also irregular, suggesting osteophyte formation.

narily seen in hyaline cartilage. Ulcerations, fissures, and cracks appear on the surface and at times may be so extensive as to disclose the underlying sclerotic and eburnated subchondral bone.

Histologic examination of the tissues from an osteoarthritic joint reflect the changes seen on gross examination. The histologic changes are equally as variable as the gross changes. At times some parts of a heavily involved joint may appear histologically normal, yet other sites may show extensive changes. As might be anticipated, the major alterations are observed in the cartilage (providing some cartilage remains) but all periarticular tissues participate in the process and usually show alterations in structure.

Histologic examination of the capsule, particularly in advanced disease, is likely to demonstrate thickening, focal areas of inflammatory infiltrate (which at times dominates the picture[214,230]), neovascularity, and in some areas hyalinization, amyloid deposition and sparse cellularity.[219,220,225,231] Histologic study of the synovium often shows a markedly variable pattern ranging from nearly normal (only slight thickening of the subsynovial tissues and reduplication of the synovial layer) to tissues with such severe inflammatory alterations as to suggest the diagnosis of rheumatoid arthritis.[222,230,232,233] Histologic examination of the bone often shows considerable variation depending on the site examined. Early in the course of the disease, the subchondral area shows gross thickening of the cortex, bony sclerosis, and prominent cement lines and dilated vascular spaces, some of which penetrate the lower layers of the cartilage.[219,221,234] Later in the course after total denudation

of the cartilage occurs, one often sees a dense sclerosis with fibrous and fibrocartilaginous plugs and some evidence for new bone formation.[216,218,224,225] The marrow cavities are often replaced by fibrous tissue and endosteal remodeling, osteoblastic rimming, and evidence for active new bone formation can be observed.[227] Periosteal new bone formation may be evident along the metaphyseal cortex. Despite the now well-documented osteoarthritic subchondral hypervascularity, strongly supported by angiography and bone scans of this region,[221,227,235,236] frequently small and sometimes large segments of osteonecrotic bone are seen.[14,218,225,228] Cysts of the bone appear as loose, sparsely cellular amorphous regions that stain poorly with hematoxylin and eosin.[14,218,224,225,228]

The cartilage histology has been the best studied.[22,23,34,35,41] The first changes seen in osteoarthritic cartilage are those of surface erosion and irregularities (Fig. 2-16). At this early stage, the matrix of the cartilage shows some mild alterations in the staining quality. When identifiable, the tidemark often shows irregularities, reduplication, discontinuous areas, and penetration with blood vessels.[218,224,237,238] This finding first pointed out decades ago by Trueta[239] is thought by many to be one of the major factors associated with the mechanism of osteophyte formation.

As the disorder progresses, the surface layer becomes more fragmented and short vertical clefts are noted often descending through the gliding zone of the cartilage into the transitional zone (see Fig. 2-16A). The matrix shows greater irregularity in staining even with hematoxylin and eosin. With metachromatic stains such as toluidine blue or Alcian blue or an orthochromatic one such as safranin-O, a progressive, patchy depletion of color and heterogeneity can be noted, initially in the surface areas then deeper, and involving first the interterritorial areas and subsequently the territorial regions.[218,224,240,241] This color alteration closely parallels the progressive depletion of PG described below. With advancing disease, the focal fragmentation of the joint surface becomes greater, the clefts become deeper (descending now as far as the calcified zone), and the matrix staining appears even more irregular and depleted (see Fig. 2-16B). Finally at end stage, only wisps of cartilage are left clinging to the denuded eburnated sclerotic subchondral bone (Fig. 2-14C)

The cellular complement of the cartilage shows some remarkable alterations. One of the most extraordinary changes in this disorder and, in fact pathognomonic, is the increased numbers of cells seen in the disease.[216,220,225,241] At first the change is that of a diffuse mild hypercellularity but with disease progression, the cells are found in clones or "brood capsules," which sometime contain a hundred or more chondrocytes.[14,228] Eventually in moderately severe disease the majority of the cells are in such formations, some of which seem to be metabolically active while others are not.[242,243] Although DNA synthesis has been documented in the osteoarthritic chondrocytes by tritiated thymidine studies,[243] (none are found in cells from

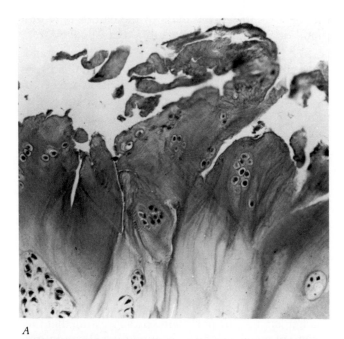

A

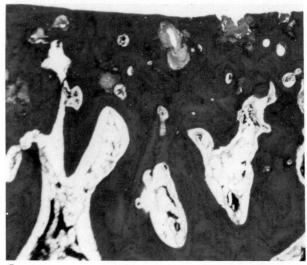

B

FIGURE 2-16
Histological picture of osteoarthritic cartilage in an early phase. Note the fragmented surface of the cartilage and the clefts that descend into the substance of the tissue. Note especially the increased numbers of cells in clones. H&E, ×180. *B.* End-stage disease with no cartilage remaining. The bone at the surface is eburnated and shows evidence of focal osteonecrosis. H&E, ×40. (Reprinted with permission of the publisher from Mankin HJ: The articular cartilages, cartilage healing and osteoarthritis, in *Adult Orthopaedics,* edited by RL Cruess, WRJ Rennie. New York, Churchill-Livingstone, 1984, 163–270.)

normal joints) mitotic figures are remarkably rare, which suggests to some that the clones arise by a process of "amitotic division."[12] As the disease progresses the chondrocytes appear less active and in late stage disease show signs of cell death and auto-digestion.[12,244] These histologic studies are supported by ultrastructural observations of a number of investigators using both SEM and transmission electron microscopy.

Causes of Osteoarthritis

Because the cause(s) of idiopathic osteoarthritis remain(s) unknown considerable speculation exists as to the various factors that may play a role in either the initiation of the disorder, its perpetuation, or its pathogenesis. Among the significant factors are:

1. Aging. Perhaps the most tantalizing aspect of the osteoarthritis puzzle is the relationship to aging. There is little doubt that osteoarthritis predicts the elderly and is virtually unknown in children and rare in young adults. With advancing years the incidence climbs precipitously[245–249] until data from autopsy studies[216,229] suggest that at age 60, over 60 percent of the population probably have some degree of cartilage abnormalities in many of their major joints. These observations and others that support the increased prevalence of osteoarthritis with advancing age[245,250,251] raise several questions. Is osteoarthritis a natural consequence of aging or are the changes of aging (see above) prerequisite?[14] Is the evolution of the process so slow that an insult sustained at an early age can only manifest the disease in the elderly? Ample evidence exists that aging alone is not a cause of osteoarthritis, but the remaining two theories are both tenable and likely.[252,253]

2. Alterations in matrix structure. Although secondary changes occur in matrix structure during the progress of osteoarthritis (see below), little or no support is offered for the concept that such changes are "primary" and lead to the development of the disease.[12,14] However, some interesting possible exceptions (or perhaps better termed special cases) include alkaptonuric ochronosis, hemachromatosis, and, more recently and perhaps much more relevantly, crystal deposition disease.[2,92–95]

3. Alterations in cellular activity. Little doubt exists that the metabolic activity of the osteoarthritic chondrocyte differs from the normal and that the changes are phenotypic and independent of the environment.[240,260] The question arises, however, are these "changes" primary or are they alterations (presum-

ably permanent) that occur when the cells are stimulated either acutely or chronically by some initiating factor for the disease?

4. Alterations in mediators. Humoral-, synovial-, and cartilage-derived chemical mediators and mechanical stimuli surely play major roles in regulation of synthetic processes. Ample evidence exists to support the notion that such materials as the IGF-I, EGF, b-FGF, TGF-β, and even insulin[261–264] have an effect on the cartilage. In addition, qualitative and quantitative changes in the chemical constituents of the substrates, electrolyte pool, mineral concentrations, and mechanical forces[28,240,265] can all alter the rates of synthesis or degradation (or both) of the matrix by normal chondrocytes. Of perhaps greater current interest are the recently assigned roles of the synovial and cartilaginous prostaglandins,[265–267] heat shock proteins,[268,269] synovially derived neutral proteases,[271,273–276] and the most recent additions to the growing list of cytokines and low molecular weight mediators, stromelysin,[271,273–276] phospholipase A_2,[171] and PAI-1.[277] Are some or any of these primary in the causation of the disease or are they simply responses to an overall alteration in metabolism associated with some occult injury to the cell? What is the role of synovial inflammation and production of IL-1 (see below)?

5. Trauma. It seems obvious that an unreduced patellar fracture that leaves the joint incongruent will in a short period of time lead to classic osteoarthritis; and such chronic states as recurrent dislocation of the patella, joint alterations as a result of osteonecrotic collapse, etc. will ultimately lead to an osteoarthritic lesion.[278–281] The role of trauma in the causation of the more occult forms of the disease, however, is far less evident. Does chronic malalignment or repetitive trauma (or both) over a lifetime initiate the cascade of biochemical and metabolic events leading to the disease.[278,282] Does stiffening of the subchondral bone plate result in increases in cartilage wear[58,59] or perhaps the reduplication of the tidemark and ultimate violation of that region by blood vessels?[238,283]

6. Immune responses. Perhaps one of the more provocative theories related to the cause of alterations in the articular cartilages in idiopathic osteoarthritis is the suggestion that because of the aneural and avascular state of the cartilages, the remainder of the body is unaware of their existence. Of perhaps greater importance is the possibility that some of the proteins of the matrix are unrecognized by the immune system as autogenous and when they or fragments of them escape from the cartilage into the synovial fluid, the local lymphocytic elements see them as antigens. This theory espoused by Cooke and co-workers[284–287] and more recently Revell and colleagues[230] and others[288] provides a hypothetical explanation for the method by which even a minor injury to the cartilage may serve as the initiating event in a local (synovial) autoimmune causation or perpetuation mechanism that over time becomes sufficiently severe so as to destroy parts of the cartilage by humoral or cellular cytotoxic antibody responses.[289]

7. Secondary causes. These are numerous and some are only infrequently associated with the disorder. There is little doubt that osteoarthritis can occur as a result of acute or chronic trauma to the joints.[278,282,290,291] and perhaps unrecognized trauma or long-standing injury based on a malalignment may be one of the causes of the idiopathic form of the disease. Similarly, congenital or acquired variations in childhood or young adulthood can result in osteoarthritis. The relationship between such entities as Legg-Calve-Perthes disease, congenital dislocation of the hip, or slipped capital femoral epiphysis and the subsequent development of osteoarthritis of the hip are so common in occurrence as to challenge the existent of an idiopathic form of that disease.[291,293,294]

An equally obvious presumptive pathogenetic mechanism may be postulated by suggesting that the variety of metabolic diseases including alkaptonuric ochronosis, hemachromatosis, and CPPD (see above) affect the cartilage by altering the physical properties of the tissue as a result of deposition of crystalline material in the matrix or causing some change in the collagen cross-linking.[254,295]

Still other forms of osteoarthritic disease give credence to the theory that osteoarthritis is in fact the final common pathway for diseased cartilage. Many patients with gout, rheumatoid arthritis, infection, Paget's disease, and osteonecrosis of various causes develop as their end-stage condition a classical osteoarthritis, indistinguishable from disorders of idiopathic or other secondary cause.[279] One must presume that the altered mechanics of the bone or joint or the changes in the cartilage lead ultimately to the process described above.

Biochemical Alterations in Osteoarthritic Cartilage

As stated above, it should be emphasized that measurements of the biochemical changes seen in osteoarthritis are not a truly scientific exercise. The reasons for these problems are the high degree of variability observed in the disease, the lack of appropriate controls, and the absence of a comparable animal model. Nevertheless, some characteristic features of the disorder stand out and are more or less agreed on by the osteoarthrologists. These include changes in the DNA content, water concentrations, PG concentration and composition, collagen structure, and anabolic and metabolic activities.

1. DNA content. Cell counts and measurements of the quantity of DNA per unit tissue show considerable variation in osteoarthritis, depending on the site tested and the degree of the disease. Usually, however, DNA concentrations have been reported to be near normal and occasionally increased in osteoarthritis.[241,296–298] This supports the concept that despite a reduction in the volume of tissue, the cell count is reasonably well maintained. Some of the chondrocyte clones show intense activity when studied autoradiographically using tritiated thymidine and cytidine,[243] whereas others, and indeed entire clones, may show little or no evidence of RNA metabolism and are probably dead or dying.[244] As the disease worsens, the tissue becomes hypocellular, and eventually all cellular substance is lost.

2. Water. The water content of osteoarthritic articular cartilage has been the subject of a number of studies in the past few decades, which have consistently shown a significant increase in water when compared with normal tissues.[30,31,38,299,300] This finding seems inconsistent with the fact that the concentration of "hydrophilic" PGs, which constitute almost 50 percent of the dry weight of normal cartilage, is significantly reduced in osteoarthritic articular cartilage. It further belies the concept that osteoarthritis is a degenerative disease in which the cartilages become "dried out." Several possible explanations are offered for this change. The first of these suggests that perhaps PG removal opens up binding sites on the collagen that are otherwise obscured and that hold water with greater avidity than the PG–collagen gel. A second and more logical possibility is that removal of the PG allows the remainder of the material to uncoil and increase its negatively charged domain and its hydrophilic character.[29,301] A more important finding than just increased water is that osteoarthritic cartilage shows increased swelling as compared with normal tissues.[301] The swelling pressure observed in these studies is significantly different from that of normal controls and implies some alteration in the collagen network.[244]

3. Proteoglycan. The PGs of osteoarthritic articular cartilage have received the greatest amount of investigative attention. It was well established decades ago that the PG content of osteoarthritic cartilage is diminished and that the decrease appears to be directly proportional to the severity of the disease.[38,241,265,298–304] Since these initial studies, additional investigations have been performed to define the nature of the PG macromolecule present in osteoarthritic articular cartilage, particularly in relation to aggregation, GAG chain length, and distribution of the GAGs. Evidence clearly demonstrates a marked increase in chondroitin sulfate concentration (especially chondroitin 4-sulfate) with a diminution in the concentration of keratan sulfate.[75,184,296,305,306] One explanation for this alteration is that the articular chondrocyte in osteoarthritic cartilage is synthesizing an "immature" PG.[303] Another is the possibility that an asymmetric degradation of the aggrecan moiety could selectively attack the hyaluronate binding region of the macromolecule or possibly the keratan sulfate chains. Still a third is supported by the finding of two populations of PG in cartilage—a larger one, rich in chondroitin sulfate, and a smaller one with increased concentrations of keratan sulfate that could be selectively degraded.[44,45,57]

As indicated above, most of the aggrecan in normal cartilage is in the form of large aggregates in which subunits are linked at specific binding sites to a long-chain filament of hyaluronic acid in the presence of link proteins. The PG of osteoarthritic cartilage appears to be considerably more extractable than from normal cartilage, and it is evident that a considerable percentage of the PG does not aggregate even in the presence of an excess of hyaluronic acid.[299,307–309] With advancing disease the ability to aggregate is reduced even further until virtually no PG is in that form. These changes suggest that increased proteolytic activity first attacks the G1 N-terminal end of the subunit followed by the G2 PG-rich region, thus producing a marked diminution in chain length.[310] Ultimately sufficient damage must occur to the hyaluronate binding region of the core protein, so that even if additional hyaluronate is added, no aggregation occurs (Fig. 2-17). Link proteins appear to be normal in character and in concentration in osteoarthritic cartilage, whereas hyaluronate is highly variable.[186,311,321]

4. Collagen. The collagen of articular cartilage from osteoarthritic joints may show some marked variations in the size and arrangement of the fibers, usually demonstrating a much less orderly and competent "felt-work" which allows for swelling of the surface with increased water (Fig. 2-18).[29,301] Despite this finding, numerous studies have demonstrated no change in the concentration of the collagen.[138,241,299,302,303] In severe disease, when the cartilage

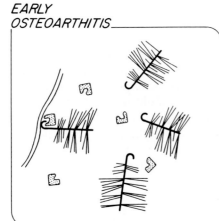

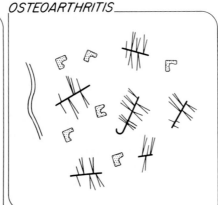

FIGURE 2-17
Diagrammatic representation of the changes in the proteoglycan molecules with advancing arthritis. Compare these with Figs. 2-3 and 2-5. With mild osteoarthritis, the subunits are smaller and aggregate poorly. With advanced disease they are badly clipped and short and probably do not aggregate at all.

is almost totally destroyed, the collagen content must fall (along with that of other constituents), but the relative concentration in relation to total mass (wet weight, dry weight, or per microgram of DNA) is not altered materially until the end stages of the disease.

One of the questions that has arisen in recent years has been whether the collagen of osteoarthritic cartilage remains as type II. Conflicting evidence exists, but the consensus suggests that the newly formed cartilage collagen, which attempts to repair the defect created by the disease, is mostly type II rather than type I[138,302,314] although type I may be somewhat increased in concentration, particularly in the region of the osteophytes. It should also be noted that scientists are just beginning to assess the variation in types IV, V, IX, and X in osteoarthritis. Such alterations may explain some of the characteristics of the disease and perhaps may have an influence on both water content and PG distribution.

5. Other materials. Severe osteoarthritis-like changes occur in patients with alkaptonuric och-

ronosis or hemachromatosis. Both of these seem to occur in relation to a "tanning" of the collagen fiber as a result of the deposition of the molecules homogentisic acid or hemosiderin in the substance of the cartilage.[256,258] A more subtle form of chemical disorder has been suggested recently by investigators who noted the markedly increased frequency of joint cartilage calcification (chondrocalcinosis articularis) in osteoarthritis.[257,259,315] Considerable data have demonstrated increased calcium pyrophosphate in the joint, increased numbers of membrane-bound calcium-containing vesicles, and increased alkaline phosphatase concentration in cartilage from some patients with osteoarthritis.[112,113,257,315,316] The relationship of these alterations to the pathogenesis of the disease is obscure but one theory at least suggests that the mid zones of the tissue are stiffened and more prone to mechanical injury.

The Metabolism of Osteoarthritic Cartilage

1. Proteoglycans. Perhaps the most controversial set of issues in the biochemical study of osteoar-

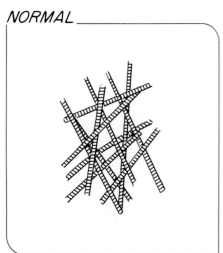

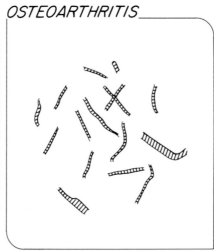

FIGURE 2-18
Diagram shows the alterations in the structure of the collagen fibers with osteoarthritis. The normal tight fibrillar structure is destroyed. The fibers vary in size, some smaller and some larger than normal.

thritic cartilage has been the assessment of the metabolic rate of the tissue as compared with that of normal. The early concept of the disease suggested that the process consisted of a passive mechanical erosion by "wear and tear" of a relatively inert tissue. It would, therefore, seem logical that the cells would show signs of degeneration and of decreased synthetic activity as the disease progressed. It was with some surprise, then, that scientists greeted the observation that articular chondrocytes from osteoarthritic human joints are considerably more metabolically active than normal articular cartilage.[241,298,317,318] Furthermore, regardless of which material is used as a tracer of PG synthesis (sulfate or glucosamine), the rates of incorporation are not only higher but appear to parallel the severity of the disease process.[241] In a recent study, hyaluronate synthesis was found to be excessively increased in osteoarthritis, which seems usual in view of the decreased aggregation and the diminished concentration of hyaluronate.[306] Considering the data, it seems reasonable that either the hyaluronate synthesized is abnormal and hence does not allow aggregation or that the excess synthesis is in response to a rapid degradation of the synthesized product.

2. Collagen synthesis. The collagen of articular cartilage is considered to be much more stable than the PG, but several metabolic studies have shown that collagen synthesis in osteoarthritic human cartilage is greater than normal and that the rate of collagen synthesis varies with the severity of the disease. Further studies have shown at least in several animal models that the material synthesized is type II rather than type I, supporting the concept that the "repair tissue" in osteoarthritis is hyaline cartilage rather than fibrocartilage.[138,302] One of the other minor constituent proteins of cartilage, fibronectin, has been recently discovered to show significant increments in both concentration and rate of synthesis in osteoarthritis.[98–100] The significance of this finding is currently unknown.

3. DNA synthesis. Studies of DNA synthesis in osteoarthritic articular cartilage have shown both mitotic activity and increased tritiated thymidine incorporation,[242,243] particularly in the cells of the chondrocyte clones, a finding supported by electron microscopic studies of the cartilage.[244] These data point to the likelihood that the articular chondrocyte in osteoarthritis "turns on the switch" for DNA synthesis and makes new cells that presumably become metabolically active. The rate of DNA synthesis appears to vary directly with the morphologic severity of the process up to a point of "failure," after which the rates falls.[241]

4. Degradative enzymes. Despite the findings that the rates for synthesis of PG, collagen, and DNA are all increased, the fact that osteoarthritis is a disorder in which the cartilage is inexorably and sometimes rapidly degraded strongly speaks for the fact that catabolic activity of the tissue is extraordinarily high and ultimately dominates the picture. Although "wear" may be a factor in the loss of articular cartilage, strong evidence supports the concept that lysosomal and extralysosomal enzymes account for the majority of the loss of substance. Over the past few years, there have been numerous demonstrations of proteolytic enzymes within the cells and matrix of articular cartilage in health and in certain pathologic states (see above). A number of studies have shown that acid cathepsins present in the lysosome of the chondrocytes have a powerful hydrolytic action on the protein core of the PG macromolecule.[153,154,156] Cathepsin D levels are elevated in osteoarthritic articular cartilage and acid phosphatase activity is markedly increased and varies with the severity of the disease.[153] In addition, neutral protease, a metal-dependent enzyme, is present in increased concentrations in articular cartilage from osteoarthritic joints and may be the principal agent in the degradation of PG.[137–159]

Perhaps the most virulent of the proteolytic materials in cartilage is collagenase, which has been noted to be increased in concentration in osteoarthritic cartilage in approximate concordance with the severity of the disease.[163,319,320] It is obvious that cathepsins, neutral protease, and collagenase are present in normal as well as osteoarthritic articular cartilage, but they are probably controlled by potent inhibitors in normal tissue. As noted in the section under the enzymes of articular cartilage above, a degradative cascade has been described and is now an accepted mechanism not only to explain normal turnover of the cartilage but the increased destruction of cartilage in osteoarthritis and other disorders in which the cartilage is damaged. In brief reiteration, the principle mover of the system appears to be IL-1 (formerly catabolin).[321–325] Although this material may be coming from the inflamed joint of monocytes, it also has been found to be synthesized by chondrocytes as a paracrine activity. IL-1 enhances the synthesis and activates a number of enzyme systems in the cartilage including a latent collagenase, a latent stromelysin, a latent gelatinase, and a TPA (see Fig. 2-9).[321–324] Plasminogen is presumed to be synthesized by the chondrocyte or is contributed by the synovial cell transudation to enter the matrix.[164,168] It should be evident that these materials are potentially destructive to the cartilage but the balance of the system lies with at least two inhibitors, TIMP and PAI-1 both of which are activated by TGF-β and diminish the degradative activity at least for a period of time.[166,167,169] If these two materials are destroyed, both stromelysin and plasmin are released. The stromelysin is believed to act in two ways: first as a cathepsin to destroy the protein core of the PG and second, and more importantly, as one part of the activation process for the collagenase. The second part of this "two-hit system" is plasmin, which also appears to act on the partially activated precursor molecule to release the completely activated and destructive collagenase (see Fig. 2-9).

The Biochemical Pathogenesis of Osteoarthritis

Although several studies have suggested that the primary lesion in osteoarthritis may be in the subchondral bone, most investigators believe that the disorder begins in the cartilage. These can be summarized by stating that the cartilage is slowly but progressively and inexorably destroyed. The changes are associated biochemically with an early loss of PG, increased water content, and no alteration in collagen content but a probable highly significant change in the arrangement and size of the collagen fibers, particularly in the middle zone. Of considerable importance is the reduction of PG aggregation. It is probable that an alteration occurs in the hyaluronate binding region of the aggrecan subunit that decreases the number of aggregates formed.

Another issue in the pathogenesis of the disease is the evident relationship of the process to low molecular weight mediators, cytokines and inhibitors. As indicated above, synovial, monocyte, and chondrocyte IL-1 appear to play a major role in the disease process and specifically in calling up the degradative cascade. Stromelysin, TPA, plasmin, collagenase, gelatinase, acid cathepsins, etc. all must play roles in the failure of the cartilage. The cartilage is not without defenses in this system, however. TIMP and PAI-1 stabilize the degradative system and mitogens such as IGF-1, TGF-β, and b-FGF must surely help to initiate a brisk repair response. The chondrocytes undergo cell replication to produce new cells, some of which appear to be active metabolically, producing increased quantities of PG, collagen,and hyaluronic acid. These new materials are probably abnormal in the sense that they do not aggregate well, and there is a significant alteration in the GAG distribution within the newly synthesized PGs.

Despite the fact that degradation and repair are noted in the cartilage (and probably the reason why the disease may take so long to evolve), the repair process appears only to keep pace with the disease for a time. The products seem to be inadequate to repair the collagen feltwork and slowly, inexorably the degradative process far exceeds the reparative one, and the individual progresses to end-stage disease, with total loss of cartilage, eburnation of bone, and severe clinical symptoms. It is the responsibility of the cartilage chemist as well as the clinician to determine if some methods of surgical, chemical, or pharmaceutical treatment can either enhance the repair process or limit the degradative one. Thus far little that we do has any real effect, but with earlier diagnosis and better understanding of the process, we stand on the threshold of dealing more effectively with this highly prevalent disorder.

REFERENCES

1. Simon WH: Scale effects in animal joints I: Articular cartilage thickness and compression strength. *Arthritis Rheum* 13:244, 1970.
2. Simon WH: Scale effect in animal joints II: Thickness and elasticity in the deformability of articular cartilage. *Arthritis Rheum* 14:493, 1971.
3. Hall FM, Wyshok G: Thickness of articular cartilage in the normal knee. *J Bone Joint Surg* 62A:408, 1980.
4. Hass GM: Studies of cartilage: A morphologic and chemical analysis of aging human costal cartilage. *Arch Pathol* 35:275, 1943.
5. Meachim G, Stockwell RA: The matrix. In *Adult Articular Cartilage,* edited by MAR Freeman. New York, Grune & Stratton, 1973, pp 1–50.
6. Van der Krost JK, Sokoloff L, Miller EJ: Senescent pigmentation of cartilage and degenerative joint disease. *Arch Pathol* 86:40, 1968.
7. McCall CJ, Norby DP, Sokoloff L: Explant of human and rabbit articular chondrocytes. *Connect Tissue Res* 6:171, 1978.
8. Walker PS, Sikorski J, Dowson D, et al: Behavior of synovial fluid on surfaces of articular cartilage. A scanning electron microscope study. *Ann Rheum Dis* 28:1, 1969.
9. Clarke IC: Surface of human articular cartilage—A scanning electron microscope study. *J Anat* 108:23, 1971.
10. Ghadially FN, Ghadially JA, Oryschak AF et al: The surface of dog articular cartilage: A scanning electron microscope study. *J Anat* 123:527, 1977.

11. Weiss C, Rosenberg L, Helfet AJ: An ultrastructural study of normal young adult human articular cartilage. *J Bone Joint Surg* 50A:663, 1968.

12. Mankin HJ: The articular cartilage, cartilage healing and osteoarthritis, in *Adult Orthopaedics,* edited by RL Cruess, WRJ Rennie. New York, Churchill-Livingstone, 1984, pp 163–270.

13. Barnett CH, Davies DV, MacConnaill MS: *Synovial Joints: Their Structure and Mechanics.* Springfield, Ill, Thomas, 1961.

14. Collins DH: *The Pathology of Articular and Spinal Disease.* London, Arnold, 1949.

15. Redler I, Mow VC, Zimny ML, et al: The ultrastructure and biomechanical significance of the tidemark of articular cartilage. *Clin Orthop* 112:357, 1975.

16. Redler I: A scanning electron microscope study of human normal and osteoarthritic articular cartilage. *Clin Orthop* 103:262, 1974.

17. Lane JM, Weiss C: Current comment: Review of articular cartilage collagen research. *Arthritis Rheum* 18:553, 1975.

18. Strangeways TSP: Observations in the nutrition of articular cartilage. *Br Med J* 1:661, 1920.

19. Brower TD, Akahoshi Y, Orlic P: Diffusion of dyes through articular cartilage *in vivo. J Bone Joint Surg* 44A:456, 1962.

20. McKibben B, Maroudas A: Nutrition and metabolism, in *Adult Articular Cartilage,* 2d ed, edited by MAR Freeman. New York, Grune & Stratton, 1979, pp 461.

21. Ekholm R: Articular cartilage nutrition. *Acta Anat* 11 (suppl) 15:1, 1951.

22. Agata K, Whiteside LA, Lesker PA: Subchondral route for nutrition of articular cartilage in the rabbit. Measurement of diffusion with hydrogen gas in vitro. *J Bone Joint Surg* 60A:905, 1978.

23. Ropes MW, Bauer W: Synovial Fluid Changes in Joint Disease. Cambridge, Harvard University Press, 1953.

24. Swann DA: Macromolecules of synovial fluid, in *The Joints and Synovial Fluid,* vol 1, edited by L Sokoloff. New York, Academic Press, 1978, pp 407–432.

25. Maroudas A: Distribution and diffusion of solutes in articular cartilage. *Biophys J* 10:365, 1970.

26. Maroudas A: Physiochemical properties of articular cartilage, in *Adult Articular Cartilage,* edited by MAR Freeman. New York, Grune & Stratton, 1973, pp 131–170.

27. Maroudas A: Transport of solutes through cartilage: Permeability to large molecules. *J Anat* 122:335, 1976.

28. Lippiello L, Kaye C, Neumata T, Mankin HJ: *In vitro* metabolic response of articular cartilage segments to low levels of hydrostatic pressure. *Connect Tissue Res,* 13:99, 1985.

29. Maroudas A, Katz EP, Wachtel EJ et al: Physiochemical properties and functional behavior of normal and osteoarthritic human cartilage, in *Articular Cartilage Biochemistry,* edited by KE Kuettner, Schleyerbach R, Hascall VC. New York, Raven Press, 1986, pp 311–330.

30. Mankin HJ, Thrasher AF: Water binding in normal and osteoarthritic cartilage. *J Bone Joint Surg* 57A:76, 1975.

31. Miles JS, Eichelberger J: Biochemical studies of human cartilage during the aging process. *J Am Geriatr Soc* 12:1, 1964.

32. Campo RD, Tourtelotte DC: The composition of bovine cartilage and bone. *Biochim Biophys Acta* 141:614, 1967.

33. Palmoski M, Perricone R, Brandt KD: Development and reversal of a proteoglycan aggregation. *Arthritis Rheum* 22:508, 1979.

34. Palmoski M, O'Connor B, Brandt KD: Interruption of articular nerves impairs macromolecular organization of articular cartilage. *Arthritis Rheum* 22:644, 1979.

35. Palmoski M, Coyler RA, Brandt KD: Joint motion in the absence of normal loading does not maintain normal articular cartilage. *Arthritis Rheum* 23:325, 1976.

36. Brocklehurst R, Bayliss MT, Maroudas A, et al: The composition of normal and osteoarthritic articular cartilage from human knee joints. With special reference to unicompartmental replacement and osteotomy of the knee. *J Bone Joint Surg* 66:95, 1984.

37. Jaffe FF, Mankin HJ, Weiss C, Zarins A: Water binding in the articular cartilage of rabbits. *J Bone Joint Surg* 56A:1031, 1974.

38. Venn MF, Maroudas A: Chemical composition and swelling of normal and osteoarthritic femoral head cartilage. I. Chemical composition. *Ann Rheum Dis* 36:121, 1977.

39. Oldberg A, Antonsson P, Hedbom E, Heinegard D: Structure and function of extracellular matrix proteoglycans. *Biochem Soc Trans* 18:789, 1990.

40. Hardingham T, Bayliss M: Proteoglycans of articular cartilage: Changes in aging and in joint disease. *Sem Arthritis Rheum* (suppl 1) 20:12, 1990.

41. Muir H: The coming of age of proteoglycans. *Biochem Soc Trans* 18:787, 1990.

42. Dodge K, Sasaki M, Horigan E, et al: Complete primary structure of the rat cartilage proteoglycan core protein deduced from cDNA clones. *J Biol Chem* 262:17, 757, 1988.

43. Halberg DF, Proulx G, Dodge K, et al: A segment of the cartilage proteoglycan core protein has lectin-like activity. *J Biol Chem* 261:8108, 1986.

44. Adams ME, Grant MD, Ho A: Cartilage proteoglycan changes in experimental canine osteoarthritis. *J Rheumatol* 14:107, 1987.

45. Roughley PJ: Structural changes in the proteoglycans of human articular cartilage during aging. *J Rheumatol* 14:14, 1987.

46. Lohmander S, DeLuca S, Nilsson B, et al: Oligosaccharides of proteoglycans from the Swarm rat chondrosarcoma. *J Biol Chem* 255:6084, 1980.

47. Thonar EJ, Sweet MB: An oligosaccharide component in proteoglycans or articular cartilage. *Biochim Biophys Acta* 584:353, 1979.

48. Muir H: Biochemistry. In *Adult Articular Cartilage,* edited by MAR Freeman. New York, Grune & Stratton, 1976, pp 100–131.

49. Muir H, Hardingham TE: Structure of proteoglycan, in *MTP International Review of Science, Biochemistry, Series One, Vol. 5: Biochemistry of Carbonhydrates,* edited by WJ Whelan. Baltimore, University of Park Press, 1975, pp 153–222.

50. Serafini-Francassini A, Smith JW: *The Structure and Biochemistry of Cartilage.* London, Churchill-Livingstone, 1974.

51. Hjertquist SO, Wasteson A: The molecular weight of chondroitin sulphate from human articular: Effect of age and osteoarthritis. *Calcif Tissue Res* 10:31, 1972.

52. Helting T, Roden L: The carbohydrate-protein linkage region on chondroitin 6-sulphate. *Biochim Biophys Acta* 170:301, 1968.

53. Lindahl U, Roden L: The chondroitin 4-sulphate-protein linkage. *J Biol Chem* 241:2113, 1966.

54. Heingard D: Hyaluronidase digestion and alkaline treatment of bovine tracheal cartilage proteoglycans. Isolation and characterization of different keratan sulfate proteins. *Biochim Biophys Acta* 285:193, 1972.

55. Rosenberg L, Pal S, Beale RJ: Proteoglycans from bovine proximal humeral articular cartilage. *J Biol Chem* 248:3681, 1973.

56. Rosenberg L: Structure of cartilage proteoglycan, in *Dynamics of Connective Tissue Macromolecules,* edited by PMC Burleigh, AP Poole. New York, American Elsevier Publishing, 1975, pp 105–128.

57. Inerot S, Heinegard D, Andell L, Olsson S-E: Articular cartilage proteoglycans in aging and osteoarthritis. *Biochem J* 169:143, 1978.

58. Muir IHM: The chemistry of ground substance of joint cartilage, in *The Joints of Synovial Fluid, vol II,* edited by L Sokoloff. New York, American Press, 1980, pp 27–94.

59. Hardingham TE, Muir H: The specific interaction or hyaluronic acid with cartilage proteoglycans. *Biochim Biophys Acta* 279:401, 1972.

60. Hascall VC, Heingard D: Aggregation of cartilage proteoglycans. I. The role of hyaluronic acid. *J Biol Chem* 249:4232, 1974.

61. Holmes MW, Bayliss MT, Muir H: Hyaluronic acid in human articular cartilage. Age related changes in content and size. *Biochem J* 250:435, 1988.

62. Rosenberg L, Hellman W, Kleinschmidet AK: Electron microscopic studies of proteoglycan aggregates from bovine articular cartilage. *J Biol Chem* 250:1877, 1975.

63. Hardingham TE: The role of link-protein in the structure of cartilage proteoglycan aggregates. *Biochem J* 177:237, 1979.

64. Caterson B, Baker JR: The link proteins as specific components of cartilage proteoglycan aggregates in vivo. *J Biol Chem* 254:2394, 1979.

65. Caterson B, Baker JR, Christner JE, et al: Monoclonal antibodies as probes for determining the microheterogeneity of the link proteins of cartilage proteoglycans. *J Biol Chem,* 260:11348, 1985.

66. Hering TM, Sandell LJ: Biosynthesis and cell-free translation of Swarm rat chondrosarcoma and bovine cartilage link proteins. *J Biol Chem* 263:1030, 1988.

67. Hering TM, Sandell LJ: Biosynthesis and processing of bovine cartilage link proteins. *J Biol Chem* 265:2375, 1990.

68. Perkins SJ, Nealis AS, Dudhia J, Hardingham TE: Immunoglobulin fold and tandem repeat structures in proteoglycan N-terminal domains and link protein. *J Mol Biol* 206:737, 1989.

69. Williams AF, Barcley AN: The immunoglobulin superfamily—domains for cell surface recognition. *Annu Rev Immunol* 6:381, 1988.

70. Mow VC, Lai VM: Recent developments in synovial joint biomechanics. *SIAM Rev* 22:275, 1980.

71. Shepard N, Mitchell N: The localization of proteoglycan by light and microscopy using safranin-O. *J Ultrastruct Res* 54:451, 1976.

72. Bjelle AO: Variations in content and composition of glycosaminoglycans within the articular cartilage of the lower femoral epiphysis of an adult. *Scand J Rheumatol* 3:81, 1973.

73. Lemperg RK, Larsson SI, Hjertquist S-O: The glycosaminoglycans of bovine articular cartilage. I. Concentration and distribution in different layers in relation to age. *Calcif Tissue Res* 15:237, 1974.

74. Rosenberg L: Chemical bases for the histological use of safranin-O in the study of articular cartilage. *J Bone Joint Surg* 53A:69, 1972.

75. Bjelle AO, Antonopoulos CA, Engfeldt B, Hjertquist S-O: Fractionation of the glycosaminoglycans of human articular cartilage on ectiolacellulose in aging and in osteoarthritis. *Calcif Tissue Res* 8:237, 1972.

76. Lipshitz H, Etheredge R III, Glimcher MJ: Changes in hexosamine content and swelling ratio of articular cartilage as a function of depth from the surface. *J Bone Joint Surg* 58A:1149, 1976.
77. Maroudas A, Evans H, Almeida L: Cartilage of the hip joint: Topographical variation of glycosaminoglycan content in normal and fibrillated tissue. *Ann Rheum Dis* 32:1, 1973.
78. Rosenberg L: Structure and function of dermatan sulfate proteoglycans in articular cartilage, in *Articular Cartilage Biochemistry and Osteoarthritis,* edited by KE Kuettner, R Schleyerback, JG Peyron, VC Hascall. New York, Raven Press, in press.
79. Stanescu V: The small proteoglycans of cartilage matrix. *Semin Arthritis Rheum* 20 (3 suppl 1):51, 1990.
80. Hausser H, Kresse H: Binding of heparin and of the small proteoglycan decorin to the same endocytosis receptor proteins leads to different metabolic consequences. *J Cell Biol* 114:45, 1991.
81. Winnemoller M, Schmidt G, Kresse H: Influence of decorin on fibroblast adhesion to fibronectin. *Eur J Cell Biol* 54:10, 1991.
82. Breuer B, Schmidt G, Kresse H: Non-uniform influence of transforming growth factor-beta on the biosynthesis of different forms of small chondroitin sulphate/dermatan sulphate proteoglycans. *Biochem J* 269:10608, 1991.
83. Kahari VM, Larjava H, Uitto J: Differential regulation of extracellular matrix proteoglycan (PG) gene expression. Transforming growth factor-beta 1 up-regulates biglycan (PGI), and versican (large fibroblast PG) but down-regulates decorin (PGII) mRNA levels in human fibroblasts in culture. *J Biol Chem,* 266:10608, 1991.
84. McDevitt CA: Biochemistry of articular cartilage: Nature of proteoglycans and collagen of articular cartilage and their role in aging and in osteoarthritis. *Ann Rheum Dis* 32:364, 1973.
85. Mayne R, Irwin MH: Collagen types in cartilage, in *Articular Cartilage Biochemistry,* edited by KE Kuettner, R Schleyerback, VC Hascall. New York, Raven Press, 1986, pp 23–39.
86. Eyre DR, Wu JJ, Apone S: A growing family of collagens in articular cartilage: Identification of five genetically distinct types. *J Rheumatol* 14:25, 1987.
87. Miller EJ: The structure of fibril-forming collagens. *Ann NY Acad Sci* 460:1, 1985.
88. Shimokomaki M, Wright DW, Irwin MH et al: The structure and micromolecular . . . of type IX collagen in cartilage. *Ann NY Acad Sci* 580:1, 1990.
89. Chu ML, Pan T-C, Conway D, et al: The structure of type VI collagen. *Ann NY Acad Sci* 580:55, 1990.
90. Schmid TM, Popp RG, Linsenmayer TF: Type X collagen, supramolecular assembly and calcification. *Ann NY Acad Sci* 580:64, 1990.
91. Duance VC, Wolton SF, Young RD: Type IX collagen function and articular cartilage. *Ann NY Acad Sci* 580:480, 1990.
92. Weiss C: Ultrastructural characteristics of osteoarthritis. *Fed Proc* 32:1459, 1973.
93. Eyre DR, Muir H: Characterization of the major CNBr-derived peptides of procine type II collagen. *Connect Tissue Res* 3:105, 1975.
94. Fugimoto D, Motiguchi T: Pyridinoline, a non-reducible cross-link of collagen. *J Biochem* 83:863, 1978.
95. Miller, EJ, Lunde LG: Isolation and characterization of the cynogen bromide peptides from the alpha I (II) chain of bovine and human articular cartilage collagen. Biochemistry 12:3153, 1973.
96. Hewitt AT, Varner HH, Silver MH, et al: The isolation and partial characterization of chondronectin, an attachment factor for chondrocytes. *J Biol Chem* 257:2330, 1982.
97. Hewitt AT, Kleinman HK, Pennypacker JP, Martin GR: Identification of an adhesion factor for chondrocytes. *Proc Natl Acad Sci* 77:385, 1980.
98. Burton-Wurster N, Horn VJ, Lust G: Immunohistochemical localization of fibronectin and chondronectin in canine articular cartilage. *J Histiochem Cytochem* 36:581, 1988.
99. Brown RA, Jones KL: The synthesis and accumulation of fibronectin by human articular cartilage. *J Rheumatol* 17:65, 1990.
100. Burton-Wurster N, Lust G: Deposition of fibronectin in articular cartilage of canine osteoarthritis joints. *Am J Vet Res* 46:2542, 1985.
101. von der Mark K, Hollenhaver J, Pfaffle M, et al: Role of anchorin CII in the interaction of chondrocytes with extracellular collagen, in *Articular Cartilage Biochemistry,* edited by KE Kuettner, R Schleyerbach, VC Hascall. New York, Raven Press, 1986, pp 125–138.
102. Paulsson M, Heinegar D: Noncollagenous cartilage proteins. Current status of an emerging research field. *Coll Relat Res* 4:219, 1984.
103. Fife RS, Brandt KD: Extracellular matrix of cartilage. C Glycoproteins. In preparation.
104. Fife RS, Palmoski MJ, Brandt KD: Metabolism of a cartilage matrix glycoprotein in normal and osteoarthritic canine articular cartilage. *Arthritis Rheum* 29:1256, 1986.
105. Rabinowitz SL, Gregg JR, Nixon JE, Schumacher HR: Lipid composition of tissue of human knee joints. *Clin Orthop* 143:260, 1973.
106. Stockwell RA: Lipid content of human costal and articular cartilage. *Ann Rheum Dis* 26:481, 1967.
107. Kincaid SA, Rudd RG, Evander SA: Lipids of normal and osteochondritic cartilage of the immature canine humeral head. *Am J Vet Res* 46:1060, 1985.

108. Ohira T, Ishikawa K, Masuda I, et al: Histologic localization of lipid in the articular tissues in calcium pyrophosphate dihydrate crystal deposition disease. *Arthritis Rheum* 31:1057, 1988.

109. Pryzanki W, Boguch, Wloch M, et al: Human articular chondrocytes synthesize phospholipase A$_2$. *Arthritis Rheum* 73:8112, 1990.

110. Pryzanki W, Boguch E, Wloch M, et al: Synthesis and release of phospholipase A$_2$ by human articular chondrocytes. *J Rheumatol* 17:1386, 1990.

111. Pryzanski W, Vadas P: Phospholipase A$_2$ in articular cartilage. *J Rheumatol* 17:569, 1990.

112. Ali SY: Mineral containing matrix vesicles in human osteoarthritic cartilage, in *Aetiopathogenesis of Osteoarthritis,* edited by G. Nuki. Tunbridge Wells, Pitman Medical Publishing, 1980, pp 105–116.

113. Rees JA, Ali SY: Ultrastructural localization of alkaline phosphatase activity in osteoarthritic human articular cartilage. *Ann Rheum Dis* 47:747, 1988.

114. Lane JM, Brighton CT, Minkowitz BT: Anaerobic and aerobic metabolism in articular cartilage. *J Rheumatol* 4:334, 1977.

115. Tushan FS, Rodnan GP, Altman M, Robin ED: Anaerobic glycolysis and lactate dehydrogenase LDH isoenzymes in articular cartilage. *J Lab Clin Med* 73:549, 1969.

116. Marcus RE: The effect of low oxygen concentration on growth glycolysis and sulphate incorporation by articular chondrocytes in monoculture. *Arthritis Rheum* 16:646, 1973.

117. Campo RD, Dziewiatkowski DD: Intracellular synthesis of protein polysaccharides by slices of bovine coastal cartilage. *J Clin Invest* 55:1373, 1976.

118. Mankin HJ: The metabolism of articular cartilage in health and disease, in *Dynamics of Connective Tissue Macromolecules,* edited by PMC Burleigh, AR Poole. New York, American Elsevier Publishing, 1975, pp 327–353.

119. Mankin HJ: The reaction of articular cartilage to injury and osteoarthritis. *N Engl J Med* 291:1285, 1335, 1974.

120. Mankin HJ, Boyle CJ: The acute effects of lacerative injury of DNA and protein synthesis in articular cartilage, in *Cartilage Degradation and Repair,* edited by CAL Basseet. Washington DC, NAS-NRC, 1967, PP 185–199.

121. Schwartz ER, Kirkpatrick RR, Thompson TC: The effect of environmental pH on glycosaminoglycan metabolism by normal human chondrocytes. *J Lab Clin Med* 87:198, 1976.

122. Palmoski J, Brandt KD: Effect of calcipenia on proteoglycan metabolism and aggregation in normal articular cartilage in vitro. *Biochem J* 182:399, 1979.

123. Brighton CT, Lane JM, Koh JK: In vitro rabbit articular cartilage organ model. II. ^{35}S incorporation at various oxygen tensions. *Arthritis Rheum* 17:245, 1974.

124. Sandy JD, Brown HL, Lowther DA: Control of proteoglycan synthesis. Studies on the activation of synthesis observed during culture of articular cartilage. Bio.

125. Smith TWD, Duckworth T, Bergenholtz A, Lemberg RK: Role of growth hormone in glycosaminoglycan synthesis by articular cartilage. *Nature* 253:269, 1975.

126. Osborne KD, Trippel SB, Manking HJ: Growth factor stimulation of adult articular cartilage. *J Clin Orthop Res* 7:35, 1989.

127. Schwartz EF, Adamy L: Effect of ascorbic acid on arylsulfate activities and sulfated proteoglycan metabolism in chondrocyte cultures. *J Clin Invest* 60:96, 1977.

128. Brighton CT, Shadle CA, Jiminez SA, et al: Articular cartilage preservation and storage. I. Application of tissue culture techniques in the storage of viable articular cartilage. *Arthritis Rheum* 22:1093, 1979.

129. Kent L, Malemud CJ, Moskowitz RW: Differential response of articular chondrocyte population to thromboxane B$_2$ and analogs of prostaglandin cyclic endoperoxidases. *Prostaglandins* 19:391, 1980.

130. Palmoski MJ, Brandt KD: Effects of salicylate and indomethacin on glycosaminoglycan and prostaglandin eS synthesis in intact canine knee cartilage ex vivo. *Arthritis Rheum* 27:398, 1984.

131. Palmoski MJ, Brandt KD: Effects of some nonsteroidal anti-inflammatory drugs on proteoglycan metabolism and organization in canine articular cartilage. *Arthritis Rheum* 23:1010, 1980.

132. Brandt KD, Slowman-Kovacs S: Nonsteroidal anti-inflammatory drugs in treatment of osteoarthritis. *Clin Orthop* 213:84, 1986.

133. Brandt KD: Effects of nonsteroidal anti-inflammatory drugs on chondrocyte metabolism in vitro an din vivo. *Am J Med* 83:29, 1987.

134. Pelletier JP, Cloutier JM, Martel-Pelletier J: In vitro effects of tiaprofenic acid, sodium salicylate and hydrocortisone on the proteoglycan metabolism of human osteoarthritic cartilage. *J Rheumatol* 16:646, 1989.

135. Ehrlich MG, Mankin HJ, Treadwell BV, Jones H: Uridine diphosphate (UDP) stimulation of protein-polysaccharide production: A preliminary report. *J Bone Joint Surg* 56A:1239, 1974.

136. Mankin HJ, Lippiello L: The turnover of adult rabbit articular cartilage. *J Bone Joint Surg* 63A:131, 1981.

137. Repo RU, Mitchell N: Collagen synthesis in mature articular cartilage of the rabbit. *J Bone Joint Surg* 53B:541, 1971.

138. Lippiello L, Hall D, Mankin HJ: Collagen synthesis in normal and osteoarthritic human cartilage. *J Clin Invest* 59:593, 1977.

139. Dehm P, Prockop DJ: Biosynthesis of cartilage procollagen. *Eur J Biochem* 35:159, 1973.

140. Miller EJ: Isolation and characterization of a collagen from chick cartilage containing three identical chains. *Biochemistry* 10:1652, 1971.

141. Kivirikko KI, Ristell: Biosynthesis of collagen and its alteration in pathological states. *Med Biol* 54:159, 1976.

142. Hill DJ, Milner RD: Platelet derived growth factor and multiplication stimulating activity II, but not multiplication stimulating activity II-2 stimulate $_3$H-thymidine and $_{35}$S sulfate incorporation by fetal rat costal cartilage in vitro. *J Endocrinol* 103:195, 1984.

143. Howes R, Bowness JM, Grotendorst GR, et al: Platelet derived growth factor enhances demineralized bone matrix-induced cartilage and bone formation. *Calcif Tissue Int* 42:34, 1988.

144. Cuevas P, Burgos J, Baird A: Basic fibroblast growth factor (FGF) promotes cartilage repair in vivo. *Biochem Biophys Res Commun* 156:611, 1988.

145. McQuillan DJ, Handley CJ, Campbell MA, et al: Stimulation of proteoglycan biosynthesis and insulin-like growth factor-I in cultured bovine articular cartilage. *Biochem J,* 240:423, 1986.

146. Luyten FP, Hascall VC, Nissley SP, et al: Insulin-like growth factors maintain steady-state metabolism of proteoglycan in bovine articular cartilage explants. *Arch Biochem Biophys* 267:416, 1988.

147. Morales TI, Roberts AB: Transforming growth factors beta regulates the metabolism of proteoglycan in bovine cartilage organ cultures. *J Biol Chem* 263:12828, 1988.

148. Hiraki Y, Inoue H, Hirae R, et al: Effect of transforming growth factor beta on cell proliferation and glycosaminoglycan synthesis by rabbit growth plate chondrocytes in culture. *Biochim Biophys Acta* 969:91, 1988.

149. Joyce ME, Terek RM, Jingushi S, Bolander ME: Role of transforming growth plate factors-beta in fracture repair. *Ann NY Acad Sci* 593:107, 1990.

150. Vivien D, Galera P, Lebrun E, et al: Differential effects of transforming growth factor-beta and epidermal growth factor on the cell cycle of cultured rabbit articular chondrocytes. *J Cell Physiol* 143:534, 1990.

151. Fell HB, Thomas L: Comparison of the effects of papain and vitamin A on cartilage. I. The effects on organ culture of embryonic skeletal tissue. *J Exp Med* 111:719, 1960.

152. Fell HB, Dingle JT: Studies on the mode of action of excess of vitamin A. 6. Lysosomal protease and the degradation of cartilage matrix. *Biochem J* 87:403, 1963.

153. Ehrlich MG, Mankin HJ, Treadwell BV: Acid hydrolase activity in osteoarthritic and normal human cartilage. *J Bone Joint Surg* 55A:1068, 1973.

154. Howell DS, Woessner JF Jr: Enzymes in articular cartilage, in *Studies in Joint Disease,* edited by A Maroudas, EJ Holoborow. Tunbridge Wells, Pitman Medical Publishing, 1980, pp. 160–169.

155. Stack MT, Brandt KD: Identification and characterization of articular cartilage hyaluronidase. *Arthritis Rheum* 25:S100, 1982.

156. Sapolsky AI, Altman RD, Woessner JF Jr, Howell DS: The action of cathepsin D in human articular cartilage on proteoglycans. *J Clin Invest* 2:624, 1973.

157. Sapolsky AI, Howell DS, Woessner JF Jr: Neutral proteinases and cathepsin D in human articular cartilage. *J Clin Invest* 53:1044, 1974.

158. Ehrlich MG, Armstrong AL, Newman RG, et al: Patterns of proteoglycan degradation by a neutral protease from human growth plate epiphyseal cartilage. *J Bone Joint Surg* 63A:1350, 1982.

159. Ehrlich MG, Armstrong A, Mankin HJ: Isolation and partial purification and characterization of growth plate neutral proteoglycanase. *Trans Orthol Res Soc* 6:109, 1981.

160. Murphy G, Cockett MI, Stephens PE, Smith BJ: Stromelysis is an activator of procollagenase. *Biochem J* 248:265, 1987.

161. Harris ED Jr: Role of collagenase in joint destruction, in *The Joints of Synovial Fluid,* vol. 1, edited by L Sokoloff. New York, Academic Press, 1978, pp 243–272.

162. Harris ED Jr, Krane SM: Collagenases. *N Engl J Med* 291:557, 605, 1974.

163. Ehrlich MG, Mankin HJ, Jones H, et al: Collagenase and collagenase inhibitors in osteoarthritic and normal human cartilage. *J Clin Invest* 59:226, 1977.

164. Mochan E, Keler T: Plasmin degradation of cartilage proteoglycan. *Biochim Biophys Acta* 800:312, 1984.

165. Campbell AK, Piccoli DS, Butler DM, et al: Recombinant human interleukin-1 stimulates human articular cartilage to undergo resorption and human chondrocytes to produce both tissue and urokinase-type plasminogen activator. *Biochim Biophys Acta,* 967:183, 1988.

166. Yamada H, Stephens RW, Nakagawa T, McNicol D: Human articular cartilage contains an inhibitor of plasminogen activator. *J Rheumatol* 15:1138, 1988.

167. Dean DD, Azzo W, Martel-Pelletier J, et al: Levels of metalloproteases and tissue inhibitor of metalloproteases in human osteoarthritic cartilage. *J Rheumatol* 14:43, 1987.

168. Ollivierre F, Gubler U, Towle CA, et al: Expression of IL-1 genes in human and bovine chondrocytes: A mechanism for autocrine control of cartilage matrix degradation. *Biochem Res Commun* 141:904, 1986.

169. Murphy G, Docherty AJP: Molecular studies on the connective tissue metalloproteinases and their inhibitor TIMP, in *The control of tissue damage,* edited by AM Galuert. Oxford, Elsevier, 1988, pp 223–241.

170. Morales TI: Cartilage proteoglycan homostasis: Role of growth factors, in *Cartilage changes in osteoarthritis,* edited by KD Brandt. Indianapolis, Indiana University School of Medicine, 1990, pp 17–21.

171. Vignon E, Mathiew P, Louisot P, et al: Phospholipase A_2 activity in human osteoarthritic cartilage. *J Rheum* (suppl) 18:35, 1989.

172. Meachim G: Effect of age on the thickness of adult articular cartilage at the shoulder joint. *Ann Rheum Dis* 30:43, 1971.

173. Mankin HJ: The calcified bone (basal layers) of articular cartilage of rabbits. *Anat Rec* 14:73, 1963.

174. Mankin HJ: The effect of aging on articular cartilage. *Bull Acad Med* 44:545, 1968.

175. Stockwell RA, Meachim G: The chondrocytes, in *Adult Articular Cartilage,* edited by MAR Freeman. New York, Grune & Stratton, 1973, pp 51–99.

176. Stockwell RA: The inter-relationship of cell density and cartilage thickness in mammalian articular cartilage. *J Anat* 109:411, 1971.

177. Mankin HJ: Localization of tritiated thymidine in articular cartilage in rabbits. III. Mature articular cartilage. *J Bone Joint Surg* 45A:529, 1963.

178. Roughley PJ, White RJ: Age related changes in the structure of the proteoglycan subunits from human articular cartilage. *J Biol Chem* 255:217, 1980.

179. Buckwalter JA, Keuttner KE, Thonar EJ: Age-related changes in articular cartilage proteoglycans: Electron microscopic studies. *J Orthop Res* 3:251, 1985.

180. Murata K, Bjelle AO: Age dependent constitution of chondroitin sulfate isomers in cartilage proteoglycans under associative conditions. *J Biochem (Tokyo)* 86:371, 1979.

181. Hjertquist S-O, Lamperg R: Identification and concentration of the glycosaminoglycans of human articular cartilage in relation to age and osteoarthritis. *Calcif Tissue Res* 10:223, 1972.

182. Simunek Z, Muir H: Changes in the protein-polysaccharides of pig articular cartilage during prenatal life, development and old age. *Biochem J* 126:515, 1972.

183. Benmaman JD, Ludoweig JJ, Anderson CE: Glucosamine and galactosamine distribution in human articular cartilage. Relationship to age and degenerative joint disease. *Clin Biochem* 2:461, 1969.

184. Mankin HJ, Lippiello L: The glycosaminoglycans of normal and arthritic cartilage. *J Clin Invest* 50:1712, 1971.

185. Roughley PJ: Structural changes in the proteoglycans of human articular cartilage during aging. *J Rheumatol* 14:14, 1987.

186. Plaas AH, Sandy JD: Age-related decrease in the link-stability of proteoglycan aggregates formed by articular chondrocytes. *Biochem J* 220:337, 1984.

187. Front P, Aprile F, Mitrovic DR, Swann DA: Age-related changes in the synthesis of matrix macromolecules by bovine articular cartilage. *Connect Tissue Res* 19:121, 1989.

188. Mankin HJ: Localization of triatiated thymidine in articular cartilage of rabbits. II. Repair in immature cartilage. *J Bone Joint Surg* 44A:688, 1962.

189. Mankin HJ: The reaction of articular cartilage to injury and osteoarthritis. *N Engl J Med* 291:1285, 1335, 1974.

190. Calandruccio RA, Gilmer WS Jr: Proliferation, regeneration and repair of articular cartilage of immature animals. *J Bone Joint Surg* 44A:431, 1962.

191. Campbell CJ: The healing of cartilage defects. *Clin Orthop* 64:45, 1969.

192. Cheung HG, Cottrell WH, Stephenson K, et al: In vitro collagen biosynthesis in healing and normal rabbit articular cartilage. *J Bone Joint Surg* 60A:1076, 1978.

193. DePalma DF, McKeever CD, Subin SK: Process of repair in articular cartilage demonstrated by histology and autoradiography with tritiated thymidine. *Clin Orthop* 48:229,1966.

194. Fuller JA, Ghadially FN: Ultrastructural observations on surgically produced partial-thickness defects in articular cartilage. *Clin Orthop* 86:193, 1972.

195. Ghadially FN, Thomas I, Oryshak AF, et al: Long term results of superficial defects in articular cartilage. A scanning electron microscope study. *Virchows Arch [B]* 25:125, 1977.

196. Hunter W: Of the structure and diseases of articulating cartilage. *Philos Trans R Soc Lond* 42:514, 1743.

197. Cheung HS, Lynch KL, Johnson RP et al: In vitro synthesis tissue specific type II collagen by healing cartilage. I. Short term repair of cartilage of mature rabbits. *Arthritis Rheum* 23:211, 1980.

198. Convery FR, Akeson WK, Keown GH: The repair of large osteochondral defects in experimental study in horses. *Clin Orthop,* 82:253, 1972.

199. Meachim G, Roberts C: Repair of the joint surface from subarticular tissue in the rabbit knee. *J Anat* 109:317, 1971.

200. Mitchell N, Shepard N: The resurfacing of adult rabbit articular cartilage by multiple perforations through the subchondral bone. *J Bone Joint Surg* 58A:230, 1976.

201. Mitchell N, Shepard N: Healing of articular cartilage in intra-articular fractures in rabbits. *J Bone Joint Surg* 62A:628, 1980.

202. O'Driscoll SW, Keeley FW, Salter RB: The chondrogenic potential of free autogenous periosteal grafts for biological resurfacing of major full-thickness defects in joint surfaces under the influence of continuous passive motion: An experimental study in the rabbit. *J Bone Joint Surg* 68A:1017, 1986.

203. O'Driscoll SW, Salter RB: The induction of neochondrogenesis in free intra-articular periosteal autografts under the influence of continuous passive motion: An experimental study in the rabbit. *J Bone Joint Surg* 68A:1248, 1986.

204. Schultz RJ, Krishnamoorthy S, Thelmo W, et al: Cellular origin and evolution of neochondrogenesis in major full-thickness defects of a joint surface treated by free autogenous periosteal grafts and subjected to continuous passive motion in rabbits. *Clin Orthop* 5:577, 1985.

205. Itay S, Abramovici A, Nevo Z: Use of cultured embryonal chick epiphyseal chondrocytes as grafts for defects in chick articular cartilage. *Clin Orthop* 220:284, 1987.

206. Aaron RK, Ciober DM, Jolly G: Modulation of chondrogenesis and chondrocytes differentiation by pulsed electromagnetic fields. *Trans Orthop Res Soc* 12:272, 1987.

207. Syftestad G, Caplan A: A 31,000 dalton bone matrix protein stimulates chondrogenesis in chick limb and gut cell cultures. *Trans Orthop Res Soc* 11:278, 1986.

208. Sporn MB, Roberts A, Wakefield LM, et al: Transforming growth factor-b. Biological function and chemical structure. *Science* 233:532, 1986.

209. Radin EL, Paul IL, Lowy M: A comparison of the dynamic force transmitting properties of subchondral bone and articular cartilage. *J Bone Joint Surg* 52A:444, 1970.

210. Repo RU, Finlay JB: Survival of articular cartilage after controlled impact. *J Bone Joint Surg* 59A:1068, 1977.

211. Radin EL, Ehrlich MG, Chernack BJ, et al: Effect of repetitive impulsive loading on the knee joints of rabbits. *Clin Orthop* 131:288–293, 1978.

212. Dekel S, Weissman SL: Joint changes after overuse and peak overloading of rabbit knees in vivo. *Acta Orthop Scand* 49:519, 1978.

213. Moskowitz RW, Howell DS, Goldberg VM, Mankin HJ: *Osteoarthritis: Diagnosis and Management,* Philadelphia, Saunders, 1984.

214. Lindblad S, Hedfors E: Arthroscopic and immunohistologic characterization of knee joint synovitis in osteoarthritis. *Arthritis Rheum* 30:1081, 1987.

215. Mankin HJ, Brandt KD, Shulman LE: Workshop on etiopathogenesis of osteoarthritis. *J Rheum* 13:1127, 1986.

216. Sokoloff L: *The Biology of Degenerative Joint Disease,* Chicago, University of Chicago Press, 1969.

217. Sokoloff L: The pathology of osteoarthritis and the role of aging, in *The Aetiopathogenesis of Osteoarthrosis,* edited by G Nuki. Tunbridge Wells, Pitman Medical Publishing, 1980, pp 1–15.

218. Jaffe HD: *Metabolic Degenerative and Inflammatory Disease of Bones and Joints,* Philadelphia, Lea & Febiger, 1972.

219. Ferguson AB Jr: The pathology of degenerative arthritis of the hip and the use of osteotomy in its treatment. *Clin Orthop* 77:84, 1971.

220. Lloyd-Roberts GC: The role of capsule changes in osteoarthritis of the hip. *J Bone Joint Surg* 35B:627, 1953.

221. Arnoldi CC, Reimann I: The pathomechanism of human coxarthrosis. *Acta Orthop Scand* (suppl) 181, 1979.

222. Gordon GV, Villaneuva T, Schumacher HR, Gobel V: Autopsy study correlating degree of osteoarthritis, synovitis and evidence of articular calcification. *J Rheum* 11:681, 1984.

223. Peter SB, Pearson CM, Marmor L: Erosive osteoarthritis of the hands. *Arthritis Rheum* 9:365, 1966.

224. Meachim G, Brooke G: The pathology of osteoarthritis, in *Osteoarthritis: Diagnosis and Management,* edited by RW Moskowitz, DS Howell, VM Goldberg, HJ Mankin. Philadelphia, Saunders, 1984, pp 29–42.

225. Lloyd-Roberts GC: Osteoarthritis of the hip. Study of the clinical pathology. *J Bone Joint Surg* 37B:8, 1955.

226. Cameron HU, Fornasier VL: Fine detail radiography of the femoral head in osteoarthritis. *J Rheum* 6:178, 1979.

227. Jeffrey AK: Osteogenesis in the osteoarthritic femoral head. *J Bone Joint Surg* 55B:272, 1973.

228. Sokoloff L: Osteoarthritis, in *The Human Joint in Health and Disease,* edited by WH Simon. Philadelphia, University of Pennsylvania Press, 1978, pp 91–111.

229. Byers P, Contemponi CA, Farkas TA: Post-mortem study of the hip joint. *Ann Rheum Dis* 29:15, 1970.

230. Revell PA, Mayson V, Lalor P, Mapp P: The synovial membrane in osteoarthritis: A histological study including the characterization of the cellular infiltrate present in inflammatory osteoarthritis using monoclonal antibodies. *Ann Rheum Dis* 47:300, 1988.

231. Ladefoged C: Amyloid in osteoarthritic hip joint: Deposits in relation to chondromatosis, pyrophosphate, and inflammatory cell infiltrate in the synovial membrane and fibrous capsule. *Ann Rheum Dis* 42:659, 1983.

232. Ehrlich GE: Inflammatory osteoarthritis. I. The clinical syndrome. *J Chronic Dis* 25:317, 1972.

233. Ehrlich GE: Erosive inflammatory and primary generalized osteoarthritis, in *Osteoarthritis: Diagnosis and Management,* edited by RW Moskowitz, DS Howell, VM Goldberg, HJ Mankin. Philadelphia, Saunders, 1984, pp 199–211.

234. Layton MW, Goldstein SA, Goulet RW, et al: Examination of subchondral bone architecture in experimental osteoarthritis by microscope computed axial tomography. *Arthritis Rheum* 31:1400, 1988.

235. Christiansen SB, Arnoldi CC: Distribution of ^{99m}Tc compounds in osteoarthritic femoral heads. *J Bone Joint Surg* 62A:90, 1980.

236. Hutton CW, Higgs ER, Jackson PC, et al: ^{99m}Tc HMDP bone scanning in generalized nodal osteoarthritis. I. Comparison of the standard radiograph and four hour bone scan image of the hand. *Ann Rheum Dis* 45:617, 1986.

237. Fazzalari NL, Vernon-Roberts B, Darracott J: Osteoarthritis of the hip. Possible protective and causative roles of trabecular microfractures in the head of the femur. *Clin Orthop* 216:224,233, 1987.

238. Inoue H: Alterations in the collagen framework of osteoarthritic cartilage and subchondral bone. *Int Orthop* 5:47, 1981.

239. Trueta J: *Studies of the Development and Decay of the Human Frame,* Philadelphia, Saunders, 1968.

240. Mankin HJ, Brandt KD: Biochemistry and metabolism of cartilage in osteoarthritis, in *Osteoarthritis: Diagnosis and Management,* edited by RW Moskowitz, DS Howell, VM Goldberg, HJ Mankin. Philadelphia, Saunders, 1984, pp 43–79.

241. Mankin HJ, Dorfman HD, Lippiello L, Zarins A: Biochemical and metabolic abnormalities in articular cartilage from osteoarthritic human hips. II. Correlation of morphology with metabolic data. *J Bone Joint Surg* 53A:523, 1971.

242. Hulth A, Lindberg L, Telhag H: Mitosis in human osteoarthritic cartilage. *Clin Orthop* 88:247, 1972.

243. Telhag H: Nucleic acids in human normal and osteoarthritic articular cartilage. *Acta Orthop Scand* 47:585, 1976.

244. Weiss C, Morow S: An ultrastructural study of osteoarthritic changes in articular cartilage of human knees. *J Bone Joint Surg* 54A:954, 1972.

245. Peyron JG: The epidemiology of osteoarthritis, in *Osteoarthritis: Diagnosis and Management,* edited by RW Moskowitz, DS Howell, VM Goldberg, HJ Mankin. Philadelphia, Saunders, 1984, pp 9–27.

246. Bergstrom G, Bjelle A, Sorenssen L, et al: Prevalence of rheumatoid arthritis, osteoarthritis, chondrocalcinosis and gouty arthritis at age 79. *J Rheum* 13:150, 1986.

247. Bjelle A: Epidemiological aspects of osteoarthritis—an interview survey of the Swedish population and a review of previous studies. *Scand J Rheum* (suppl) 43:35, 1982.

248. Nilsson BE, Danielsson LB, Hernborg SA: Clinical features and natural course of coxarthrosis and gonarthrosis. *Scand J Rheum* 43:12, 1982.

249. Brandt KD, Fife RS: Aging in relation to the pathogenesis of osteoarthritis. *Clin Rheum Dis* 12:117, 1986.

250. Peyron JG: Osteoarthritis: The epidemiologic viewpoint. *Clin Orthop* 213:13, 1986.

251. Valkenberg HA: Clinical versus radiological osteoarthrosis in the general population, in *Epidemiology of Orthoarthrosis,* edited by JG Peyron. Basel, Ciba-Geigy, 1981, pp 53–58.

252. Verstraeton A, Van Ermen H, Haghebaert G, et al: Osteoarthrosis retards the development of osteoporosis: Observation of the coexistence of osteoarthrosis and osteoporosis. *Clin Orthop* 264:169, 1991.

253. Cushnaghan J, Dieppe P: Study of 500 patients with limb joint osteoarthritis. I. Analysis by age, sex and distribution of symptomatic joint sites. *Ann Rheum Dis* 50:8, 1991.

254. Howell DS: Etiopathogenesis of osteoarthritis, in *Osteoarthritis: Diagnosis and Management,* edited by RW Moskowitz, DS Howell, VM Goldberg, HJ Mankin. Philadelphia, Saunders, 1984, pp 129–146.

255. Mankin HJ, Treadwell BV: Osteoarthritis in 1987: A review. *Bull Rheum Dis,* in press, 1987.

256. Schumacher HR: Ochronosis, hemochromatosis and Wilson's disease, in *Arthritis and Allied Conditions,* edited by DJ McCarty. Philadelphia, Lea & Febiger, 1979, pp 1262–1275.

257. Dieppe P, Watt I: Crystal deposition in osteoarthritis: An opportunistic event? *Clin Rheum Dis* 11:367, 1985.

258. de Jong Bok JM, MacFarlane JD: The articular diversity of early heamochromatosis. *J Bone Joint Surg* 69:41, 1987.

259. Mitrovic DR, Stankovic A, Iriarte-Borda O, et al: The prevalence of chondrocalcinosis in the human knee joint. An autopsy survey. *J Rheumatol* 15:633, 1988.

260. Teshima R, Treadwell BV, Trahan CA, Mankin HJ: Comparative rates of proteoglycan synthesis and size of proteoglycans in normal and osteoarthritic chondrocytes. *Arthritis Rheum* 26:1225, 1983.

261. Towle CA, Mankin HJ, Avruch J, Treadwell BV: Insulin promoted increase in the phosphorylation of protein synthesis initiation factor eIF-2. *Biochem Res Commun* 121:134, 1985.

262. Mankin HJ, Jennings LC, Treadwell BV, Trippel SB: Growth factors and articular cartilage. *J Rheumatol* 18:66, 1991.

263. Pujol J-P, Galer P, Redini F, et al: Role of cytokines in OA: Comparative effects of IL-1 and TGF-B on cultured rabbit articular chondrocytes. *J Rheumatol* 18:76, 1991.

264. Franchmont P, Bassleer C: Effects of hormones and local growth factors on articular chondrocyte metabolism. *J Rheumatol* 18:68, 1991.

265. Treadwell BV, Mankin HJ: The synthetic processes of articular cartilage. *Clin Orthop* 213:50, 1986.

266. Mitrovic D, Lippiello L, Gruson F, et al: Effects of various prostanoids on the in vitro metabolism of bovine articular chondrocytes. *Prostaglandins* 22:499, 1981.

267. DiBattista JA, Martel-Pelletier J, Cloutier J-M Pelletier J-P: Modulation of glucocorticoid receptor expression in human articular chondrocytes by cAMP and prostaglandins. *J Rheumatol* 18;102, 1991.

268. Madreperla SA, Louwerenburg B, Mann RW, et al: Induction of heat shock protein synthesis in chondrocytes at physiological temperatures. *J Orthop Res* 3:30, 1985.

269. Kubo T, Towle CA, Mankin HJ, Treadwell BV: Stress induced proteins in chondrocytes from osteoarthritic patients. *Arch Rheum* 28:1140, 1985.

270. Martel-Pelletier J, Zafarullah M, Kodama S, Pelletier J-P: In vitro effects of Il-1 on the synthesis of metalloproteases, TIMP, plasminogen activators and inhibitors in human articular cartilage. *J Rheumatol* 18:80, 1991.

271. Woessner JF Jr, Gunja-Smith Z: Role of metalloproteinases in human OA. *J Rheumatol* 18:99, 1991.

272. Treadwell BV, Gray DH, Mankin HJ: Anabolic and catabolic activities associated with osteoarthritic chondrocytes, in *Osteoarthritis,* edited by JG Peyron, Basel, Ciba-Geigy, 1985, pp 299–306.

273. Shinmei M, Masuda K, Kikuchi T, et al: Production of cytokines by chondrocytes and its role in proteoglycan degradation. *J Rheumatol* 18:89, 1991.

274. Roughley PJ, Nguyen Q, Mort JS: Mechanisms of proteoglycan degradation in human articular cartilage. *J Rheumatol* 18:52, 1991.

275. Treadwell BV, Towle CA, Ishizue K, et al: Stimulation of the synthesis of collagenase activator protein in cartilage by a factor present in synovial conditioned medium. *Arch Biochem Biophys,* 251:724, 1986.

276. Treadwell BV, Neidel J, Pavia M, et al: Purification and characterization of collagenase activator protein synthesized by articular cartilage. *Arch Biochem Biophys* 251:715, 1986.

277. Treadwell BV, Pavia M, Towel CA, et al: Cartilage synthesizes the serine protease inhibitor PAI-1: Support for the involvement of serine protease in cartilage. *J Orthop Res* 9:309, 1991.

278. Bentley G, Dowd G: Current concepts of the etiology and treatment of chondromalacia patellae. *Clin Orthop* 189:209, 1984.

279. Schumacher HR: Secondary osteoarthritis, in *Osteoarthritis: Diagnosis and Management,* edited by RW Moskowitz, DS Howell, VM Goldberg, HJ Mankin. Philadelphia, Saunders, 1984, pp 235–264.

280. Funk FJ: Trauma and osteoarthritis of the knee. Some implications of change in surgical practice, in *Epidemiology of Osteoarthrosis,* edited by JG Peyron. Basel, Ciba-Geigy, 1991, pp 236–242.

281. Hadler NM, Gillings DB, Imbus HR, et al: Hand structure and function in an industrial setting. Influence of three patterns of stereotyped repetitive usage. *Arch Rheum* 21:210, 1978.

282. Chrisman OD, Ladenbauer, Bellis IM, et al: 1981 Nicolas Andry Award. The relationship of mechanical trauma and the early biochemical reactions of osteoarthritic cartilage. *Clin Orthop* 161:275, 1981.

283. Donohue JM, Oegema TR Jr, Thompson RC Jr: The zone of calcified cartilage: The focal point of changes following blunt trauma to articular cartilage. *Trans Orthop Res Soc* 11:233, 1986.

284. Cooke TD: Immune pathology in polyarticular osteoarthritis. *Clin Orthop* 213:41, 1986.

285. Moskowitz RW, Kresina TF: Immunofluorescent analysis of experimental osteoarthritic cartilage and synovium: Evidence for selective deposition of immunoglobin and complement in cartilaginous tissues. *J Rheumatol* 13:391, 1985.

286. Cooke TD: Pathogenetic mechanisms in polyarticular osteoarthritis. *Clin Rheum Dis* 11:203, 1985.

287. Cooke TD, Bennet EL, Ohno O: Identification of immunoglobins and complement components in articular collagenous tissues of patients with idiopathic osteoarthrosis, in *The Aetiopathogenesis of Osteoarthrosis,* edited by G Nuki. Tunbridge Wells, Pitman Medical Publishing, 1980, pp 144–155.

288. Kennedy TD, Plater ZC, Partridge TA, et al: Morphometric comparison of synovium from patients with osteoarthritis and rheumatoid arthritis. *J Clin Pathol* 41:847, 1988.

289. Goldberg VM: The immunology of articular cartilage, in *Osteoarthritis: Diagnosis and Management,* edited by RW Moskowitz, DS Howell, VM Goldberg, HJ Mankin. Philadelphia, Saunders, 1984, pp 81–92.

290. Peyron JG: Review of the main epidemiologic-etiologic evidence that implies mechanical forces as factors in osteoarthritis. *Eng Med* 15:77, 1986.

291. Genti G: Occupation and osteoarthritis. *Ballieres Clin Rheumatol* 3:193, 1989.

292. Harris WH: Etiology of osteoarthritis of the hip. *Clin Orthop* 213:20, 1986.

293. Danielson L, Lindberg H, Nilsson B: Prevalence of coxarthrosis. *Clin Orthop* 191:110, 1984.

294. Ordeberg G, Hansson LI, Sandstrom S: Slipped femoral capital femoral epiphysis in Southern Sweden. Long-term result with no treatment or symptomatic primary treatment. *Clin Orthop* 191:95, 1984.

295. Mankin HJ: Speculation regarding the biochemical pathogenesis of generalized osteoarthritis. *J Rheumatol* 10:7, 1983.

296. Mankin HJ, Johnson ME, Lippiello L: Biochemical and metabolic abnormalities in articular cartilage from osteoarthritic human hips. II. Distribution and metabolism of amino sugar containing macromolecules. *J Bone Joint Surg* 51A:1591, 1969.

297. Meachim G, Collins DH: Cell counts of normal and osteoarthritic cartilage in relation to the uptake of sulfate ($^{35}SO_4$) in vitro. *Ann Rheum Dis* 221:45, 1962.

298. Thompson RC Jr, Oegema TR Jr: Metabolic activity of articular cartilage in osteoarthritis. An in vitro study. *J Bone Joint Surg* 61A:407, 1979.

299. McDevitt CA, Gilbertson F, Muir H: An experimental model of osteoarthritis: Early morphological and biochemical changes. *J Bone Joint Surg* 59B:24, 1977.

300. Sweet MBE, Thonar EJ, Immelman AR, Soloman L: Biochemical change in progressive osteoarthritis. *Ann Rheum Dis* 36:387, 1977.

301. Maroudas A, Venn M: Chemical composition and swelling of normal and osteoarthritic femoral head cartilage. II. Swelling. *Ann Rheum Dis* 36:399, 1977.

302. Floman Y, Eyre DR, Glimcher MJ: Induction of osteoarthrosis in the rabbit knee joint: Biochemical studies on the articular cartilage. *Clin Orthop* 147:288, 1980.

303. Muir H: Molecular approach to the understanding of osteoarthritis. *Ann Rheum Dis* 36:199, 1977.

304. Lust G, Pronsky W: Glycosaminoglycan content of normal and degenerative articular cartilage from dogs. *Clin Chim Acta* 39:281, 1972.

305. Brockelhurst R, Maroudas A: Comparative studies of the composition and sulfate uptake of normal and osteoarthritic cartilage from the knee, hip and the ankle, in *Epidemiology of Osteoarthritis,* edited by JG Peyton. Paris, Geigy, 1981, pp 124–135.

306. Ryu T, Treadwell BV, Mankin HJ: Biochemical and metabolic abnormalities in normal and osteoarthritic human articular cartilage. *Arthritis Rheum* 27:613, 1984.

307. Brandt KD, Palmoski MJ, Pericone E: Aggregation of cartilage proteoglycans. I. Evidence for the presence of a hyaluronate binding region in proteoglycans from osteoarthritic cartilage. *Arthritis Rheum* 19:1308, 1976.

308. Brandt KD: Enhanced extractability of articular cartilage proteoglycans in osteoarthritis. *Biochem J* 143:475, 1974.

309. Moskowitz RW, Howell DS, Goldberg VM, et al: Cartilage proteoglycan abnormalities in an experimentally induced model of rabbit osteoarthritis. *Arthritis Rheum* 22:155, 1979.

310. Hughs CE, Fosang AJ, Murphy G, et al: Proteoglytic digestion of cartilage proteoglycans involves destruction of the second globular domain. *J Bone Joint Surg* 1992, in press..

311. Mort JS, Poole AR, Roughley PJ: Age-related changes in the structure of proteoglycan link proteins present in normal human articular cartilage. *Biochem J* 214:269, 1983.

312. Palmoski MJ, Brandt KD: Hyaluronate binding by proteoglycans: Comparison of mildly and severely osteoarthritic regions of the human femoral cartilage. *Clin Chim Acta* 79:87, 1976.

313. Mankin HJ, Lippiello L: Biochemical and metabolic abnormalities in articular cartilage from osteoarthritic human hips. *J Bone Joint Surg* 52A:424, 1970.

314. Eyre DR, McDevitt CA, Muir H: Experimentally induced osteoarthritis in the dog collagen. Biosynthesis in control and fibrillated cartilage. *Ann Rheum Dis* (suppl) 34:138, 1975.

315. Ali SY, Griffiths S: Formation of calcium phosphate crystals in normal and osteoarthritic cartilage. *Ann Rheum Dis* (suppl) 42:45, 1983.

316. Dieppe PA, Hukesson EC, Crocker P, Willoughby DA: Apatitic deposition diseases: A new arthropathy. *Lancet* 1:266, 1976.

317. Mitrovic D, Gruson M, Demignon J, et al: Metabolism of human femoral head cartilage in osteoarthrosis and subcapital fracture. *Ann Rheum Dis* 40:18, 1981.

318. Eronen I, Videman T, Freeman MAR, Michelsson JE: Glycosaminoglycan metabolism in experimental osteoarthritis caused by immobilization. *Acta Orthop Scand* 49:329, 1978.

319. Ehrlich MG, Howle PA, Vigliani G, Mankin HJ: Correlation between articular cartilage collagenase activity and osteoarthritis. *Arthritis Rheum* 21:761, 1978.

320. Pelletier JP, Martel-Pelletier J, Altman RD, et al: Collagenolytic activity and collagen matrix breakdown of the articular cartilage in the Pond-Nuki model of osteoarthritis. *Arthritis Rheum* 26:866, 1983.

321. Kandel RA, Dinarell CA, Biswas C: The stimulation of collagenase production in rabbit articular chondrocytes by interleukin-1 is increased by collagens. *Biochem Int* 15:1021, 1987.

322. Pujol JP, Loyau G: Interleukin-1 and osteoarthritis. *Life Sci* 41:1187, 1987.

323. Dodge GR, Poole AR: Immunohistochemical detection and immunochemical analysis of type II collagen degradation in human normal, rheumatoid, and osteoarthritic articular cartilages and in explants of bovine articular cartilage cultured with interleukin-1. *J Clin Invest* 83:647, 1989.

324. Blanckaert A, Mazieres B, Eeckjout Y, Vaes G: Direct extraction and assay of collagenase from human osteoarthritic articular cartilage. *Clin Chim Acta* 185:73, 1989.

325. Ratcliffe A, Tyler JA, Hardingham TE: Articular cartilage cultured with interleukin-1: Increased release of link protein, hyaluronate-binding region and other proteoglycan fragments. *Biochem J* 238:571, 1986.

CHAPTER 3

Patellofemoral Biomechanics

Freddie H. Fu
Michael J. Seel
Richard A. Berger

INTRODUCTION

Orthopaedic surgeons evaluating and treating patellofemoral dysfunction must have a coherent understanding of the normal function of the patellofemoral joint. Knowledge of patellofemoral biomechanics is a prerequisite for correct application of operative as well as conservative therapy. Postoperative and rehabilitative therapy should be based on sound biomechanical principles. Programs not based on these principles may worsen rather than improve the initial pathology.

Biomechanical analysis of the patellofemoral joint is complex. As a result, reported "normal" biomechanical analyses of the patellofemoral joint have varied widely in the literature. No general agreement has yet been reached on the best methods to elucidate the fundamental biomechanical properties of the patellofemoral joint.

In both engineering and nature, form follows function. Thus, detailed understanding of the anatomy of the patellofemoral joint is required before embarking on a clinically useful biomechanical analysis. Based on a firm anatomic foundation, this chapter focuses on normal patellofemoral biomechanics. Patellar function as well as kinematics and dynamics are emphasized. Finally, the biomechanics of surgical procedures affecting the patellofemoral joint are analyzed. This chapter is intended to provide a broad, clinically relevant overview of patellofemoral biomechanics. Where possible, complex mathematical relationships and detailed engineering principles have been deliberately avoided.

THE FUNCTION OF THE PATELLA

The primary function of the patella is to act as a fulcrum, effectively increasing the lever arm of the quadriceps. The patella is aptly suited to act as a pivot surface for the quadriceps tendon. This fulcrum action requires a surface adapted to bearing high compressive loads with minimal friction forces. The hyaline cartilage of the patella, the thickest in the body, provides this environment. The viscoelastic properties of cartilage allow it to deform to distribute the contact load over a large area. This load distribution and resulting reduction in pressure are vital to protect the underlying innervated bone.

Cartilage damage or loss of the patella can have devastating consequences. For example, in chondromalacia, the loss of mechanical integrity of the cartilage causes large localized contact pressures and leads to significant pain. When the patella is absent, the quadriceps tendon is subjected to the high compressive loads normally borne by the patella. The tendon cannot accommodate this compressive force well and large frictional forces result.

The patella also acts as a site of convergence for the four quadriceps muscles (Fig. 3-1). Through articular congruency with the patellofemoral groove, it produces stability of these four muscles under load. Finally, the patella also protects the underlying femoral condyles from trauma.

Patellar Contribution to Quadriceps Extension Torque

Early clinical follow-up studies of patients after patellectomy cited excellent extensor function.[1,2] Con-

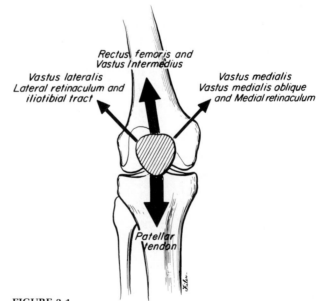

FIGURE 3-1
Forces and constraints on the patella during function.

currently, some early investigators believed that the patella actually inhibited knee extensor function and efficiency.[3,4] We now know through theoretical calculations,[5,6] experimental works,[7,8] and clinical studies[9–11] that the patella is an important component of extensor function, significantly contributing to knee extension torque.

Knee extension torque or moment is the product of the quadriceps force multiplied by the length of the moment arm through which it acts. The *moment arm*, the distance between the joint center of rotation and the quadriceps mechanism, is increased if the quadriceps mechanism is moved anteriorly and decreased if it is moved posteriorly. The patella more effectively increases the moment arm of the quadriceps as the knee is extended. The maximum effect is at a knee flexion angle of approximately 20 degrees.[12,13] This is due to the prominent anterior position of the patella at low flexion angles as it rests high in the trochlear. In this prominent position, the patella accounts for nearly one-third of the extension moment arm at full extension[7,14] (Figs. 3-2 and 3-3). The patella becomes less prominent with flexion as it sinks posteriorly into the intercondylar notch. Subsequently the patella only contributes about one-sixth of the moment arm between 60 and 120 degrees flexion.[7]

Transmission of the Quadriceps Force to the Patellar Tendon

The patella was once thought to act as a simple "pulley." From this assumption it followed that the forces in the quadriceps tendon and patellar tendon should be equal. This is now known to be incorrect. A complex relationship exists between the force in the quadriceps tendon and the force in the patellar tendon.[15–17] The relative force in each tendon varies with knee flexion angle. At small angles, the patellar tendon force is larger, whereas at large flexion angles, the quadriceps tendon force is larger. The relative changes in the ratio of forces in each tendon are due to variations in the moment arm of each tendon with knee flexion angle (Fig. 3-4).

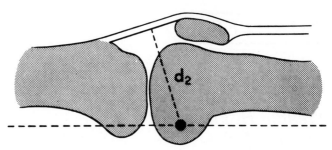

FIGURE 3-3
The patella lengthens the extension moment arm of the knee at full extension. Note from Fig. 2, $d_2 > d_1$. (Reprinted with permission from Kaufer H: Mechanical function of the patella. *J Bone Joint Surg* 53A:1551–1560, 1971.)

Huberti and colleagues[15] were among the first to demonstrate experimentally this complex relationship theorized by Maquet[5] many years earlier. At a knee flexion angle of 30 degrees, Huberti found that the force in the patellar tendon exceeds the force in the quadriceps by 30 percent, while at 50 degrees flexion, the two forces are equal. As knee flexion is continued beyond 90 degrees, the force in the patellar tendon is 30 percent less than the force in the quadriceps tendon (Fig. 3-5).

The results of Buff and coworkers[16] paralleled those of Huberti. They concluded that the patellofemoral joint acts more like a balance beam than a pulley, noting that because the patella is unconstrained in the sagittal plane, it is free to rock or tilt in this plane.

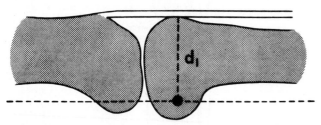

FIGURE 3-2
Without a patella the knee at full extension has a small moment arm. (Reprinted with permission from Kaufer H: Mechanical function of the patella. *J Bone Joint Surg* 53A:1551–1560, 1971.)

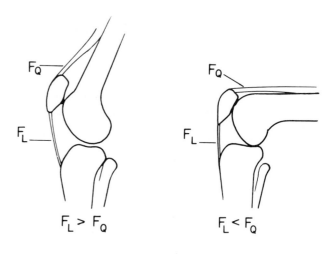

FIGURE 3-4
Shifting location of patellofemoral contact area at different flexion angles determines the force ratio. *A.* At 30 degrees knee flexion, the contact area is located distally. The quadriceps (F_Q) acts as a mechanical advantage and generates a greater ligamentum force (F_L). *B.* At 90 degrees of knee flexion, the opposite situation occurs. (Reprinted with permission from Huberti HH, Hayes WC, Stone JL, Shybut GT: Force ratios in the quadriceps tendon and ligamentum patellae. *J Orthop Res* 2:49–54, 1984.)

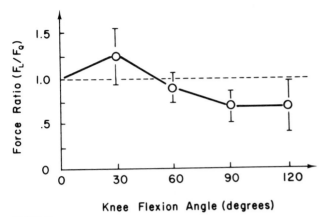

FIGURE 3-5
Force ratio (F_L/F_Q) of ligamentum patellae force (F_L) of quadriceps tendon force (F_Q) as function of flexion angle. At 30 degrees knee flexion, F_L is approximately 30 percent greater than F_Q. At > 90 degrees knee flexion, F_L is approximately 30 percent < F_Q. (Reprinted with permission from Huberti HH, Hayes WC, Stone JL, Shybut GT: Force ratios in the quadriceps tendon and ligamentum patellae. *J Orthop Res* 2:49–54, 1984.)

The torque generated by the quadriceps tendon and the patellar tendon is balanced by the tilting of the patella. The amount of tilt in the sagittal plane varies as a function of flexion angle. The lever arms for the quadriceps tendon and patellar tendon are different and vary directly with patellar tilt and, therefore, with flexion angle. The lever arms of each tendon are different while the torques must be balanced; therefore, the patellar tendon must be subjected to a different force than the quadriceps tendon (Fig. 3-6).

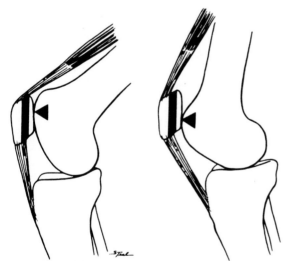

FIGURE 3-6
The patella as a balancing beam. The torque from the quadriceps tendon and the patellar tendon is balanced by the patella. The arrow identifies patellofemoral contact. The striped bar shows the balance beam effect. Note the difference in the lever arm length between the patella tendon and quadriceps tendon as a function of knee flexion angle. (Reprinted with permission from Buff HU, Jones LC, Hungerford DS: Determination of forces transmitted through the patellofemoral joint. *J Biomech* 21:17, 1988)

DYNAMICS

The term *dynamics* refers to the forces on an object. In this section, we analyze the forces on the patellofemoral joint and the contact pressure that results from these forces. To obtain the relationship between force and pressure, we must also analyze the contact area of the patellofemoral joint.

Anatomic Adaptations

In 1941, Wiberg[18] was one of the first to evaluate patellofemoral contact areas. He transversely sectioned cadaveric knees at various flexion angles and determined valuable information about the contact areas. He also postulated loading conditions from osseous structure (Fig. 3-7). A transverse section, or axial computed tomography (CT) view through the knee, shows the subchondral bone to have increased density on the lateral patellar facet as compared to the medial facet. This suggests that the lateral facet is subjected to higher forces. The trabecular orientation of the patellofemoral joint also provides information about the joint loading pattern. The trabeculae of the patella are parallel, all aligned in the sagittal plane. The femoral trabeculae are similarly aligned, but appear to be perpendicular to the articular surface.

Patellofemoral Compression Force

The resultant patellofemoral compression force is due to the component of the force in the quadriceps tendon and patellar tendon perpendicular to the articular surface of the patellofemoral joint (Fig. 3-8).

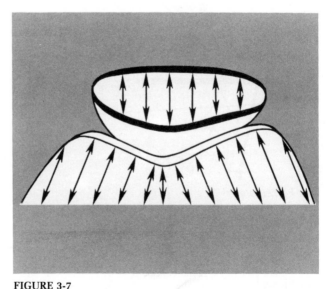

FIGURE 3-7
Osseous structure of the patellofemoral joint as seen in cross section demonstrating the contact forces carried by the patellofemoral joint.

These components hold the patella in contact with the femur. The resultant patellofemoral force depends on two factors—knee flexion angle and the force in the quadriceps and patellar tendons.

Increasing knee flexion angle decreases the angle between the quadriceps tendon and patellar tendon, thus increasing the proportion of the force in the quadriceps and patellar tendons that acts on the patellofemoral articular surface. Theoretically, then, increasing knee flexion increases the resultant patellofemoral force. In the actual case, this increase in force with flexion is limited at flexion angles beyond 70 to 80 degrees by contact between the quadriceps tendon and the distal femur.[14,19] The resultant patellofemoral force is significantly reduced due to load sharing from the tendofemoral contact point. Hehne[14] found that at 130 degrees knee flexion, the tendofemoral contact carries as much force as the patellofemoral joint, reducing the patellofemoral contact force by one-half. This confirms earlier work by Huberti and coworkers[19] who found that the tendofemoral force reduces the resultant force on the patella by one-third at 120 degrees knee flexion. Investigators disagree on the precise flexion angle that corresponds to the maximum patellofemoral resultant force. Although the range of reported values is between 60 and 130 degrees,[6,12,20–22] recent authors suggest that this angle is between 70 and 80 degrees for most activities.[14,19,20]

Increased force in the quadriceps tendon will result in increased force in the patellar tendon, as discussed above. Increased force in the quadriceps tendon and patellar tendon, in turn, results in increased resultant patellofemoral force.

The torque generated by the quadriceps muscle during walking, climbing stairs, and other normal activities is the product of the weight of the subject multiplied by the distance between the center of mass of the upper body and the center of the knee joint. Therefore, hip flexion, which brings the center of mass of the upper body closer to the center of rotation of the knee, reduces the torque generated by the quadriceps muscle. This reduction in torque causes similar decreases in the quadriceps force and the resultant patellofemoral force. Patients with knee joint pathology or pain compensate by modifying their body position.[23] For example, when ascending stairs these patients will use more hip flexion and less knee extension, reducing the resultant patellofemoral force[23,24] (Fig. 3-9). In activities such as skiing, where the center of mass of the upper body may be moved far behind the center of rotation of the knee (i.e., as the skier leans back in his boots), the resultant patellofemoral force may be increased significantly.

A large range in magnitude of the resultant patellofemoral force has been reported. This resultant

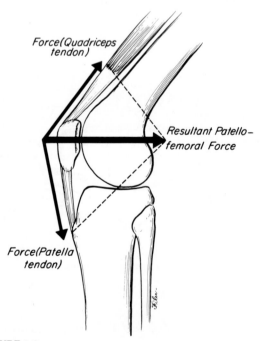

FIGURE 3-8
The resultant patellofemoral force compresses the patella against the femur. This compressive force is the consequence of the quadriceps tendon force and patella tendon force.

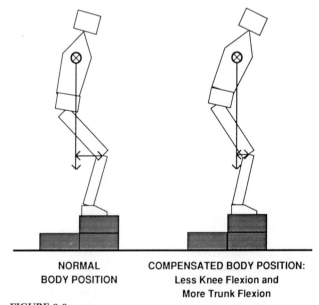

NORMAL BODY POSITION   **COMPENSATED BODY POSITION: Less Knee Flexion and More Trunk Flexion**

FIGURE 3-9
Ascending stairs with less knee flexion and more trunk flexion reduces the torque on the knee. This compensated body position moves the center of mass of the trunk closer to the knee, thereby reducing the knee moment arm and the knee torque.

force varies based on the method of analysis, knee flexion angle, and type of activity considered. For example, Bishop's early work with theoretical models found the resultant patellofemoral force to be 10 times body weight at 90 degrees flexion.[21] Rielly and Martens[25] reported a resultant patellofemoral force of 0.5 times body weight for walking and 7.8 times body weight for squatting using theoretical calculation applied to experimental data. Bandi[26] reanalyzed the work of Rielly and Martens, accounting for hip flexion. This modification resulted in a reduction of the resultant patellofemoral force during squatting to 3.8 times body weight. More recently, authors used newer experimental data, accounted for inequality in quadriceps and patellar tendon forces, and considered the changes in the center of mass of the upper body with activity. These factors have resulted in a reduction in the estimated maximum resultant patellofemoral force to 2 to 3 times body weight.[12–14,27] These newer studies agree that the maximum resultant patellofemoral force occurs between 70 and 80 degrees knee flexion.

The resultant patellofemoral force is not distributed equally over the medial and lateral patellar facets. As theorized by Wiberg[18] from the morphology of the patella, the lateral facet carries more of the resultant force than the medial facet. This was reinforced by Hehne[14] who demonstrated that the force on the lateral facet was approximately 60 percent more than the force on the medial facet throughout most of knee flexion.

Patellofemoral Contact Area

The patella begins to contact the femur with quadriceps muscle recruitment without knee flexion. This contact begins on the inferior patella at full extension and moves superiorly with increasing knee flexion. At 90 degrees, the contact area has reached the superior patella[17,28] (Fig. 3-10). Throughout this range, from 0 to 90 degrees, the contact area extends transversely across the patella.[14,19,28] All areas of the lateral facet and medial facet proper contact the femur in this flexion range (Fig. 3-11). Hehne[14] found that the lateral facet contact area was approximately 60 percent greater than the medial facet contact area throughout most of the knee flexion range. (This contact area inequality correlates with the difference in force distribution between the lateral facet and medial facet.) The total contact area increases with flexion angle, reaching a maximum at about 90 degrees[19,29] (Fig. 3-12). Beyond 90 degrees, the contact area diminishes slightly, as only the lateral and medial edges of the patellar facets are in contact with the femur (see Fig. 3-11). Huberti and colleagues discovered that at high flexion angles the quadriceps

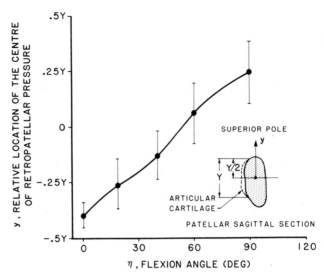

FIGURE 3-10
The effect of knee flexion on the location of the center of pressure on the patella. The center of pressure moves superiorly from the inferior articular surface with knee flexion. (Reprinted with permission from Ahmed AM, Burke DL, Hyder A: Force analyses of the patellar mechanism. *J Orthop Res* 5:69–85, 1987.)

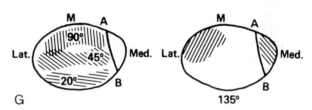

FIGURE 3-11
Patellofemoral contact location of the patella with flexion. (M: location of the medial ridge. A-B: Ridge separating the medial facet proper and the "odd" facet.) (Reprinted with permission from Hungerford DS, Barry BS: Biomechanics of the patellofemoral joint. *Clin Orthop* 144:9–15, 1979.)

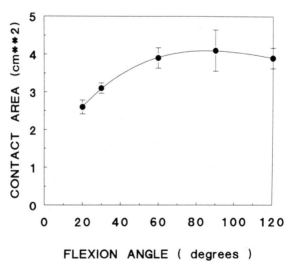

FIGURE 3-12
Patellofemoral contact area with flexion on normal knees. (Reprinted with permission from Hayes WC, Huberti, HH, Lewallen DG, Riegger CL, Myers ER: Patellofemoral contact pressure and the effects of surgical reconstruction procedures, in Ewing JW (ed): *Articular Cartilage and Knee Joint Function: Basic Science and Arthroscopy,* edited by JW Ewing. New York, Raven Press, 1990.)

tendon contacts the femur. They found that the tendofemoral contact area was 75 percent of the patellofemoral contact area at 120 degrees. Later, Hehne[14] demonstrated that tendofemoral contact begins at 70 degrees and increases as a function of increased knee flexion angle.

Patellofemoral Contact Pressure

Patellofemoral contact pressure is defined as the normal (perpendicular) force per unit contact area. Proper assessment and characterization of patellofemoral contact pressure during knee motion requires consideration of both force and contact area. When considering contact pressure, two different mechanical situations must be analyzed: physiologic flexion and extension against resistance.

Physiologic flexion may be defined as flexing or extending the knee with the weight of the upper body being supported by the knee joint. Activities of daily living involving physiologic flexion include walking, raising from a chair, and squatting. In physiologic flexion, knee torque and therefore, quadriceps force, increase with increasing knee flexion angle. The resultant patellofemoral force also increases with flexion angle to a maximum at 70 to 90 degrees flexion.[19,29] The increase in patellofemoral force would markedly increase the contact pressure if not for the accompanying increase in contact area with flexion to 90 degrees (see Fig. 3-12). The increase in contact area protects the patellofemoral joint by limiting the increase in the contact pressure with increasing patellofemoral force. The resultant patellofemoral force does, however, increase disproportionately to the contact area, causing the contact pressure to increase modestly with flexion[14,19] (Fig. 3-13).

The patella is further protected by the articular cartilage thickness. The thickness of the articular cartilage varies with the functional needs of the patella. Figure 3-14*A* is a cross section of the patella that articulates at 30 degrees knee flexion. At 30 degrees, the patellofemoral contact pressure is low. Figure 3-14*B* is a cross section of the patella that articulates at 60 degrees knee flexion. At 60 degrees, the contact pressure is almost double the pressure at 30 degrees; hence the cartilage is much thicker in this area (see Fig. 3-13).

The contact pressure is distributed over both the medial and lateral facets. In the flexion range from 0 through 90 degrees, the entire articular surface of the patella comes into contact with the femur. The resultant patellofemoral force and the contact area are greater on the lateral facet than the medial facet throughout this flexion range. The ratio of both these

parameters from 0 through 90 degrees is approximately equal.[14] This results in an equality in the contact pressure on the medial and lateral facets, even though the lateral facet is subjected to greater force than the medial facet. In fact, Hehne[14] found experimentally that the pressure on the medial facet was actually 6 to 10 percent higher than that on the lateral facet. The increase in pressure on the medial facet as compared to the lateral facet may account for the higher incidence of chondromalacia of the medial facet despite the fact that the lateral facet is subjected to more force.

A different contact pressure profile is obtained during extension against resistance. Extension against resistance, extending (or flexing) the lower leg against gravity, occurs in the sitting position when a weighted lower leg is raised (or lowered) against gravity. This motion is typical of quadriceps strengthening exercises used in knee rehabilitation programs. In this situation, the torque generated at the knee increases with extension because the weight is moved farther from the center of rotation of the knee. This increase in torque with extension is supplied by increasing the quadriceps force, and hence, increasing the resultant patellofemoral force. Therefore, unlike physiologic flexion where the resultant patellofemoral force increases with flexion, in extension against resistance the resultant patellofemoral force increases with extension. This situation concentrates the maximum patellofemoral force over the smaller

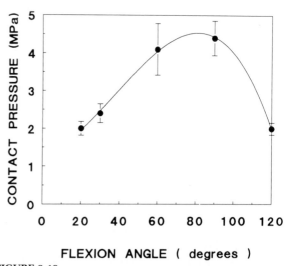

FIGURE 3-13
Patellofemoral contact pressure with flexion on normal knees. (Reprinted with permission from Hayes WC, Huberti HH, Lewallen DG, Riegger CL, Myers ER: Patellofemoral contact pressure and the effects of surgical reconstruction procedures, in *Articular Cartilage and Knee Joint Function: Basic Science and Arthroscopy,* edited by JW Ewing. New York, Raven Press, 1990.)

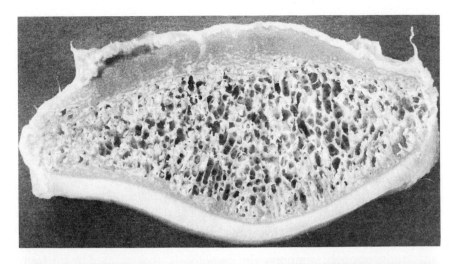

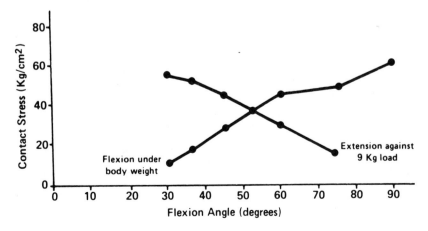

FIGURE 3-14
Cross section through the patella at the *(A)* 30 degree and *(B)* 60 degree contact zones.

B

contact area present at low flexion angles. The high force on a small area leads to large contact pressures on the patella. Hungerford and coworkers[28] calculated the normal patellofemoral contact pressure during extension against resistance with a 20-lb weight (Fig. 3-15). At 30 degrees flexion, the pressure is four times that found under conditions of physiologic flexion. During extension against resistance exercises with larger weights (100 lb), the physiologic contact pressure on the patella may be exceeded by more than an order of magnitude. Rehabilitation programs using these exercises should be applied cautiously because of potential worsening of patellofemoral problems.

FIGURE 3-15
Comparison of contact pressure with flexion for flexion under body weight (physiologic flexion) and extension against resistance. (Reprinted with permission from Hungerford DS, Barry BS: Biomechanics of the patellofemoral joint. *Clin Orthop* 144:9–15, 1979.)

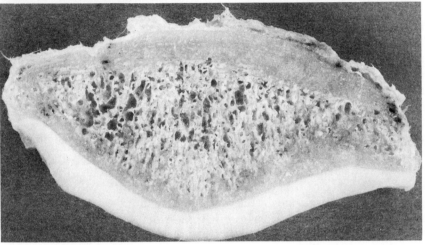

CONTACT PRESSURE IN PATHOLOGIC KNEES

The pathogenesis of patella chondromalacia remains somewhat controversial. Many investigators of chondromalacia have made the implicit assumption that excessive patellofemoral contact pressure is related to the etiology of chondromalacia. Ohno and colleagues recently investigated this theory.[30] They analyzed biopsies of 12 young patients with early chondromalacia and found that the collagen fiber network of the superficial matrix had deteriorated. They concluded that this was consistent with a pathogenesis associated with mechanical overloading. This elegant study strongly supports the hypothesis that chondromalacia is due to mechanical breakdown of the articular cartilage.

In knees with chondromalacia, the pressure over the lesions is significantly reduced due to the loss of mechanical integrity of the cartilage. Lewallen and colleagues[29] found that the pressure directly over grade I and II lesions was 50 percent less than normal (Fig. 3-16). Over grade III and IV lesions, the pressure was reduced by more than 90 percent. Interestingly, the cartilage immediately adjacent to the lesions was subjected to significantly higher contact pressure than the normal cartilage. This increased pressure in the adjacent cartilage may be the reason for the rapid spread of the chondromalacia lesion. In addition, the transmission of high pressure directly to the bone is probably responsible for the pain associated with this disease.

KINEMATICS

Kinematics refers to motion of an object without reference to the forces acting on the object. In this section we will quantify the motion of the normal patella with respect to the femur.

Q Angle

The *Q angle* is the angle between the quadriceps tendon and patellar tendon at full extension (Fig. 3-17). Normal knee valgus would generate a small Q angle. The major contribution to the Q angle is created by the terminal external rotation of the tibia, the "screw-home" effect. This laterally rotates the tibial tubercle, the attachment of the patellar tendon, greatly accentuating the Q angle. At full extension, the Q angle produces a valgus force on the patella. In this situation, the patella is free from the restraints of the trochlea and this valgus force must be resisted by the medial retinaculum and vastus medialis.

Patellofemoral Motion

At full extension with the quadriceps contracted, the patella lies in the supratrochlear fat pad. From full

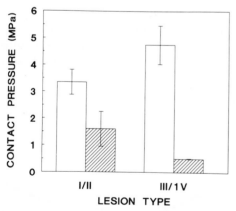

FIGURE 3-16
The average contact pressure over lesions in chondromalacic knees *(hashed bar)* compared to corresponding areas in normal knees *(white bar)*. There is a 50 percent reduction over grade I to II lesions and a 90 percent reduction over grade II to IV lesions. (Reprinted with permission from Hayes WC, Huberti HH, Lewallen DG, Rieger CL, Myers ER: Patellofemoral contact pressure and the effects of surgical reconstruction procedures, in *Articular Cartilage and Knee Joint Function: Basic Science and Arthroscopy,* edited by JW Ewing. New York, Raven Press, 1990.)

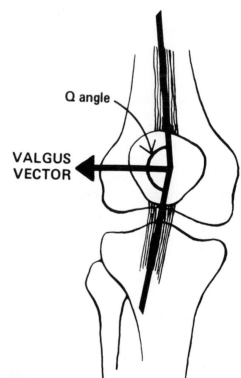

FIGURE 3-17
The angle between the quadriceps tendon and the patella tendon forms the Q angle. The Q angle produces a valgus force on the patella. (Reprinted with permission from Hungerford DS, Barry BS: Biomechanics of the patellofemoral joint. *Clin Orthop* 144: 9–15, 1979.)

extension through about 20 degrees flexion the patella is not yet firmly entrenched in the patellofemoral groove of the femur. In this early stage of flexion, the stability of the patella is maintained by the tension of the quadriceps. The lack of firm stability in early flexion is reflected by the relatively high frequency of tracking problems in this range. After 20 degrees flexion, the stability of the patella is maintained by congruity with the trochlea. This congruity accounts for the consistent tracking patterns encountered after 20 to 30 degrees flexion.

Because of the angle of the quadriceps mechanism (Q angle), the patella enters the patellofemoral groove from the lateral side as flexion is initiated. The patella continues to move medially to about 30 degrees flexion as the tibia derotates, releasing the valgus force produced by the Q angle. Concurrently, the patella assumes a prominent position on the trochlea. In this prominent position, the quadriceps lever arm is greatest. At this stage, patellar tracking is ensured by congruity with the femur. After 40 degrees of flexion, the patella begins to return to a centered position as it sinks posteriorly into the trochlea. It reaches a central position at roughly 80 degrees and remains centered throughout the remainder of flexion.[31]

The patella normally exhibits a slight tilt with flexion. The patella, initially level, slowly tilts medially until it reaches about 4 degrees medial tilt at 40 degrees flexion. At this point, it reverses and begins to tilt laterally, reaching a neutral tilt at a knee flexion angle of 70 degrees. The patella continues to tilt laterally, attaining 4 degrees lateral tilt at a knee flexion angle of 100 degrees. Further flexion returns the patella to a neutral position at 120 to 140 degrees.[31]

The patella also rotates about its center with knee flexion. Defining neutral rotation as the patella position at full extension, the patella steadily internally rotates to reach a maximum of 12 degrees internal rotation with full flexion.[31]

BIOMECHANICS OF SURGICAL PROCEDURES

Although other chapters will address the indications, techniques, and clinical outcomes of various surgical procedures, a biomechanical manuscript of the patellofemoral joint would be incomplete without analyzing the biomechanical effects of common surgical procedures for patellar problems. A wide variety of procedures have been advocated for the treatment of anterior knee pain. The goal of most procedures is to reduce or redistribute the patellofemoral contact pressure. Four of the most common surgical procedures are elevation of the tibial tuberosity, lateral release or medial plication, decreasing the Q angle of the quadriceps mechanism, and patellectomy. In this section we analyze the biomechanical consequences of these procedures on patellofemoral contact pressure.

Elevation of the Tibial Tuberosity

Cadaveric studies on normal knees have demonstrated that as the tibial tuberosity is displaced anteriorly, the patellofemoral contact pressure decreases. Ferguson and coworkers[32] demonstrated that the decrease in patellofemoral contact pressure is proportional to the amount of anterior displacement up to 1 cm. Further displacement results in minimal pressure reduction (Fig. 3-18). More recently, Ferrandez and colleagues[33] also found that anterior displacements > 1 cm reduced the contact pressure only slightly (Fig. 3-19). With displacements > 1 cm, however, they discovered that certain zones were subject to increased pressures, reaching values higher than those seen initially. The localized increase in pressure with > 1 cm elevation was most significant on the superior part of the patella where pressures were concentrated on the lateral facet (Fig. 3-20). Hehne[14] also noted this superior redistribution of pressure. He demonstrated that the resultant patellofemoral pressure is reduced in part by diverting a part of the resultant force superiorly to tendofemoral contact.

Most recently, Lewallen and coworkers[29] studied the biomechanical effects of tibial tubercle elevation on both normal knees and knees with chondromalacia. They concluded that knees with chondromalacia had a different biomechanical response to tibial tuberosity elevation. In contrast to the fact that the pressure on the normal knees is reduced with elevation, they found no significant reduction in either peak or mean pressure on the knees with chondromalacia (Fig. 3-21). As in normal knees, knees with chondromalacia had a pressure redistribution superiorly following elevation.

Lateral Release or Medial Plication

Lewallen and colleagues[29] studied four procedures on cadaveric knees with chondromalacia: lateral release, bilateral release, lateral plication, and medial plication. They found that medial plication and lateral plication resulted in increased contact pressure on the medial and lateral facets, respectively. This was due to increased force on the facet without a compensatory increase in contact area. Neither procedure had an effect on the contralateral facet. They also

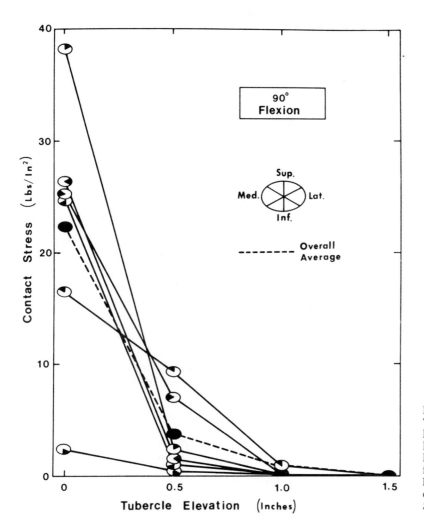

FIGURE 3-18
The effects of tibial tubercle elevation in normal knees on the patella contact pressure (stress). The local pressure in each zone of the patella is analyzed separately. (Reprinted with permission from Ferguson AB, Brown T, Fu F, Rutkowski R: Relief of patellofemoral contact stress by anterior displacement of the tibial tubercle. *J Bone Joint Surg* 61A:159–166, 1979.)

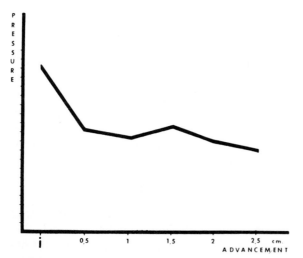

FIGURE 3-19
The overall effects of tibial tubercle elevation in normal knees on the patella contact pressure. (Reprinted with permission from Ferrandez L, Usabiaga J, Yubero J, Sagarra KJ, No LD: An experimental study of the redistribution of patellofemoral pressure by the anterior displacement of the anterior tuberosity of the tibia. *Clin Orthop* 238:183–189, 1989.)

studied lateral release with medial plication and found that the addition of the lateral release did not change the effects of the medial plication.

Similar results were noted for the lateral and bilateral capsular release procedures. Both procedures demonstrated unpredictable and inconsistent effects on the patellofemoral contact pressure. Neither procedure reduced the resultant patellofemoral force or contact pressure (see Fig. 3-21). In some specimens the contact pressure was redistributed to different areas of the patella in a highly variable fashion. Lateral release did not consistently unload the lateral facet as empirically assumed. The authors concluded that this variability in redistribution may account for the variability in clinical results following these procedures for chondromalacia.

Altering the Q Angle

Huberti and colleagues[19] experimentally analyzed the effects of changing the Q angle on cadaveric knees with normal Q angles. They discovered that either increasing or decreasing the Q angle redistributed the

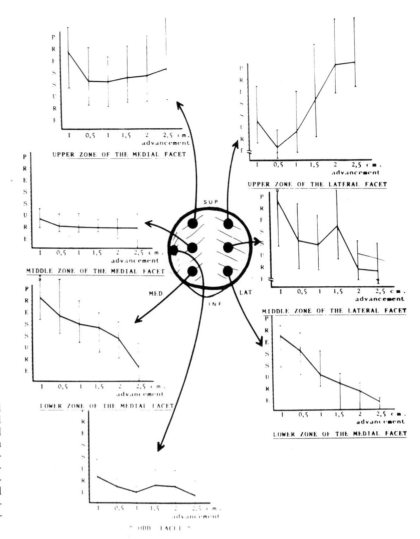

FIGURE 3-20
The effects of tibial tubercle elevation in normal knees on the patella contact pressure. The local pressure in each zone of the patella is analyzed separately. Note the elevation in pressure with large elevation on the superior lateral facet. (Reprinted with permission from Ferrandez L, Usabiaga J, Yubero J, Sagarra KJ, No LD: An experimental study of the redistribution of patellofemoral pressure by the anterior displacement of the anterior tuberosity of the tibia. *Clin Orthop* 238:183–189, 1989.)

contact pressure over the surface of the patella. With both increased and decreased Q angle, the central area of the patella was unloaded, shifting the pressure to the periphery. This redistribution decreased the total contact area, resulting in an increase in the con-

tact pressure since the resultant patellofemoral force was unchanged (Fig. 3-22). The authors concluded that any change to the normal Q angle increases the contact pressure (Fig. 3-23), while redistributing it.

Hehne[14] also experimentally studied changes in

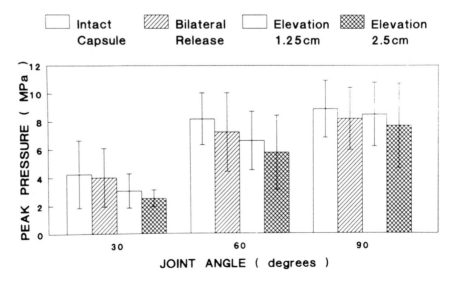

FIGURE 3-21
Average peak patellofemoral contact pressures in chondromalacic knees at three flexion angles for specimens with intact capsule and then following bilateral retinacular release and tibial tubercle elevation of 1.25 and 2.50 cm. None of these procedures resulted in statistically significant reductions in average pressure. (Reprinted with permission from Lewallen DG, Riegger CL, Myers ER, Hayes WC: Effects of retinacular release and tibial tubercle elevation in patellofemoral degenerative joint disease. *J Orthop Res* 8:856–862, 1990.)

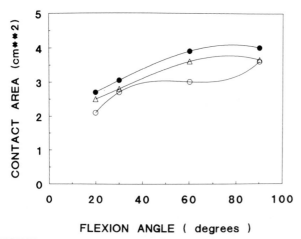

FIGURE 3-22
Patellofemoral contact area of normal knees with normal Q angles is shown with black dots (●). Alternating the normal Q angle, +10 degrees (△), reduces the contact area. (Reprinted with permission from Lewallen DG, Riegger CL, Myers ER, Hayes WC: Effects of retinocular release and tibial tubercle elevation in patellofemoral degenerative joint disease. *J Orthop Res* 8:856–862, 1990.)

the Q angle on normal knees with normal Q angles. He confirmed Huberti's analysis,[19] demonstrating that as the Q angle decreased, the overall pressure decreased slightly while the medial facet pressure increased significantly. He concluded that while decreasing the Q angle may be useful for lateral facet problems, it was not useful and may aggravate medial facet pathology.

Patellectomy

As previously described, the patella is an important contributor to the extensor mechanism. Patellectomy

directly reduces the extension moment arm by allowing the extensor mechanism to sink posteriorly in the patellar groove. This reduction in the quadriceps moment arm causes loss of knee extension torque, particularly at low flexion angles. The patella accounts for nearly one-third of the extension moment arm at full extension.[7,14] Thus, patellectomy results in the reduction of the extension moment arm by one-third at full extension[7,14,22] (see Figs. 3-2 and 3-3). The consequence of patellectomy is less severe at increasing knee flexion angles, with only a one-sixth reduction between 60 and 120 degrees.

The method of repair of the patellectomy has been found to affect the residual extension torque (Fig. 3-24). A longitudinal repair improves the extensor torque only marginally due to diversion of part of the quadriceps pull to the medial and lateral retinacula. Diverting the quadriceps pull in this manner reduces extension torque because the lateral and medial retinacula have shorter moment arms than the patellar tendon and contribute little to extensor torque. In contrast, a transverse repair results in very little diverting effect and allows more force to be transmitted to the patellar tendon. Despite the improvement in knee extension torque afforded by a transverse repair, a 25 percent torque deficiency at full extension remains.[7]

Patellectomy may also result in instability of the quadriceps mechanism as the stabilizing effect of the patella in the patellar groove has been lost. Finally, some authors have recommended tibial tubercle elevation after patellectomy to restore extension torque.

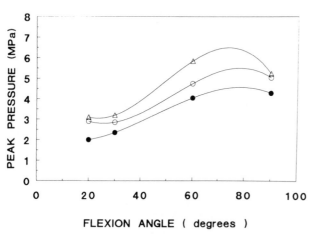

FIGURE 3-23
Patellofemoral contact pressure of normal knees with normal Q angles is shown with black dots (●). Alternating the normal Q angle, +10 degrees (o) or −10 degrees (△), increases the contact pressure. (Reprinted with permission from Lewallen DG, Riegger CL, Myers ER, Hayes WC: Effects of retinacular release and tibial tubercle elevation in patellofemoral degenerative joint disease. *J Orthop Res* 8:856–862, 1990.)

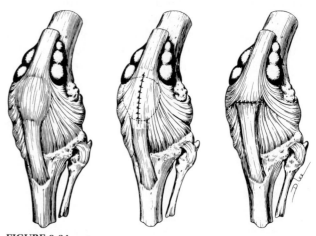

FIGURE 3-24
In an intact knee, the patella provides a secure connection between patella tendon and quadriceps tendon. After patellectomy and longitudinal closure, there is some separation of the quadriceps tendon and the patella tendon. The patella tendon relaxes a little and some quadriceps pull is diverted to the retinacula. After transverse repair, full tension is restored to the patella tendon and no pull is diverted to the retinacula. (Reprinted with permission from Kaufer H: Mechanical function of the patella. *J Bone Joint Surg* 53A:1551–1560, 1971.)

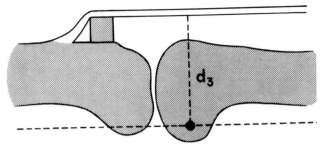

FIGURE 3-25

Tibial tubercle elevation following patellectomy increases the extension moment arm and reestablishes the normal extension torque at full extension. (Reprinted with permission from Kaufer H: Mechanical function of the patella. *J Bone Joint Surg* 53A:1551–1560, 1971.)

This increase in extension torque occurs because the extension moment increases as the patellar tendon is moved anteriorly with the tubercle (Fig. 3-25).

Kaufer[7] demonstrated a full recovery of extension torque after patellectomy with tibial tubercle elevation.

Summary of Surgical Procedures

The common surgical procedures discussed above affect the patellofemoral joint uniquely. No one procedure is a panacea for reducing contact pressure. There are many different causes of anterior knee pain and many sites of chondromalacia patella. As arthroscopy, CT, and magnetic resonance imaging become standard evaluation tools for the patellofemoral joint, the surgeon will be better able to choose the procedure that may most benefit the patient based on individual needs. The proper choice must be based on correct application of sound biomechanical principles.

REFERENCES

1. Boucher HH: Patellectomy in the geriatric patient. *Clin Orthop* 11:33, 1958.
2. West FE: End results of patellectomy with quadricepsplasty. *J Bone Joint Surg* 40A:386, 1958.
3. Brooke R: The treatment of fractured patella by excision. A study of morphology and function. *J Bone Joint Surg* 24:733, 1937.
4. Hey Groves EW: A note on the extension apparatus of the knee joint. *J Bone Joint Surg* 24B:747, 1937.
5. Maquet P: *Biomechanics of the knee. With Application to the Pathogenesis and the Surgical Treatment of Osteoarthritis.* Berlin, Springer-Verlag, 1976.
6. Yamaguchi GT, Zajac FE: A planar model of the knee joint to characterize the knee extensor mechanism. *J Biomech* 22:1, 1989.
7. Kaufer H: Mechanical function of the patella. *J Bone Joint Surg* 53A:1551, 1971.
8. Haxton H: The function of the patella and the effects of its excision. *Surg Gynecol Obstet* 80:389, 1945.
9. Lewis MM, Fitzgerald PF, Jacobs B, Install J: Patellectomy, an analysis of one hundred cases. *J Bone Joint Surg* 58A:1551, 1971.
10. Symposium on Total Knee Replacement. *Clin Orthop* 94:2, 1973.
11. Instell JN: Intra-articular surgery for degenerative arthritis of the knee. A report of the work of the late K.H. Pride. *J Bone Joint Surg* 48B:221, 1967.
12. Reithmeyer, E, Plitz W: A theoretical and numerical approach to optimal positioning of the patellar surface replacement in a total knee endoprosthesis. *J Biomech* 23:883, 1990.
13. Perry J, Antonelli D, Ford W: Analysis of knee joint forces during flexed knee stance. *J Bone Joint Surg* 57A:961, 1975.
14. Hehne HJ: Biomechanics of the patellofemoral joint and its clinical relevance. *Clin Orthop* 258:73, 1990.
15. Huberti HH, Hayes WC, Stone JL, Shybut GT: Force ratios in the quadriceps tendon and ligamentum patellae. *J Orthop Res* 2:49, 1984.
16. Buff HU, Jones LC, Hungerford DS: Determination of forces transmitted through the patellofemoral joint. *J Biomech* 21:17, 1988.
17. Ahmed AM, Burke DL, Hyder A: Force analysis of the patellar mechanism. *J Orthop Res* 5:69, 1987.
18. Wiberg G: Roentgenographic and anatomic studies of the femoro-patellar joint. *Acta Orthop Scand* 12:319, 1941.
19. Huberti HH, Hayes WC: Patellofemoral contact pressures. *J Bone Joint Surg* 66A:715, 1984.
20. Ziebelman MS, Colwell, CW, Irby SE, Walker RH: Dynamic in-vitro patellofemoral forces: Intact and after tibial tubercle osteotomy. *Trans Orthop Res Soc* 15 (2):500, 1990.
21. Bishop RED: On the mechanics of the human knee. *Engin Med* 6:46, 1977.
22. Denham RA, Bishop RED: Mechanics of the knee and problems in reconstructive surgery. *J Bone Joint Surg* 60B:345, 1978.
23. Berger RA, Elbaum LH, Hodge WA: Advantages in total body performance of unicompartimental knee replacement over total knee replacement. *Orthop Trans* 14:406, 1990.

24. Andriachi TP, Galante JO, Fermier RW: The influence of total knee-replacement design on walking and stair-climbing. *J Bone Joint Surg* 64A:1328, 1982.

25. Rielly DJ, Martens M: Experimental analysis of the quadriceps force and patellofemoral joint reaction force for various activities. *Acta Orthop Scand* 43:126, 1972.

26. Bandi W: Chondromalacia patellae und femor-patellare arthrose. *Helv Chir Acta* (suppl)1:3, 1972.

27. Seedhom BB, Terayama K: Knee forces during the activity of getting out of a chair with and without the aid of arms. *Biomed Engin*:278, August 1976.

28. Hungerford DS, Barry BS: Biomechanics of the patellofemoral joint. *Clin Orthop* 144:9, 1979.

29. Lewallen DG, Riegger CL, Myers ER, Hayes WC: Effects of retinacular release and tibial tubercle elevation in patellofemoral degenerative joint disease. *J Orthop Res* 8:856, 1990.

30. Ohno O, Naito J, Iguchi T, et al: An electron microscopic study of early pathology in chondromalacia. *J Bone Joint Surg* 70A:883, 1988.

31. Rhoads DD, Noble PC, Reuben JD, et al: The effect of femoral component position on patellar tracking after total knee arthroplasty. *Clin Orthop* 260:43, 1990.

32. Ferguson AB, Brown T, Fu F, Rutkowski R: Relief of patellofemoral contact stress by anterior displacement of the tibial tubercle. *J Bone Joint Surg* 61A:159, 1979.

33. Ferrandez L, Usabiaga J, Yubero J, et al: An experimental study of the redistribution of patellofemoral pressure by the anterior displacement of the anterior tuberosity of the tibia. *Clin Orthop* 238:183, 1989.

34. Hayes WC, Huberti HH, Lewallen DG, et al: Patellofemoral contact pressure and the effects of surgical reconstruction procedures, in *Articular Cartilage and Knee Joint Function: Basic Science and Arthroscopy*, edited by JW Ewing. New York, Raven Press, 1990.

35. Fulkerson JP, Hungerford DS: *Disorders of the Patellofemoral Joint*. 2d ed. Baltimore, Williams & Wilkins, 1990.

SECTION II
Clinical

CHAPTER 4

Extensor Mechanism Examination

Jack C. Hughston

EXAMINATION WITH THE PATIENT SITTING

When I have a new patient coming in for knee examination, I like to begin with the patient sitting on the examining table with his or her legs hanging loose off the side of the table. The patient should be wearing shorts or be draped so that at least the distal two-thirds of the thighs are exposed. This allows me an immediate glancing inspection of the lower limbs as I enter the room (Fig. 4-1). I may note comparative thigh atrophy, patella alta, or even a lesser prominence of the tibial tuberosity on one leg as opposed to the other, indicating a 1+ posterior instability.

After this initial brief glance, I sit down in a chair facing the patient and carry on a conversation to find out generally what's going on in the patient's world. I've always enjoyed people and their interests. I'm sure I do this as much for my pleasure as for their comfort. However, having a sincere interest in the patient is the fun of orthopaedics. The resultant relaxation and appreciation of the patient is phenomenal. Patients always remember that you sat down and took time with them, that you didn't just rush in and out.

Furthermore, sitting across from the patient allows the orthopaedist a good opportunity and vantage point from which to inspect the knees and lower limbs (Fig. 4-2). From this position, the patient's

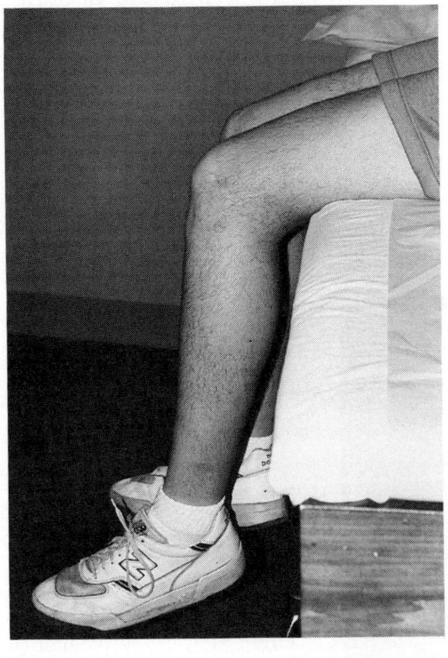

FIGURE 4-1
On entering the examining room, with the patient sitting on the examining table with his legs hanging loosely off the side, the physician can immediately see some aspects of the patellofemoral joint. In this case, there is obviously slight patella alta and the resultant mild prominence of the tibial tuberosity indicative of acute or chronic Osgood-Schlatter's disease in the left knee.

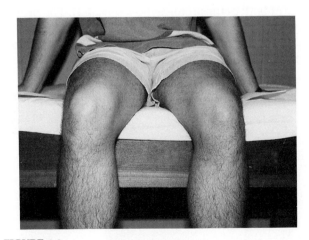

FIGURE 4-2
By sitting down in a chair across from the patient, with the patient sitting on the examining table, one can carry on a general conversation with the patient while at the same time observing the two lower limbs. As in this case, one may notice a comparative flattening of the patient's left thigh, as compared with the right, indicating some atonia. Also, there is less fullness of the vastus medialis obliquus on the left as compared with the right, and less definition of the adductor muscles on the left.

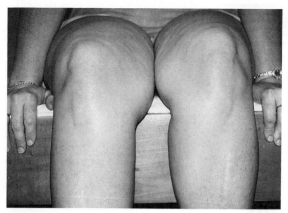

FIGURE 4-3
Even a mild amount of lateral posture of the patella may be noted with the patient sitting.

thigh contours are evident. In one thigh, the quadriceps region and the soft tissue areas outlining the abductors and adductors may be well rounded, with good definition between the muscles. In contrast, the quadriceps region of the involved thigh may appear comparatively flat, with the medial and lateral surfaces of the thigh appearing flabby and without the contour of healthy, underlying muscles. The vastus medialis obliquus (VMO) is also evaluated at this stage of examination for its bilateral fullness. The position of the patella is noted for a possible lateral posture. Even a mild amount of lateral facing of the patella can be appreciated (Fig. 4-3). The Q angle should appear to be about 0 degrees and can be measured at this time, if desired.

The normal concavities to either side of the patellar tendon can be noted, with even a minimal swelling of the knee joint evident on observing and feeling one or both of these concavities (Fig. 4-4). The prominence or lack thereof of the tibial tuberosity can be noted and, depending on the amount of protrusion, may indicate the presence or previous presence of

Osgood-Schlatter disease (Fig. 4-5). The pes anserinus is inspected, and if the region appears a bit prominent on one side as compared to the other, it can then be palpated for tenderness. Not infrequently, the pes bursa will be involved in an extensor mechanism problem. This is because the patient, on experiencing pain during contraction of the muscles of the extensor mechanism, unconsciously tends toward an excessive use of the medial hamstrings while walking.

From your seated position, have the patient extend and flex each knee separately and repeatedly so that you may evaluate the tracking of the patella, its rhythm, and the possibility of its demonstrating a jump or snap or perhaps a snapping of soft tissue medially or over the medial or lateral retinaculum. With the patient actively extending and flexing, palpate lightly over the patella to feel if the excursion in the patellofemoral joint is smooth or to recognize any grating that may be present. Palpate the femoral condyles, especially medially, for any abnormal prominence indicative of arthritic overgrowth of the medial femoral condyle in the patellofemoral region.

Stand up, and again note the contours of the quadriceps, the adductors, and the vastus lateralis for possible atrophy. Grasp a handful of one thigh at about the midthird region and then grasp a handful from the contralateral side. The relaxed quadriceps resulting from the patient's seated position make it easy to appreciate considerable atonia or atrophy when performing this test. So, I prefer to perform this part of the examination while the patient is sitting with knees and hips flexed, rather than having them in a supine position.

Once you have evaluated muscle tone, stand to one side or the other of the patient and inspect the patella posture laterally for patella alta or possible patella baja (Fig. 4-6); also check for associated mild concavity of the quadriceps tendon region immedi-

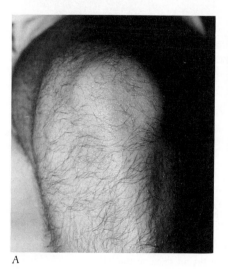

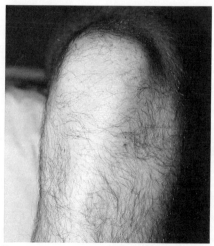

A   *B*

FIGURE 4-4
The normal dimples or concavities to either side of the patellar tendon may be noted with the patient in the sitting position. In the case of a minimal swelling within the knee joint, these concavities on one knee may be absent as compared with the opposite normal knee. *A* shows a normal knee and *B* demonstrates minimal swelling.

64

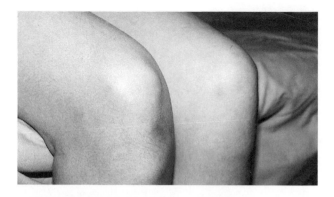

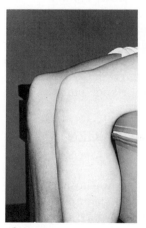

B

FIGURE 4-5
Observing the flexed knees with the patient sitting may easily demonstrate the presence of Osgood-Schlatter's disease in one knee as compared with the other, such as is present in this right knee (A). Or Osgood-Schlatter's may be present in both knees (B).

ately proximal to the patella. This concavity is another subtle sign of patella alta. If an accessory center of ossification of the patella is present, the superior and lateral prominence and abnormal shape of the patella are easily noted. Now, again judge the patellar

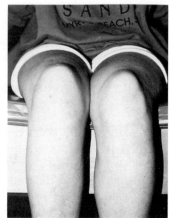

FIGURE 4-6
Patella alta is easily visualized by standing to the side of the patient and observing the patellae to see if they are sitting down on the end of the femur, or if they are sitting too high. In this moderate case of patella alta, we notice both in the side view (lateral view) and in the front view (anterior view) a concavity of the thigh immediately proximal to the patella. This concavity is a subtle sign of patella alta; however, it is sometimes not present with the milder degrees of patella alta.

rhythm by dorsal inspection while the patient flexes and extends the knee.

At this point, measure the Q angle by having the patient first hold one lower limb, and then the other, in 30 degrees to 40 degrees extension against gravity (Fig. 4-7A–C). Previous operative experience has shown that in patients who had a prior dislocated patella and osteochondral fracture of the lateral femoral condyle, the disrupted surface of the patella and the osteochondral fracture site always fit together at some point between 30 degrees and 45 degrees flexion. This is the reason the Q angle is measured with the quadriceps under tension and the knee flexed approximately 30 degrees to 40 degrees. This position recreates the functional angle of patellar tendon alignment at the time of subluxation or dislocation.

Next, with the patient again holding the leg extended 30 degrees to 40 degrees against gravity, evaluate the VMO (Fig. 4-8). When dysplastic, there will be a concavity proximal and medial to the patella. In a patient blessed with a little extra adipose tissue in the distal thighs, the concavity will not be as obvious; palpation of the area will disclose the lack of muscle mass. Often this sign is not reliable in the 10- to 14-year-old patient. A patient noted with concavity at this age often demonstrates a good fullness of the VMO at 18 years of age. Why? I don't know. Does the VMO develop late in growth, or does growth keep the muscles stretched out so that the VMO doesn't develop mass? True atrophy of the thigh muscles, for whatever reason, causes loss of mass of the VMO and

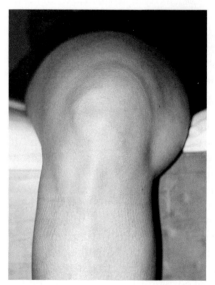

FIGURE 4-7A
With the patient sitting, the legs hanging loosely off the side of the table, the alignment of the patellar tendon should be 0 degrees. It should not deviate, either medially or laterally. In this case, the mild lateral deviation of the patellar tendon is evident, indicating that we will find a measurable increase of the Q angle in partial extension and in full extension.

65

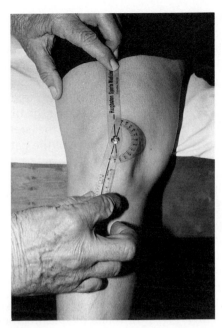

FIGURE 4-7B
Probably the most meaningful measurement of the Q angle is with the patient sitting and holding the leg extended with the knee at about 30 degrees to 40 degrees. I say meaningful because this approach is the functional position of the knee in the process of cutting, twisting, and pivoting. The goniometer is aligned with its central point over the center of the patella, its distal arm centered over the patellar tendon, and its proximal arm centered over the quadriceps tendon pointing toward the superior iliac spine. The proper placement of the goniometer over the patellar tendon is facilitated by grasping the patellar tendon with the forefinger and thumb and having the distal arm of the goniometer fit between these two fingers.

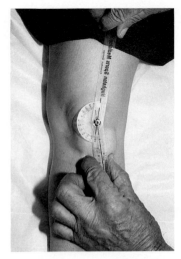

FIGURE 4-7C
The Q angle is also measured with the knee in full extension and the quadriceps contracted. Some investigators consider that the quadriceps should be relaxed when measuring the Q angle in extension, because contraction of the quadriceps causes some slight lateral deviation of the patella because in this position the patella is resting proximal to the confines of the patellofemoral sulcus. However, contraction of the quadriceps represents the functional Q angle, whether the knee is in full extension or in 30 degrees to 40 degrees flexion.

Over the years, in the process of performing extensor mechanism reconstructions, we have routinely measured the Q angle with the knee joint open and with simulating quadriceps contraction by pulling proximally on the quadriceps tendon with a towel clip. The comparisons between the preoperative clinical measurements and the operative measurements have demonstrated that the clinical technique of measuring the Q angle is rarely the same as the operative measurement.

a relative concavity. However, in this situation, the VMO on the opposite thigh should be normal.

Although a dysplastic VMO does not produce patellar subluxation, it is almost always associated. Anyway, beware of diagnosing patellar subluxation in the presence of a normal, or especially a prominent, VMO.

The hip flexor strength is tested at this time by having the patient lean slightly forward on the table, using the table edge as a brace, and then lift one thigh and try to hold it against your attempts to force the thigh back down to the table top (Fig. 4-9). Test the strength on both sides. A comparative weakness is almost always noted, and even a bilateral weakness can be appreciated once this test has become an accustomed part of the knee examination.

With the patient still in the sitting position, extend the knees passively to grasp the foot and examine for heel cord tightness (Fig. 4-10). You may notice, additionally, a little hamstring tightness if the patient leans a little backward during the extension. It still amazes me to see heel cord tightness prove to be the only explanation for anterior knee pain (extensor mechanism malfunction). Tight heel cords may make

the patient walk with a slightly flexed knee, thereby putting more stress on the extensor mechanism about the knee and producing anterior knee pain. Or, the patient may walk with slight recurvatum to compensate for the heel cord tightness, or with a mild slew foot or pronation, thus causing passive stress along the anteromedial retinacular region of the knee. The patient with tight heel cords who walks with a bouncing gait rarely develops anterior knee pain.

EXAMINATION WITH THE PATIENT LYING DOWN

At this point, have the patient assume a supine position. Begin your examination by inspecting the alignment of the lower limbs with the patellae pointing straight up (vertical; Fig. 4-11). You may note tibia vara, or internal tibial torsion. This is known as the "bayonet sign" (Fig. 4-12), wherein the patellar tendon appears to deviate laterally to a considerable degree. Ask the patient to contract the quadriceps and measure the Q angle with the knee in extension (see Fig. 4-7C). The small pocket goniometer is conve-

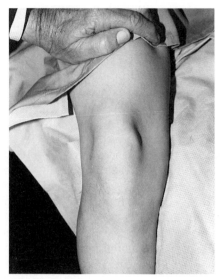

FIGURE 4-8
With the patient's leg resting off the side of the table at 30 degrees to 40 degrees knee flexion and the quadriceps contracted, a dysplasia of the VMO will be noted by an excess concavity medial to the proximal third of the patella. I consider VMO dysplasia to be the most significant factor in the possible presence of lateral patellar subluxation. Again, in the process of performing extensor mechanism reconstructions, it is important to observe the thickness or thinness of the VMO. The dysplasia is a true pathology with most cases demonstrating a real comparative deficit of muscle fiber thickness as compared with that seen in the normal knee in the process of doing other types of knee operations.

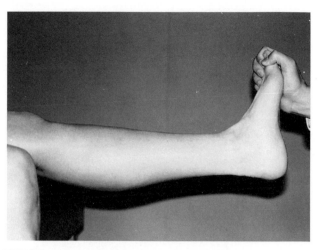

FIGURE 4-10
Heel cord tightness must be a routine evaluation in examination of the lower limb, particularly in patellofemoral disorders. Different examiners become accustomed to evaluating heel cord tightness in various manners. The important thing is that the examiner be consistent from one patient to another so that he or she develops a baseline of normal evaluation. I like to examine the heel cord tightness from a sitting position with the patient's knee extended and then test the active and passive dorsiflexion of the foot at the ankle and measure and record it. This position puts the gastrocnemius portion under tension. Then, with the knee and hip flexed, the heel cord tightness can be evaluated wherein the gastrocnemius portion is relaxed.

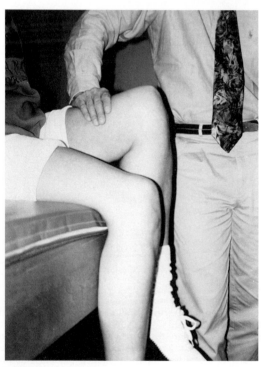

FIGURE 4-9
Hip flexor strength is tested by having the patient sit erect on the examining table, not leaning backward, and lift one thigh, and then the other with the examiner attempting to push the thigh back to the table top. If there is any pathologic involvement in the lower extremity, the presence of a comparative hip flexor weakness is usual. Thus, improvement of the strength of the hip flexors is necessary in the rehabilitation of the patellofemoral joint.

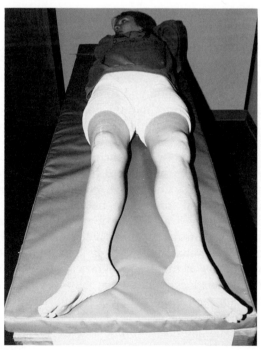

FIGURE 4-11
The alignment of the lower limbs is extremely important. Alignment should be evaluated with the patient standing as well as supine. Have the legs positioned so that the patellae point straight up and then note the alignment of the patellae. With internal femoral torsion, or external tibial torsion, or usually a combination of the two, the feet will point outward when the patellae are pointing straight forward. When the feet are pointing straight forward, the patellae will point in toward one another. In this photograph, the patient's right ankle and foot are turned outward while the patella points straight forward.

67

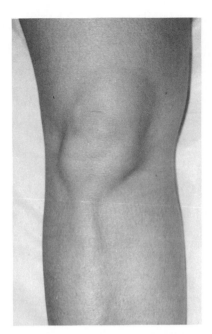

FIGURE 4-12
With the patient supine and the knee in extension, one may note a so-called bayonet sign, wherein there is a mild degree of tibia vara and possibly an excess degree of external tibial torsion. This sign has been often equated with the probability of a painful patellofemoral joint, even patellar subluxation, because of the increased Q angle. However, observation of very agile athletes with no patellofemoral pain will sometimes demonstrate this bayonet phenomenon.

nient for these measurements. The center of the goniometer should rest over the patella. The distal arm is placed over the surface of, and in line with, the patellar tendon. The thumb and forefinger should grasp the patellar tendon to hold the goniometer in place. The proximal arm of the goniometer is aligned with the quadriceps tendon, pointing toward the anterior superior iliac spine. In measuring the Q angle with the patient's leg extended and the quadriceps contracted, we are all accustomed to accepting 10 degrees valgus as normal for a male patient and approximately 13 degrees as normal for a female patient. These clinical measurements have proved to be very accurate in comparison with our routine operative measurements of the same angle with the extensor mechanism exposed and a towel clip in the quadriceps tendon, pulling proximally to simulate quadriceps contraction.

With the patellae pointing straight up, you may note that the tibiae and the feet are externally rotated. This is particularly noticeable with associated internal femoral torsion. Also, in cases of patella alta, the fat pad appears as a double hump. Some years ago, we labeled this the "camel sign."

Next, examine each hip by rotating the tibia internally and externally with the hip in extension. Oddly, a hip may sometimes have limited rotation in extension but have no similar limitation in 90 degrees

flexion. Since we walk with the hip in relative extension, a rotation limitation may strain the extensor mechanism at the knee joint. Each hip is then flexed and its rhythm of flexion noted, as well as its range. We are all familiar with the slipped capital femoral epiphysis producing an external rotation of the lower limbs as the hip is flexed toward 90 degrees. This may be the major sign of an early slipping. Certainly we are well aware of hip disorders producing referred pain along the obturator nerve to the anterior region of the knee. With the hips flexed to 90 degrees, each hip is rotated internally and externally and then abducted. These ranges of motion are noted in each hip and compared for equivalency.

With the patient's hip flexed 70 degrees to 90 degrees, flex the knee acutely, noting if this produces pain, either anterior or posterior, or neither. Then flex and extend the patient's knee, rotating the tibia internally and adducting the femur. While flexing and extending the knee, place a mild medial pressure on the patella with the butt of your hand. As the knee nearly reaches extension, the patient may complain bitterly and you may feel the patella subluxating medially as a result of a prior lateral release (Fig. 4-13).

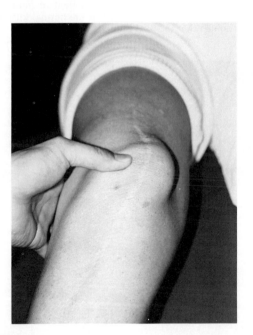

FIGURE 4-13
Medial patellar subluxation is evaluated by flexing and extending the patient's knee and exerting mild medial pressure and compression over the lateral side of the patella. If the medial patellar subluxation is secondary to prior lateral release, the patient will usually exhibit and express considerable discomfort with this maneuver. (This patient had a painful medial patellar subluxation after arthroscopic lateral retinacular release. I saw this patient after a subsequent attempt at correction by an extensor mechanism reconstruction. The patella was still subluxating medially with pain and disability. The lateral patellotibial ligament was apparently not reconstructed at the time of the extensor mechanism reconstruction. In cases of congenital patellar subluxation of the loose retinacular type, a patella may subluxate medially; however, it is rarely painful, as in the iatrogenic case.

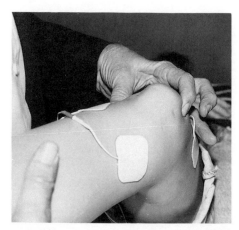

FIGURE 4-14
While flexing and extending the knee, palpate along the medial border of the patella to see if you may feel a snapping of the suprapatellar plica between the patella and the medial femoral condyle. This is often painful, as it proved to be in this patient who had had a prior lateral retinacular release.

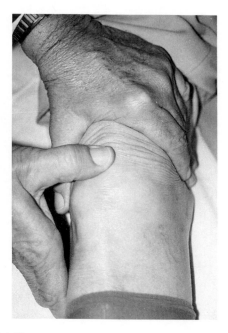

FIGURE 4-15
To check for effusion within the knee joint, one hand compresses the suprapatellar pouch to cause the fluid in the knee joint to gather in the region of the patella and then the patella is palpated (balloted) with the other hand to see if it bounces against the femoral condyles. Though inspection often distinguishes between a swollen suprapatellar bursa and swelling within the knee joint (effusion), ballottement of the patella is sometimes necessary for distinguishing between the two conditions.

In this case, a defect is usually palpable in the region of the lateral patellotibial ligament.

While flexing and extending the knee with mild medial pressure on the patella, you may also feel a snapping or jumping. This may or may not be audible and can sometimes cause considerable pain and arouse apprehension or other reactions from the patient (Fig. 4-14). The snapping could be a catching of the plica between the patella and the medial femoral condyle. An inflamed and fibrotic plica will be painful. When patients have complained of the patella slipping or jumping out of place and immediately jumping back into place, they often relate that the sensation created by this test is what they have been feeling.

Using the same passive motion of flexion and extension, continue by lightly pressing the patella onto the femur to evaluate the smoothness or roughness in the congruity of the patellofemoral joint. Although this is evaluated during examination of the patient in the sitting position, with active flexion and extension, it is important to check to see if the result is the same under passive flexion and extension. Next, palpate the medial and lateral edges of the patellofemoral joint and the synovium around these edges during the process of flexion to extension. The medial area is often tender in the case of an irritated plica.

With the lower limbs resting in an extended position on the examining table, note any swelling in the suprapatellar pouch, and compress the pouch to "float" the patella, which can be balloted if there is excess fluid in the knee joint (Fig. 4-15). Of course, swelling in this area would have been noted earlier, first during examination of the patient in the sitting position and second with the patient supine, when

attempts to acutely flex the knee would have proved limited and uncomfortable over the anterior knee area.

Now, with the knee still extended on the table, press the proximal pole of the patella and palpate the distal pole for tenderness indicative of patellar tendinitis (Fig. 4-16). Then press the distal pole and palpate the quadriceps tendon insertion to evaluate tenderness of the quadriceps. Palpate the fat pad to either side of the patellar tendon, primarily to elicit any tenderness and excessive firmness (fibrosis), but also to see if it is overly thick.

Compress the patella to the femoral condyle and rock the patella proximally and distally, then laterally and medially. Any one of these movements may produce discomfort if a fold of synovium is trapped between the patella and the femur. However, roughness of the patellar surface (chondromalacia) or a roughness or defect of the intercondylar sulcus can rarely be correctly evaluated by these tests.

Palpation of the edge of the patella may elicit acute tenderness secondary to synovial irritation along the edges of the patella. Palpation of the suprapatellar pouch may reveal masses or a fibrotic cord-like mass superior to the patella, representing a thickened and fibrotic suprapatellar plica. Sometimes this mass is more prominent laterally and superiorly in

69

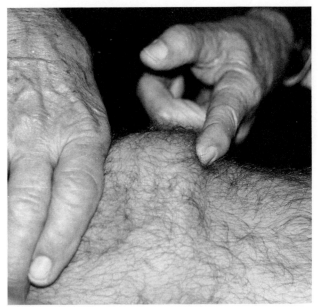

FIGURE 4-16
Patellar tendon tendinitis is most easily determined by compressing the suprapatellar pouch region and forcing the proximal pole of the patella against the femur, thereby elevating the distal pole, and then palpating the distal pole of the patella with the finger of the other hand. This will disclose comparative tenderness in this region if there is even a mild degree of patellar tendon tendinitis.

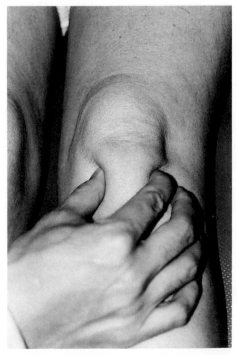

FIGURE 4-17
This represents palpation to either side of the patellar tendon to determine the consistency of the infrapatellar fat pad and to determine whether or not there is discomfort on firm palpation of the fat pad. A fibrotic fat pad is a frequent cause of patellofemoral pain.

the pouch. It may be quite tender. Patients may relate to you that this is the exact location and type of pain they have been having, whereas before, they could not localize it for you.

At this point, palpate to either side of the patellar tendon, feeling the fat pad and its consistency with the knee extended (Fig. 4-17). A fibrotic fat pad can produce considerable patellofemoral discomfort. Such fibrosis is usually the result of prior arthroscopic intervention in the knee; however, this is not necessarily true. Fibrosis can occur as a result of trauma.

Once again, with the patient supine, inspect the contours of the thighs, carefully observing the adductors, abductors, and quadriceps for roundness or flatness. Grasp a handful of the quadriceps at about midthigh and compare one side with the other for tone (Fig. 4-18).

Carefully measure the circumference of the thigh at a point 7 inches (17 cm) above the lateral tibial plateau. This landmark gives us a constant point of departure. Mark the site where the circumference is to be measured on each thigh. Have the patient keep the muscles relaxed, not contracted (Fig. 4-19).

It has been my experience that one thigh may appear to be 1 inch or 1.5 inches atrophic, whereas actual measurements prove the thighs to be of equal circumference. I consider this to be a characteristic point of differential diagnosis for disorders of the extensor mechanism in which there is considerable

loss of tone and no atrophy, as compared with disorders of the tibiofemoral joint, in which there is usually measurable atrophy. I cannot explain this phenomenon; it just constitutes a consistent finding.

Tight hamstrings are such a frequent singular finding in our experience with patellofemoral pain

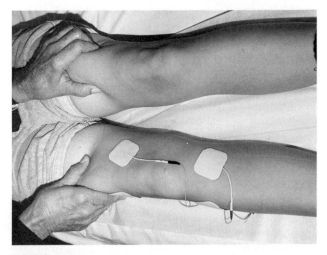

FIGURE 4-18
It is important to check the tone of the thigh muscles by grasping a "handful" of the tissue. It is rather easy to determine the increased muscle tone of the uninvolved lower limb as compared to the involved one. The tone may be considerably decreased and yet when you subsequently measure the circumference of the thighs you may find them equal.

70

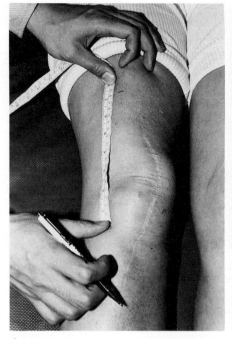

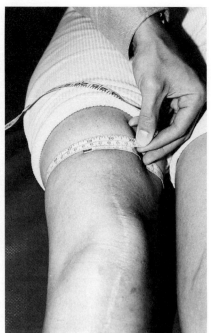

FIGURE 4-19
A. The circumference of the thighs is measured at a point 7 inches (17 cm) proximal to the prominence of the lateral tibial plateau. This landmark is used because it is not variable, whereas the measurement from the proximal pole of the patella can vary. *B.* The circumference is then measured on each lower limb at the determined point and compared to help determine the presence or absence of atrophy rather than merely atonia.

A

B

that we have a special diagnostic category termed the "hamstrung knee." While extending the patient's flexed knee with the hip flexed 90 degrees, we test and record, with a goniometer reading, the degree of hamstring tightness (Fig. 4-20). When hamstring tightness is the only possible etiology that we can find for patellofemoral pain, the two knees are usually equally uncomfortable. However, the patellofemoral pain can be unilateral in some cases where the hamstrings are equally tight bilaterally. We place these patients on hamstring stretching exercises and maintain a close follow-up as to their subsequent relief of pain and loss of disability. If the patient is not relieved, then we reevaluate at intervals until we can come up with another explanation of the patellofemoral pain. It is amazing how often tight hamstrings are the singular cause of disabling patellofemoral pain, especially in well-conditioned athletes participating in karate, competitive tennis, and similar activities.

Next, roll the patient over on his or her side. Have the patient abduct the lower limb into the air against gravity and hold it there while you exert pressure at the level of the knee in an attempt to force the lower limb down toward the examining table. Test the opposite side in a similar manner. Do not pass over the importance of hip abductor strength in the function of the extensor mechanism (Fig. 4-21).

Rehabilitation of weak hip abductors has relieved pain and disability of the knee in many of my patients, including recreational athletes, joggers, marathon runners, and a few professional athletes, thus allowing them to resume their desired activities. Generally, these patients have not been impressed

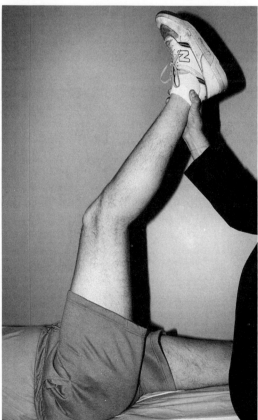

FIGURE 4-20
Tight hamstrings are a frequent singular cause of disabling patellofemoral pain, especially in the well-conditioned athlete. We evaluate tightness of the hamstrings by flexing the hip to 90 degrees and then bringing the knee into as great a degree of nonforceful extension as possible. When tight hamstrings are the singular cause of patellofemoral pain, the pain is relieved by diligent hamstring stretching exercises over a period of 1 to 2 months.

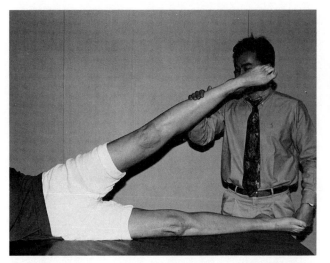

FIGURE 4-21
The strength of the hip abductors is evaluated by having the patient lie on one side and then the other while attempting to hold the lower limb elevated in abduction and holding against the resistance of the examiner. Weak hip abductors are a frequent component of patellofemoral disease and may sometimes be the sole etiology of the patellofemoral pain. Weak hip abductors certainly need to be rehabilitated in cases of patellofemoral disorder.

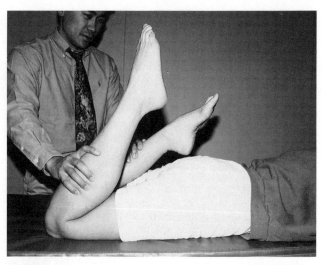

FIGURE 4-22
With the patient prone, comparison of quadriceps tightness secondary to pathologic contracture or physiologic overdevelopment can be determined by flexing both knees to their maximum. Also, such limitation of motion can be the result of effusion in the knee joint or the result of a painful patellofemoral joint with the patient not allowing you to flex the involved knee to as great an extent as the uninvolved.

with this treatment. Their transportation for the initial visit and then follow-up often costs them a great deal more than the clinical evaluation and our recommendations or rehabilitation. They remain curious as to my interest and why I give them a follow-up call 3, 6, or 12 months later, when operation was not even necessary. So, finding hip abductor weakness as the sole cause of the extensor mechanism pain and malfunction may not make you a hero. Some people are not going to appreciate your talents unless you cut their skin. However, you may save yourself and the patient a considerable amount of misery from having operated and gotten an unsatisfactory result.

For the next part of the examination, have the patient roll onto the abdomen. Note the gluteus maximus development and tone. Sometimes you will see apparent atrophy or atonia evidenced by the lack of protrusion of one buttock as compared to the other. Also test the hip extension at this time. Even in the presence of atonia of one buttock as compared to the other, the hip extensor strength is often equivalent and cannot be broken by the examiner.

While the patient is still on the abdomen, flex the knees to a maximum to examine for quadriceps tightness (Fig. 4-22). If this were a routine with trainers, particularly in the gymnastics divisions, the cause of a considerable number of cases of anterior knee pain could be recognized and corrected. It might even eliminate some of the quadriceps tendon ruptures.

Now return the patient to the supine position for the last part of the examination on the table. I examine

for patellar subluxation last to avoid jumping to conclusions and thereby not being thorough in the rest of the examination (Fig. 4-23). The technique of evaluating patellar subluxation is important.

First, seat yourself on the examining table, abducting the patient's lower limb. In the case of the right lower extremity, place the patient's distal right thigh over your right thigh. Then on the dorsum of the distal end of your left thigh, which is mobile, rest the calf or proximal ankle region. This resting of the patient's right ankle on your left thigh is extremely important, because it is the only way you can ensure that the extensor mechanism is relaxed when you are checking patellar mobility. You will notice that as you drop your left thigh, discontinuing support of the patient's right leg, the patient not infrequently continues to hold the leg in extension, with contraction of the quadriceps muscle. With your right thigh resting under the patient's, you can note, or sense, any cocontraction of the hamstrings. If cocontraction occurs, advise the patient to relax the muscles in the right thigh and allow the right ankle to rest on your left knee.

Once you have gained this point of relaxation, then you may evaluate passive patellar mobility at 30 degrees to 45 degrees. Place your hands in such a fashion that the fingers of both hands are to the outer (lateral) aspect of the distal thigh and upper tibia and your thumbs are resting on the medial aspect of the patella. With gentle, repetitious pressure in the lateral direction, you can ascertain the mobility or hypermobility of the patella with a fair degree of cer-

72

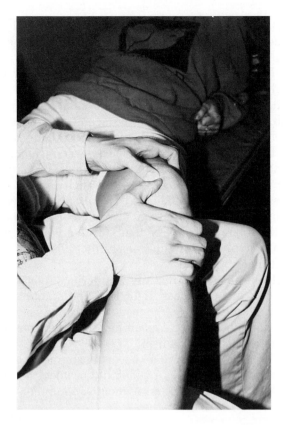

FIGURE 4-23
Examine for possible lateral patellar subluxation by sitting on the examining table, placing the patient's thigh over your thigh, and having the patient's leg rest on your opposite thigh with the knee flexed approximately 30 degrees to 40 degrees. Then, grasping above and below the knee, apply repetitious lateral pressure to the medial side of the patella. In the case of patellar subluxation, the patella will have an abnormal lateral excursion and may almost dislocate. Or this may elicit a snapping sensation, which the patient states is the pain being experienced. If so, and if there is no increased lateral motion of the patella, you may become suspicious of a plica being the cause of the patient's complaint of the patella slipping out of place.

tainty. If there is a so-called apprehension sign (a tightening of the muscles), it is easy to quiet the patient by advising that you are not going to cause any undue pain. Once again, evaluate lateral hypermobility of the patella, at the functional position of 30 degrees to 45 degrees knee flexion. You and the patient may feel some snapping under the medial aspect of the patella. The patient may have some related discomfort or pain. In such a case, you may not be able to demonstrate simultaneous patellar hypermobility. The wisest course is to consider this apprehension and snapping to be caused by a plica, rather than a subluxating patella.

The opposite lower extremity is examined in a similar manner.

If the patient has true lateral patellar subluxation, you will most often be able to note it objectively in the process of this examination. If no passive hypermobility is found during this part of the examina-

tion, I would rule out patellar subluxation in the patient until subsequent evaluation proves otherwise. Furthermore, attempts should be made to correlate a negative finding in this lateral subluxation examination with the possible finding of crepitation, pain, apprehension, snapping, and so forth discovered in the previous examination for medial patellar mobility and medial plica irritation.

I have not discussed a few clinical signs. One is lateral compression syndrome. I have not seen this. I may be blind; however, I have looked for it diligently. I cannot recognize it clinically or radiographically. In view of the considerable comparative absence of chondromalacia of the lateral patellar facet, I cannot agree that compression produces deterioration with resultant pain.

EXAMINATION WITH THE PATIENT STANDING

The examination is not complete yet. Ask the patient to stand and make sure that the patellae point straight ahead. Note the direction of the feet; they too may point straight ahead. On the other hand, even with the patellae pointing straight ahead, the feet may point into slew footedness (external rotation posture). If so, have the patient stand with the feet touching and parallel and pointing straight ahead. Note the posture of the patellae. Are they pointing toward one another acutely, looking one another in the eye, so to speak (Fig. 4-24)? If so, what is the cause? Is there a severe internal femoral torsion? Or, is there severe external tibial torsion? Is there a combination of the two? Or, perhaps there is an internal rotation contracture of the hips secondary to an habitual sitting posture.

Now have the patient walk down the hall outside the examining rooms. Evaluate the gait. Is the patient extending the knees, hyperextending the knees, or walking with the knees in a bit of flexion? Is there any evidence in the gait of abductor weakness of the hip (a dropping of the pelvis on the unaffected side)? Is there an adduction of the thigh toward the midline, and an internal rotation of the thigh to place the weight-bearing foot on the involved side under the center of the pelvis? Recognition of this alone may solve the disability of the lower limb as regards extensor mechanism function. Unfortunately, an abnormality of gait, whatever its cause, is sometimes recognized only after the patient has been through four or five operations on the extensor mechanism.

Thus, problems relative to the extensor mechanism may test your patience. They may necessitate repeated evaluations. The problems may be resolved only after a year of intermittent and repeated evalua-

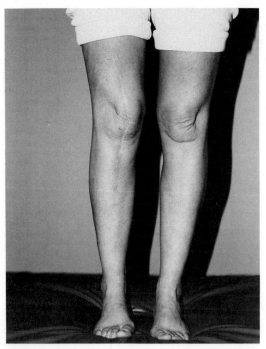

FIGURE 4-24
With the patient standing with both feet pointing straight ahead, note the posture of the patellae. Are they pointing toward one another as in this picture? If so, this represents internal femoral torsion or external tibial torsion or a combination of the two; the resultant gait in this patient may be the sole cause of the patellofemoral pain. This is because of the abnormal stresses placed on the patella in the process of walking.

tions and rehabilitation of the patient. If operations are considered, each operation then adds another element of complexity.

If you cannot arrive at an etiology that you are comfortable with on your initial evaluation, do not hesitate to have the patient come back for further evaluation after a few more weeks, and after a period of rehabilitative exercises. If such a program does not suit these patients, if they have come a considerable distance and are unwilling to make the trip again, if they have even the slightest bit of such concern for your sincerity and dedicated interest to their well being and, thus, desire to go elsewhere, be gracious, bid them farewell, and be thankful that you did not end up involved with them at a further postoperative point down the road.

I can only hope that my wanderings relative to abductor hip weakness, tight heel cords, and such create a resolve within the readers to be dedicated in their complete physical examination and evaluation of the extensor mechanism.

Good luck! Perform a knee extensor mechanism examination according to a definite protocol, with a checklist, and you will rarely be disappointed.

CHAPTER 5

Imaging of the Patellofemoral Joint: Emphasis on Advanced Techniques

Andrew L. Deutsch
Frank G. Shellock
Jerrold H. Mink

INTRODUCTION

The past decade has seen significant interest in the application of advanced imaging techniques such as magnetic resonance imaging (MR) and computed tomography (CT) toward evaluation of the knee and patellofemoral joint. Because of their direct multiplanar imaging capabilities, these new diagnostic methods have provided insights regarding both normal and aberrant patellofemoral alignment and tracking that in many instances have challenged long-standing conceptions. Rapidly developing technical advances including ultrafast imaging have brought us to the precipice of true dynamic joint imaging with the potential of a wealth of even greater information. Much of this new data and their implications have yet to be assimilated by the orthopaedic community. This chapter reviews patellofemoral joint imaging, with particular emphasis on the recent developments in advanced imaging methods and their potential implications for patient management.

CONVENTIONAL RADIOGRAPHY

The orthopaedic literature is replete with studies devoted to conventional radiographic analysis of the patellofemoral joint.[1–22] The majority of these are devoted to methods of tangentially imaging the joint to obtain an axial projection. From these images, a large number of indices have been generated to distinguish normal from abnormal patellofemoral alignment. With the advent of direct axial imaging accomplished using CT or MR, certain limitations of these conventional techniques have become increasingly apparent.[23–30] Additionally, confusion and imprecision regarding definitions of terms, such as malalignment, subluxation, instability, and chondromalacia, have significantly complicated critical analysis of the clinical utility of these various methods.[9,13] These conventional methods have been the subject of several recent excellent reviews.[9,11,22] In this chapter, salient aspects of these conventional methods are discussed

to provide the background for further consideration of the newer advanced imaging techniques.

Anteroposterior View

The anteroposterior (AP) projection, one of the standard radiographic views for evaluation of the knee,[19,31] is used primarily for assessment of the tibiofemoral articulation. For this purpose, it may be performed with the patient supine or erect (weight-bearing). The projection is most optimally obtained with a 5 degree caudal tube tilt to accommodate the posterior tilt of the tibial articular surface and best profile the joint space. With regard to the patellofemoral joint, the AP projection is of greatest value in assessing trauma and in demonstrating variants in development (e.g., multipartite patella). Beyond this function, the AP projection is of little aid in the assessment of the functional relationship of the patella and distal femur.[9] However, certain relationships that may influence patellofemoral dynamics, including knee varus/valgus, patella height, patellar and condylar measurements, can be obtained.[31]

Lateral Projection

The standard lateral view is accomplished with the patient in a lateral decubitus position and the knee flexed 20 to 30 degrees. The x-ray tube is perpendicular to the tibiofemoral articulation. The femoral condyles are superimposed but can usually be differentiated. The lateral condyle is characterized by a flatter contour and the condylopatellar sulcus separating the articular surface for the patella from that for the tibia is located in approximately the middle of its curve.[32] A similar groove is located on the medial aspect of the medial femoral condyle at the junction of its anterior and middle thirds, allowing its identification.[31,33]

The lateral projection has had a more prominent role in assessment of the patellofemoral joint; particularly for evaluation of the vertical position of the patella. Several investigators have proposed different indices for the assessment of patella alta. Blumensaat described a dense white line representing the surface of the intercondylar notch tangential to the x-ray beam.[34] Elevation of the distal pole of the patella above this line with the knee flexed 30 degrees was considered indicative of patella alta. There is common agreement today, however, that this measurement is not accurate.[1] In the method of Insall and Salvati, the length of the patellar tendon (LT) measured from the tibial tubercle to the lower pole is compared with the greatest diagonal length of the patella (LP)[5] (Fig. 5-1). Usually these measurements are equal. An LT:LP ratio of > 1.3:1 is considered abnormally high. The ratio has been used to define patella alta and its relationship to the presence of patellar malalignment, subluxation, or chondromalacia. The technique requires a lateral radiograph of the knee to be taken at 30 degrees flexion.

Blackburne and Peel modified this technique using the tibial articular surface as the reference level for patellar height and the length of the articular surface for patellar length.[3] The ratio of the patellar articular length to the distance between the tibial articular surface and caudad extent of the patellar articular surface should be 0.8 in normal knees at 30 degrees flexion. Labelle and Laurin have described a method requiring a lateral radiograph to be taken with the knee at 90 degrees flexion.[9] A line projected along the anterior aspect of the femoral shaft passes above the

superior pole of the patella in all but 3 percent of normal knees. Alta exists when this line passes through the patella. If, however, patella alta is considered to represent an abnormally high position of the patella in relation to the developed trochlear sulcus, all of these proposed indices fall short of this characterization compared with that depicted on direct axial CT or MR images. This introduces the concept of "functional" patella alta that will be further described in subsequent sections.

The lateral projection may also be used for assessing the depth of the proximal trochlear in patients being evaluated for patellar instability.[7] Trochlear depth is assessed by measuring the mean distance from the trochlear groove to the anterior borders of both femoral condyles measured perpendicular to the femoral surface. A trochlear depth of < 5 mm in the proximal portion of the groove (level of the physeal line) was found to greatly increase the risk for patellar instability.

Tangential (Axial) Patellar Views

Tangential or axial (e.g., "sunrise") views of the patella have been used extensively by clinicians for assessment of the patellofemoral joint, and these studies have been the hallmark for radiographic analysis of the patellofemoral joint. Multiple methods have been proposed by different investigators, and from these, innumerable indices have been developed in an attempt to define normal patellofemoral relationships and identify subtle derangements in alignment.[6,8] During the past decade, since the introduction of CT and now MR imaging, significant limitations in the information provided by these projections are becoming increasingly apparent.[23,25,27,28,35,36] Principal among these shortcomings is the inability of all the conventional techniques to image the patellofemoral joint at < 20 degrees (and more commonly at < 30 to 40 degrees) of knee flexion. Both CT and MR, unfettered by these constraints, have convincingly demonstrated alignment aberrations in the initial degrees of flexion that were no longer apparent on the conventional views obtained at greater degrees of knee flexion.[23,27,28,36] Additionally, as single static images of a dynamic articulation, the implications of the findings on conventional radiographs may potentially be misleading. In contrast, ultrafast imaging with both CT and MR is approaching virtual "real-time" imaging of the patellofemoral joint with the potential for evaluation of the true dynamic state of this articulation.[37]

In 1921, Settagast produced the first conventional axial images of the patellofemoral joint.[9,22] The

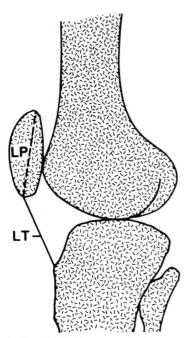

FIGURE 5-1
Patella alta. Method of Insall and Salvati. The ratio of patella tendon length (LT) to the greatest diagonal length of the patella (LP). The upper limit of normal is 1.2 at the 90 percent confidence level.

diagnostic value of these images, however, was significantly limited by marked distortion of patella shape and inadequate visualization of the proximal trochlear.[9] In 1924, Jaroschy described a different technique, later modified by Hughston. These images are also limited by distortion resulting from the x-ray beam striking the cassette at an approximate 45 degree angle.[9,11] In 1941, Wiberg and Knuston, working independently, described techniques that reversed the direction of the x-ray beam as compared to the prior methods with the cassette resting on the anterior tibia and the beam parallel to it.[10] In 1970, Ficat described a method for simultaneous imaging of both patellofemoral joints with the knees in 30, 60, and 90 degrees flexion.[20] The 30 degree position was advocated to detect subluxation that might be reduced on views obtained with increased flexion. The 60 degree projection purported to demonstrate the central contact area best.[9] The technique is performed with the patient seated on a chair or platform placed on the x-ray table with legs flexed to the desired degree and resting on a cushion. The x-ray beam is directed from the feet, angled at 10 degrees toward the tibia; the cassette is held by the patient on the thighs perpendicular to the beam. The knees and feet are held together to control rotation and the feet are plantar flexed. The technique is technically demanding and increased patient radiation exposure results from the direction of the x-ray beam.[31]

In 1974, Merchant and associates developed a technique that has become widely used in the United States.[8] The examination is performed with the patient supine and the knees flexed 45 degrees over the edge of the table. A fixed angle frame is available to ensure the angle of the knee flexion at 45 degrees. The legs are strapped to prevent rotation. The beam is directed toward the feet with a beam-to-femur angle of 30 degrees. The cassette is held on the shins in a specially constructed holder and the beam is incident upon the film at 90 degrees.

To evaluate patellofemoral relationships in earlier degrees of flexion, Laurin developed a technique creating an axial image with the knee flexed 20 degrees.[6] With this method the patient is supine, knees flexed 20 degrees, legs together, quadriceps relaxed, and beam perpendicular to the cassette. The Laurin view is technically demanding but valuable in detecting more subtle tracking abnormalities. Laurin showed that the patella is well into the trochlear sulcus in 97 percent of normal individuals by 20 degrees knee flexion; these data further emphasize the need for assessment of the initial degrees of flexion before a potentially malaligned patella is brought into more normal alignment as the patella is brought further into the deepening sulcus by increasing degrees of knee flexion. These concerns have been underscored by the findings observed with CT and MR.

Malghem and Maldague introduced the 30 degree axial radiograph with lateral rotation of the knee and described it as useful in the assessment of patellar subluxation.[38] Teitge has advocated the application of direct stress to supplement the tangential radiograph of the patellae analogous to stress examinations routinely performed of other articulations.[21] In the stress examination used by Teitge, the Merchant projection is utilized and ideally is perfomed at the angle of knee flexion at which the greatest instability or pain is detected on physical examination. Stress is applied with a rubber padded wooden pusher. Teitge demonstrated gross abnormal motion when comparing right/left stress views in patients with normal Merchant angles. Additionally, Teitge documented medial subluxation of the patella using the stress examination.[21]

PATELLA CONFIGURATION

The upper three-fourths of the posterior surface of the patella is covered by hyaline cartilage, which in the central portion is thicker (5 to 6 mm) than in any other articulation.[22,32] The articular surface, roughly oval in shape, is divided into medial and lateral facets by a vertical ridge oriented along the long axis of the patella. The medial facet demonstrates considerable anatomic variation. It is subdivided by a small vertical ridge (secondary ridge) into the medial facet proper and a smaller "odd" facet along its medial border. The medial facet is usually flat or convex with considerable variation related to the thickness of the articular cartilage.[22] The odd facet is concave or flat. The lateral facet is both longer and wider than the medial and is concave in both vertical and transverse planes.

In his classic paper, Wiberg proposed a three-part classification to encompass the majority of patellar facet configurations[10] (Fig. 5-2). The system was based on the configuration of the subchondral bone of the facets as depicted on a tangential conventional radiograph. In the type I configuration, both facets appear gently concave, symmetrical, and nearly equal in size. This is the least commonly encountered form. In type II the medial facet is smaller than the lateral. The lateral facet remains concave; the medial is flat or convex. This is the most common form, accounting for up to 65 percent of patellae.[39] The changes from type I to II represent a continuum and may be subtle. In the type III configuration, the medial

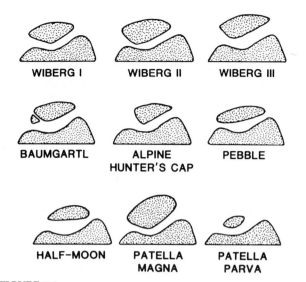

FIGURE 5-2
Schematic diagram demonstrates the more common variations in patella configuration. (Modified with permission from Fulkerson JP, Hungerford DS: *Disorders of the Patellofemoral Joint*, 2d ed. Baltimore, William & Wilkins, 1990.)

facet is distinctly smaller with marked lateral prominence. This configuration accounted for 25 percent of patellae in Hennsge's series.[39] Type III was considered dysplastic by Wiberg although he was unable to demonstrate a higher incidence of chondromalacia than with the other forms. This lack of association of type III with chondromalacia has also been noted by other investigators.[24] Studies using the tomographic capabilities of CT and MR have demonstrated a change in apparent patella configuration between proximal and distal sections, an observation further questioning the value of the classification system.[24] In addition, in contrast to radiography, MR affords direct depiction of the articular cartilage of the subchondral outline.

Ficat proposed an alternate classification system based on the angle subtended by the two major facets[20] (see Fig. 5-2). The so-called pebble-shaped patella is characterized by an angle > 140 degrees. An angle of 90 to 100 degrees most closely corresponds to the Wiberg type III. The Alpine hunter's cap deformity is characterized by a patella approaching a single articular facet with the angle 90 degrees. This hemipatella configuration with one articular facet is commonly observed with lateral instability and is associated with hypoplasia of the vastus medialis and decreased depth of the trochlear sulcus.[22] The half-moon patella is characterized by an acute angle with a single articular facet. It is associated with permanent subluxation/dislocation of the patella.

PATELLOFEMORAL INDICES

A large number of indices have been developed based on the various axial projections in an attempt to define normal and detect and quantify abnormal patellofemoral relationships. A compilation of the earlier morphologic indices is provided in the textbook of Fulkerson and Hungerford.[22] These measurements are based on tangential projections obtained at 60 degrees and are summarized in Fig. 5-3. Of these indices, the trochlear depth ratio and sulcus angle may have the greatest implications with respect to patellar instability.

The congruence angle of Merchant and the lateral patellofemoral angle, patellofemoral index, and lateral patellar displacement of Laurin have been among the measurements receiving the broadest general application.[6,8] The congruence angle was developed in an attempt to detect subtle patellar subluxation.[8] The congruence angle is determined by initially bisecting the sulcus angle to obtain a reference line. A second line is then drawn from the most posterior

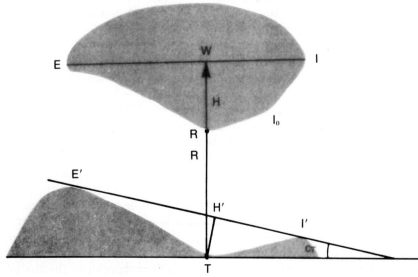

FIGURE 5-3
Normal patellofemoral indices.

I. Patella
    1. Facet ratio:
       Brattsom   1 $<RE / RI>$ 1.75
       Ficat-Bizou   1 $<RE / RI>$ 3.0

    2. Depth index   3.6 $<W / H>$ 4.2

    3. Facet angle   ERI $= 130 +/- 10$

II> Trochlea
    Depth index   E'I' / TH' $= 5.3 +/- 1.2$
    Sulcus angle   E'TI' $= 140 +/- 5$

Angle of inclination cт $= 4$ degree 95' $+/- 1$ degree 45' (Reprinted with permission from Fulkerson JP, Hungerford DS: *Disorders of the Patellofemoral Joint*, 2d ed. Baltimore, Williams & Wilkins, 1990.)

point of the patella to the apex of the sulcus angle. The angle between the reference line and the patellar line is the congruence angle (Fig. 5-4). Medial patellar deviation is considered negative and lateral deviation positive. In their original study, Merchant reported an average sulcus angle of 138 degrees, which correlated well, given differences in technique, with that of Brattstrom's angle of 142 degrees.[8] The congruence angle averaged −6 degrees in asymptomatic knees; +16 degrees was determined to be abnormal at the 95th percentile. Aglietti and coworkers, in repeating Merchant's work, determined the normal congruence angle to be −8 degrees but with a standard deviation of 6 degrees, nearly 50 percent smaller than that in the original series of Merchant.[40] In Merchant's series, control subjects without history of knee complaints were assumed to be normal and were not examined. In contrast, Aglietti examined all normal controls and excluded those with physical abnormalities as well as a history of knee problems. Merchant believes that this accounts for the difference between the two series and that it underscores the prevalence of asymptomatic patellofemoral dysplasia in the general population.[13,18] Merchant has indicated his belief that the values obtained by Aglietti are more accurate. Accordingly, subluxation with a congruence angle of > +4 to +6 should be considered abnormal at the 95th percentile.

Multiple studies have been performed to further investigate the clinical implication of the congruence angle. In the report of Moller, a total of 64 patients, 39 with unilateral chondromalacia and 25 with uni-

lateral recurrent subluxation, were studied by the method of Merchant.[9,12] The asymptomatic side was the control. The mean angle for the subluxation group was +6 with a wide range from −6 to +32, compared with a mean angle of −2 for the control group. Although the congruence values for the symptomatic group were often within normal limits according to the original Merchant criteria, they differed significantly from the patient's contralateral asymptomatic side. The investigators suggested that in the case of unilateral complaints, side-to-side comparison to normative values is necessary. In 1986, Dowd and Bentley studied 118 patients, 35 with arthroscopically confirmed chondromalacia, 33 with instability confirmed under anesthesia, and 50 normal volunteers.[2] They evaluated multiple indices including the congruence angle, sulcus angle, patellofemoral angle, and Insall-Salvati index. Only 20 percent of their instability patients demonstrated congruence angles beyond two standard deviations of normal (original Merchant criteria). In part these discordances may reflect the use of Merchant's original criteria rather than those of Aglietti and likely in part can be accounted for by differences in definition of instability or determination of its magnitude. These latter concerns underlie the difficulty in comparing the multiple published reports on assessment of patellofemoral disorders and in extracting clinically significant information from them.[9]

Laurin and colleagues described three patellofemoral indices[6] (Fig. 5-5). The *lateral patellofemoral angle* is defined by two lines, one drawn along the lateral patellar facet and the other joining the apices of the femoral condyles. The angle should normally be open laterally. In Laurin's series, 97 percent of controls demonstrated a lateral patellofemoral angle open laterally. Sixty percent of patients with patellar subluxation demonstrated parallel lines and 40 percent had an angle open medially. Fulkerson and Hungerford suggest that this measurement is more appropriate for assessment of patellar tilt rather than patellar subluxation and that other indices, such as the congruence angle, be used for this latter determination.[22]

The *patellofemoral index* is the ratio of the medial and lateral patellofemoral interspaces (see Fig. 5-5). The medial interspace is measured as the shortest distance between the lateral patellar facet and the lateral femoral condyle. The lateral interspace is the shortest distance between the lateral facet and lateral condyle. The upper limit of normal for this index is 1.6. According to the authors, an abnormal patellofemoral index relates to an abnormal tilt of the patella with widening of the medial interspace rather than

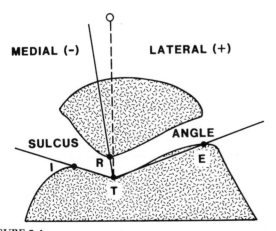

FIGURE 5-4
Congruence angle. The sulcus angle ETI is bisected by a neutral reference line TO. The apex of the medial patellar ridge is connected to the lowest point of the trochlear sulcus. When this line (RT) is medial to the neutral reference line, the angle is given a negative value; when lateral, a positive value. (Modified from Merchant AC, Mercer RL, Jacobsen RH, Cool CR: *J Bone Joint Surg* 56A:1391-1396, 1974.)

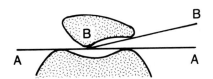
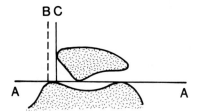
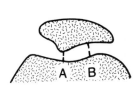

FIGURE 5-5
Patella relationships after Laurin. (*Top*) Lateral patellofemoral angle. Two lines, one connecting the apices of the femoral condyles (AA) and the other along the lateral facet of the patella (BB) are defined. The angle of intersection usually opens laterally; less commonly the lines are parallel. (*Bottom Left*) Lateral patellar displacement. A line is drawn connecting the highest points of the medial and lateral femoral condyles (AA). A perpendicular to that line at the medial edge of the medial femoral condyle (B) normally lies 1 mm or less medial to the patella (line C). (*Bottom Right*) Lateral patellofemoral index. This represents the ratio between the narrowest medial patellofemoral distance measured at the lateral edge of the medial facet (A) and the narrowest lateral patellofemoral distance (B). The ratio is normally one or less. (Modified from Laurin CA, Dussault R, Levesque HP: *Clin Orthop* 144:16-26, 1979.)

reduction of the lateral interspace.[6] An index of 1.6 was seen in 93 percent of patients with a diagnosis of chondromalacia. The criteria, however, used to establish the diagnosis of chondromalacia were not specifically defined, a fact which undermines the implied association.

Laurin undertook a study of *lateral patellar displacement* in an attempt to distinguish patients with chondromalacia and those with subluxation from normals. A line is drawn through the highest points of the medial and lateral femoral condyles (see Fig. 5-5). A perpendicular to that line, at the medial edge of the medial femoral condyle, normally lies 1 mm or less medial to the patella. One-third of patients with chondromalacia and approximately one-half of patients with subluxating patellae had lateralized patellae. As discussed by Minkoff and Fein in their review article, failure to define the diagnostic criteria for chondromalacia and subluxation preludes any conclusion about using the lateral patellar displacement for distinguishing between idiopathic chondromalacia and chondromalacia secondary to entities such as malalignment or instability.[9] Additionally, subluxation was not defined in this study with regard to its physical manifestations, and no distinction was made between subluxation in the sense of malposition and subluxation in conjunction with instability.[9]

COMPUTED TOMOGRAPHY

The introduction of CT to the evaluation of the patellofemoral joint by Delgado-Martins in 1979 allowed axial plane assessment of patellofemoral relationships in extension and in the initial degrees of flexion for the first time.[25] The findings obtained from this and subsequent studies have challenged many longstanding conceptions regarding normal patellofemoral dynamics and have paved the way for a more sophisticated approach to the determination of nor-

mal patellofemoral dynamics and assessment of patellofemoral disorders.

In the study of Delgado-Martins, 24 normal knees were examined by CT in the extended position and compared with axial radiographs obtained with the knee in 30, 60, and 90 degrees knee flexion.[25] While 96 percent of the patients demonstrated patellar centering at 90 degrees flexion, this number decreased to 29 percent at 30 degrees. On CT, obtained in extension, only 13 percent were centered with the quadriceps relaxed, and only one patient demonstrated a centered patella with quadriceps contracted. In extension, contact of the patella with the lateral condyle was observed with the crest of the patella alone or with the crest and lateral facet. The medial patella surface was rarely observed to be in contact with the medial femoral condyle.

Boven and colleagues subsequently reported data on 71 patients who underwent CT of their symptomatic patellofemoral joints following conventional double contrast knee arthrography.[35] Conventional axial radiographs were preliminarily obtained at 30, 60, and 90 degrees. CT was performed with the knee at 15 degrees flexion with six 5-mm CT sections obtained through the patella. Using the criteria of Ficat, 43 percent of the patellae were considered subluxated on CT compared with 34 percent on axial radiographs. Using Laurin's criteria, 40 percent of the patellae were considered tilted on CT compared with 17 percent on conventional tangential radiographs. This study further substantiated the ability of CT to detect malalignment not depicted with conventional methods. Additionally, the CT following contrast was significantly more sensitive to depiction of articular cartilage abnormalities than the conventional arthrogram.

Schutzer and colleagues used CT to evaluate patients with patellofemoral pain and described three basic tracking abnormalities.[27,41] Patients were positioned in the CT gantry in the lateral decubitus position using bolsters to reproduce the patients' normal standing alignment as closely as possible. Axial sections were obtained at the level of the midtransverse plane at 0, 15, 30, 45, and 60 degrees knee flexion. The images were analyzed based on the authors' modification of the technique of Merchant. The posterior femoral condyles provided a more reliable reference plane for the determination of patellar tilt as compared to that obtainable using the anterior femoral trochlear, the anatomy of which changes considerably as the patella moves through flexion.[22,27] The patellar tilt angle is defined by the angle obtained between a line drawn along the lateral patellar facet and posterior femoral condyle reference line (see Fig. 5-5). The angle should always be > 7 degrees on the image obtained at 20 degrees knee flexion.[22] The congruence angles are determined using the same image for which patellar tilt was determined (see Fig. 5-4). In a preliminary CT study, the congruence angle became 0 or negative by 10 degrees knee flexion in 10 asymptomatic volunteers. Fulkerson and Hungerford consider a patella to be congruent when it centers in the trochlea (as determined by CT) by 15 to 20 degrees flexion.[22]

Schutzer and colleagues described three malalignment patterns based on the patellar tilt and congruence angles obtained using CT[27] (Fig. 5-6). Type 1 represents a subluxated but nontilted patella. The

MALALIGNMENT PATTERNS

45 PATIENTS

Type 1 - Sublux without tilt

18 Patients, 21 Knees

Type 2 - Sublux with tilt

14 Patients, 19 Knees

Type 3 - Tilt without sublux

19 Patients, 25 Knees

FIGURE 5-6
Malalignment patterns determined by CT in 45 patients. Using this classification, tilt may occur with or without patellar subluxation. From Schutzer SF, Ramsby GR, Fulkerson JP: *Orthop Clin North Am.* 17:235–248, 1986. (Reprinted with permission from Fulkerson JP, Hungerford DS: *Disorders of the Paellofemoral Joint,* 2d ed. Baltimore, Williams & Wilkins, 1990.)

trochlear depth was shallower than that seen in controls but deeper than that observed in patients with type 2 pattern. The type 2 pattern is characterized by subluxation associated with a tilted patella. The trochlear depth was significantly more shallow, representing apparent trochlear dysplasia. The third group (type 3) was characterized by isolated patellar tilting unassociated with subluxation. Patients in this group demonstrated patellar tilt angles within the low-normal range in extension that progressively decreased with further flexion to 30 degrees. The essential difference between the type 1 and 2 categories is the dysplastic trochlear anatomy characteristic of type 2.[22] Of particular note is the observation that nearly 40 percent of the patients with a type 1 or type 2 malalignment pattern were completely reduced at a knee flexion angle of 30 degrees. This finding further underscores the limitations of conventional axial radiographs (rarely technically obtainable at < 30 degrees flexion) in assessing patellofemoral alignment. The type 3 pattern correlated with the findings expected in the excessive lateral pressure syndrome initially described by Ficat.[22]

This entity is characterized clinically by anterior knee and peripatellar pain and radiographically by patellar tilting. It is speculated this entity arises in the presence of a tight lateral retinaculum. Marginal patellar osteophytes, presumably reflective of excessive traction from the tight lateral retinaculum were observed in 35 percent of type 3 patients but in no type 1 (e.g., subluxation without tilt) or normal controls. In patients with this malalignment pattern, the lateral patellar facet is forced into the femoral trochlear causing excessive lateral loads that are potentially damaging to patellar cartilage. Evaluation of the status of cartilage may have important management implications.

CT may also be used effectively in the postoperative assessment of patients having undergone either lateral release or realignment surgery. Fulkerson and colleagues found a mean decrease in congruence angle of 5 degrees on midpatellar CT sections obtained on six patients following lateral release.[26,42] In a smaller group of patients with isolated patellar tilt (type 3), a direct correlation with the degree of preoperative tilt and postoperative lateral release improvement was observed. In patients after anterior tibial tubercle transfer, a two- to threefold improvement in patellar tilt was documented. Both lateral release and anterior tibial tubercle transfer had less effect on congruence angle. Fulkerson correlated the CT findings with clinical findings before and after surgery and assessment of the patellar articular cartilage at the time of surgery. This correlation indicated that patients with CT types 1 and 2 malalignment may not respond as well to lateral release as patients with isolated patellar tilt (type 3).[22] Additionally, in the presence of more severe patellar cartilage degeneration, lateral release was less effective in restoring normal tracking and obtaining good clinical results. Fulkerson suggests that patients with type 1 and 2 malalignment who have not responded to lateral release may be candidates for anteromedial tibial tubercle transfer.[22] Patients with excessive lateral pressure (type 3) in whom extensive facet articular erosion has occurred may also be candidates for anterior tibial tubercle transfer to unload the lateral or central patellar rather than simple lateral release.

Recent technical advances have allowed patellofemoral motion to be evaluated by ultrafast CT methods.[43] This technique offers the opportunity for objective observations of the dynamic influences of muscle contraction on the patellofemoral joint as the knee is actively moved through a range of motion from extension to 90 degrees flexion. Using the technique of Stanford and colleagues, ten images at each of eight levels encompassing an 8-cm length of the knee can

be acquired in 7 s as the knee is moved from 90 degrees flexion to full extension and back to 90 degrees flexion.[43] The processed images can be played back in a closed-loop movie format that allows for visualization of real-time axial images of patellofemoral motion during muscle contraction and leg movement (Fig. 5-7). Additionally, single frame measurements can be obtained at any point in the imaging sequence.

Two patterns of patellar movement based on observation of the cine CT have been described.[43] In one pattern, the patella remained centered throughout the range of motion (90 degrees flexion to full extension). In the second pattern, the patella was centered within the patellofemoral groove until the last 20 degrees extension, at which point it would sublux into a lateral position. The authors termed this latter pattern "J" subluxation. In their quantitative data analysis, Stanford and colleagues corroborated the initial CT observations of Delgado-Martins that the patella often lies laterally and incongruently in contact with the lateral femoral condyle in full extension. They observed lateral subluxation to become most apparent

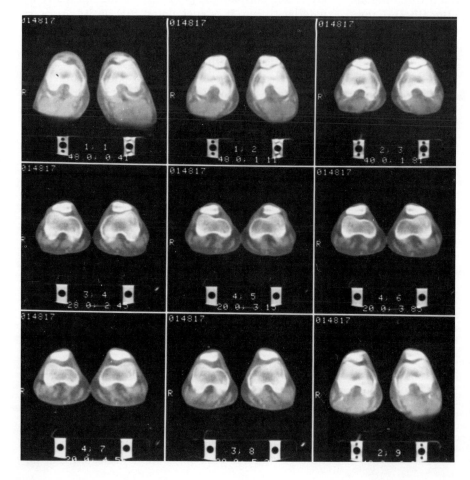

FIGURE 5-7
Cine CT of the patellofemoral joint. This composite of selected images shows the patella during movement from 90 degrees flexion to full extension and back to 90 degrees flexion. Image 1,1 is 90 degrees flexion. Images 1,2 and 2,9 are about 60 degrees flexion. Images 2,3 and 4,7 are about 45 degrees flexion. Images 3,4 and 4,6 are about 30 degrees flexion, and image 4,5 is at full extension. (Reprinted with permission from Stanford W, Phelon J, Kathol MH, et al: *Skeletal Radiol* 17:487–492, 1988.)

in the final 20 degrees knee extension as the patella rode proximally out of the anterior intercondylar groove. Of significant note, the authors reported frequent difficulty in determining multiple parameters including the sulcus angle, congruence angle, patellar tilt, and lateral patellofemoral angle with the knee in full extension. This related to the extension of the patella above the level at which the condyles could be defined. As a consequence of this observation, the authors urged caution in depending on measurements of these parameters in extension and advocated use of qualitative assessment of patellofemoral motion using the cine capability of their technique.[43]

Computed Arthrotomography (CT Arthrography)

The role of conventional arthrography was, at most, limited in the assessment of the patellar articular cartilage.[44] The introduction of CT, however, with its tomographic capability and improved visualization of the articular surface allowed an enhanced role for arthrographic evaluation of chondromalacia.[24,35,44] Boven and colleagues reported on the ability of CT to assess chondromalacia in 67 patients who underwent double contrast CT arthrography.[24] A scoring system was devised based on the regularity and congruity of the cartilage as well as the degree of imbibition of contrast material. Surgical correlation was available in only 25 of the 67 patients. CT correctly depicted the presence of chondromalacia in 8 of 11 patients and correctly excluded it in 11 of 14 patients. Two studies were equivocally positive and four indeterminant. CT demonstrated a clearly enhanced capability compared with conventional arthrography. In assessment of potentially related parameters, no correlation with patella configuration based on the Wiberg classification could be detected. In addition, the shape of the patella changed in appearance between more proximal and distal sections, a finding that has been corroborated on other cross-sectional imaging studies. Lateral subluxation of the patella was noted in 82 percent of the patients with chondromalacia compared with 31 percent with normal cartilage. CT arthrography is also capable of depiction of synovial plica and is an excellent technique in assessment of osteochondral injuries and loose osteochondral bodies within the joint[44] (Fig. 5-8).

MAGNETIC RESONANCE

Magnetic resonance (MR) represents the only diagnostic method capable of directly and noninvasively depicting all components of the extensor mechanism including the patella and patella articular cartilage,

trochlear sulcus, quadriceps muscle and tendon, and patella tendon and retinaculum. The principal advantages of MR as compared to CT for assessment of the musculoskeletal system are markedly increased soft tissue contrast resolution, direct multiplanar imaging capability, and lack of ionizing radiation or any known biologic risk at this time.

Basic Principles

Although a discussion of the physical basis of the MR signal and the manner in which it is collected is beyond the scope of this text, a brief consideration of certain fundamentals which have an impact on image contrast may be useful. The signal generated from a clinical MR pulse sequence primarily results from the interaction of hydrogen nuclei with radiofrequency waves in the presence of an external magnetic field.[45,46] The signal generated will be influenced by the density of hydrogen nuclei in the body part being examined, as well as by unique properties representing the interaction of these nuclei with the surrounding molecular environment known as the relation times T1 and T2.

The relative contrast of a tissue in an MR image will depend on the intensity or strength of the MR signal generated at the time of scan production.[47,48] A bright or white area on an MR scan demonstrates high signal intensity, whereas a dark area denotes an area of low signal intensity. The strength of the signal received from a tissue depends on the T1 and T2 relaxation times of the tissue, the density of protons

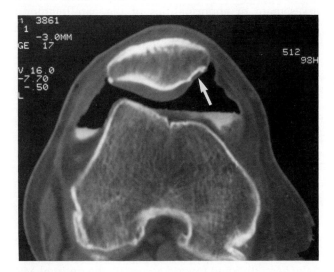

FIGURE 5-8
Computed arthrotomography. Axial CT section obtained following a double contrast knee arthrogram. The articular cartilage along the lateral facet and medial ridge is well defined. A localized area of osteochondritis dissecans involving the medial facet is depicted (arrow).

within the tissue, and on a complex number of instrument parameters under the control of the operator. In conventional MR spin-echo imaging, fat appears of high signal intensity (bright) on pulse sequences emphasizing T1 relaxation times (T1 weighted images) and of slightly lower signal intensity (darker) on pulse sequences emphasizing T2 relaxation times. Thus, adipose tissue and fatty bone marrow will have a bright appearance on T1 weighted images. In contrast, muscle has a relatively short T2 relaxation time and will appear of lower signal intensity (darker) on T2 weighted images. Tendons and fibrous tissue such as the patellar retinaculum demonstrate low signal intensity (appear darker) on all MR pulse sequences. In general, pathologic processes are characterized by relatively increased free water and thus increased hydrogen proton density. MR pulse sequences are designed to maximize image contrast between the tissue of interest and suspected pathology. Thus in tendons, T2 weighted images are useful, because they contrast most pathologic processes such as tumor and edema, which appear bright on these pulse sequences compared to the lower signal intensity background of the tendon.

Patellofemoral Joint

The application of MR toward the assessment of the menisci and cruciate ligaments of the knee has become one of the most widely accepted musculoskeletal applications of this new imaging technique.[49] The tomographic capability and high soft tissue contrast resolution of MR also allow its application toward assessment of abnormalities of the patellofemoral joint including articular cartilage assessment and evaluation of patella alignment and motion. Indeed, MR is the only technique capable of direct assessment of all constituent components of the extensor mechanism including quadriceps muscle and tendon, patella tendon, patella, and supporting soft tissue structures including the patellar retinaculum. These applications will be reviewed and comparisons made to other imaging techniques where appropriate.

Articular Cartilage

MR is unique among noninvasive imaging methods in its ability to directly depict articular cartilage.[50–56] The appearance of articular cartilage depends on the MR pulse sequence used to image it. Multiple studies have been directed toward assessing the optimal MR pulse sequences for depiction of patellar chondromalacia and articular cartilage defects in general. Before their consideration, certain unique features of articular cartilage merit brief review because knowledge of the composition and structure of normal articular cartilage provides a rational basis for optimizing the application of MR pulse sequences designed to depict cartilage abnormalities.

Articular cartilage consists of cells (e.g., chondrocytes) embedded in an abundant extracellular matrix. In contrast to other parenchymal tissues, the cellular component contributes relatively little (< 10 percent) to the total volume of cartilage.[57] Water constitutes the largest component of the matrix with tissue fluid accounting for 60 to 80 percent of the wet weight of cartilage. This high water content distinguishes articular cartilage from most other connective tissues.[58] Approximately 90 percent of the water is extracellular. The water content of articular cartilage is generally highest next to the articular surface, although its variation in successive layers is not large. Structural macromolecules contribute 20 to 40 percent of the wet weight of cartilage and include collagens, proteoglycans, and noncollagenous proteins or glycoproteins.[58–60] Collagens form the fibrillar meshwork that gives cartilage its tensile strength and form. Proteoglycans and noncollagenous proteins bind to the collagen meshwork or become mechanically trapped within it.[58]

The physical and chemical properties of the proteoglycans are important to the resiliency of the articular cartilage. One of the unique features of articular cartilage, in distinction to other hyaline cartilages, is the highly ordered structure that changes from joint surface to subchondral bone.[58,61,62] Four distinct layers or zones have been described and are referred to as the superficial zone, the middle or transitional zone, the deep or radial zone, and the zone of calcified cartilage. Within these zones, distinct matrix regions or compartments can be identified, including the pericellular matrix, the territorial matrix, and the interterritorial matrix.[58]

The mechanical properties of articular cartilage are governed by both the composition of the tissue and the movement of the interstitial fluid within the tissue.[58,60,63] When loaded in compression, articular cartilage exudes its interstitial fluid and is compressed. The negatively charged proteoglycan macromolecules are also compressed and exert a resistive force because of electrostatic charge repulsion ultimately resulting in a state of equilibrium whereby the matrix-resistive force caused by tissue consolidation balances the applied compressive forces. The movement of fluid through the tissue, which depends on the frictional interactions between the fluid and the "branches" of the proteoglycan macromolecules, governs both the rate and absolute amount of deformation.[58] In compression and fluid expression experiments, a higher permeability for fluid flow has been found in the superficial cartilaginous zone than in the deep zone likely reflecting the lower concentration of proteoglycans in the former.[63] Thus, as a consequence of its higher hydraulic permeability and fluid flow to non–weight-bearing areas, the superficial layer appears to act as a cushion, initially absorbing and distributing the impact of compressive force. Only with higher or prolonged strain is the compressive force also translated to the deeper cartilage zones. In contrast, surface fibrillated cartilage demonstrates far greater deformation as a consequence of permeability increases secondary to cartilage disruption with resulting decreased resistance to fluid motion.

The appearance of normal articular cartilage, using a number of different MR imaging strategies, has been reported in several investigations. Leher and colleagues, in an experimental study using bovine patella, demonstrated a bilaminar appearance to the patellar articular cartilage.[63] A superficial zone, characterized by longer T1 and T2 values, correlated with the tangential and transitional zones of normal articular cartilage. A second MR imaging zone, with shorter T1 and T2 values, was identified in the depth of the articular cartilage. On heavily T1 weighted inversion recovery sequences, the superficial cartilaginous layer demonstrated lower signal intensity than the deeper slightly higher signal intensity zone. This zonal signal intensity pattern was inverted on heavily T2 weighted spin-echo sequences. The findings correlated with differences between the better hydrated superficial zone and lower water content of the deeper zone. In investigating other pulse sequences, however, Leher and coworkers were not able to demonstrate the bilaminar appearance using T1 weighted spin-echo sequences or with T1 and T2 weighted gradient echo sequences. Hayes and colleagues, using fresh cadaver patellae and a strongly T1 weighted spin-echo sequence, also described a bilaminar appearance to the patella articular cartilage.[55] In this work, the basal two-thirds of the cartilage demonstrated a lower signal intensity than the superficial one-third. This appearance was more pronounced in disarticulated cadaver patellae than in in vivo studies in which the cartilage most commonly demonstrated a uniform intermediate signal intensity with this pulse sequence. In a clinical series using spin-echo sequences, Yulish and colleagues described a homogeneous appearance to the articular cartilage that was of intermediate signal intensity.[53] The authors of this article have used a specialized inversion recovery sequence in which the signal from fat is nullified and that from water accentuated. On this sequence, bone appears nearly black secondary to suppression of sig-

nal from marrow fat. The patellar articular cartilage is intermediate in intensity and is well contrasted between low signal intensity subchondral bone and high signal intensity synovial fluid (see Fig. 5-9).

The ability of MR to depict relative differences in hydration has been used experimentally to assess the response of normal and degenerated articular cartilage to compression.[63] With the application of a low compressive strain, MR detected an impression on the load-bearing superficial lamina and fluid flow within the lamina toward adjacent nonloaded areas. With prolonged pressure, an increase in signal intensity within the deep cartilaginous layer was demonstrated on T1 weighted inversion recovery sequences indicating a loss of fluid in the deep zone of the burden bearing cartilage. After release of pressure, the MR appearance of normal hyaline cartilage returned to its initial appearance within 20 min. Four specimens with macroscopic fibrillation were evaluated to assess morphologic features of early degeneration as depicted by MR. These areas demonstrated increased signal intensity within the superficial zone on T2 weighted images and decreased intensity on T1 weighted inversion recovery sequences, changes consistent with increased hydration compared with normal. When subject to compression, the zonal pattern demonstrated delayed reconstitution in the specimens with early degeneration. This early work underscores the potential of MR in the study of articular surfaces.

Chondromalacia

Current concepts suggest that patella chondromalacia develops most commonly secondary to abnormal patellar alignment and the consequent increased loading of the patellar articular cartilage and increased contact stresses.[9,18,22] Less commonly, direct trauma may precipitate immediate cartilage degradation.[22] Patella chondromalacia is thought rarely to develop on an idiopathic basis.[18] The voluminous literature on the subject of chondromalacia is replete with contradictory observations, largely because of a lack of precise terminology. Numerous investigators have decried the confusion surrounding the subject of chondromalacia and have emphasized the need for the determination of the underlying pathoanatomy and altered knee mechanics responsible for the cartilage degradation in the majority of cases.[9,13,22] Both CT and MR can be used to advantage for such purposes.

Histologic and ultrastructural studies suggest that the initial changes of chondromalacia occur within the matrix below the articular surface.[58,64] This contrasts with the pathogenesis of osteoarthritis in

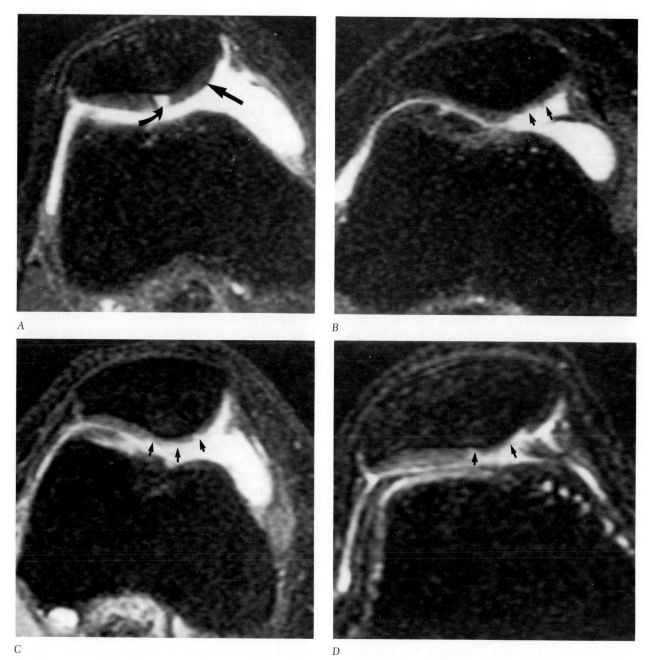

A

B

C

D

FIGURE 5-9

Chondromalacia patella. Axial STIR (TR 2200 TE 35 T1 160) images from four different patients demonstrating the ability of MR to grade different degrees of chondromalacia. *A.* Normal articular cartilage appears of relatively homogeneous intermediate signal intensity (arrow) and is well contrasted against the high signal intensity (white) synovial fluid. A prominent focus of altered increased signal within the cartilage along the medial ridge (curved arrow) correlated with an area of softening at arthroscopy. *B.* A subtle serrated appearance to the articular cartilage is noted along the medial facet (arrows). At arthroscopy this correlated with early surface fibrillation. *C.* Focal areas of altered signal are seen within the cartilage and in association with surface irregularity along the median ridge in this patient with grade 2 to 3 chondromalacia (small arrows). Irregularity of the cartilage along the lateral trochlear surface is also demonstrated. *D.* Grade 4 chondromalacic changes are seen along the medial ridge in this individual. The cartilage is completely denuded with exposure of subchondral bone (small arrows). Subchondral erosion is also depicted along the lateral trochlear.

which the earliest changes are observed at the cartilage surface with fraying of the bundles of collagen fibers in the superficial zone.[65,66] In the earliest stages of closed chondromalacia (e.g., softening), the initial findings are seen in the transitional zone.[22] The surface tangential network of collagen fibers is spared at this stage. The soft, edematous quality of this cartilage may be explained by the loss of an intact collagen network allowing proteoglycan aggregates to expand into a larger molecular domain.[58]

The surface appearance of patellar chondromalacia has been described by multiple investigators and numerous classification systems have been proposed.[67–73] Outerbridge described the earliest finding in chondromalacia as the change in appearance of the articular cartilage from its normal bluish white smooth glistening surface to a dull and even slightly yellowish white appearance.[70] On probing, the cartilage was soft and readily depressed. Outerbridge described chondromalacia as most common along the medial facet and attributed this to the presence of an abnormal ridge at the superior margin of the articular surface of the femur at the junction of the epiphysis and metaphysis. This macroscopic stage of chondromalacia correlates with the initial stage of "closed chondromalacia" described by Ficat and Hungerford.[20] This stage may progress to the development of a localized surface swelling or blister with the overlying cartilage remaining grossly intact. According to these investigators, the lesion predominates along the lateral facet and results secondary to excessive lateral pressure. Insall and coworkers also described the initial stages of chondromalacia as swelling and softening ("closed"), but described the most common location, based on the observation of 105 patellae, as occurring at the midpoint of the medial ridge with extension equally onto the medial and lateral patellar facets.[74] More than 70 percent of the lesions were located within an ellipse located transversely across the cental area of the patella, with the upper and lower thirds of the patellar articular surface nearly always spared. Goodfellow and colleagues differentiated two types of chondromalacia.[67,69] The macroscopic stage of cartilage softening followed by blister formation correlates with the process they termed basal degeneration and represents a localized posttraumatic form of cartilage injury that usually occurs in younger patients. This process was most commonly observed along the inferior part of the central ridge separating medial and lateral facets.

The initial stages of closed or surface intact chondromalacia may progress toward the loss of surface integrity with the development of cracks, fissures, fibrillation, and eventually gross ulceration extending into subchondral bone.[22] Outerbridge did not distinguish between grades II and III with regard to surface appearance, both of which are characterized by fissuring and fragmentation, but rather differentiated them on the basis of extent (diameter) of involvement. Ficat and Hungerford distinguish between closed (grade I) and open (grade II) chondromalacia. In open (grade II) chondromalacia, a distinction is made between fissures and ulcerations, both of which may be superficial or extend to subchondral bone and are not further subclassified. Insall distinguishes

between fissuring (grade II) and fibrillation (grade III), although the criteria are qualitative.[74] Goodfellow and coworkers distinguish between basilar degeneration and superficial degeneration, a second type of chondromalacia most commonly encountered along the odd facet of the patella and thought related to decreased contact. In superficial degeneration, initial changes were manifested at the surface with flaking progessing to fibrillation and fissure formation.[67] Although the early stages of these two entities differ, the more advanced stages are similar at gross examination with ulceration and gross fibrillation (grade III) and crater formation and subchondral eburnation (grade IV) predominating.

The utility of MR in the assessment of chondromalacia and in general of articular cartilage has been the subject of multiple investigations. Of particular interest and of considerable practical importance has been the evaluation of different MR pulse sequences in their ability to depict changes in cartilage. With the continued introduction of new MR pulse sequences, this is an area abundant in potential and much in evolution.

Wojyts and colleagues studied experimentally produced chondral lesions of the patella and femoral condyles, as well as arthroscopically confirmed lesions in 10 patients.[56] In the clinical group, using a T2 weighted spin-echo sequence, MR successfully identified 15 of 18 lesions involving at least partial thickness hyaline cartilage defects (grades II and III) but only 1 of 5 lesions confined to the surface with no cartilage substance loss (grade I). The lesions ranged in size from 1×1 cm to 3×3 cm. In the cadaver group in which discrete cartilage defects were created, MR demonstrated 15 of 16 lesions that were 4 mm or greater in width and all those 3 mm and greater in depth. In addition 7 of 9 lesions 1 mm in depth were identified in this group. An important point to be considered, however, is that sharp borders created by experimentally produced drill holes may well have enhanced their identification compared with naturally occurring chondral lesions. Despite technical considerations limiting spatial resolution and signal to noise in this early investigation (0.35T imager, 30-cm coil, 5-mm section thickness, 0.95 mm/pixel in plane resolution), this study clearly documented the ability of MR to detect relatively small (> 3 mm) partial thickness articular cartilage defects.

Yulish and coworkers compared the MR and arthroscopic findings in 19 patients (12 with MR before arthroscopy and 7 with MR following arthroscopy).[53] Agreement between MR and arthroscopy occurred in 17 of the 19 cases. MR was unable to demonstrate changes in one patient in whom cartilage softening was noted on arthroscopy and was false positive for an apparent cartilage fracture in another patient. The authors described areas of "hypointensity with swelling" on relatively T1 weighted images, which they speculate might represent the MR correlates of early basal degeneration as described by Goodfellow. The arthroscopic effect of T2 weighted images was useful for depiction of more advanced cartilage changes with fluid extending into surface fissures that otherwise would have been difficult to detect on T1 weighted images.

Handelberg and colleagues compared the utility of MR, CT, and arthroscopy in detecting chondral lesions of the patella using both a cadaveric model as well as in a prospective clinical series.[54] MR detected all experimentally created lesions, which ranged from 0.8 to 5 mm in diameter and 1 to 2 mm in depth. The images were obtained on a high field strength system (1.5T) using a T2 weighted spin-echo sequence, and the superficial defects were sharply contrasted against high signal intensity joint fluid. Double contrast CT arthrography, performed after the MR examination, missed 50 percent of the 1.5- and 2-mm lesions and detected none of the 0.8-mm holes. Despite this impressive demonstration by MR, the same caveat mentioned in regard to conspicuity of experimentally produced drill holes versus naturally occurring chondral lesions mentioned in the discussion of the work of Wojyts and coworkers must be considered. In a prospective clinical series including 54 knees examined by MR before arthroscopy, the same investigators reported an overall accuracy for MR of 81.5 percent with a sensitivity of 100 percent but a specificity of only 50 percent due to false-positive examinations. The false-positive MR diagnosis related to the depiction of linear areas of decreased signal intensity within the deep zones of the articular cartilage, which the authors suggest may represent the correlates of early histologic aberrations. Arthroscopically, however, these findings did not even correlate with mild softening. Other investigators have described similar findings and considered them normal variants and thus clarification awaits further MR-histologic correlation. The authors suggested a four-stage system for classifying patellar chondral lesions. Stage 1 lesions are manifest on MR by round areas of low signal intensity within the cartilage on both intermediate and T2 weighted sequences. The arthroscopic correlates of this stage are softening to probing the small surface fibrillations. MR stage 2 lesions appear as zones of low signal surrounded by high signal within the cartilage on T2 weighted sequences. These correspond to fissures into which synovial fluid can penetrate and sometimes are asso-

ciated with flap lesions. Stage 3 lesions are readily demonstrated as superficial or deep defects of the cartilage surface filled by synovial fluid appearing bright (high signal) on T2 weighted images. Stage 4 lesions represent degenerative arthritis and marked thinning and irregularity of the cartilage contour.

Hayes and coworkers, in a study of naturally occurring chondral lesions in 14 cadavers, found MR to be an accurate means for detecting and staging moderate and advanced patellar cartilage lesions.[55] Fourteen cadaver knees were studied using high spacial resolution T1 weighted images. A smaller subgroup of knees were additionally studied with T2 weighted sequences, which despite the desirable arthrogram effect, were not preferred by the authors because of less satisfactory spatial resolution, decreased contrast between subchondral bone and cartilage, and decreased conspicuity of internal cartilage signals. Lesions were classified by a modification of the system proposed by Shahiaree to include cartilage lesions reflective of both basal degeneration and superficial degeneration as described by Goodfellow, and colleagues.[55,67,68] In this system stage 1 lesions are manifest grossly as either palpable softening (basal degeneration) or as minor surface fibrillation (superficial degeneration). Six specimens were considered stage 1 on gross inspection and MR was unable to detect lesions in any of the six. All specimens in this group demonstrated changes more consistent with superficial degeneration and thus no examples of softening were available for evaluation. Five specimens were considered normal and demonstrated a bilaminar appearance with lower signal intensity within the basal layer and slightly higher signal intensity in the superficial layer. Of the remaining nine specimens, all demonstrated at least one lesion graded as stage 2 or higher and all of these specimens demonstrated corresponding MR changes.

Gylys-Morin and coworkers examined the detectability of experimentally produced cartilage lesions and in contrast to other investigations found that T1 weighted and "balanced" images alone were inadequate for detecting focal lesions.[50] In this investigation, drill holes ranging in diameter from 1 to 5 mm were made in the femoral condyles of six cadaveric knees. No patellar lesions were made. In this study, saline and gadolinium-DTPA were investigated as potential intra-articular contrast agents. In the presence of saline, the smallest lesion that could be detected was 3 mm (using a T2 weighted sequence). With gadolinium, lesions 2 mm or greater could be detected on all pulse sequences investigated. For enhanced diagnostic capability and shorter imaging times, the authors recommended the use of intra-articular gadolinium for assessment of articular cartilage.

The authors of this review have used a specialized MR pulse sequence for assessment of the patella. In this pulse sequence, known as short tau inversion recovery (STIR), the signal from fat is nullified, accounting for the dark appearance of bone (e.g., suppression of signal from fatty marrow that comprises the predominant source of signal within cancellous bone). The effects of T1 and T2 relaxation are additive, contributing to increased lesion conspicuity. This pulse sequence allows sensitive depiction of the subchondral bone, articular cartilage, and articular surface, which is particularly well delineated in contrast to the high signal intensity of synovial fluid. Normal articular cartilage demonstrates a homogeneous intermediate intensity appearance. Early changes of closed chondromalacia are demonstrated by focal areas of increased signal within the articular cartilage, reflecting the histologically known increase in water content (Fig. 5-9). Early surface fibrillation can also be demonstrated, particularly when a joint effusion is present (Fig. 5-9B). The more advanced changes of ulceration extending into subchondral bone are readily demonstrated and can be precisely mapped (Fig. 5-9C). In a comparative study, this sequence was found far more sensitive than T1 weighted sequence.[75]

Patellofemoral Motion Studies

Shellock and coworkers described a method of analysis of patellofemoral dynamics using MR imaging that has been widely applied toward the evaluation of patellar alignment and tracking. In a manner similar to that described for cine CT,[43] axial images are obtained at selected locations through the patellofemoral joint, and subsequently displayed both as static images and as simulated real-time images[28,76–78] (Fig. 5-10). Termed kinematic MRI, the technique uses a special patient-activated positioning device designed to allow simultaneous axial plane imaging of both knees from extension to 30 degrees flexion at 5-degree increments. The patient is placed in a prone position on the device with special care taken to position the lower extremities to ensure that the individual's alignment is maintained. This positioning scheme is unique because it does not inhibit rotational movements of the lower extremities, which may be partially responsible for abnormal patellar tracking,[10,69,79] during flexion of the patellofemoral joint.[77,80] Shellock and colleagues have reported that prone positioning of the patient does not alter the kinematics of

the patellofemoral joint during flexion when compared with the supine position.[77]

Three to four different slice locations through the femoral trochlear groove (depending on the height of the patella) are chosen, which depict the path of excursion of the patella during flexion. As a consequence of disagreement on the normal position of the patella with the knee extended[27,29,81] only the images obtained with the patellofemoral joint flexed from 5 to 30 degrees are analyzed for the kinematic study. While static images are obtained,[82,83] these investigators[28,76–78,80,82–84] have considered it more appropriate and practical to use qualitative rather than quantitative criteria to describe the patella in relation to the femoral trochlear groove during flexion of the patellofemoral joint. The preference of dynamic image display has also been advocated by Stanford, using ultrafast CT[43] and Kujala using MR.[81,85] This may, in part, be accounted for by the observation that in contrast to static conventional radiographs, the changes in anatomic configuration of the patella and trochlear seen with the tomographic capabilities of MR and CT, preclude simple application of the previously described parameters developed for conventional radiographs.[28,76–78,80,82–84]

The configurations of the patella and femoral trochlear groove are well-demonstrated on the kinematic MRI study by the sequential axial plane images obtained through the patellofemoral joint during extension. Abnormalities of patella alignment related to dysplasia of either the patella or trochlear sulcus, as well as related to patella height, can be readily demonstrated. Normal patellar height is considered to appear on the kinematic MR examination when the inferior pole of the patella is positioned in the superior aspect of femoral trochlear groove with the knee in extension.[10,69,86] Patella alta is present when the inferior pole of the patella is positioned above the superior aspect of the femoral trochlear groove with the joints extended, and patella baja, an abnormally low position of the patella, is present when the entire patella is positioned in or below the femoral trochlear groove with the joint extended. This determination often differs from that accomplished using the conventional criteria developed for lateral radiographs,[6,8–10,11,69,79] and introduces the concept of "functional" patella alta or baja relating patella position to the trochlea sulcus directly through the use of axial tomographic techniques.

Normal patellar alignment and tracking is present when the medial ridge of the patella is positioned in the femoral trochlear groove as it travels in a vertical plane during flexion of the knee, without transverse displacement of the medial or lateral facets of

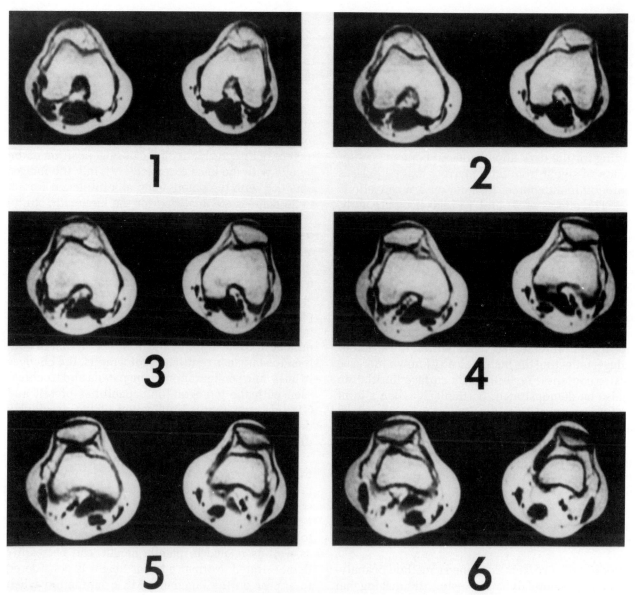

FIGURE 5-10

Bilateral lateral subluxation (TR-400 ms, TE-20 ms, 5-mm slice thickness). Sequential axial images at 5 degree increments obtained through the patellofemoral joint demonstrate lateral subluxation of the patella bilaterally. The midplane of the patella is significantly cephalad to the developed trochlear sulcus with most of the articulation occurring in the early degrees of flexion between the patella and supratrochlear femur. The findings are reflective of "functional" patella alta. Additionally, these selected images from the dynamic examination demonstrate the difficulty often encountered in applying the standard measurements of patella position such as the congruence angle to tomographic images obtained in the initial degrees of flexion. As a consequence of the dysplastic anatomy, no clearly defined landmarks are present and a qualitative approach is preferred.

the patella.[28,76,77] This orientation causes the patella to appear "centered" in the femoral trochlear groove. Any deviation of this normal pattern of patellar alignment or tracking seen on or more slice locations at 5 degrees flexion or greater on the kinematic MRI study is regarded as an abnormality.[1–3,11–15] Shellock and colleagues have defined five patterns of patella malalignment using MR.[28,76–78,80,82–84]

LATERAL SUBLUXATION OF THE PATELLA

On the kinematic MRI study, lateral subluxation of the patella is diagnosed when the medial ridge of the patella is laterally displaced relative to the femoral trochlear groove and the lateral facet of the patella overlaps the lateral aspect of the femoral trochlear.[28,76–78,80,82–84] This is the most common form of patellar malalignment and occurs with varying degrees of severity[4,10] (see Fig. 5-10). MR may demonstrate abnormalities of articular cartilage at the impact site between the patella and femoral trochlear groove as a result of chronic hyperpressure that develops from contact stress due to lateral subluxation of the patella.[10,12,20,67,87] One of the unique observations afforded by the high soft tissue contrast resolution of kinematic MRI has been the presence of a redundant lateral retinaculum associated with lateral subluxation of the patella. This may have important implications regarding the consideration of surgical release of the lateral retinaculum.[82,84]

EXCESSIVE LATERAL PRESSURE SYNDROME

Excessive lateral pressure syndrome, or ELPS, was first described by Ficat.[4] This form of patellar malalignment is characterized by patellofemoral pain and tilting of the patella with functional patellar lateralization usually toward a dominant lateral facet.[20] With ELPS, a small amount of lateral subluxation of the patella may also be seen during knee flexion on the kinematic MRI study (see Fig. 5-10). Because the patellar tilting that occurs with ELPS has a tendency to worsen with increasing degrees of joint flexion, kinematic MRI of the patellofemoral joint is particularly suited for identifying this abnormality.[76-78]

MEDIAL SUBLUXATION OF THE PATELLA (PATELLA ADENTRO)

Medial subluxation of the patella, or patella adentro, is distinguished by a medial displacement of the medial patellar ridge relative to the femoral trochlear groove.[76-78] Medial subluxation has been reported as a complication of prior surgical realignment procedures for presumed lateral subluxation and has been reported as well in patients with no prior surgery (Fig. 5-11). Similar to other forms of abnormal patellar alignment, medial subluxation of the patella may cause localized hyperpressure and, therefore, may be associated with MR demonstrable cartilage abnormalities along the medial patellar facet.[76-78]

Various causative mechanisms are thought to be responsible for medial subluxation of the patella that exist either individually or in combination, including an insufficient lateral retinaculum, overtaut medial retinaculum, abnormal patellofemoral anatomy, and unbalanced quadriceps muscles.[76] In addition, excessive internal rotation of the lower extremities is a common clinical finding with medial subluxation of the patella (Fig. 5-12). The presence of medial subluxation of the patella is especially important to identify and to distinguish from lateral or tilting forms of

patellar subluxation because various surgical stabilization techniques (e.g., medial transposition of the extensor mechanism, lateral retinacular release, etc.) can further increase medial subluxation of the patella and not only lead to failure of the procedure, but can also exacerbate the patient's symptoms.[88] Of additional importance is that most physical rehabilitation techniques, including the use of patellofemoral braces and McConnell taping, are usually implemented to correct lateral subluxation of the patella[89] and need to be modified when treating patients with medial subluxation of the patella.

LATERAL-TO-MEDIAL SUBLUXATION OF THE PATELLA

Lateral-to-medial subluxation of the patella is a pattern of abnormal patellar tracking whereby the patella is in a slightly laterally subluxated position during the early increments of knee flexion, moves across the femoral trochlear groove or femoral trochlea as flexion continues, and displaces medially at the higher increments of flexion (Fig. 5-13). This type of abnormal patellar tracking is commonly exhibited by the patellofemoral joint that tends to have patella alta, a poorly developed femoral trochlear groove or a misshaped patella.[76,78] Again, no mechanical restraint is provided by the bony anatomy and patellofemoral instability results when these structural abnormalities exist. The actual mechanisms responsible for lateral-to-medial subluxation of the patella are complicated and not well understood. Multiple disordered or uncoordinated forces apparently act on the patella to produce this form of abnormal patellar movement. As with other patellar malalignment syndromes, kinematic MRI is particularly suited to identify this unusual type of patellar tracking because it shows the various positions and movements of the patella at several different increments of flexion of the joint.

Ultrafast MRI of the Patellofemoral Joint

Recently, several new MRI techniques have been developed that allow rapid imaging with sufficient image quality to permit the evaluation of physiologic motion.[90,91] Similar to ultrafast CT,[43] Shellock and colleagues, in preliminary studies, have demonstrated that ultrafast MRI may be used to obtain multiple images at a temporal resolution suitable for examining the patellofemoral joint during active movement.[92-94] This provides a more physiologic and realistic assessment of the kinematic aspects of this joint because of the activated contribution of the activated muscles and soft tissue structures[92-94] (see Fig. 5-12).

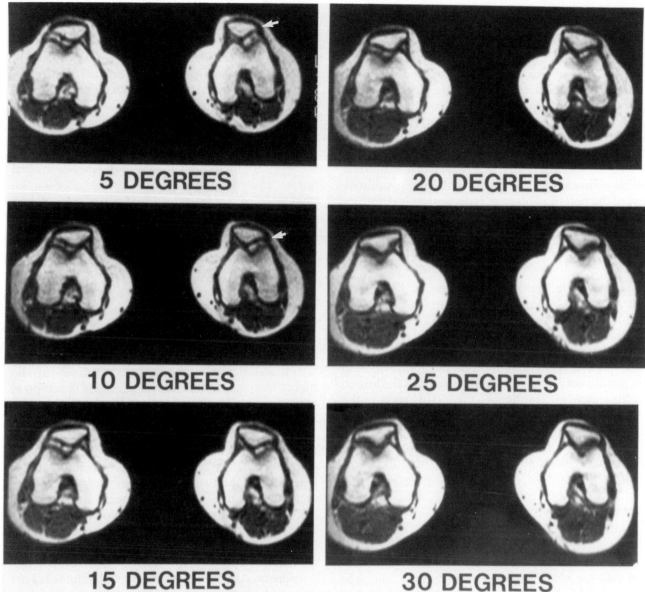

5 DEGREES **20 DEGREES**

10 DEGREES **25 DEGREES**

15 DEGREES **30 DEGREES**

FIGURE 5-11
Medial subluxation of the patella (TR-400 ms, TE-20 ms, 5-mm slice thickness). Serial axial MR images obtained at 5 degree increments through the patellofemoral joint. There is evidence of medial subluxation of the patella bilaterally. A lateral release had previously been performed on the left knee. The lateral retinaculum is thickened as a result of the surgery (arrows). The right knee had not been previously operated on and is also strikingly medial. Medial subluxation can occur not only following overzealous lateral release, but may exist before any surgical intervention, an observation underscoring the need to depict clearly the altered patellar tracking before therapy is initiated.

Extensor Mechanism Injuries

The extensor mechanism of the knee is comprised of the quadriceps femoris muscles and tendon, the patella, and the patella tendon and is excellently depicted using MR. Tears of the extensor mechanism may occur from either direct or indirect trauma, with complete loss of extension most commonly associated with indirect causes.[95-100] Disruption may occur at one of multiple sites including tendo-osseous junction, intratendinous, intramuscular, myotendinous,

and tendo-osseous. Tears may be complete or incomplete.

Quadriceps tendon ruptures most often occur at the tendo-osseous junction.[95,97] Patients are most commonly elderly and rupture is generally associated with one of several conditions contributing to tendon weakness, including chronic renal disease, diabetes mellitus, steroid therapy, collagen vascular disease (systemic lupus erythematosus), obesity, and gout.[31,34] The central and anterior segment of the tendon usually tears first at a level approximately 2 cm above the patella. Diagnosis may be difficult on physical examination, particularly in the presence of a severe hemarthrosis.[101,102] In patients with partial tears and in whom the retinaculum may be intact, active extension may be possible. Delay in diagnosis may complicate repair or reconstruction, underscoring the need for an accurate means of evaluation.

Conventional radiographic findings are nonspecific and diagnosis is difficult.[97] Findings include hemarthrosis, blurring of distal quadriceps tendon, suprapatellar soft tissue mass, and low patellar position (not invariable). Arthrography has been used in quadriceps disruption. Injection of contrast into the suprapatellar bursa may allow detection of full thickness tears with extension of contrast into the soft tissues anteriorly.[103,104] MR is an exceptional diagnostic

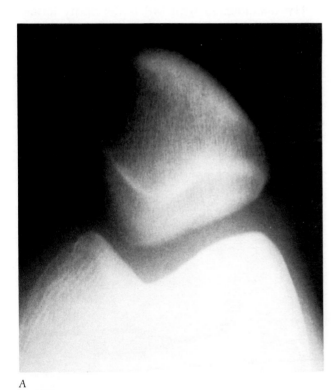

A

FIGURE 5-12
A. Plain radiograph "skyline view" of the patellofemoral joint obtained at approximately 45 degrees flexion showing congruency between the patella and femoral trochlear groove. *B.* Axial plane images. Six images obtained with ultrafast spoiled GRASS technique in 9 s while the patient actively moved the knee joint from extension (image #1) to approximately 40 degrees flexion (image #6). The patella is tilted and initially lateralized. The degree of lateral subluxation decreases during flexion with the patella nearly centralized although persistently tilted at 30 degrees. (TR-8 ms, TE-2 ms, 7-mm slice thickness). This case further illustrates the value of imaging during the initial degrees of flexion to not miss alignment abnormalities that are no longer manifest at angles of flexion 35 to 40 degrees, the range most typical of conventional radiographs.

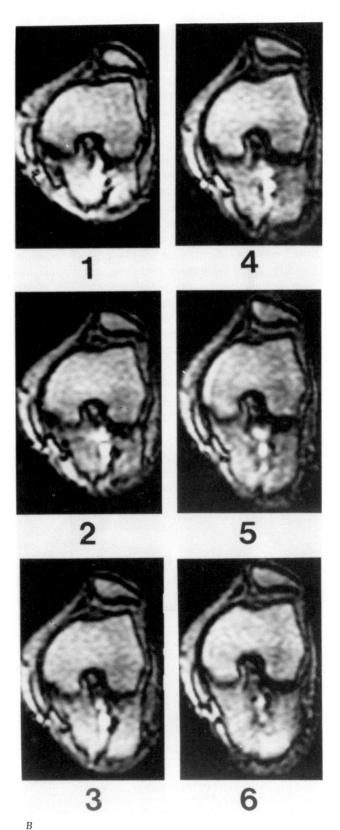

B

method for evaluation of these patients. The technique is capable of direct depiction of the tendon as well as the retinaculum. The precise extent of the tear and degree of separation can be quantitated. T1 weighted sequences suffice for depiction of abnormal tendon morphology (see Fig. 5-13). T2 weighted sequences are used for complete depiction of the extent of surrounding edema and soft tissue injury.

Ruptures of the patellar tendon are the least common cause of extensor mechanism disruption.[95,97] In contrast to patients with quadriceps rupture, patients with patellar tendon disruption are typically younger, athletic individuals.[105] The tendon usually ruptures at its origin on the lower pole of the patella or less commonly at the level of the tibial tubercle. On conventional radiographs, elevation of the patella, indistinctness of the tendon, and at times an avulsion fracture at the inferior pole may be present.[37,97] More recently, high resolution real-time ultrasound has been used to assess the patellar tendon.[106–111] This technique is capable of directly depicting the tendon and demonstrating areas of contained abnormalities including tendonitis and partial tears. The method, however, is greatly operator dependent, a significant factor limiting its wider use. Abnormalities of the patellar tendon are most precisely demonstrated using MR.[112] As a consequence of their low water content, normal tendons demonstrate a low signal intensity (appear dark) on all MR pulse sequences. Abnormalities ranging from foci of tendinitis to partial and complete disruption can be readily demonstrated. On MR, uncomplicated patellar tendinitis is manifest by tendon thickening without significant signal changes. Complications such as chronic tears, necrosis, and inflammation cause intratendinous foci of increased signal on both T1 and T2 weighted images. Chronic tears, which are associated with ingrowth of synovium and accompanied by fibrinoid necrosis and inflammation, contribute to foci of increased signal intensity. Complete tendon disruption is readily demonstrated and the extent of injury and degree of apposition of torn edges can be directly evaluated. T2 weighted spin-echo, and STIR sequences are optimal for portraying these signal changes.

One form of chronic patellar tendon stress that can be documented with MR is the entity termed "jumper's knee." This condition, commonly observed in certain activities associated with patellar tendon stress related to jumping (e.g., basketball, volleyball), is manifest clinically by pain and on examination by tenderness to palpation.[113] The stress creates microtearing; the tissue response results in ingrowth of bone, synovium, or cartilage within the tear. MR demonstrates localized tendon thickening

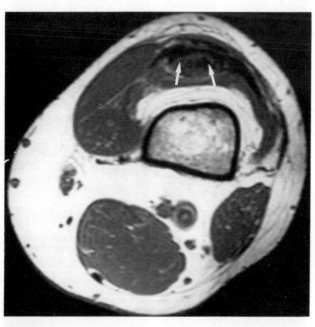

FIGURE 5-13
Quadriceps tear. Axial TR2000 TE 20 scan through the distal femur. There is complete disruption of the rectus femoris muscle at the muscle tendon junction (arrows). The remainder of the quadriceps mechanism was intact.

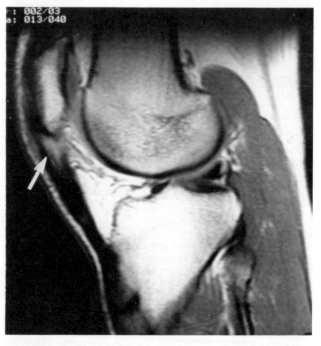

FIGURE 5-14
Jumper's knee. Sagittal TR2000 TE 20 image of the knee demonstrates increased signal within the patella tendon just inferior to the lower pole of the patella (arrow). The tendon is focally increased in girth in this professional basketball player.

and signal alternation within the tendon, most commonly seen just beneath the lower pole[114] (Fig. 5-14). Osgood-Schlatter disease represents another type of stress injury common in adolescents up to age 18. This condition results from an avulsive force on the tibial apophysis transmitted via the patellar tendon secondary to quadriceps contraction. On MR, signal and morphologic changes within the distal tendon are seen in association with osseous changes in the region of the tibial tubercle.

In the adult, the patella itself is the weakest link in the quadriceps mechanism. Patella fracture may be secondary to direct or indirect trauma. With indirect trauma, the degree of separation of the fragments relates to the extent of associated disruption of the medial and lateral retinaculum. With patellar fracture secondary to direct trauma without retinacular disruption, the fragments are not widely displaced. Conventional radiography is generally insufficient for diagnosis, although MR can directly demonstrate the status of the articular surface. Additionally, radiographically occult trauma including bone bruises secondary to direct contusion and occult fractures can be demonstrated with MR (Fig. 5-15).

Patellar Dislocation

The natural history of most acute dislocations is for the patella to relocate before the patient's clinical presentation. Physical findings vary widely and cases can at times be difficult to diagnose.[101,102] Many patients present with a relocated patella but a large tense hemarthrosis. Tenderness or a defect in the

vastus medialis obliquus (VMO) may be demonstrable or a medial retinacular hematoma may be present. Other patients may have only mild swelling that is predominantly periarticular and no palpable medial defect may be present. Lateral patellar hypermobility accompanied by apprehension and pain is usually demonstrable.

Lateral patellar dislocation results in demonstrable injury to both soft tissue and bony structures. The medial capsule and retinaculum along with the medial patelloepicondylar and patellotibial ligaments may be ruptured. In addition to the static supporting structures, the VMO, which contributes dynamic medial patellar support, may be ruptured. VMO rupture may occur at one of several sites: at the level of insertion into the patella, interstitial rupture in its midportion, or tear from its origin at the adductor tubercle.[22] Articular cartilage injury is common and occurs typically along the medial edge of the patella and lateral femoral trochlea as the patella impacts at the time of spontaneous reduction. Loose purely chondral or osteochondral fragments may result.

Considerable controversy surrounds the question of optimal treatment of acute patellar dislocation.[101,102] Advocates for both conservative care as well as those suggesting early operative intervention agree on the need for comprehensive assessment of the injured joint to provide a basis for clinical decision-making. Analysis of potential conditions that might predispose to recurrent dislocation (e.g., shallow sulcus angle, abnormal patellar configuration, patella alta) are considered important by many inves-

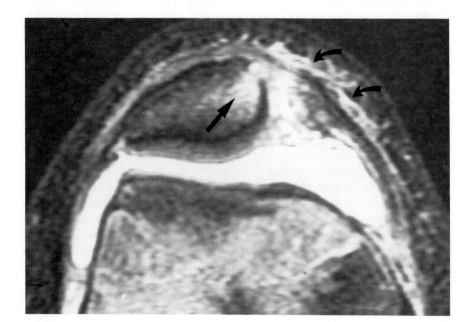

FIGURE 5-15
Patellar dislocation. Axial STIR (TR2200 TE 30 T1 160) sequence through the midplane of the patella. There is increased signal intensity within the subchondral bone of the medial facet most consistent with a bone "bruise" or osteochondral impaction injury (arrow). Edema is seen superficial and deep to the medial retinaculum, which is partially disrupted (curved arrows).

tigators in devising optimal therapy. Additionally, accurate determination of the extent of current injury, including damage to soft tissue structures (e.g., retinaculum) as well as to bone and cartilage, is important to management. In patients with acute knee injuries, limitations to both physical examination and conventional roentgenographic evaluation are well recognized. Axial views of the patella may be particularly difficult to obtain and under any circumstances are not able to diagnose purely chondral injuries. In contrast, however, MR is particularly well suited toward evaluation of all the constituent components of the extensor mechanism that might be potentially injured in patellar dislocation. In addition, MR can be easily obtained even in the acute setting. MR can precisely delineate and characterize anatomic features of the patellofemoral joint that might underlie and predispose to recurrent subluxation and dislocation (e.g., trochlear sulcus angle and depth, patellar configuration and height (alta). In a recent study, Lance and colleagues reported data on 22 patients with a final diagnosis of acute patellar dislocation who underwent MR examination.[115] In 10 of the 22 patients (46 percent), the diagnosis was unsuspected by the referring orthopaedist at the time of referral for the MR examination and the diagnosis was established based on the MR findings. MR demonstrated hemarthrosis in 21 patients (96 percent) and disruption of the medial retinaculum in 18 (82 percent). Abnormal subchondral and cancellous bone signal was detected within the lateral femoral condyle in 18 of 22 (82 percent) patients and within the medial facet of the patella in 9 (44 percent) patients (see Fig. 5-15). This signal presumably reflects trabecular microdisruption and edema and hemorrhage occurring secondary to direct impaction. Loose osteochondral fragments were detected in nearly half the cases. No cruciate ligament abnormalities were detected, although meniscal tears were detected in 2 patients and confirmed at surgery in both cases.

Synovial Plicae

Synovial plicae are remnants of synovial tissue that in early development originally divided the joint into three separate compartments and which may be found normally in the adult knee.[116,117] Although often of no clinical significance, these structures may become pathologically thickened and produce symptoms that mimic other causes of internal derangement such as meniscal tears. In addition, persistence of these structures in their embryonic form, as complete septa, may create a variety of intra-articular compartment syndromes.

The three most common plicae are classified according to the partitions from which they took origin, as suprapatellar, medial patellar, and infrapatellar. The medial patella plica is the most common of these remnants to become pathologically thickened and symptomatic.[44,116] This remnant has been variably referred to as a wedge, band, or shelf and has its origin on the medial wall of the knee joint near the suprapatellar plica. It courses obliquely downward relative to the patella, to insert into the synovium that covers the infrapatellar fat pad. Pathologic thickening of the plica may occur secondary to a number of postulated initiating events. The resulting less elastic and thickened plica no longer glides normally, but rather snaps against the underlying femoral condyle. Repeated irritation and abrasion result in erosive changes of the articular cartilage of the condyle or even the patella. A dull aching pain medial to the patella aggravated by flexion or a clicking sensation without locking or giving way are common clinical complaints. A palpable or audible snap may occur on knee movement, and a symptomatic plica may be palpated as a tender bandlike structure parallel to the medial border of the patella. A pathologic plica has been reported to simulate a monarticular arthritis.

Synovial plicae may be identified on conventional arthrography, CT arthrography, and MR imaging. The decided advantage of MR is the lack of need for an intra-articular contrast agent, direct multiplanar image acquisition, and direct depiction of the articular cartilage and potential damage to the articular surface. The normal plica on MR is visualized as a thin linear low signal intensity band most optimally contrasted against joint fluid on pulse sequences in which joint fluid is depicted as high signal intensity. Thickening of the synovial shelf is readily demonstrated as are changes in adjacent articular cartilage.

ULTRASOUND

High resolution real-time ultrasound has been increasingly used to characterize a wide spectrum of disorders involving the musculoskeletal system.[106–111] In the region of the knee, reported applications of ultrasound include articular cartilage evaluation, assessment of tendons and ligaments, and evaluation of menisci, synovial cysts, adjacent vessels, and muscles. Advantages of sonography include its noninvasive nature, lack of ionizing radiation, high patient acceptance, and relatively low cost. The technique, however, is highly operator dependent and the lack of diagnostic expertise in musculoskeletal applications potentially limits the availability of this diagnostic method.

As a consequence of their superficial location, both the quadriceps and patellar tendons are readily accessible to ultrasound examination. Normal tendons and ligaments appear as moderately echogenic structures with well-defined margins on ultrasound examination. The appearance, however, may vary depending on the orientation of the scan beam in relation to the long axis of the tendon.[108] Oblique imaging of the tendon may produce artifactual hypoechogenicity leading to false-positive diagnosis of tendon pathology. Fornage and associates described the ultrasound findings in 32 normal patellar tendons and in 33 patients with focal degenerative tendinitis, diffuse dystrophic changes, intratendinous hematoma, or mucoid degeneration.[110] In cases of acute tendinitis, tendon volume is increased, echogenicity decreased, and contours blurred. In chronic tendinitis the tendon is thickened, inhomogeneous, and focally hypoechoic. Ultrasound is highly sensitive in detecting even minute calcifications associated with chronic tendinitis. Partial tears of the patellar tendon may appear as hypoechoic areas or as discontinuities in the tendon. They frequently are observed at the patellar apex as partial detachments giving rise to small, relatively well-defined encysted hematomas. In complete tears, the extent of tendon retraction can be visualized directly.

Sonography has also been applied toward evaluation of the patellar plica syndrome. In a recent study comparing sonography with arthroscopy in the detection of patellar plica, Derks and coworkers found a sensitivity for sonography of 92 percent, a specificity of 73 percent, and accuracy of 85 percent. In their study, the plica appeared as a strongly echogenic zone that moved into the patellofemoral space as the knee moved from extension to 30 degrees flexion. Several studies have described the application of ultrasound in the evaluation of the hyaline cartilage of the knee.[107] In particular, the femoral condylar cartilage can be reliably visualized in patients who can adequately flex their knees. The patellar articular surface, however, is blocked from the ultrasound beam by the osseous portion of the patella and cannot be imaged using sonography.

RADIONUCLIDE IMAGING

Scintigraphic methods provide a sensitive albeit nonspecific means for detecting abnormalities of bone.[118,119] Anecdotal experience with the use of bone scans for localizing patellofemoral pathology have been reported. Dye and Boll performed both quantitative and qualitative analysis of bone scans in patients with anterior knee pain and normal Merchant and Laurin axial radiographs.[120] In the quantitative analysis, the investigators defined a percentage of patellar activity (PPA) as the patellar counts divided by the patellar counts and femoral counts. In this study, scintigraphy was found useful for differentiating patients with parapatellar symptoms (negative scan) from those with patellar symptoms (positive scan). Quantitative assessments basically confirmed the qualitative impressions. Sequential scanning demonstrated a progression of positive conversions in patients with persisting symptoms and diminution in activity in patients whose symptoms resolved. The basis for positive scans was attributed by the authors to bone remodeling rather than increased blood flow.

Hejgaard and Diemer evaluated 80 patients with retropatellar pain using bone scintigraphy, intraosseous pressure determination, radiography, physical examination, and arthroscopy.[121] On scintigraphy, 48 percent of the painful knees demonstrated increased patellar uptake compared to 9 percent of the asymptomatic knees. Bone scan activity was correlated with the extent of chondromalacia using the grading system of Hungerford and Ficat. Increased activity (e.g., "hot patella") was more common in patients with advanced (e.g., grade 2, 3) chondromalacia than with normal cartilage. Fifteen of 38 patients with normal cartilage, however, had positive scans, and 14 of 41 patients with grade 2 chondromalacia had normal scans, findings questioning the overall specificity and sensitivity of the method. In addition, in this investigation, the sensitivity of bone scintigraphy for the detection of increased intraosseous pressure (intraosseous engorgement-pain syndrome) was < 50 percent.

The nonspecificy of augmented patellar uptake on bone scintigraphy has been addressed by other investigators.[122] Lin and colleagues, reported an overall incidence of "hot patellae" of 38 percent of 130 patients undergoing bone scans for reasons other than patellofemoral pain. Kipper and coworkers, in a prospective study of 100 patients undergoing scintigraphy predominantly for staging of malignancy, demonstrated increased patella uptake in 20 patients. Only 3 patients gave a history of symptomatic knees, and the authors concluded that the findings were nonspecific and likely multifactorial. Fogelman and coworkers, in a study of 409 bone scans, found the overall incidence of hot patella to be 31 percent in 200 routine scans, 26 percent in patients with various metabolic disorders, and 31 percent in patients undergoing scans for malignant disease. The authors

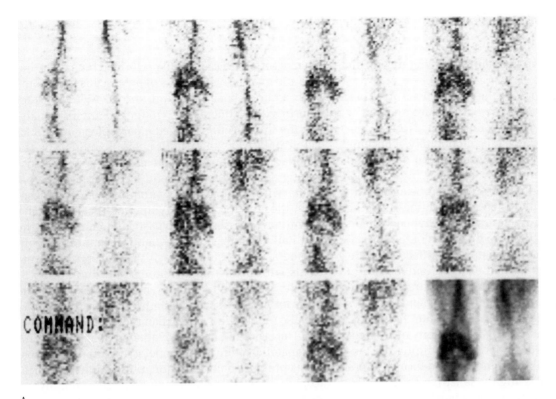

A

B

FIGURE 5-16
Reflex sympathetic dystrophy syndrome (RSDS); three-phase bone scan. *A.* Sequential images obtained over both knees at 3-s intervals following the bolus injection of the isotope. There is asymmetric increased flow to the right knee. The final image in the lower right is the "blood pool" phase also demonstrating striking increased activity. *B.* Lateral view from the delayed bone scan demonstrates markedly increased activity involving the right knee. The activity also involves the patella, which is typical of RSDS.

concluded that patella uptake was nonspecific and of limited diagnostic value. The study, however, did not include either radiographic or arthroscopic evaluation of the knee joints.

A potential role for scintigraphic evaluation is in assessment of patients with suspected reflex sympathetic dystrophy syndrome (RSDS).[123,124] RSDS represents a distinct clinical entity characterized by pain and swelling, vasomotor instability, soft tissue swelling, and dystrophic skin changes. Any neurally related visceral, musculoskeletal, neurologic, or vascular condition is a potential cause for RSDS, although an incipient etiology is frequently not identified. The syndrome is most classically associated with the upper extremity with involvement of the shoulder and hand. In cases involving the knee joint, the patella is uniformly involved.

The most characteristic radiographic findings in RSDS are soft tissue swelling and regional osteoporosis. The findings many mimic a primary articular disorder, although preservation of the joint space is a hallmark of the condition allowing differentiation from the primary arthridities.[44] Quantitative CT for bone mineral assessment has confirmed the profound bone mineral loss. Scintigraphy with technetium-labeled agents typically demonstrates increased periarticular uptake. Radionuclide flow studies demonstrate asymmetric blood flow in the extremities, increased on the affected side (Fig. 5-16). In the series of Kozin and colleagues, bone scans were positive in

60 percent of cases of RSDS.[123] The introduction of the more sophisticated techniques has revealed that RSDS is a bilateral process although the abnormalities are much more marked on one side than the other.[44]

Single photon emission computed tomography (SPECT) represents a technique in which tomographic sections of bone scans can be obtained.[119] Multiple studies have demonstrated the increased sensitivity of this method for lesion detection. Advocates of SPECT have described its potential value in localizing knee pathology, although no critical series have been performed. Anecdotal reports have described the value of the SPECT scan in localizing knee pathology that had previously defied depiction using other methods.[119] With the advent of MR, however, and its enhanced capability of directly depicting abnormalities of articular cartilage as well as subchondral bone, it is unlikely that scintigraphy, particularly considering its nonspecificity, will be widely used in the diagnosis of patellofemoral disorders.

CONCLUSION

Advances in diagnostic imaging during the past decade have provided the orthopaedic surgeon with a wealth of information regarding the patellofemoral joint. Much of this information, and particularly that obtained from the new cross-sectional imaging methods of CT and MR, has challenged several previously held conceptions regarding the patellofemoral joint and has provided new insights regarding patella alignment and tracking. To a considerable degree these new data have yet to be assimilated into clinical orthopaedic practice. As the impact of these newer concepts becomes increasingly manifest, it is anticipated that the demand for the newer and more sophisticated imaging techniques will increase.

REFERENCES

1. Brattstrom H: Shape of the intercondylar groove normally and in recurrent dislocation of patella. *Acta Orthop* 68(suppl):134, 1964.
2. Dowd GSE, Bentley G: Radiographic assessment in patellar instability and chondromalacia patellae. *J Bone Joint Surg* 68B:297, 1986.
3. Blackburne J, Peel T: A new method of measuring patellar height. *J Bone Joint Surg* 58B:241, 1977.
4. Ficat RP, Phillipe J, Hungerford DS: Chondromalacia patellae: A system of classification. *Clin Orthop* 144:55, 1979.
5. Insall J, Salvati E: Patella position in the normal knee joint. *Radiology* 101:101, 1971.
6. Laurin CA, Dussault R, Levesque HP: The tangential x-ray investigation of the patellofemoral joint: X-ray technique, diagnostic criteria and their interpretation. *Clin Orthop* 144:16, 1979.
7. Malghem J, Maldague B: Patellofemoral joint 30 degree axial radiograph with lateral rotation of the leg. *Radiology* 170:566, 1989.
8. Merchant AC, Mercer RL, Jacobsen RH, et al: Roentgenographic analysis of patellofemoral congruence. *J Bone Joint Surg* 56A:1391, 1974.
9. Minkoff J, Fein L: The role of radiography in the evaluation and treatment of common anarthritic disorders of the patellofemoral joint. *Clin Sports Med* 8:203, 1989.
10. Wiberg G: Roentgenographic and anatomic studies on the femoro-patellar joint. With special reference to chondromalacia patellae. *Acta Orthop Scand* 12:319, 1941.
11. Carson WGJ, James SL, Larson RL, et al: Patellofemoral disorders: Physical and radiographic evaluation. Part II. Radiographic examination. *Clin Orthop* 185:178, 1984.
12. Moller BN, Krebs B, Jurik AG: Patellofemoral incongruence in chondromalacia and instability of the patella. *Acta Orthop Scand* 57:232, 1986.
13. Merchant AC: Classification of patellofemoral disorders. *Arthroscopy* 4:235, 1988.
14. Bentley G, Dowd G, Orth MC: Current concepts of etiology and treatment of chondromalacia patellae. *Clin Orthop* 189:209, 1984.
15. Bradley WG, Ominsky SH: Mountain view of the patella. *AJR* 136:53, 1981.
16. Hille E, Schulitz, KP: Rotational instability of the patella on radiographic images. *Arch Orthop Trauma Surg* 104:74, 1985.
17. Egund N: The axial view of the patello-femoral joint. *Acta Radiol* 27:101, 1986.
18. Merchant AC: Patellofemoral malalignment and instabilities, in *Articular Cartilage and Knee Joint Function: Basic Science and Arthroscopy,* edited by JW Ewing. New York, Raven Press, 1990, pp 79–91.
19. Sartoris D, Resnick D: Plain film radiography: Routine and specialized techniques and projections, in *Diagnosis of Bone and Joint Disorders,* 2d ed, edited by D Resnick, G. Newayama. Philadelphia, Saunders, 1988, pp 2–54.
20. Ficat RP, Hungerford DS: *Disorders of the Patellofemoral Joint.* Baltimore, Williams & Wilkins, 1977.

21. Teitge RA: Radiology of the patellofemoral joint. *Orthopedic Surgery Update Series*, 3, 1985.

22. Fulkerson JP, Hungerford DS: *Disorders of the Patellofemoral Joint*. 2d ed. Baltimore, Williams & Wilkins, 1990.

23. Kujala UM, Osterman K, Kormano M, et al: Patellofemoral relationships in recurrent patellar dislocation. *Radiology* 175:886, 1990.

24. Boven F, Belleman MA, Geurts J, et al: The value of computed tomography scanning in chondromalacia patella. *Skeletal Radiol* 8:183, 1982.

25. Delgado-Martins H: A study of the position of the patella using computerized tomography. *J Bone Joint Surg* 61:443, 1979.

26. Fulkerson JP, Schutzer SF, Ramsby GR, et al: Computerized tomography of the patellofemoral joint before and after lateral release or realignment. *Arthroscopy* 3:19, 1987.

27. Schutzer SF, Ramsby GR, Fulkerson JP: Computed tomographic classification of patellofemoral pain patients. *Orthop Clin North Am* 17:235, 1986.

28. Shellock FG, Mink JH, Fox JM: Patellofemoral joint: Kinematic MR imaging to assess tracking abnormalities. *Radiology* 168:551, 1988.

29. Kujala UM, Osterman K, Kormano M, et al: Patellar motion analyzed by magnetic resonance imaging. *Acta Orthop Scand* 60:13, 1989.

30. Martinez S, Korobkin M, Fondren FB, et al: A device for computed tomography of the patellofemoral joint. *AJR* 140:400, 1983.

31. Weissman BN, Sledge CB: The knee, edited by BN Weissman, CB Sledge. *Orthopedic Radiology*, Philadelphia, Saunders, 1986, pp 497–587.

32. Resnick D, Niwayama G: Anatomy of individul joint, in *Diagnosis of Bone and Joint Disorders*, edited by D Resnick, G Newayama. Philadelphia, Saunders, 1988, pp 647–755.

33. Harrison RB, Woods MB, Keats TE: The grooves of the distal articular surface of the femur—a normal variant. *AJR* 126:751, 1976.

34. Blumensaat C: Die Lageabweichungen und Verrunkungen der Kneischeibe. *Ergeg Chir Orthop* 31:149, 1938.

35. Boven F, Bellemans MA, Geurts J, et al: Comparative study of the patello-femoral joint on axial roentgenogram, axial arthrogram, and computer tomography following arthrography. *Skeletal Radiol* 8:179, 1982.

36. Inoue M, Shino K, Hirose H, et al: Subluxation of the patella: Computed tomography analysis of patellofemoral congruence. *J Bone Joint Surg* 70A:1331, 1988.

37. Hehne HJ: Biomechanics of the patellofemoral joint and its clinical relevance. *Clin Orthop* 258:73, 1990.

38. Malghem J, Maldague B: Correspondence. *J Bone Joint Surg* 71A:1575, 1989.

39. Hennsge J: Arthrosis deformans des patella gleitweges. *Zentabl Chir* 32:1381, 1962.

40. Aglietti P, Insall JN: Patellar pain and incongruence. *Clin Orthop* 176:217, 1983.

41. Schutzer SF, Ramsby GR, Fulkerson JP: The evaluation of patellofemoral pain using computerized tomography. A preliminary study. *Clin Orthop* 204:286, 1986.

42. Fulkerson JP, Schutzer SF: After failure of conservative treatment for painful patellofemoral malalignment: Lateral release or realignment? *Orthop Clin* 17:283, 1986.

43. Stanford W, Phelan J, Kathol MH, et al: Patellofemoral joint motion: Evaluation by ultrafast computed tomography. *Skeletal Radiol* 17:487, 1988.

44. Resnick D, Niwayama G: *Diagnosis of Bone and Joint Disorders*. 2d ed. Philadelphia, Saunders, 1988.

45. Deutsch AL, Herfkens RJ: Technical consideration in musculoskeletal MRI, in *MRI of the Musculoskeletal System: A Teaching File*, edited by JH Mink, AL Deutsch. New York, Raven Press, 1990.

46. Crues JV, Shellock FG: Technical consideration, in *Magnetic Resonance Imaging of the Knee*, edited by JH Mink. New York, Raven Press, 1987.

47. Haacke E: Image behavior: Resolution, signal-to-noise, contrast and artifacts, in *Magnetic Resonance Imaging of the Spine*, edited by M Modic, T Masaryk Chicago, Mosby Year Book Medical Publishers, 1989, pp 1–34.

48. Mitchell DG, Burk DL Jr, Vinitski S, Rifkin MD: The biophysical basis of tissue contrast in extracranial MR imaging. *AJR* 149:831, 1987.

49. Mink JH, Deutsch A: The knee, in *MRI of the Musculoskeletal System: A Teaching File*, edited by JH Mink, AL Deutsch. New York, Raven Press, 1990.

50. Gylys-Morin VM, Hajek PC, Sartoris DJ, et al: Articular cartilage defects: Detectability in cadaver knees with MR. *AJR* 148:1153, 1987.

51. Konig H, Sauter R, Deimling M, et al: Cartilage disorders: Comparison of spin-echo, CHESS and FLASH sequence MR images. *Radiology* 164:753, 1987.

52. Reiser MF, Bongartz G, Erlemann R, et al: Magnetic resonance in cartilaginous lesions of knee joint with three-dimensional gradient-echo imaging. *Skeletal Radiol* 17:465, 1988.

53. Yulish BS, Montanez J, Goodfellow DB, et al: Chondromalacia patella: Assessment with MR imaging. *Radiology* 164:763, 1987.

54. Handleberg F, Shahabpour M, Castelyn PP: Chondral lesions of the patella evaluated with computed tomography, magnetic resonance imaging, and arthroscopy. *J Arthroscopy* 6:24, 1990.

55. Hayes CW, Sawyer RW, Conway WF: Patellar cartilage lesions: In vitro detection and staging with ME imaging and pathologic correlation. *Radiology* 176:479, 1990.

56. Wojtys E, Wilson M, Buchwalter K, et al: Magnetic resonance imaging of knee hyaline cartilage and intraarticualr pathology. *Am J Sports Med* 15:455, 1987.

57. Mankin HJ: The water of articular cartilage, in *The Human Joints in Health and Disease,* edited by WH Simon. Philadelphia, University of Pennsylvania Press, 1978, pp 37–42.

58. Buckwalter JA, Rosenberg LC, Hunziker EB. Articular cartilage: Comparison, structure, response to injury, and methods of facilitating repairs, in *Articular Cartilage and Knee Joint Function: Basic Science and Arthroscopy,* edited by JW Ewing. New York, Raven Press, 1990, pp 19–54.

59. Kempson GE: The mechanical properties of articular cartilage, in *The Joints and Synovial Fluid,* edited by R Sokoloff. New York, Academic Press, 1980, pp. 177–238.

60. Buckwalter JA: Articular Cartilage. American Academy of Orthopaedic Surgeons Instructional Course lectures. St. Louis, Mosby, pp. 349–370, 1983.

61. Schnenck RK, Eggli PS, Hunziker EB: Articular cartilagemorphology, in *Articular Cartilage Biochemistry,* edited by KE Kuettner, R Schleyerback, VC Hascall. New York, Raven Press, 1986, pp 3–22.

62. Poole CA, Flint MH, Beaumont BW: Morphological and functional interrelationships of articular cartilage matrices. *J Anat* 138:13, 1984.

63. Lehner KB, Rechl HP, Gmeinwieser JK, et al: Structure, function, and degeneration of bovine hyaline cartilage: Assessment with MR imagining in vitro. *Radiology* 170:495, 1989.

64. Ohno O, Naito J, Iguchi T, et al: An electron microscopic study of early pathology in chondromalacia of the patella [see comments]. *J Bone Joint Surg* 70A:883, 1988.

65. Mankin HJ: The response of articular cartilage to mechanical injury. *J Bone Joint Surg* 64A:460, 1982.

66. Mankin H: Current concepts review: The response of articular cartilage to mechanical injury. *J Bone Joint Surg* 64A:460, 1982.

67. Goodfellow J, Hungerford DS, Woods C: Patello-femoral joint mechanics and pathology. II: Chondromalacia patella. *J Bone Joint Surg* 58B:291, 1976.

68. Shahriaree H: Chondromalacia. *Contemp Orthop* 11:27, 1985.

69. Goodfellow JW, Hungerford DS, Zindel M: Patello-femoral joint mechanics and pathology: I: Functional anatomy of the patello-femoral joint. *J Bone Joint Surg* 58B:287, 1976.

70. Outerbridge RE: The etiology of chondromalacia patellae. *J Bone Joint Surg,* 43B:752, 1961.

71. Outerbridge RE: Further studies on the etiology of chondromalacia patellae. *J Bone Joint Surg* 46B:179, 1964.

72. Noyes FR, Stabler CL: A system for grading articular cartilage lesions at arthroscopy. *Am J Sports Med* 17:505, 1989.

73. Shahriaree H: Chondromalacia patellae, in *O'Connor's Textbook of Arthroscopic Surgery,* edited by EP Lowe. Philadelphia, Lippincott 1984, pp 237–262.

74. Insall J, Falvo KA, Wise DW: Chondromalacia patellae. A prospective study. *J Bone Joint Surg* 58A:1, 1976.

75. Deutsch AL, Fox J, Mink JH: MR imaging of chondromalacia patella (submitted for publication), 1991.

76. Shellock FG, Mandelbaum B: Kinematic MRI of the joints, in *MRI of the Musculoskeletal System. A Teaching File,* edited by JH Mink, AL Deutsch. New York, Raven Press, 1990.

77. Shellock FG, Mink JH, Deutsch AL, et al: Evaluation of patellar tracking abnormalities using kinematic MR imaging. Clinical experience in 130 patients. *Radiology* 172:799, 1989.

78. Shellock FG, Mink JH, Deutsch AL: Kinematic MRI of the joints. *Mag Res Q* 1991, in press.

79. Larson RL: Subluxation-dislocation of the patella, in *The Injured Adolescent Knee,* edited by JC Kennedy. Baltimore, Williams & Wilkins, 1979, pp 161–204.

80. Shellock FG, Mink JH, Deutsch AL, et al: Kinematic magnetic resonance imaging for evaluation of patellar tracking. *Physician Sports Med,* 17:99, 1989.

81. Kujala U: Knee injuries in athletics. *Sports Med* 3:447, 1986.

82. Shellock FG, Mink JH, Fox JM, et al: Kinematic MRI evaluation of symptomatic patients following two or three patellar realignment surgeries. *JMRI* 1991, in press.

83. Shellock FG, Deutsch AL, Mink JH, et al: Identification of medial subluxation of the patella in a dancer using kinematic MRI of the patellofemoral joint: A case report. *Kinesiology Med for Dance* 1991, in press.

84. Shellock FG, Mink JH, Deutsch AL, et al: Evaluation in patients with persistent symptoms after lateral retinacular release by kinematic magnetic resonance imaging of the patellofemoral joint. *Arthroscopy* 6:226, 1990.

85. Kujala U: Knee exertion injuries in adolescents and young adults. A study with special reference to anatomic predisposition. Publications of the Social Insurance Institution, 64, 1986.

86. Nordin M, Frankel VH: *Basic Biomechanics of the Musculoskeletal System.* 2d ed. Philadelphia, Lea & Febiger, 1989.

87. Insall J, Falvo KA, Wise DW: Patellar pain and incongruence. II: Clinical application. *Clin Orthop* 176:225, 1983.

88. Hughston J, Deese M: Medial subluxation of the patella as a complication of lateral retinacular release. *Am J Sports Med* 16:383, 1988.

89. DeHaven KE, Solan WA, Mayer PJ: Chondromalacia patellae in athletes. Clinical presentation and conservative management. *J Sports Med* 7:5, 1979.

90. Haake EM, Tkach JA: Fast MR imaging: Techniques and clinical applications. *AJR* 155:951, 1990.

91. Foo TKF, Bernstein MA, Holsinger AE, et al: Ultra-fast spoiled gradient recalled (SPGR) image acquisition. *Society of Magnetic Resonance in Medicine, Book of Abstracts* 1:1308, 1990.

92. Shellock FG, Foo T, Mink JH: Dynamic imaging of the joints by ultrafast MRI techniques. *Proc Eur Cong Radiol* 1991, in press.

93. Shellock FG, Cohen MS, Brady T, et al: Evaluation of patellar alignment and tracking: Comparison between kinematic MRI and true dynamic imaging by hyperscan MR. *JMRI* 1991, in press.

94. Shellock FG, Foo TK, Deutsch AL, et al: Evaluation of the patellofemoral joint during active flexion by ultra-fast spoiled GRASS MR imaging. *Radiology* 1991 (submitted).

95. Siwek CW, Rao JP: Ruptures of the extensor mechanism of the knee joint. *J Bone Joint Surg* [*AM*] 63A:932–937, 1981.

96. Larsen E, Lund PM: Ruptures of the extensor mechanism of the knee joint. Clinical results and patellofemoral articulation. *Clin Orthop* 213:150, 1986.

97. Nance EPJ, Kaye JJ: Injuries of the quadriceps mechanism. *Radiology* 142:301, 1982.

98. Mac Eachern AG, Plewes PL: Bilateral simultaneous spontaneous rupture of the quadriceps tendons. Five case reports and a review of the literature. *J Bone Joint Surg* 66:81, 1984.

99. Chekofsky KM, Spero CR, Scott WN: A method of repair of the late quadriceps rupture. *Clin Orthop* 147:190, 1980.

100. Jelaso DV, Morris GA: Rupture of the quadriceps tendons: Diagnosis by arthroscopy. *Radiology* 116:621, 1975.

101. Cash JD, Hughston JC: Treatment of acute patellar dislocation. *Am J Sports Med* 16:244, 1988.

102. Hawkins RJ, Bell RH, Anisette G: Acute patellar dislocations. *Am J Sports Med* 14:117, 1986.

103. Aprin H, Broukhim B: Early diagnosis of acute rupture of the quadriceps tendon by arthrography. *Clin Orthop* 195:185, 1985.

104. Resnick D: Arthrography, tonography, and bursography, in *Diagnosis of Bone and Joint Disorders,* edited by D Resnick, G Niwayama. Philadelphia, Saunders, 1988.

105. Kricun R, Kricun ME, Arangio GA, et al: Patellar tendon rupture with underlying systemic disease. *AJR* 135:507, 1980.

106. Mourad K, King J, Guggiana P: Computed tomography and ultrasound imaging of jumper's knee-patellar tendinitis. *Clin Radiol* 39:162, 1988.

107. Richardson ML, Selby B, Montana MA, et al: Ultrasonography of the knee. *Radiol Clin North Am* 26:63, 1988.

108. Fornage BD, Rifkin MD: Ultrasound examination of tendons. *Radiol Clin North Am* 26:87, 1988.

109. Dillehay GL, Deschler T, Rogers LF, et al: The ultrasonographic characterization of tendons. *Invest Radiol* 19:338, 1984.

110. Fornage BD, Rifkin MD, Touche DH, et al: Sonography of the patellar tendon: Preliminary observations. *AJR* 149:179, 1984.

111. Laine HR, Harjula A, Peltokallio P: Ultrasound in the evaluation of the knee and patellar regions. *J Ultrasound Med* 6:33, 1987.

112. Gould ES, Taylor S, Naidich JB, et al: MR appearance of bilateral, spontaneous patellar tendon rupture in systemic lupus erythematosus. *J Comput Assist Tomogr* [*Am*] 11:1096, 1987.

113. Blazina M, Kerlan R, Jobe F, et al: Jumper's knee. *Orthop Clin North Am.* 4:665, 1973.

114. Bodne D, Quinn S, Murray W, et al: Magnetic resonance imaging of chronic patellar tendinitis. *Skeletal Radiol* 17:24, 1988.

115. Lance E, Deutsch AL, Mink JH: MR imaging of patella dislocation. Radiology 1991 (submitted).

116. Patel D: Arthroscopy of the plical-synovial folds and their significance. *Am J Sports Med* 6:217, 1978.

117. Deutsch AL, Resnick D, Dalinka MK, et al. Synovia plicae of the knee. *Radiology* 141:627, 1981.

118. Alazraki N: Radionuclide techniques, in *Diagnosis of Bone and Joint Disorders*, 2d ed, edited by D Resnick, G Niwayama. Philadelphia, Saunders, 1988, pp 460–505.

119. Holder LE: Clinical radionuclide bone imaging. *Radiology* 176:607, 1990.

120. Dye S, Boll D: Radionuclide imaging of the patellofemoral joint in young adults with anterior knee pain. *Orthop Clin* 17:249, 1986.

121. Hejgaard N, Diemer H: Bone scan in the patellofemoral pain syndrome. *Int Orthop* 11:29, 1987.
122. Fogelman I, McKillip JH, Gray HW: The "hot patella" sign: Is it any clinical significance? Concise communication. *J Nucl Med* 24:312, 1982.
123. Kozin F, Soin JS, Ryan LM, et al: Bone scintigraphy in the reflex sympathetic dystrophy syndrome. *Radiology* 138:437, 1981.
124. Tietjen R: Reflex sympathetic dystrophy of the knee. *Clin Orthop* 209:234, 1986.

CHAPTER 6

Patellofemoral Disorders in Children

Lyle J. Micheli

INTRODUCTION

Disorders of the patellofemoral joint are frequently encountered in the care of children and adolescents. The pediatrician, pediatric orthopaedist, or physician dealing with athletically active children must have a clear understanding of the etiology of these disorders and, in particular, steps that may be taken early to minimize symptoms and to prevent progression of tissue injury and anatomic derangement. A number of different classifications of patellofemoral disorders have been proposed. The most recent attempt to unify these classifications was that of Alan Merchant in 1988.[1] The focus of his classification is that of disorders encountered in physically active individuals (Table 6-1). Thus, there is no discussion of congential disorders or disorders of the patellofemoral mechanism related to genetic conditions, such as Down syndrome or nail–patella syndrome.

Merchant has divided the traumatic disorders into two broad classifications: painful conditions resulting from trauma in otherwise normal knees and painful conditions occurring in individuals with evidence of patellofemoral dysplasia. He has used further subdivisions of idiopathic chondromalacia patella and has classed osteochondritis dissecans separately, presumably because of the lack of consensus at this time on its etiology, and has similarly placed synovial plica in a separate classification.

Although this is a useful structure and framework for helping to understand painful patellofemoral disorders, we have also included a discussion of conditions such as neoplasm and special problems encountered in children, such as dysfunction of the patellofemoral mechanism in association with below-knee amputation and prosthetic treatment to this structure.

We will therefore divide our discussion of these disorders in pediatric and adolescent patients into congenital disorders or those that occur in association with defined genetic syndromes; acquired conditions, either as a result of repetitive microtrauma, acute trauma, or direct sequela of either of these mechanisms; and, finally, certain other rare conditions that may present as patellofemoral pain in this age group.

CONGENITAL AND GENETIC DISORDERS

Congenital disorders are defined as conditions present and detectable at birth. This strict definition has been modified in certain situations in which the clinical detection of the abnormality, because of difficulties in diagnosis, is not made for some years. We have included conditions present at birth and those diagnosed then or within the first decade of life. This expanded definition can be justified with disorders of the patellofemoral mechanism because detection at birth of frank dislocation of the patellofemoral mechanism is often not possible.

Ossification of the patella usually begins in the third year and is often well advanced by late in the fourth year of life.[2] However, in certain conditions, ossification may be delayed into the adolescent period. Newer imaging techniques, such as magnetic resonance imaging (MRI), may indeed aid in early diagnosis if derangements of the extensor mechanism are suspected at birth or in the neonatal period.

Stanisavljevic and colleagues[3] have suggested dividing congenital dislocations of the patella into those that are permanent and irreducible versus those that show a dislocatable or unstable patellofemoral mechanism at birth. They have suggested that the etiology of this condition is due to failure of internal rotation of the myotome, which contains the quadriceps femoris and patella in the fetus. In their initial report on this condition and survey of the literature, they recommended an operative intervention that has as its foundation a subperiosteal dissection of the quadriceps mechanism off the femur and a complete medial displacement of the entire quadriceps mechanism on the femur. They suggested that other procedures recommended for this early derangement, which were patterned after the initial description by Goldthwaite in 1889[4], were inadequate because they only addressed the patella itself.

They recommended early intervention in particular before associated anatomic abnormalities such as genu valgum and external rotation of the tibia became severe and rendered treatment much more difficult. It is noteworthy that in this initial report of seven knees operated in six patients, four of the children were afflicted with Down syndrome.[3]

TABLE 6-1

Classification of Patellofemoral Disorders[1]

I.   Trauma (conditions caused by trauma in the otherwise normal knee)
    A.   Acute trauma
        1.   Contusion (hematoma)
        2.   Fracture
            a.   Patella (bipartite)
            b.   Femoral trochlea
            c.   Proximal tibial epiphysis (tubercle)
        3.   Patellar dislocation
        4.   Rupture
            a.   Quadriceps tendon
            b.   Patellar tendon
    B.   Repetitive trauma (overuse syndromes)
        1.   Patellar tendinitis (jumper's knee)
        2.   Quadriceps tendinitis
        3.   Peripatellar tendinitis (anterior knee pain of adolescence due to hamstring contracture)
        4.   Peripatellar bursitis
        5.   Apophysitis
            a.   Osgood-Schlatter disease
            b.   Sinding-Larsen-Johansson disease
    C.   Late effects trauma
        1.   Posttraumatic chondromalacia patellae
        2.   Posttraumatic patellofemoral arthritis
        3.   Anterior fat-pad syndrome (posttraumatic fibrosis)
        4.   Reflex sympathetic dystrophy of the patella
        5.   Patellar osseous dystrophy
        6.   Acquired patella infera
        7.   Acquired quadriceps fibrosis

II. Patellofemoral Dysplasia
    A.   Lateral patellar compression syndrome
        1.   Secondary chondromalacia patellae
        2.   Secondary patellofemoral arthritis
    B.   Chronic subluxation of the patella
        1.   Secondary chondromalacia patellae
        2.   Secondary chondromalacia arthritis
    C.   Recurrent dislocation of the patella
        1.   Associated fractures
            a.   Osteochondral (intra-articular)
            b.   Avulsion (extra-articular)
        2.   Secondary chondromalacia patellae
        3.   Secondary patellofemoral arthritis
    D.   Chronic dislocation of the patella
        1.   Congenital
        2.   Acquired

III. Idiopathic chondromalacia patellae

IV. Osteochondritis dissecans
    A.   Patella
    B.   Femoral trochlea

V.   Synovial plicae
    A.   Medial patellar (shelf)
    B.   Suprapatellar
    C.   Infrapatellar
    D.   Lateral patellar

Careful evaluation of knee motion with particular attention to loss of full knee flexion and evidence of early valgus and external rotation is mandatory. Although congenital dislocation of the extensor mechanism is often associated with babies having other stigmata of genetic derangement, it may exist as a totally independent entity in the otherwise normal child.[5]

The second congenital condition noted in the literature is that of duplication of the patellofemoral mechanism. This duplication most commonly exists in the sagittal plane and is totally consistent with normal function. Rarely, there have been reports of duplication in the coronal plane and reports of centralization of the more structurally dominant mechanism with resection realignment of the lesser one.[6,7]

There is a relatively high incidence of clinically significant derangement of the patellofemoral joint in Down syndrome. Dugdale and Renshaw[8] reported an 8.3 percent incidence in their review of 210 institutionalized patients with Down syndrome and 151 noninstitutionalized patients. They concluded in their review that although instability of the patellofemoral joint was relatively prevalent in Down syndrome, it was rarely disabling. Only eight knees seen in their series have been operated on and they felt this was an inadequate number on which to base surgical recommendations. They noted, however, that four knees operated on with an average follow-up of 15 years following surgery, had satisfactory results.

Mendez and colleagues[9] found that 20 of 252 patients with Down syndrome were hospitalized with the chief complaint of severe patellofemoral instability. They noted that no apparent correlation existed between instability of the patellofemoral joint of these patients and clinical function. They further noted, however, that a definite correlation occurred between the severity of fixed patellofemoral dislocation and the development of subsequent deformities including genu valgum, external tibial torsion, and flexion contractures about the knee. They recommended operative intervention for patients with Down syndrome who have a clear functional disability, such as frequent falls, but have not yet developed significant deformities. Late attempts to correct dislocated patellofemoral mechanism in this group when these deformities have already occurred have, in general, been unsuccessful.

The role of exercises to help balance the patellofemoral mechanism in this population group is relatively limited. In addition, patellar stabilizing braces are often not well tolerated. Conversely, some reports have noted satisfactory functional response to the use of full-length bracing in children with dislocated patellae and the associated deformities of genu valgum and external tibial rotation, which increase the knee instability.

Hereditary onyco-osteodysplasia, or nail–patella syndrome, is a another genetic disorder in which derangement of the patellofemoral mechanism may be prominent at presentation. This condition has now been identified as an autosomal dominant genetic disorder of incomplete penetrance but with variable expressivity and marked pleomorphism. This condition involves multiple systems, often with abnormalities in the hands or feet. Other characteristics include hypoplasia of the lateral aspect of the elbow, iliac horns at the anterosuperior iliac spine, often first diagnosed radiographically, and absence or hypoplasia of the patellae. The radiographic abnormalities of the patella include an ovoid or triangular shape and patella baja. Interestingly, disability from the patellofemoral abnormalities have rarely been noted in the literature, despite the prominence of this finding in the presentation of the syndrome as a whole.[10]

The fourth congenital syndrome in which patellofemoral findings may be prominent is that of dysplasia epiphysialis multiplex, or multiple epiphyseal dysplasia syndrome. This syndrome was first described by Fairbank in 1935.[11] Mansoor reviewed a series of eight cases in 1970, half of which had patellar abnormalities and disorders of the knee including loose bodies.[12] This syndrome is characterized by involvement of multiple epiphyses with associated dwarfism. In 1982, Dahners and colleagues reported the resection of a portion of a double-layer patella found in this syndrome.[6] The patellofemoral mechanism was successfully realigned after resection of the dysplastic lateral half of the mechanism.

Although there may be a hereditary aspect to some patients presenting with maltracking and dysplasia of the patellofemoral mechanism, the consensus is that these conditions are usually multifactorial. Constitutional factors, such as generalized ligamentous laxity, femoral anteversion, genu valgum, tibial vara, and pes planus, may indeed increase the likelihood of patellofemoral derangements; however, it is the interaction of these anatomic risk factors, some of which may be developmental, and the multiplicity of other intrinsic and extrinsic factors that usually result in patellofemoral pain or dysfunction occurring and becoming symptomatic (Table 6-2).

ACUTE TRAUMA

Acute trauma of the patellofemoral mechanism includes fractures of the patella, trochlea groove, or

TABLE 6-2

Risk Factors for Overuse Injury

Training error
Muscle–tendon imbalance
Anatomic malalignment
Footwear
Playing surface
Associated disease state
Nutritional factors
Cultural deconditioning
Growth factors

the tibial insertion; acute patellar dislocation; and ruptures of the quadriceps or patellar tendons.

The child or adolescent presenting with knee pain, disability, and swelling with a history of an acute blow, fall, or twist, must be carefully assessed for a variety of etiologies, including that of ligamentous disruption, internal derangement, physeal fracture of the distal femoral and proximal tibial physis, and, certainly, derangements of the extensor mechanism. History is extremely important in helping to sort this differential diagnosis. Often there is a history of a direct blow to the knee from a fall or a blow to the side of the patellofemoral joint from objects such as an opponent's stick or helmet. The child may also give a history of having a sense that the knee was out of place and then "popped" back into place or may have observed that the "knee cap looked funny."

Careful physical examination is essential even in the face of a large knee effusion or hemarthrosis. Tenderness localized to the medial retinaculum in particular or an abnormal appearance or abnormal location by palpation of the patella may also be indications of an extensor mechanism disruption.

Radiographs can be helpful in making a diagnosis. Abnormalities of patellar integrity or position and associated fractures of the trochlear margin or patella may be evident. Newer imaging techniques have been extremely helpful in diagnosing these disorders. Previously undetected osteochondral injury to the trochlear groove in particular may be evident by MRI or computed tomography (CT) scan.[13] Unfortunately, in many cases patellofemoral dislocation may have no salient indicators on history, physical examination, or imaging techniques. It must still remain high on the diagnostic scale in any child presenting with a history of acute knee injury and hemarthrosis, where disruption of the cruciate ligaments is less likely.[14]

Despite our advances in imaging techniques, arthroscopy may be imperative to diagnose or help confirm the diagnosis of an acute medial retinacular disruption or of osteochondral injury of the trochlear groove. In two instances, we have discovered large osteochondral fractures in this age group, which we treated successfully by replacement and *in situ* pinning. Neither diagnosis was made despite preoperative radiographic and MRI imaging of the knees.

Traumatic fractures of the patella, as seen in the adult, are not encountered in this population. Diebold found that only 1 percent of patellar fractures involve patients under 15 years of age in his series.[15] Although rare, careful radiographs must be obtained, even in a child as young as 2 years, to rule out the possibility of patellar fracture. If displacement of the fracture fragments is evident, open reduction is indicated. Belman and colleagues reported a case of transverse fracture of the patella in an 11-year old boy following a direct blow to the knee.[16] Surgical exploration revealed the fragments to be separated by a portion of the retropatellar articular cartilage.

The sleeve fracture is a patellar fracture unique to children. An extensive sleeve of cartilage and capsule may be avulsed from the main body of the osseus patella, sometimes with only a small fragment of bone evident radiographically. The functional result is a patellar tendon avulsion analogous to a tibial spine avulsion. Houghton and Ackroyd reported on three cases and recommended open reduction and surgical repair.[17]

Avulsion fractures of the tibial tuberosity have been most commonly reported in boys between the ages of 14 and 16 years. These avulsions were originally described by Watson-Jones and more recently reclassified by Ogden into the three major classes based on the site and size of the fragment and the extent of involvement of the articular surface of the tibial proximal.[18]

Treatment of this injury involves mechanical restoration of the fragment in its bed and immobilization sufficient to allow bony healing. Because this injury occurs near the end of physeal growth, premature growth arrest rarely occurs, although some authors have suggested that genu recurvature may be a potential complication.[19]

Marginal fractures of the patella, either of the inferior pole or lateral portions, have been reported in children. Some confusion has occurred, however, when a marginal fragment is noted radiographically and classed as an accessory ossification center or bipartite patellae by the radiologist, yet the clinician caring for the child notes that this site is painful and tender, suggesting a traumatic origin of the anomaly rather than a developmental one.

Green first reported three cases of painful bipartite patellae in 1975 and reported complete recovery by excision of the accessory ossification center.[20]

In 1977 Weaver reported data on 21 cases of athletically active individuals with activity-related pain, pain with pressure over the patella, or painful catching or swelling, who all had bipartite patellae radiographically.[21] Sixteen of these 21 patients were treated by excision of the accessory fragment with complete relief of symptoms. He further noted that the 5 who had not had surgery all still had pain when training vigorously, but not enough for them to consider surgery.

He noted that the incidence of bipartite patellae in the population at large is estimated to be 2 percent to 3 percent and that given the population of his area of practice, one would have expected 2000 people with radiographic evidence of bipartite patellae. He therefore suggested that less than 2 percent of patients with bipartite patellae suffer pain and disability, the majority of these, apparently, in association with athletic activities and possible superimposed athletic trauma.

Prior to Weaver's report in 1977, most authorities looked on accessory or bipartite patellae as a normal variant unrelated to knee symptoms.

An anatomic classification of patellar abnormalities based on radiographic appearance has been proposed by Saupe (Fig. 6-1)[22] This includes lesions of the distal patellar pole (type I), lateral margin (type II), and supralateral pole (type III). Although Weaver noted that all of his symptomatic cases were of type III,[21] it has been our experience that patients may present with pain-related type I lesions also. This has also been the experience of Schmidt and Henry.[23]

Ogden and colleagues reviewed data on a series of children with painful bipartite patellae and suggested that the etiology of the type III lesion might represent a chondralosseus disruption secondary to chronic stress and, in effect, represent a chronic stress fracture of the patella that then renders it more susceptible to injury (Fig. 6-2)[24].

OVERUSE INJURY OF THE EXTENSOR MECHANISM

As with acute injuries, disorders of the patellofemoral mechanism must play a prominent part in the differential diagnosis of knee pain of gradual onset

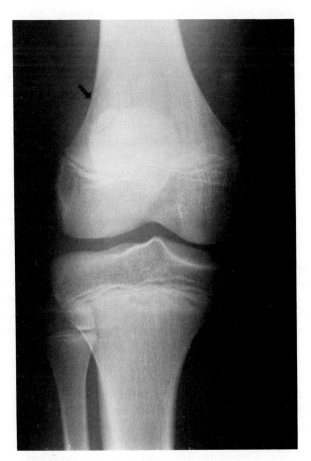

FIGURE 6-2
Typical radiograph of a type III bipartite patellae in an adolescent. This child was symptomatic and ultimately required resection.

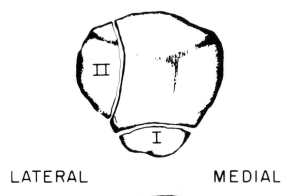

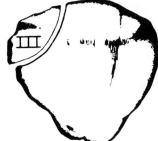

LATERAL   MEDIAL

FIGURE 6-1
Saupe's classification of bipartite patellae.[20]

in children and adolescents. Consistent with Merchant's overview of patellofemoral disorders, it is useful to divide overuse injuries of the extensor mechanism that occur primarily independent of alignment or constitutional mechanical characteristics from those that appear to be primarily associated with mechanical derangements of the extensor mechanism or in which anatomic malalignment plays a predominant part.[1] In the former category are included Osgood-Schlatter disease, Sinding-Larsen-Johansson disease, and osteochondritis dissecans of the patella or trochlea groove. In addition, and although relatively uncommon in this age group, tendinitis of the quadriceps insertion of the patella and of the patellar tendon itself may be encountered.

An adolescent complaining of low-grade aching pain associated with activity, insidious in onset, and localized to the area of the tibial tubercle most probably has Osgood-Schlatter disease. This condition, the most common traction apophysitis, was independently noted by Osgood and Schlatter in 1903.[25,26] In Osgood's original paper, entitled "Lesions of the tibial tubercle appearing during adolescence," he hypothesized trauma as the etiology of this condition, as did Schlatter. More recently, Ogden has provided anatomic evidence that suggests repetitive microtrauma to the tubercle at the time of formation of the secondary ossification center as the most probable explanation for the occurrence of this entity.[27] His anatomic dissections provide histologic evidence of repetitive healing and avulsion at the tubercle, resulting in bone and cartilage accretion and formation of a prominent tibial tubercle, characteristic of the full-blown condition.

The association between this condition and sports activity during adolescence is well known. Kujala and colleagues found an incidence of Osgood-Schlatter disease of 21.2 percent in athletically active boys, whereas the nonathletic controls had an incidence of 4.5 percent.[28]

It has been our experience that the population affected by this condition is changing, as more and more girls are also participating in repetitive sports training, particularly in sports such as gymnastics or soccer. Whereas formerly the typical patient was an athletically active boy, aged 13 or 14 years, we now have a second population developing this condition: athletically active girls, aged 10 or 11 years. The 10- or 11-year old girl, of course, is at a stage of skeletal maturation equivalent to that of the 13- or 14-year old boy. Therefore, this presentation is expected.

A child with this condition will usually demonstrate a tender tibial tubercle, often with an obvious bony and cartilaginous prominence, pain on resisted extension of the knee from the 90 degree flexed position, and a positive Ely test, reflecting quadriceps contracture. Quadriceps atrophy may also be present, with decreased thigh circumference.

Assessment should include anteroposterior and lateral radiographs. These radiographs are done to rule out other conditions such as neoplasms or infections. Lateral radiographs may demonstrate simple prominence of the bony portion of the tubercle, fragmentation of the ossific nucleus, or a free bony fragment proximal to the tubercle.

Management of the child with Osgood-Schlatter disease is individualized and depends on the severity of symptoms. Because we believe that the primary factor in the etiology of this condition is a tight quadriceps, which then becomes weak with onset of pain, our primary emphasis is directed to therapeutic exercises to restore the strength and flexibility of the lower extremity musculature, with particular emphasis on the quadriceps.

The cornerstone of our management program is a progressive resistive straight leg raising exercise program with three sets of ten repetitions performed with each leg. Resistance is increased to the level of 12 lb, so long as the child is able to progress without pain or quadriceps lag. Three sets of ten repetitions are our usual protocol.

Knee braces may also be useful in managing this condition, allowing the child to play with reduced pain while strength and flexibility are returning. These braces can be simple because their primary function is to prevent direct mechanical impact to the tubercle.

Activity limitation may be necessary in some cases although most children can continue to pursue sports or other activities without difficulty. Rarely, a child may be so symptomatic that immobilization or crutch support may be required. We prefer a three- or four-point crutch gait, which will enable the child to continue exercises. Cylinder cast immobilization may be necessary in some cases. In the rare case where casting is required to reduce pain, we immobilize a child for a maximum of 4 weeks and then begin rehabilitation exercises.

A certain percentage of children with Osgood-Schlatter disease will remain symptomatic, with hypersensitive and easily injured tubercles, following skeletal maturation. Krause and colleagues found 60 percent incidence of continued symptoms in a follow-up of 68 knees in 50 children (Fig. 6-3).[29] These patients usually have free ossific nuclei over the tubercle or within the patellar tendon. They may require excision for full symptomatic relief.[30] It has been our experience that not only should the ossicle

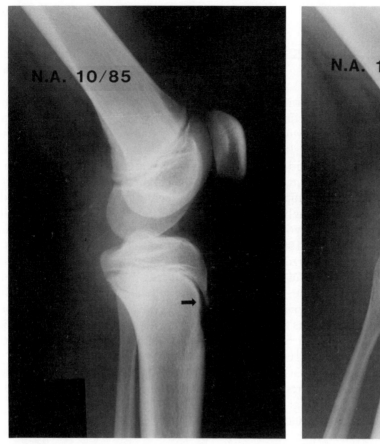
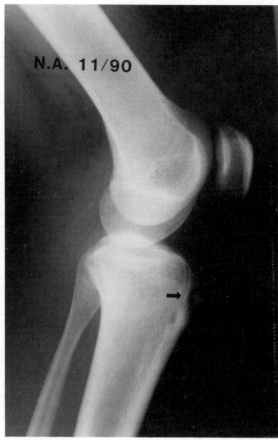

A   B

FIGURE 6-3
A. Adolescent with early Osgood-Schlatter disease shows slight fragmentation on lateral radiograph. *B.* Same patient 5 y later with painful tibial tubercle ossicle requiring resection for resolution of symptoms.

be removed, but also any underlying bony tubercle prominence, to ensure complete relief.

We have not found anti-inflammatory medication particularly useful in managing this condition. Corticosteroid injections are specifically contraindicated because it is not primarily an inflammatory condition. In addition, thinning of the skin over the prominent tubercle after cortisone injection may result in an additionally painful condition requiring plastic surgery procedures for skin coverage.[31]

SINDING-LARSEN-JOHANSSON SYNDROME

Presentation of this condition is similar to that of Osgood-Schlatter disease, but the child has tenderness over the distal pole of the patella.[32] Physical findings are similar to those of Osgood-Schlatter disease, with usually a tight and weak quadriceps mechanism. Lateral radiographs will often demonstrate elongation of the distal pole of the patella or a small avulsion ossicle at this site.

Our treatment is similar to that for Osgood-

Schlatter disease, particularly in those children who give the history of a slow progressive onset of symptoms. In children presenting with this condition in whom a history of a particular acute trauma further exacerbated or dramatically increased symptoms, such as a kick in soccer or a particular jump that increased symptoms, we will sometimes use a cylinder cast in full extension for a period of 3 to 4 weeks before beginning muscle rehabilitation.

We have, on occasion, encountered a condition similar to Sinding-Larsen-Johansson but occurring on the proximal margin of the patella and usually medially, as opposed to the accessory ossicle seen in bipartite patellae. The history of onset is often similar to Osgood-Schlatter or Sinding-Larsen-Johansson with the child often giving a history of vague knee pain in a single episode of macrotrauma increasing symptoms. Approximately half these cases have had a small ossific avulsion site proximally, which subsequently heals. In these children, a cylinder cast in full extension for a period of 3 to 4 weeks followed by rehabilitation has been successful in relieving symptoms and promoting complete healing.

111

OSTEOCHONDRITIS DISSECANS OF THE PATELLA

Osteochondritis dissecans occurs in a variety of joints and anatomic locations. Surveys of this entity have suggested that the knee is the most common site of occurrence followed by ankle, elbow, and hip. It is obviously most evident in joints that bear load or stress. Although its occurrence in the patella is relatively rare, it can be a source of significant symptoms. Fewer than 50 cases have been reported in the English literature. Two recent reviews, by Desai and coworkers in 1987 and Schwarz and colleagues in 1988, found that treatment results depended on the size of the lesion.[33,34] Of the 13 cases reviewed by Desai, 2 were treated nonoperatively with healing of the lesion with excellent results; 10 of 11 treated by operation had good or excellent results. Two patients required reoperation for persistent defect with a fair result reported. This defect was judged clinically to be quite large. Schwarz reviewed 31 operative cases in 25 patients. The most commonly performed procedures were curettage of the patella and removal of loose bodies. Only 38 percent of their knees had a good or excellent result. Persistent pain with restricted function and residual patellofemoral crepitus were common findings.

Kurzwell and colleagues described two cases of trochlear osteochondritis dissecans in 1988. Each of their cases were also identified late and required curettage and drilling for treatment.[35]

Logic would dictate against removing large pieces of articular cartilage in conditions such as osteochondritis dissecans or acute osteochondral injury. Newer imaging techniques have made early diagnosis of this condition much more possible and amenable to intervention treatment. Newer techniques such as transarticular drilling to help restore vascularity under arthroscopic control, as well as debridement of the base of the lesion and replacement with permanent pin or absorbable pin fixation, now hold much promise. It would appear much more logical, particularly in this age group, to make an early diagnosis of this condition whenever possible and to use techniques of intervention that help to maintain normal articular viability and congruity (Fig. 6-4). We have been successful in treating two cases of this condition with complete healing by cast immobilization for a period of 8 weeks. Both cases are still prepubescents with open growth plates. In addition, and since the publication of Desai and coworkers, we have successfully treated three cases of this lesion by transarticular drilling under arthroscopic control with subsequent immobilization of 4 weeks.[33] This is consistent with Guhl's earlier report and parallels similar interventions as other sites of osteochondritis dissecans in this young age group.[36]

Another overuse injury that occurs primarily in athletically active individuals and that appears to be primarily related to maltraining rather than anatomic factors is stress fracture of the patella. Schmidt and Henry, in reviewing stress injuries of the adolescent extensor mecanism, note that stress fractures of the patella have been reported with increased frequency in recent years, paralleling the increased participation of children and adolescents in running and jumping sports.[23] The first report of this entity was by Devas in 1960 who reported four cases of stress fracture occurring in the patella.[37] Subsequent reports have cited two basic clinical presentations: the first is a child or adolescent with insidious onset of dull patellar pain, whereas the second is a child who has an acute episode superimposed on a chronic history of knee pain.

Knee pain and, in particular, tenderness over the patella in the child participating in ballistic sports

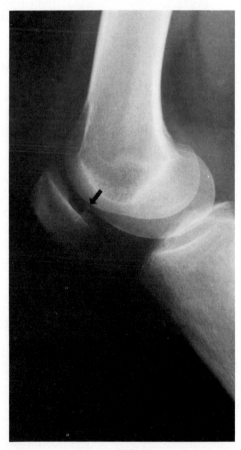

FIGURE 6-4
Symptomatic osteochondritis dissecans of the patella in older adolescent treated with transarticular drilling.

must be carefully evaluated with a complete radiographic assessment and imaging. Schmidt and Henry note that these children rarely have retropatellar grating or grinding but, rather, have tenderness directly over the patella itself often associated with atrophy of the quadriceps mechanism and loss of full flexion.[23] They note that patellar stress fractures are generally of the transverse type, suggesting longitudinal load. Other authors have reported longitudinal stress fractures. Iwaya and Takatori reported longitudinal stress fractures in two children aged 10 and one child aged 12 in association with running and fencing.[38]

As with other stress fractures, bone scanning can be confirmatory if plain radiographs are equivocal.[39]

Treatment consists of 6 to 8 weeks of immobilization to allow proper healing of the bone, followed by rehabilitation of the extensor mechanism.

ACUTE DISLOCATION OF THE PATELLA

Acute dislocation of the patella in children and adolescents is a relatively frequent occurrence. As noted above, the diagnosis of this condition may be inferential because no specific diagnostic elements of the history, physical examination, or imaging techniques absolutely confirm the diagnosis. The traditional orthopaedic treatment for this condition has been immobilization ranging from 3 to 6 weeks, followed by progressive restoration of motion and strength of the extremity. Although earlier orthopaedic studies have suggested a high preponderance of this condition in girls, with over 80 percent reported in some series being girls, more recent reviews of a primarily athletic population have actually shown a preponderance of boys, with Hawkins' study reporting 14 boys and 13 girls.[40] The study of Cash and Hughston reported 70 boys and 30 girls in the acute dislocation group.[41]

In 1986, Hawkins and colleagues presented a series of 27 cases with acute patellar dislocation and suggested that patients with acute patellar dislocation with additionally predisposing factors, such as patellofemoral malalignment, abnormal patella configuration, or a history suggesting prior instability, were more prone to recurrent dislocation and might benefit from acute operative intervention (Fig. 6-5).[40]

The natural history of acute dislocation of the patella in children has been a matter of some debate. Although the review by McManus and colleagues, based on a retrospective review of 55 cases of acute dislocation at the Toronto Children's Hospital, suggested that one-sixth of these patients will go on to recurrent dislocations, other series have suggested a much higher rate of recurrence, particularly in athletically active individuals.[42] Cofield and Bryan reported a 44 percent redislocation rate and 27 percent of these patients went on to late reconstructive surgery because of continued symptoms.[43]

Cash and Hughston, however, took exception to the recommendation for immediate operative intervention with acute dislocations.[41] They divided their series of 103 knees in 100 patients into two groups. Group 1, consisting of 69 knees, showed evidence of anatomic abnormality of the extensor mechanism in the unaffected knee. Group 2, consisting of 54 knees, showed no clinically perceptible congenital predisposition to dislocation based on examination of the unaffected knee. Nonoperative treatment of group 1 patients resulted in a 52 percent incidence of good or excellent results; nonoperative treatment in group 2 resulted in a 75 percent incidence of good or excellent results.

It has been the practice of our clinic to treat acute dislocations of the patella usually with 3 weeks of complete immobilization followed by careful progressive rehabilitation of the quadriceps mechanism and hamstrings. However, there are important exceptions to this rule. In an anatomically normal knee in which a significant amount of trauma has been associated with the dislocation, such as a hockey player hitting the sideboard directly with the side of the knee, we will frequently recommend arthroscopy and possible acute retinacular repair because of the increased amount of trauma we have encountered in such knees and the possible associated factor of

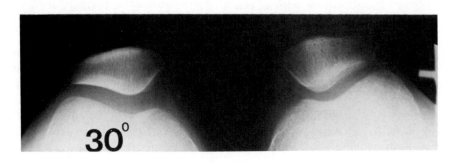

FIGURE 6-5
Adolescent girl with dislocating right patella demonstrating bilateral patellar dysplasia on the 30 degree flexion skyline view.

significant osteochondral injuries. Conversely, we have successfully treated performing athletes and artists who demonstrate high levels of constitutional laxity about the knee but with otherwise satisfactory anatomic alignment of the extremity with early rapid restoration of motion and rehabilitation without further problems or recurrent dislocations. Two patients have been able to resume ballet dance training with the adjunct of patellar taping within 3 weeks of acute injury without further problems, pain, or disability.

OVERUSE INJURIES OF THE PATELLOFEMORAL MECHANISM IN CHILDREN

Overuse injuries, the result of repetitive microtrauma to anatomic sites often in association with anatomic or physiologic predispositions, are being encountered with increased frequency in children and adolescents, particularly those involved in repetitive sports training. We have previously reported on the classification of risk factors related to overuse injuries in this age group, which is particularly useful for the assessment and subsequent treatment of these overuse injuries (Table 6-2). Interestingly, the overuse injuries of the extensor mechanism divide themselves into two major subgroups. One group of injury occurs in essentially anatomically normal individuals with maltraining appearing to be the major risk factor. These include Osgood-Schlatter disease, Sinding-Larsen-Johansson syndrome, the various described abnormalities of poles of the patella including the three accessory ossification centers, osteochondritis dissecans, and stress fractures of the patella. The second group of overuse injuries, that of patellofemoral stress syndrome or anterior knee pain, symptomatic subluxation of the patella, and chronic dislocation of the patella, appears to be encountered more frequently in children and adolescents with anatomic malalignments of the lower extremity and the extensor mechanism itself. There is an overlap between both groups, as in dislocations of the patella where reported series have indicated a certain percentage of individuals with apparently normal anatomic structure and function. In addition, muscle–tendon imbalances may be active in both general classifications, particularly insofar as a relatively tight quadriceps in association with the adolescent growth spurt can result in further lateral displacement of the extensor mechanism and relative patella lata in either group of susceptible individuals.

It is evident by now to even the most casual reader of the sports medicine and knee derangement literature that the term *chondromalacia patella* is widely condemned as a diagnostic entity and as an explanation for anterior knee pain. It has been pointed out by various authors that this term must be reserved exclusively for pathologic deterioration of the surface of the articular cartilage, including fissuring, fibrillation, and grossly evident irregularity.

Patellofemoral stress syndrome is a clinical syndrome characterized by complaints of knee pain parapatellar in location, most often associated with increased activity level, and usually associated with increased pain when ascending stairs and achiness and pain after prolonged sitting in one position. There may be associated findings on physical evaluation of patella alta, increased Q angle of the patella, femoral anteversion, genu valgum with associated external tibial torsion and tibia vara, and pronation of the feet. In addition, local examination of the extensor mechanism may reveal a relatively tight lateral retinaculum at 30 degrees of flexion.

Thanks to arthroscopy, there is now evidence that frank chondromalacic changes on the undersurface of the patella in association with this clinical syndrome are really quite rare. In particular, loss of integrity of the articular cartilage surface in children who still have open growth plates is extremely rare in our own experience, having peformed hundreds of arthroscopies on this age group. It is our hypothesis that the response of growing articular cartilage to abnormal or repetitive stress in a child with open physes, in which the articular cartilage, of course, is still a physeal plate, is the development of osteochrondritis dissecans. Clinical observation would suggest that true chondromalacia only becomes possible once the physeal plate has closed and full skeletal maturation has been attained.

To adults, there appears to be a much higher association between frank deterioration of the articular surface of the patella and symptoms and signs of patellar knee pain. In 1975, Outerbridge suggested that chondromalacia patella was the result of mechanical abnormalities of the patella in motion or articulation and further advised that the treatment of this condition should be directed at detection and correction of the abnormal mechanics, not simply shaving and debridement of the chondromalacic lesion itself.[46]

Ohno and colleagues published a landmark study on the early pathlogy of injury of the patellar articular cartilage.[47] His group was given the opportunity to perform biopsies of the articular cartilage in 12 patients with symptomatic patellofemoral pain. As a result of these pathologic specimens, they hypothesized two different stages of deterioration of the patellar articular cartilage. Stage 1 they characterized as the closed stage in which there were already detectable changes in the matrix, specifically, in the ground substance of the matrix. Stage 2 lesions were characterized as open lesions in which there was frank fissuring and opening of the surface of the articular cartilage to the ground substance (Fig. 6-6).

Based on their detection of a variety of apparent progressive changes in the articular cartilage, depending on their proximity to the most severe, clinically detectable lesion, they suggested that reversibility may be a unique quality of early chondromalacia patella in young patients. In essence, they have suggested that the child or adolescent with parapatellar pain and intact surface articular cartilage may have ground substance changes evident only by electron microscope analysis, which might have potential for reversibility and healing if mechanical factors related to their occurrence are altered.

They further suggested that chondromalacic changes seen in areas of apparent unloading or disuse may again be related to an increased weakness of the matrix, making the surface more susceptible to single traumatic events.

Summarizing the literature on this subject to the present day, there appear to be two general schools of thought related to patellofemoral stress syndrome in children and adolescents. One group believes this is a relatively serious condition that may progress to further deterioration of the patella, insofar as this pain reflects early tissue injury and maltracking of the patella or abnormal pressures on the patellar surface.

A second group dismisses this as a serious clinical entity and suggests that it is self-limited and does not go on to aggressive deterioration of the patella or osteoarthritis of the patellofemoral mechanism. In 1985, Sandow and Goodfellow performed a retrospective review of 54 adolescent girls who had been seen for "anterior knee pain" in the outpatient clinic of the Nuffield Orthopaedic Centre in Oxford.[48] On initial evaluation, the patients were all told their condition would improve with time and were essentially treated with benign neglect. At the follow-up, 2 to 17 years following initial assessment, 95 percent of these patients still had pain, but the authors noted that only 13 percent of these patients said that the pain was worse. They further reported that 48 percent of these patients had no restriction from sports activities. Based on this review, the authors suggested that their initial hypothesis that this was a benign, self-limiting condition had indeed been confirmed and that no treatment was required for this condition. It must be noted that the results of this series, when compared with the usual criteria used to judge the success of operative or nonoperative interventions, would be generally considered disappointing by most practitioners, the authors' sanguine conclusions notwithstanding.

By contrast, many other observers think that anterior knee pain in this group appears to persist unless steps are taken to restore normal function to the joint. It has been our experience that the entity of anterior knee pain in children and adolescents without dramatic associated anatomic abnormalities does indeed exist. Intervention aimed at decreasing the stress on the patellofemoral joint and attempting to centralize the patella in this groove, specifically with a progressive resistance program of static leg raising, has been consistently successful. We have found that the majority of these patients will respond to physical therapy techniqes and exercises with disappearance of pain and restoration of full function. Early therapeutic intervention in patellofemoral pain syndrome, even when extremity alignment is normal, is therefore recommended.

This observation has been shared by a number of other observers. DeHaven and colleagues noted a satisfactory response with cessation of pain in over 80 percent of adolescents placed on a progressive straight leg raising exercise regimen with associated flexibility exercises as needed.[49]

It is our belief that part of the confusion and disagreement between different observers is a matter of overlapping treatment groups and semantics. In particular, failure to separate anterior knee pain in children or adolescents with relatively normal ana-

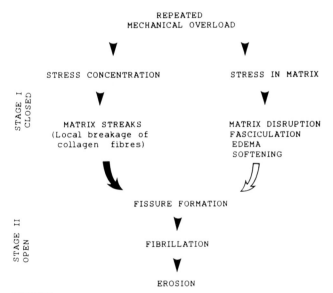

FIGURE 6-6
Hypothetical pathway for degradation of matrix in chondromalacia patellae.[47]

tomic structures from those with anatomic abnormalities sufficient to result in recurrent subluxation of the patella is a major cause of confusion and disagreement in the literature.

In 1984, Fairbank and coworkers published the results of a prospective study in which 446 children complaining of anterior knee pain were compared with age-matched controls.[50] These symptomatic children and asymptomatic controls were carefully assessed for parameters of variability of joint mobility, Q angle, genu valgum, and femoral anteversion. No significant differences could be determined between the symptomatic children and the asymptomatic controls. The only significant difference was found in the amount of sports participation between the two groups, and the conclusion of the authors was that training error with repetitive overload from increased sports participation was the major etiologic factor in this condition and not faulty lower extremity mechanics.

Conversely, in 1981, Reider and colleagues published the clinical characteristics of patellar disorders in young athletes.[51] Using eight anatomic and physiologic parameters, including alignment, quadriceps balance, and measurements of universal laxity, they concluded that there was a progressive continuum of abnormality from those children complaining only of anterior knee pain through those having evidence of patellofemoral dislocation. The greatest occurrence of abnormal findings was in those children with episodes of recurrent dislocation of the exterior mecanism. It is noteworthy that their category of chondromalacia patellae consisted of patients who complained of parapatellar pain but who denied swelling.

More recently Fulkerson has hypothesized that the anterior knee pain in these patients results from chronic injury to the lateral parapatellar retinaculum, with neuromatous degeneration of small retinacular nerves and resultant pain.[52]

PATELLOFEMORAL SUBLUXATION

Review of the recent and even more historic literature of parapatellar knee pain in the young patient suggests that there has been a great deal of overlap between the concept or entity of anterior knee pain and that of patellofemoral subluxation. In 1968, Hughston defined a clinical entity of subluxation of the patella which he distinguished from historic patellar dislocation.[53] He noted, "Many surgeons have expressed disbelief that subluxation of the patella appears in athletes, because they have not seen the condition in an athlete. It is more correct to say that they have not

recognized the condition in an athlete." He noted that a high percentage of these patients gave a history of parapatellar pain, swelling, intermittent giving out or popping, and, occasionally, grating of the patella. He further described associated objective signs of lateral posture of the patella, ease of passive subluxation of the patella from medial to lateral with the knee flexed 30 degrees, tenderness over the medial retinaculum, patellofemoral crepitus, dystrophy of the vastus medialis muscle, external tibial torsion, lateral insertion of the patellar tendon on the tibia, genu valgum, patella alta, and general atrophy of the thigh muscles. This entity has been more recently reviewed by Henry and colleagues, who have further noted a high success rate with conservative management of patellofemoral subluxation using immobilization and exercises.[54] They noted success rates in the range of 80 percent with these nonoperative techniques.

There is some debate in the literature regarding the patients who have failed nonoperative management of patellofemoral stress syndrome or subluxation of the patella. Most series suggest that between 10 percent and 20 percent of the individuals who present initially with parapatellar pain or symptoms suggestive of subluxation of the patella will not be able to reach effective levels of strength, or, having reached these levels (12 lb straight leg raising), will still remain symptomatic.

Subcutaneous or open lateral release has been suggested to have a high degree of success in patients with parapatellar stress syndrome who have failed this conservative management program. It has been our own experience and that of a number of others that careful patient selection is indicated if this intervention is to be successful. Patients who do not have a contracted lateral retinaculum will most probably not benefit by this release and, in some instances, complications such as medial subluxation of the patella may result.[55,56]

There is further debate regarding the proper management of patients with subluxation of the patella who do not respond to conservative treatment. Again, in such patients, our recommendation is to consider a lateral retinacular release if indeed they do have primarily quadriceps and retinacular pathology contributing to the mechanical malalignment of their extensor mechanism. This view is shared by Henry, who has noted in a review of subluxating patella treated by lateral release alone, that a surprisingly high percentage of patients had attained symptomatic relief and cessation of instability symptoms using this technique.[54] Frank operative realignment of the extensor mechanism for patients with subluxation of the patella alone should be reserved for those who do not respond to the conservative management, or subsequent lateral retinacular release, or in whom there is a significant component of subpatellar malalignment such as increased Q angle with associated genu valgum. Formal extensor mechanism reconstruction, which has in the past been reserved primarily for patients with recurring dislocations of the patella, may have to be considered.

DISLOCATION OF THE PATELLA

Surgical interventions to correct dislocations or fixed dislocations of the patella date back to the nineteenth century. The first surgical intervention for a dislocated patella was described by Goldthwaite in 1899 and the first summary on this entity, entitled "Slipping or recurrent dislocation of the patella: with the report of 11 cases," was again published by Goldthwaite in 1904.[4,57] A great variety of surgical interventions have since been described for recurrent dislocation or chronic dislocation of the patella. These may be divided into three broad types: interventions that recommend primarily proximal realignment or quadriceps realignment above the patella; those that recommend primarily realignment of the distal attachment of the patella on the tibia; or combinations of the two. In addition, the relative skeletal maturity of the patient is a major determinant of the type of intervention recommended, with most authors being careful to avoid bony realignment procedures distally with open physes. In 1965, Green recommended quadricepsplasties of the proximal mechanism for dislocation of the patella in the growing child.[58] In a recent long-term review of a number of these patients who were subjected to quadriceps realignment proximally, we found that the major determinant of success was the presence of chondral changes of the patella at the time of surgery. If there was evidence of grade 2 or grade 3 chondromalacia by the time surgical intervention occurred, prognosis was uniformly fair to poor.[59]

In children with open physes in whom there is a significant contribution of distal malalignment to the dislocating mechanism, or in those in whom generalized ligamentous laxity has resulted in poor formation and modeling of the patellofemoral mechanism, we have found the Galleazzi procedure to be particularly useful as a way of realigning the extensor mechanism.[60] In addition to the proximal quadricepsplasty with lateral release, the semitendinosus is used as a tenodesis through the patella and passes in such a way as to result in a significant shift of its distal force mechanism medially. This can also be done, of course, without any insult to the proximal tibial physis.

In older adolescents with closed physes, or in those having less than 1 cm of growth remaining at the proximal tibial physis, we recommend a formal alignment consisting of proximal quadricepsplasty with lateral release and a distal osteotomy of the Elmslie-Trillat type for alignment. Our experience with this operative intervention in this age, in particular, has been particularly gratifying and parallels the reported successes of Trillat and Cox with this procedure (Fig. 6-7).[61,62]

OTHER CONDITIONS

A number of other acquired or developmental conditions may contribute to the complaint of parapatellar knee pain or dysfunction of the patellofemoral mechanism in the child. The physician dealing with these complaints must be aware of the existence of these entities. Neoplasms of the patella itself are rare. Chondroblastoma is fortunately a benign condition, which may present and occur in the patella itself. Series of this tumor have noted a 1 percent to 3 percent incidence of occurrence in the patellar bone. This tumor, of course, is normally an epiphyseal tumor that may occur in round or short bones such as the patella. Treatment has been successfully described with curettage and, in some instances, bone grafting of the lesion.[63]

Another neoplasm that may also occur in the patella is osteoblastoma. This lesion normally occurs in the metaphyseal regions of long bones, although, once again, it can be found in the round or flat bones.[64]

Disorders of the synovial plica of the knee may present as derangements of the extensor mechanism. In our experience, derangements of the synovial plica may present with a history of acute injury or as a chronic injury syndrome. Synovial shelves or plica are a frequently encountered anatomic aberrant. Their incidence has been reported as high as 20 percent of normal knees.[65] It is noteworthy that they are rarely seen in the neonate or the juvenile knee. It has been our own experience that they are rarely encountered in prepubescent knees at arthroscopy. However, the incidence in the adolescent and adult has been suggested to be as high as 20 percent, often occurring bilaterally. It is possible that these anatomic structures become more evident at the time of the adolescent growth spurt with the tightening and elongation of the extensor mechanism. The tendency toward proximal and lateral deviation of the patella may increase tension on the medial retinaculum and

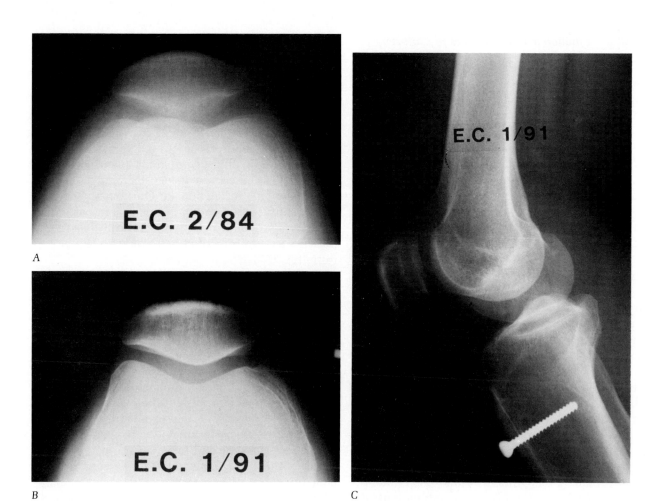

A

B   C

FIGURE 6-7
A. Adolescent girl with recurrent dislocation of the patella, treated at age 14 with lateral retinacula release, with improved symptoms and no further episodes of dislocation. Patient at age 19 was treated with Elmslie-Trillat because of reinjury and recurrent dislocations following diving accident. B and C. Radiographs 2 years postoperatively demonstrate satisfactory patellofemoral alignment. Patient has had no recurrent dislocations.

the medial retinacular synovium with shelf formation.

We have had at least six episodes in which derangements of this structure have presented as acute traumatic injury. In one case a young cheerleader came in with a locked knee that she refused to move into flexion. She was locked in full extension. Arthroscopy revealed a synovial plica, which had become completely detached from the wall of the capsule and was projecting across the joint between the patella and trochlea.

More commonly this entity will present as a chronic overuse syndrome with slow, progressive, activity-related pain. Characteristically, the patient will most often complain of medial parapatellar pain. This may be an important clinical observation in a patient whose distress is indistinguishable from the usual patellofemoral stress syndrome complaints of the adolescent.

Patel and others have reported a high level of satisfactory results from removal and surgical exci-

sion arthroscopically of this lesion.[66] It has also been our experience that when derangements of this entity appear to be the direct cause of the pain, a high rate of success may be attained. Concern must be raised when there is a high ratio of painful synovial plica made as a diagnosis for anterior knee pain in this age group with surgical intervention being recommended. Too often, this is simply an incidental finding in a young person with patellofemoral pain, or even lateral subluxation of the patella, in whom an incidental synovial plica is found. In addition, resection of a portion of the medial retinaculum and snyovium in a child or adolescent who is already subject to lateral subluxation of the patella may result in further episodes of lateral luxation and increase in symptoms, as has been pointed out by Hughston and others.[53]

Finally, as has been noted by Ficat and Hungerford in their classic text on disorders of the patellofemoral joint, in which they devote an entire chapter to its discussion, pain syndromes and, in particular,

118

reflex sympathetic dystrophy, may follow injury or surgical intervention of the knee and, in particular, be confused with pain due to patellofemoral dysfunction.[67] Reflex sympathetic dystrophy, once thought to be quite rare in children and really an adult diagnosis, is now being recognized with increased frequency in this age group. In 1990, Dietz and colleagues reported 5 additional cases of this entity and reviewed 80 cases of pediatric reflex sympathetic dystrophy in the medical literature.[68] Three of their five cases involved the knee, and in our own experience with more than 74 cases recently been reviewed at our institution, more than 50 percent involved the knee. These demonstrate findings of pain, often not conforming to anatomic or neurologic patterns, dysesthesia, and automatic dysfunction or instability. When fully established, there may be sensitivity to cold, and the involved extremity may actually be measurably colder than the opposite extremity. Surgical intervention is not useful and may be catastrophic in these children. Our own treatment techniques have involved the use of pain-blocking modalities such as transcutaneous electrical stimulation, gentle supportive physical therapy in which pain is never allowed to progress, and, in some cases, nerve blocks.

SUMMARY

Disorders of the patellofemoral mechanism are common in children and encompass a great range of clinical disorders. In conditions involving instability or malalignment of the patellofemoral joint mechanism in particular, early intervention, either with appropriate exercises and manipulations, or even surgery, to preserve the articulation of the patellofemoral joint and to prevent the development of progressive deformation of this articulation are particularly warranted because of the plasticity inherent in the child and the progressive changes associated with growth in the patellofemoral mechanism.

REFERENCES

1. Merchant AC: Classification of patellofemoral disorders. *Arthroscopy* 4:235, 1988.
2. Ogden JA: Radiology of postnatal skeletal development. X. Patella and tibial tuberosity. *Skeletal Radiol* 11:246, 1984.
3. Stanisavljevic S, Zemenick G, Miller D: Congenital, irreducible, permanent lateral dislocation of the patella. *Clin Orthop* 116:190, 1976.
4. Goldthwaite JE: Permanent dislocation of the patella. *Ann Surg* 29:62, 1899.
5. McCall RE, Lessenberry H: Bilateral congenital dislocation of the patella. *J Pediatr Orthop* 7:100, 1987.
6. Dahners LE, Francisco WD, Halleran WJ: Findings at arthrotomy in a case of double layered patellae associated with multiple epiphyseal dysplasia. *J Pediatr Orthop* 2:67, 1982.
7. Gasco J, Del Pino JM, Gomar-Sancho F: Double patella. A case of duplication in the coronal plane. *J. Bone Joint Surg* 69B:602, 1987.
8. Dugdale TW, Renshaw, TS: Instability of the patellofemoral joint in Down syndrome. *J Bone Joint Surg* 68A:405, 1986.
9. Mendez AA, Keret D, MacEwen GD: Treatment of patellofemoral instability in Down's syndrome. *Clin Orthop* 234:148, 1988.
10. Duthie RB, Hecht F: The inheritance and development of the nail-patella syndrome. *J Bone Joint Surg* 45B:259, 1963.
11. Fairbank HAT: Generalized diseases of the skeleton. *Proc R Soc Med* 28:611, 1935.
12. Mansoor IA: Dysplasia epiphysialis multiplex. *Clin Orthop* 72:287, 1970.
13. Mink JH, Reichar MA, Cures JV: *Magnetic Resonance Imaging of the Knee*. New York, Raven Press, 1987.
14. Bergström R, Gillquist J, Lysholm J, et al: Arthroscopy of the knee in children. *J Pediatr Orthop* 4:542, 1984.
15. Diebold O: Uber Kniescheibenbruche im Kindesalter. *Arch Klin Chir* 14:664, 1927.
16. Belman DAJ, Nevaiser RJ: Transverse fracture of the patella in a child. *J Trauma* 13:917, 1973.
17. Houghton GR, Ackroyd CE: Sleeve fractures of the patella in children. A report of three cases. *J Bone Joint Surg* 61B:165, 1979.
18. Ogden JA, Tross RB, Murphy MJ: Fractures of the tibial tuberosity in adolescents. *J Bone Joint Surg* 62A:205, 1980.
19. Hand WL, Hand CR, Dunn AW: Avulsion fractures of the tibial tubercle. *J Bone Joint Surg* 53A:1579, 1971.
20. Green WT: Painful bipartite patella. *Clin Orthop* 110:197, 1975.
21. Weaver JK: Bipartite patellae as a cause of disability in the athlete. *Am J Sports Med* 5:137, 1977.

22. Saupe H: Primare Knochenmark seilerung der Kniescheibe. *Dtsche Z Chir* 258:386, 1943.

23. Schmidt DR, Henry JH: Stress injuries of the adolescent extensor mechanism. *Clin Sports Med* 8:343, 1989.

24. Ogden JA, McCarthy SM, Jokl P: The painful bipartite patella. *J Pediatr Orthop* 2:263, 1982.

25. Osgood RB: Lesions of the tibial tubercle occurring during adolescence. *Boston Med J* 148:114, 1903.

26. Schlatter C: Verletzungen des Schnabel Formingen fortsatzes der oberen Tibiaepiphyse. *Beitr Klin Chir* 38:874, 1903.

27. Ogden JA, Southwick WO: Osgood-Schlatter's disease and tibial tuberosity development. *Clin Orthop* 116:180, 1976.

28. Kujala UM, Kvist M, Heinonen O: Osgood-Schlatter's disease in adolescent athletes. Retrospective study of incidence and duration. *Am J Sports Med* 13:236, 1985.

29. Krause L, Williams JPR, Catterall A: Natural history of Osgood-Schlatter disease. *J. Pediatr Orthop* 10:65, 1990.

30. Mital MA, Matza RA, Cohen J: The so-called unresolved Osgood-Schlatter's lesion. *J Bone Joint Surg* 62A:732, 1980.

31. Rostram PKM, Calver RF: Subcutaneous atrophy following methylprednisolone injection in Osgood-Schlatter epiphysitis. *J Bone Joint Surg* 61A:627, 1979.

32. Micheli LJ: The traction apophysitises. *Clin Sports Med* 6:389, 1987.

33. Desai SS, Patel MR, Micheli LJ, et al: Osteochondritis dissecans of the patella. *J Bone Joint Surg* 69B:320, 1987.

34. Schwarz C, Blazina ME, Sisto DJ, et al: The results of operative treatment of osteochondritis dissecans of the patella. *Am J Sports Med* 16:522, 1988.

35. Kuzweil PR, Zambetti GJ JR, Hamilton WG: Osteochondritis dissecans in the lateral patellofemoral groove. *Am J Sports Med* 16:308, 1988.

36. Guhl JF: Arthrosopic treatment of osteochondritis dissecans. *Clin Orthop* 167:65, 1982.

37. Devas MB: Stress fractures of the patella. *J Bone Joint Surg* 42B:71, 1960.

38. Iwaya T, Takatori Y: Lateral longitudinal stress fracture of the patella. Report of three cases. *J Pediatr Orthop* 5:73, 1985.

39. Rosen PR, Micheli LJ, Treves S: Early scintigraphic diagnosis of bone stress and fractures in athletic adolescents. *Pediatrics* 70:11, 1982.

40. Hawkins RJ, Bell RH, Anisette G: Acute patellar dislocations. The natural history. *Am J Sports Med* 14:117, 1986.

41. Cash JD, Hughston JC: Treatment of acute patellar dislocation. *Am J Sports Med* 16:244, 1988.

42. McManus F, Rang M, Heslin DJ: Acute dislocation of the patella in children. The natural history. *Clin Orthop* 139:88, 1979.

43. Cofield RH, Bryan RS: Acute dislocations of the patella: Results of conservative treatment. *J Trauma* 17:526, 1977.

44. Micheli LJ, Slater JA, Woods, E, et al: Patella alta and the adolescent growth spurt. *Clin Orthop* 213:159, 1986.

45. Micheli LJ: Overuse injuries in childen's sports: The growth factor. *Orthop Clin North Am* 14:337, 1983.

46. Outerbridge RE, Dunlop JAY: The problem of chondromalacia patellae. *Clin Orthop* 110:177, 1975.

47. Ohno O, Naito J, Iguchi T, et al: An electron microscopic study of early pathology in chondromalacia of the patella. *J Bone Joint Surg* 70A:883, 1988.

48. Sandow MJ, Goodfellow JW: The natural history of anterior knee pain in adolescents. *J Bone Joint Surg* 67B:36, 1985.

49. DeHaven KE, Dolan WA, Mayer PJ: Chondromalacia patellae in athletes. *Am J Sports Med* 7:5, 1979.

50. Fairbank JCT, Pynsent P, Van-Poorvilet, et al: Mechanical factors in the incidence of knee pain in adolescents and young adults. *J Bone Joint Surg* 66B:685, 1984.

51. Reider B, Marshall JL, Warren RF: Clinical characteristics of patellar disorders in young athletes. *Am J Sports Med* 9:270, 1981.

52. Fulkerson JP: Evaluation of the peripatellar soft tissues and retinaculum in patients with patellofemoral pain. *Clin Sports Med* 8:197, 1989.

53. Hughston JC: Subluxation of the patella. *J Bone Joint Surg* 50A:1003, 1968.

54. Henry JH, Goletz TH, Williamson B: Lateral retinacula release in patellofemoral subluxation. Indications, results, and comparison to open patellofemoral reconstruction. *Am J Sports Med* 14:121, 1986.

55. Lankenner PA, Micheli LJ, Clancy R: Arthroscopic percutaneous lateral patellar retinacula release. *Am J Sports Med* 14:267, 1986.

56. Busch MT, DeHaven KE: Pitfalls of the lateral retinacula release. *Clin Sports Med* 8:279, 1989.

57. Goldthwaite JE: Slipping or recurrent dislocation of the patella: With the report of eleven cases. *Boston Med Surg J* 150:169, 1904.

58. Green WT: Recurrent dislocation of the patella—Its surgical correction in the growing child. *J Bone Joint Surg* 47A:1670, 1965.

59. Laurencin CT, Silver SA, Tannenbaum D, et al: Late results of the Green quadricepsplasty for recurrent dislocation of the patella. *J Sport Med* 2, 1992.

60. Hall JE, Micheli LJ, McManama GB Jr: Semitendinosus tenodesis for recurrent subluxation dislocation of the patella. *Clin Orthop* 144:31, 1979.

61. Trillat A, Dejour H, Coutette A: Diagnostic et traitement des subluxations recideventes de la rotule. *Rev. Chir Orthop* 50:813, 1964.

62. Cox JS: Evaluation of the Roux-Elmslie-Trillat procedure for knee extensor realignment. *Am J Sports Med* 10:303, 1982.

63. Moser RP Jr, Brochmole DM, Vinh TN, et al: Chondroblastoma of the patella. *Skeletal Radiol* 17:413, 1988.

64. DeCoster E, Van Tiggelen R, Shahabpour M, et al: Osteoblastoma of the patella. Case report and review of the literature. *Clin Orthop* 243:216, 1989.

65. Broom MJ, Fulkerson JP: The plica syndrome: A new perspective. *Orthop Clin North Am* 17:279, 1986.

66. Patel D: Arthroscopy of the plicae—snyovial folds and their significance. *Am J Sports Med* 6:217, 1978.

67. Ficat RP, Hungerford DS: *Disorders of the Patellofemoral Joint.* Baltimore, Williams & Wilkins, 1977.

68. Dietz FR, Mathews KD, Montgomery WJ: Reflex sympathetic dystrophy in children. *Clin Orthop* 258:225, 1990.

SECTION III
Malalignment

CHAPTER 7

Acute Dislocation of the Patella

Jeffrey L. Halbrecht
Douglas W. Jackson

INTRODUCTION

An acute dislocation of the patella may be described as a primary disruption of the patellofemoral relationship where the patella is displaced out of the femoral sulcus. The direction of dislocation is most commonly lateral, although superior,[1,2] intra-articular,[3–8] and even medial dislocations have been described[9] (Fig. 7-1). This chapter will deal primarily with the acute traumatic lateral patella dislocation.

Two mechanisms of injury for acute dislocation of the patella have been proposed: quadriceps contracture or direct contact. Because of the diverging axis (quadriceps) of the lower limb, a powerful quadriceps contracture, especially when imposed on an internally rotated femur, can lead to a patella dislocation (Fig. 7-2A). A direct blow to the medial aspect of the patella would be the other more obvious mechanism (Fig. 7-2B). A combination of these two mechanisms may contribute to a single injury.

Great amounts have been written on the contribution of predisposing factors to patella dislocation, including excess femoral internal rotation, hypoplastic lateral femoral condyle, insufficiency of the vastus medialis obliquus (VMO), and increased Q angle. Table 7-1 includes a more complete list.

Many authors have demonstrated a high incidence of patellofemoral dysplasia in patients with acute dislocations of the patella.[10,11–14] Wiberg[13] has described three types of patella morphology and Baumgartl[15] has added a fourth and fifth type and correlated these with predisposition to patella instability (Fig. 7-3). Others have linked hypoplasia of the lateral femoral condyle to patella dislocation.[16] Numerous radiographic measurements have been described to objectively evaluate the patellofemoral relationship. These have been discussed elsewhere in this text.

A classification of lateral patella dislocations may be proposed that considers etiological factors, severity of soft tissue injury, and associated bony pathology (Table 7-2). This classification would differentiate dislocations with and without associated dysplasia, include the presence or absence of osteochondral fractures, and describe the condition of the medial retinaculum at the time of injury. All these factors have been suggested as contributing to the prognosis in acute patella dislocations.

NATURAL HISTORY AND DEMOGRAPHICS

The incidence of acute patella dislocations is difficult to determine and has only been addressed in a few studies. McManus and colleagues[17] reviewed the records of 94,875 pediatric visits to their emergency room over a 4-year period and found some evidence of patella dislocation in 55 (0.05 percent), although only 33 of these could be proven to be acute dislocations (0.03 percent). Cash and Hughston[10] reported treating 399 patients with this disorder over a 30-year period (13.3 percent patients yearly). More recently Casteleyn[18] and Handelberg[19] reported an incidence of acute patella dislocation of 2.44 percent in their series of knee injuries.

Most reports in the literature agree that acute patella dislocation occurs in a young population, with an average age of approximately 20 most commonly reported.[10,17] However, within this group, the actual age at dislocation may have some significance, with a higher incidence of redislocation reported in patients who dislocate before age 15[10] or 20.[20]

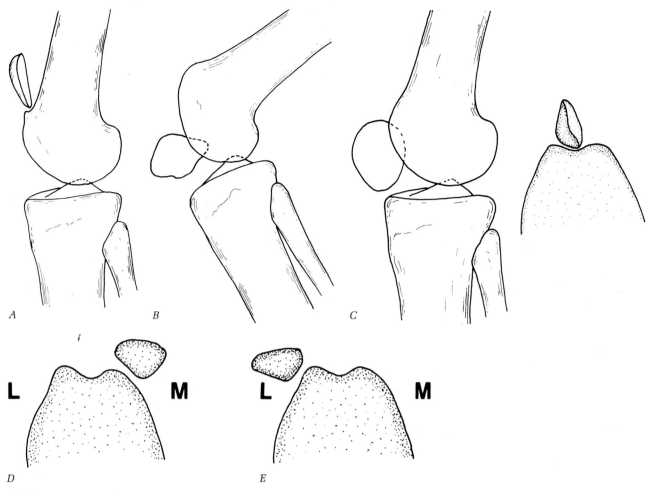

FIGURE 7-1
Five types of patella dislocation: *A.* Superior; patella caught on anterior femoral osteophytes. *B.* Horizontal intra-articular. *C.* Vertical intercondylar. *D.* Medial. *E.* Lateral; most common type.

Although recurrent dislocation of the patella tends to predominate in the female population, this gender difference does not seem to apply as consistently to acute dislocations (Table 7-3). Many studies indicate an almost equal incidence among males and females, while Hughston actually reported a much higher incidence in males.[10] Prognosis in acute dislocations also does not appear to be affected by gender.[20,24]

The natural history of acute dislocations of the patella has been addressed in a number of studies. Hawkins[12] treated 20 patients conservatively (3 weeks of immobilization). At 40 months of average follow-up, 3 had redislocated (15 percent), 4 had apprehension or complaints of instability (20 percent), and 15 had pain associated with patellofemoral crepitus. Remarkably, 100 percent were able to return to work and recreational sports. Cofield[22] studied 48

TABLE 7-1

Predisposing Factors Contributing to Patella Dislocation

1. Q angle	6. Patella alta
2. Valgus	7. Patella shape (Wiberg)
3. ER tibia	8. Insufficiency of VMO
4. IR femur	9. Patella tilt
5. Hypoplastic LFC	10. Tight lateral retinaculum
	11. Generalized ligamentous laxity

ER, externally rotated; IR, internally rotated; LFC, lateral femoral condyle; VMO, vastus medialis obliquus.

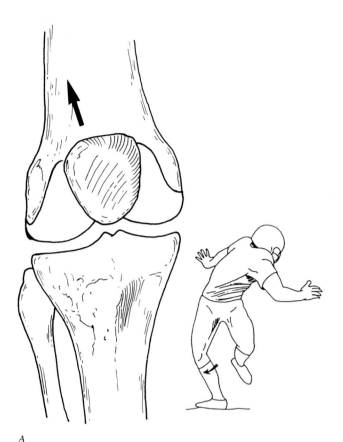

A

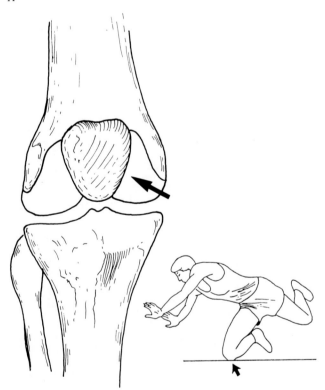

B

FIGURE 7-2
Two mechanisms for acute patella dislocation: *A.* Indirect mechanism; powerful quadriceps contracture imposed on an internally rotated femur (externally rotated tibia). *B.* Direct mechanism; direct blow to medial aspect of patella, usually by a direct fall onto the knee.

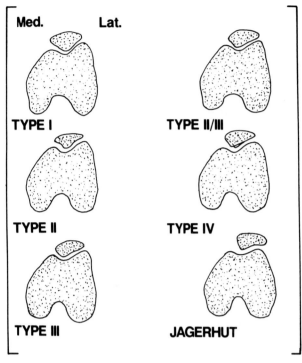

FIGURE 7-3
Patella morphology as described by Wiberg[13] and Baumgartl.[15]

patients with acute dislocations treated conservatively (closed reductions and immobilization for 1 to 6 weeks). Forty-four percent redislocated and 27 percent went on to need subsequent surgery. If subjective criteria are included, 52 percent were considered failures.[22]

McManus and coworkers[17] reviewed 28 patients with acute dislocations; 21 were treated without surgery. Five patients redislocated and 11 were considered symptomatic. Hughston[10] reported a redislocation rate of 20 to 43 percent among first time dislocators treated with immobilization alone, with the rate depending on the presence of congenital predisposition (patellofemoral dysplasia). Review of the above literature suggests that the natural history of acute patellofemoral dislocations is for a high percentage of redislocations (20 to 40 percent).

DIAGNOSIS

The diagnosis of acute dislocations of the patella is not difficult if the patella is actually dislocated at the time of presentation (Fig. 7-4). If the patella spontaneously reduces, the diagnosis can be difficult. The patient will usually present with a large hemarthrosis and will have tenderness over the medial retinaculum and under the medial facet of the patella. Rarely, a defect may be palpable in the medial reti-

125

TABLE 7-2
Classification of Acute Lateral Patella Dislocations

1. Mechanism
   A. Direct blow
   B. Quads contracture
2. Predisposition
   A. Associated dysplasia
   B. No dysplasia
3. Osteochondral fracture
   A. Yes
   B. No
4. Severity
   A. Attenuation of medial capsule
   B. Rupture of medial capsule
   C. Avulsion fracture of medial capsule

naculum (Fig. 7-5). Tenderness may also be present along the lateral femoral condyle. Often, however, the pain may be diffuse, and the diagnosis will remain in doubt.

Radiographs may be helpful if they reveal an osteochondral fracture from the medial patella facet or the lateral femoral condyle (Fig. 7-6 and 7-7). An avulsion fracture of the retinaculum off the medial border of the patella is even more diagnostic. Teittge[25] suggested the use of an axial oblique view to better visualize this avulsion. Occasionally, the diagnosis can only be made by the demonstration of a chondral defect as seen by magnetic resonance imaging (MRI) or the demonstration of a tear of the medial retinaculum by arthroscopy[18] (Fig. 7-8). Aspiration of the knee hemarthrosis may be another helpful diagnostic test if the dislocation is associated with an occult osteochondral fracture not visible on x-ray. The presence

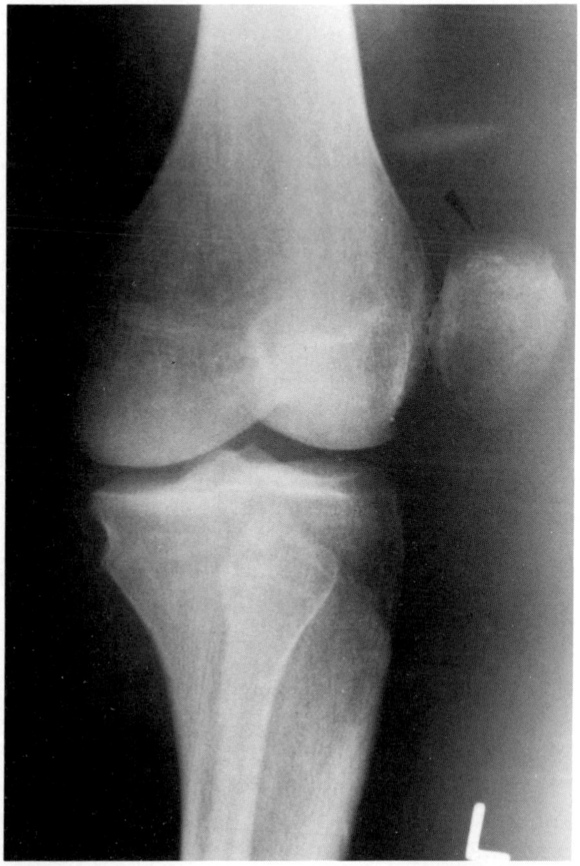

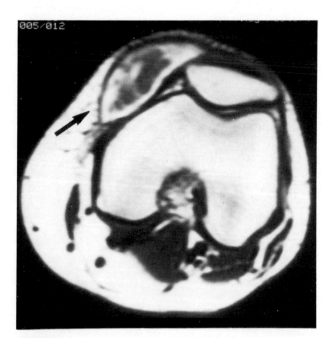

FIGURE 7-4
Anteroposterior x-ray of an acute lateral patella dislocation.

FIGURE 7-5
Magnetic resonance image of a hematoma superficial to the medial retinaculum. This may be misinterpreted on physical examination as a torn medial retinaculum.

TABLE 7-3

The Relationship of Gender to Acute Patella Dislocation

Hughston	70% males	
Hawkins	14 males	13 females
Vainionpaa	21 males	34 females
Boring	8 males	7 females
Cofield	19 males	26 females
Larsen	27 males	44 females
Rorabeck	8 males	10 females

of a hemarthrosis with fat droplets will suggest this diagnosis.

Osteochondral Fractures

Osteochondral fractures occur frequently with dislocation of the patella and may be easily missed on initial films. In an arthroscopic study on patients with acute patella dislocation, Dainer and colleagues found a "significant sized" osteochondral fragment not seen on preoperative x-rays in 40 percent of their 29 patients. In another recent study, Krodel[27] noted an incidence of osteochondral fracture of 24 of 78. Cofield[22] reported only 7 of 48 patients to have an osteochondral fracture noted on initial x-rays; but of 13 patients who went on to surgery, 6 were found to have fractures. Hawkins[12] reported 14 of 27 patients with osteochondral fractures with 4 cases missed on plain films. Similarly, Jensen[28] reported 5 of 23 patients with fractures, 4 of which were missed on preoperative x-ray. Harilainen[24] operated on 64 consecutive patients with acute patella dislocations and

noted chondral fractures in 46 percent, with loose bodies in 26 percent. Only 7 fractures and 10 loose bodies had been seen on preoperative x-rays.

It can be seen from the above data that the incidence of osteochondral fracture with patella dislocations may approach 40 to 50 percent if proper evaluation is performed. This has led some authors to recommend arthroscopy of all acute patella dislocations.[11,26,29] Computed tomography (CT) arthrography and MRI may also be helpful in detecting cartilage lesions.[19]

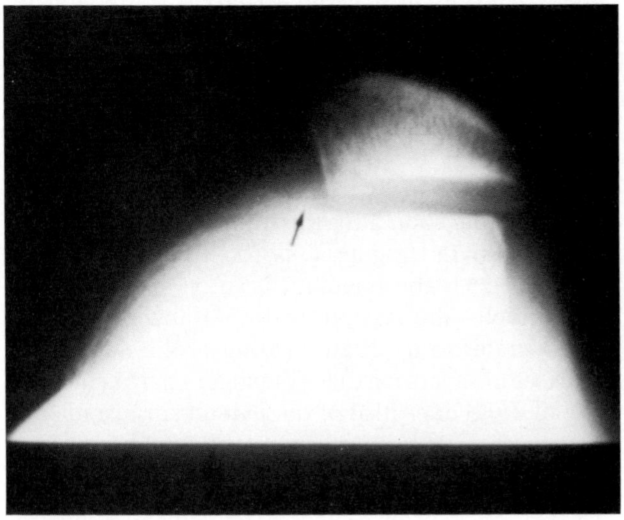

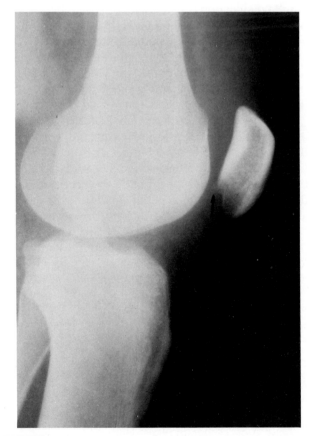

FIGURE 7-6
Sunrise view following patella dislocation reveals a small osteochondral loose body (arrow).

FIGURE 7-7
Lateral of a different patient following an acute patella dislocation demonstrates an osteochondral fracture (arrow).

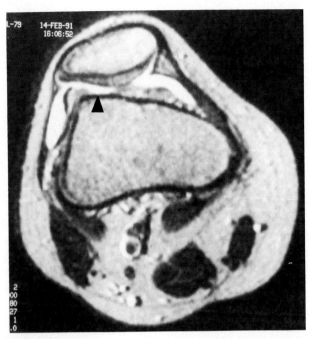

FIGURE 7-8
MRI following an acute patella dislocation demonstrates a chondral defect not seen on plain x-rays.

Three types of fracture are associated with acute patella dislocation (Fig. 7-9): an inferomedial patella fragment, a lateral femoral condyle fragment, and an avulsion fracture of the medial retinaculum.[17,23] The avulsion fragment is common and was reported in 23 of 55 patients treated surgically by Vainionpaa.[14] This fracture is nonarticular and is significant only in that it represents a disruption of the medial retinaculum.

Fractures of the inferomedial aspect of the patella and those of the lateral femoral condyle involve the articular surface and require treatment. These fractures can occur either with dislocation or relocation of the patella. Depending on the degree of knee flexion, either the lateral patella margin or the patella articular surface will act as a wedge into the lateral condyle during dislocation. This will cause either a chondral or osteochondral defect from the condyle.[30] More commonly, the medial patella facet is sheared off by the lateral femoral condyle during relocation as

the VMO contracts.[30] Fractures involving the articular surface of the patella are the most common, with Rorabeck and Bobechko[23] reporting this in 14 of 18 of their cases. Only two cases involved the lateral condyle, and importantly, a combined lesion was reported in two cases.

A further injury has been described with acute patella dislocations when a nondisplaced osteochondral fracture occurs. The undisplaced fragment may go on to desiccate, become a free fragment in the joint, and be indistinguishable from osteochondritis dissecans (OCD).[30,31]

The fracture pattern with patella dislocation may be different in adolescents and adults. In adults, articular shear fractures tend to occur along the junction of calcified and uncalcified cartilage (tidemark) and thus be mostly cartilaginous. In adolescents, where little calcified cartilage exists, the fracture tends to extend into subchondral bone presenting more as an osteochondral fracture,[32] which is easier to repair.

The treatment of osteochondral fractures remains controversial, although almost all authors agree that the fragment must be either excised or reattached. Many authors have reported excellent results with removal alone.[30,33,34] Rorabeck[23] reported excellent results after discarding 17 of 18 osteochondral fragments. The one fragment repaired measured 1.5 × 3.5 cm and was off the lateral femoral condyle. Similarly, Dainer reported 83 percent good/excellent results in 29 patients, 40 percent of whom had excision of osteochondral fractures and debridement of their craters.

Some authors are much more aggressive about fixing osteochondral fractures.[14,27,33,35] Vainionpaa[14] reported repairing 3 of 6 osteochondral fractures using absorbable suture through drill holes. Drodel[22] reported repairing 10 of 24 osteochondral fractures. Lewis[36] fixed 8 cases using a Herbert screw and reported excellent results at follow-up with no redislocations and normal knee function. Although all authors emphasize the need for an adequate-sized fragment to replace, the actual size varies among authors.

If the fragment is to be repaired, it is important that it be done soon after the injury. After more than 10 days or so, the fragment may be difficult to fit back into its bed.[9] If the fragment is to be excised, other authors have emphasized the importance of trephining the crater to facilitate healing of the defect.[31] In rare cases of severe cartilage damage, a partial facetectomy of up to one-third of the patella surface may be indicated.[9]

The Role of Arthroscopy in Diagnosis

Arthroscopy can be a valuable tool in the diagnosis of occult cases of acute patella dislocation and in

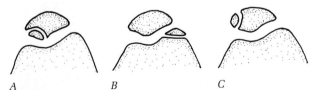

A   *B*   *C*

FIGURE 7-9
Three types of fracture associated with patella dislocation: *A.* Inferomedial patella fragment (osteochondral). *B.* Lateral femoral condylar fragment (osteochondral). *C.* Avulsion fragment (osseous-nonarticular)

128

determining the presence of osteochondral fractures not seen on initial x-rays (Fig. 7-10). In their series of knee injuries, Casteleyn and colleagues[18] reported that only 25 percent of their cases of patella dislocation were apparent without the aid of arthroscopy.

Dainer[26] reported significant osteochondral fractures in 40 percent of his series of acute patella dislocations not seen on preoperative x-rays. Similar findings have been reported by other authors.[29,37,38]

Delince and coworkers[11] have suggested an additional use of arthroscopy to aid in treatment determination. Based on the appearance of the medial capsule and the degree of fluid extravasation seen at arthroscopy, they have suggested that the integrity of the capsule may be ascertained and used to determine the need for surgical repair (Fig. 7-11).

TREATMENT OF ACUTE PATELLA DISLOCATION

Nonoperative

Nonoperative management has long been the mainstay of treatment for recurrent patellofemoral instability and subluxation.[39] Nonoperative treatment for acute dislocations, however, is not nearly as effective,[12,22] although some authors still recommend this treatment in certain patients.[9] As discussed under the section on natural history, the prognosis for redislocation or symptomatology is poor following conservative treatment. Redislocation rates of 15 to 44 per-

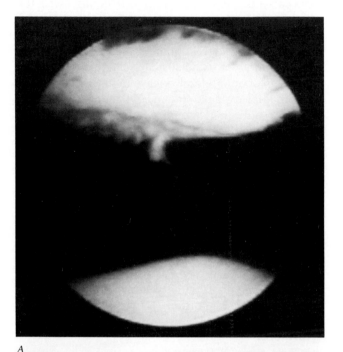

A

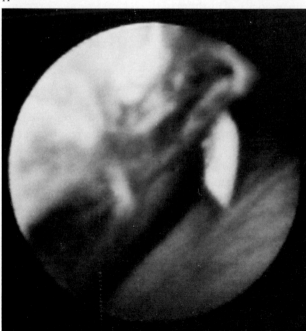

B

FIGURE 7-10
Arthroscopic view of osteochondral fracture. *A.* Damaged undersurface of patella shows origin of osteochondral fragment. *B.* Loose osteochondral fragment found in medial gutter. Disrupted medial retinaculum is to left.

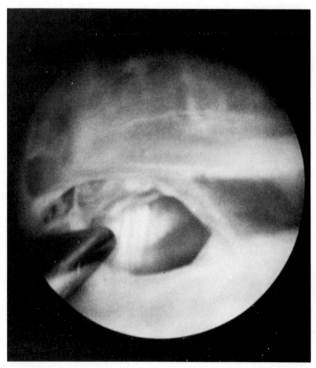

FIGURE 7-11
Arthroscopic view of ruptured medial retinaculum and capsule. Probe demonstrates that rupture is complete.

cent have been reported[12,17,22] after immobilization alone, with subjective results even worse. Hawkins[12] reported 75 percent of patients to have persistent pain, while Cofield[22] reported a 52 percent failure rate when subjective criteria were considered. Larsen[20] reported a very high incidence of redislocation but a somewhat better clinical result.

Cash and Hughston[10] attempted to differentiate patients with "congenital predisposition" to dislocate from those not predisposed based on clinical findings of lateral hypermobility of the patella or previous dislocation in the opposite knee. They found that patients without predisposition to dislocate did much better with conservative management than those predisposed, with 75 percent good/excellent results and only a 20 percent redislocation rate compared to 52 percent good/excellent results and a 43 percent redislocation rate. Other authors[12,20,22] have been unable to show a similar relationship between dysplasia and redislocation following conservative management of an acute dislocation.

Nonoperative treatment as reported in the literature for acute dislocations of the patella has usually meant some sort of immobilization followed by progressive physical therapy.[10,12,22] Interestingly, however, the benefit of immobilization for acute dislocations of the patella has not been proven, and results after immobilization and early range of motion are the same.[12,22] Furthermore, most authors agree that there is no correlation between length of immobilization and results.[10,12,22]

Operative

The role of arthroscopy in the diagnostic evaluation of acute patella dislocations has already been discussed. Arthroscopy may be used as a treatment modality as well and includes the arthroscopic removal of small osteochondral bodies with associated drilling and abrading of the crater, lateral retinacular release,[26] or arthroscopic repair of the medial capsule.[40] Although a number of authors discuss arthroscopy as a treatment modality, few reports exist in the literature evaluating the results of arthroscopic treatment alone. Dainer[26] reported on 29 patients with acute patella dislocations who underwent early arthroscopic evaluation and treatment. Patients with large osteochondral fragments that required arthrotomy for fixation were excluded from the study. Fifteen of the 29 patients had a lateral release performed somewhat arbitrarily on the basis of surgeon's perfence. Overall results were 83 percent good/excellent with 14 percent dislocations. Interestingly, all of the dislocations were in the patients who had received

lateral releases, and these patients had overall worse results than the nonreleased group (73 percent good/excellent versus 93 percent). The authors explained the higher incidence of redislocation in the released group by the initiation of earlier range of motion in these patients. This explanation is in conflict with the numerous reports showing no correlation between duration of immobilization and redislocation[10,12,22] with nonoperative treatment.

Yamamoto[40] treated 30 acute patella dislocations with arthroscopic lateral release along with arthroscopic medial capsular repair. He reported good results with only one case of redislocation (Fig. 7-12).

One of us (JLH) has developed a new technique for arthroscopic repair of the medial retinaculum. Using a suture hook and arthroscopic knot-tying techniques, the entire repair can be performed through the medial portal and avoids any medial skin puncture or incision (Figs. 7-13 and 7-14). Initial results have been quite good.

Although no one has yet compared arthroscopic and open results in a controlled randomized study, it would appear that arthroscopy has a promising role in the treatment of primary acute dislocation and should be explored further.

Arthrotomy

The majority of authors in the recent literature recommend surgical treatment for primary acute dislocations[10,14,17,21,35,41] (Fig. 7-15). In comparing their results of open medial reefing and lateral release to conservative treatment, Hawkins and colleagues[12] had no redislocations after open treatment but 15 percent after nonoperative treatment. Those treated surgically also had a lower incidence of pain, although some continued to have apprehension.[12] There was no difference in strength in the two groups as evaluated by Cybex testing. Cash and Hughston[10] also reported better results in patients who had an open repair of their medial retinaculum than in those treated with immobilization alone. Of those treated surgically, 80 to 91 percent had good/excellent results with no reported redislocations, compared to 52 to 75 percent good/excellent results and 20 to 43 percent redislocation in those treated by immobilization. The best results with immobilization alone were those patients with no predisposition to dislocate. In one of the earliest reports, Sargent and Teipner[41] reported excellent results and no dislocations following open repair of the medial retinaculum to drill holes in 11 patients.

Although most reports of surgical treatment recommend medial capsular repair and reefing, a number of other procedures have been advocated.

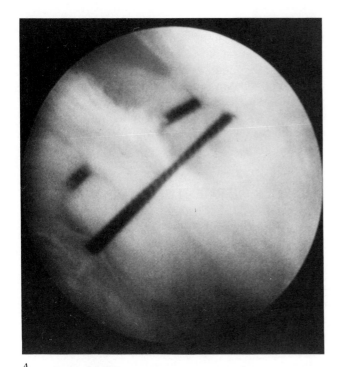

A

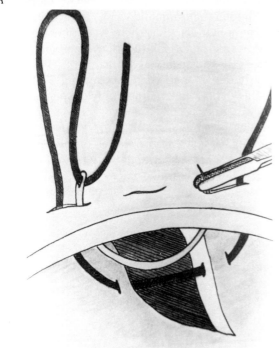

B

FIGURE 7-12
A. Arthroscopic repair of medial retinaculum. Shown are percutaneously placed sutures traversing the defect. *B.* Schematic showing techniques of suture placement.[40]

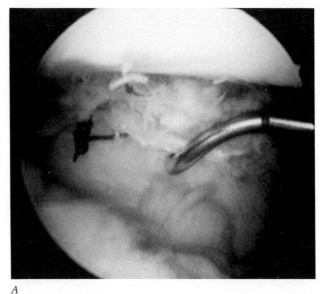

A

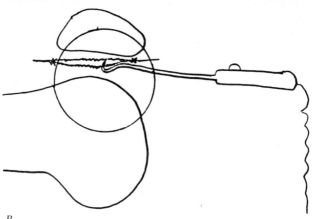

B
FIGURE 7-13
A. Authors' technique for arthroscopic repair of torn medial retinaculum. Arthroscopic view. *B.* Schematic diagram of repair technique.

McManus and Rang[17] used a semitendinosus tenodesis for some of their patients with acute dislocations, but did not report their results. Boring and O'Donoghue[21] operated on 17 patients for acute dislocations. Eight patients with normal patella alignment

had a medial reefing; 9 patients with an increased Q angle had a distal realignment. There were no redislocations, although 2 patients reported a single episode of subluxation and 12 patients had some degree of pain. The results were the same whether a reefing or realignment were performed. Vainionpaa[14] repaired the medial retinaculum in 55 cases of acute patella dislocation and added a lateral release when the lateral retinaculum was tight. Eight percent reported good/excellent results with a 9 percent redislocation rate. Harilainen[24] reported excellent results in 56 patients after medial reefing and lateral release at 1-year follow-up, with only one redislocation and a Lysholm score of 92. Seven patients were dissatisfied due to chondromalacia. Interestingly, these patients tended to have an overreduced sulcus angle postoperatively.

The addition of a lateral release is criticized by other authors. Jensen[28] reported no advantage of add-

131

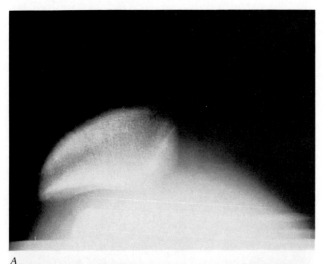

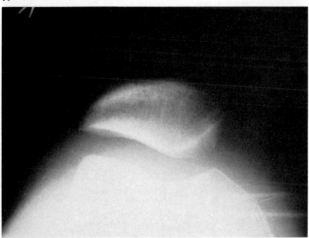

B

FIGURE 7-14
A. Reduced patella dislocation prior to arthroscopic repair. *B.* After arthroscopic repair of medial retinaculum.

ing a lateral release in a study of 23 patients who underwent medial capsulorrhaphy for acute traumatic dislocations of the patella. In an arthroscopic study, Dainer[26] actually reported worse results when a lateral release was added to medial capsular repair, with a higher incidence of redislocation and fewer good/excellent results. In a study by Vainionpaa,[14] 4 of 5 patients who redislocated had lateral releases in addition to medial capsular repair.

THE ROLE OF ROENTGENOGRAMS

Many authors have demonstrated a high incidence of patellofemoral abnormalities in radiographs of patients with acute dislocations. However, the ability to correlate x-ray findings to prognosis has been less successful. In a 5-year follow-up of 71 patients treated conservatively, Larsen[20] was unable to correlate patellofemoral incongruence, patella morphology, or patella alta to redislocation. Furthermore, patella alta was the only statistically significant predisposing radiographic abnormality found to occur more frequently among nontraumatic versus traumatic dislocators. He concluded that there was no correlation of x-ray dysplasia to classification or prognosis. In another study of conservative treatment, Hawkins[12] found only 6 of 27 patients to have patella alta and was unable to correlate radiographic dysplasia to incidence of redislocation.

Studies of surgical treatment for acute patella dislocations suggest that correlation of certain radiographic abnormalities correlate with a good clinical result. Harilainen[24] studied lateral patella displacement, Insall ratio, Wiberg morphology, sulcus angle,

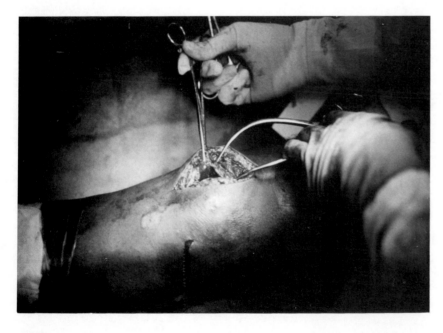

FIGURE 7-15
Surgical exposure of disrupted medial retinaculum prior to repair. Clamp is on torn edge of retinaculum.

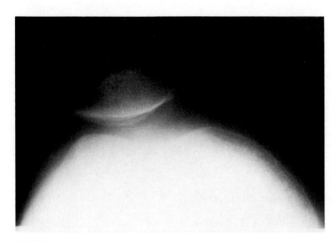

FIGURE 7-16
Sunrise view following acute patella dislocation showing lateral patella displacement and increased patella tilt. Correction of these abnormalities should be the surgical goal.

and Q angle in patients preoperatively, and then at 3 and 12 months after open repair of their dislocations. At 1 year, correction of lateral patellofemoral displacement (.0001) and patellofemoral angle (.001) correlated well with good clinical results. Interestingly, unsatisfied patients tended to have overcorrected sulcus angles. Vainionpaa[14] correlated correction of lateral patella displacement to clinical results at up to 2 years' follow-up, but found patellofemoral angle unreliable.

It would appear that when surgical treatment is undertaken, correction of lateral patella displacement should be the goal (Fig. 7-16). Although no similar prognostic radiographic criteria are available for conservatively treated patients, it might be extrapolated from the surgical data that a patient with a normal or minimally displaced patella might be expected to do well after nonsurgical treatment as well.

AUTHORS' RECOMMENDATIONS

Arthroscopic evaluation is recommended for most primary acute patella dislocations for the evaluation of chondral and osteochondral fractures. Additional surgical decisions will depend on the position of the patella as seen on the postreduction Merchant's view and as visualized arthroscopically (Fig. 7-17).

If there is persistent lateral displacement of the patella after reduction, we recommend repairing the

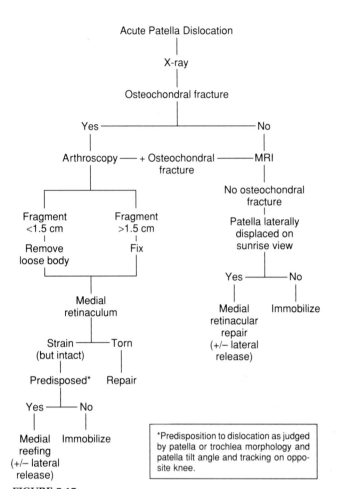

FIGURE 7-17
Decision tree for acute patella dislocation.

torn medial retinaculum. The choice of arthroscopic versus open repair remains the surgeon's choice until further studies can be done. A lateral release should be added if lateral tracking persists intraoperatively, despite medial repair, or if the patient had evidence of lateral tracking prior to the dislocation. Other procedures such as distal realignments do not appear to be necessary and have not been shown to improve the results in acute dislocations.

Nonoperative treatment of an acute primary patella dislocation should probably only be considered when a postreduction Merchant's view shows central tracking of the patella, there is no anatomic predisposition to dislocate, and there is no evidence of osteochondral fracture as verified by x-ray and MRI studies.

REFERENCES

1. Friden T: A case of superior dislocation of the patella. *Acta Orthop Scand* 58(4):429, 1987.
2. Wimsalt MH, Carey RJJ: Superior dislocation of the patella. *J Trauma* 17:77, 1977.
3. Feneley RC: Intraarticular dislocation of the patella. *J Bone Joint Surg* 50B:653, 1968.
4. Frangakes EK: Intraarticular dislocation of the patella. *J Bone Joint Surg* 56A:423, 1974.
5. Gore DR: Horizontal dislocation of the patella. *JAMA* 214:1119, 1970.
6. Kaufman I, Habermann ET: Intercondylar vertical dislocation of the patella. A case report. *Bull Hosp Joint Dis* 34:222, 1973.

7. Langendorff HU, Grabbe F, Jungbluth KH: The horizontal patella dislocation. *Unfallchirurgie* 16:80, 1990.

8. Nsouli AZ, Nahabedian AM: Intra-articular dislocation of the patella. *J Trauma* 28:256, 1988.

9. Larson RL, Jones OC: Dislocations and ligamentous injuries of the knee, in *Fractures in Adults*, edited by CA Rockwood, DP Green, 2d ed. Philadelphia, Lippincott, 1984.

10. Cash JD, Hughston JC: Treatment of acute patella dislocation. *Am J Sports Med* 16:244, 1988.

11. Delince P, Hardy D, Lafontaine M, Simons M: Initial dislocation of the patella; which treatment? *Acta Orthop Belg* 55:411, 1989.

12. Hawkins RJ, Bell RH, Anisette G: Acute patella dislocations; the natural history. *Am J Sports Med* 14:117, 1986.

13. Wiberg G: Roentgenographic and anatomic studies on the femoropatellar joint. With special reference to chondromalacia patella. *Acta Orthop Scand* 12:319, 1941.

14. Vainionpaa S, Laasonen E, Silvenoinen T, et al: Acute dislocation of the patella. A prospective review of operative treatment. *J Bone Joint Surg* 72:365, 1990.

15. Baumgartl F: *Das Knieglenk*. Berlin, Springer Verlag, 1944.

16. Anderson PT: Congenital deformities of the knee joint in dislocation of the patella and achondroplasia. *Acta Orthop Scand* 28:22, 1958.

17. McManus MB, Rang M, Heslin J: Acute dislocation of the patella in children. *Clin Orthop* 139:88, 1979.

18. Casteleyn PP, Handelberg F: Arthroscopy in the diagnosis of acute dislocation of the patella. *Acta Orthop Belg* 55:381, 1989.

19. Handelberg F, Shahabpour M, Van Betten F, et al: CT arthrography and MRI of the patella. *Acta Orthop Belg* 55:331, 1989.

20. Larsen E, Lauridsen F: Conservative treatment of patella dislocations: Influence of evident factors on the tendency to redislocated and the therapeutic result. *Clin Orthop* 171:131, 1982.

21. Boring TH, O'Donoghue DH: Acute patella dislocation: Results of immediate surgical repair. *Clin Orthop* 136:182, 1978.

22. Cofield RH, Bryan RS: Acute dislocation of the patella: Results of conservative treatment. *J Trauma* 17:526, 1977.

23. Rorabeck CH, Bobechko WP: Acute dislocation of the patella with osteochondral fracture. *J Bone Joint Surg* 58B:237, 1976.

24. Harilainen A, Myllynen P: Operative treatment in acute patella dislocation: Radiologic predisposing factors, diagnosis and results. *Am J Knee Surg* 1:178, 1988.

25. Teittge RA: Radiology of the patellofemoral joint. *Orthopedic Surgery update series*. Princeton, NJ Continuing Professional Education Center, 1985.

26. Dainer RD, Barrack RL, Buckley SL, Alexander AH: Arthroscopic treatment of acute patella dislocation. *Arthroscopy* 4:267, 1988.

27. Krodel A, Refior HJ: Patella dislocation as a cause of osteochondral fracture of the femoropatella joint. *Unfallchirurgie* 16:12, 1990.

28. Jensen CM, Roosen JU: Acute traumatic dislocations of the patella. *J Trauma* 25:160, 1985.

29. Savarese A, Lunghi E: Traumatic dislocations of the patella: Problems related to treatment. *Cir Organi Mov* 75:51, 1990.

30. Rosenberg NJ: Osteochondral fractures of the lateral femoral condyle. *J Bone Joint Surg* 46A:1013, 1964.

31. O'Donoghue DH: Chondral and osteochondral fractures. *J Trauma* 6:469, 1966.

32. Landells JW: The reactions of injured human articular cartilage. *J Bone Joint Surg* 39B:548, 1957.

33. Ahstrom JP: Osteochondral fracture in the knee joint associated with hypermobility and dislocation of the patella. *J Bone Joint Surg* 47A:1491, 1965.

34. Kennedy JC, Grainger RW, McGraw RW: Osteochondral fractures of the femoral condyles. *J Bone Joint Surg* 48B:437, 1966.

35. Smillie IS: Injuries of the knee joint in 4th ed. Baltimore, Williams & Wilkins, pp 205–223.

36. Lewis PL, Foster BK: Herbert screw fixation of osteochondral fractures about the knee. *Aust N Z J Surg* 60:511, 19.

37. Sperner G, Benedetto KP, Glotzer W: The value of arthroscopy following traumatic patella dislocation. *Sportverletz Sportschaden* 2:20, 1988.

38. Muhr G, Knopp W, Neuman K: Dislocation and subluxation of the patella. *Orthopaedics* 18:294, 1989.

39. Henry JH, Crossland JW: Conservative treatment of patellofemoral subluxation. *Am J Sports Med* 7:12, 1979.

40. Yamamoto RK: Arthroscopic repair of the medial retinaculum and capsule in acute patellar dislocation. *Arthroscopy* 2:125, 1986.

41. Sargent JR, Teipner WA: Medial patella retinacular repair for acute and recurrent dislocation of the patella—A preliminary report. *J Bone Joint Surg* 53A:386, 1971.

CHAPTER 8

Chronic Patellar Instability: Subluxation and Dislocation

John P. Fulkerson
Richard A. Cautilli

Paramount to understanding patellofemoral malalignment is a differentiation of those patients who have patellar subluxation or dislocation from those who have chronic tilt in the coronal plane. Furthermore, in patients with patellofemoral pain, those patients with pain related to malalignment must be differentiated from those with pain *not* related to patellar malalignment. This chapter focuses on patellar malalignment problems in which the patella is chronically or recurrently displaced out of the femoral trochlea.

CLASSIFICATION

Our classification (Table 8-1) has been most helpful in differentiating alignment patterns (Fig. 8-1) associated with patellofemoral dysfunction and pain. In this classification, patients with patellar instability (subluxation and dislocation) were categorized as either type I malalignment (subluxation alone) or type II malalignment (subluxation with tilt). Merchant[1] has provided another classification that is helpful in characterizing patellofemoral problems, including those not related to malalignment (Table 8-2). In general, the clinician should know that characterization of each patient with patellofemoral pain according to these classifications will improve the accuracy and overall quality of treatment (particularly when nonoperative measures fail). There is no short-cut to understanding patellofemoral malalignment and patellofemoral pain. Historically these problems have been difficult to understand and, therefore, it is important to be specific about each patellofemoral disorder, using an appropriate classification to identify each problem. By so doing, the clinician will use realignment surgery techniques (including lateral release) only to correct a specific alignment problem, as determined by careful clinical and radiographic evaluation.

TABLE 8-1
Fulkerson-Schutzer Classification of Patients with Patellofemoral Pain

Type I	A)	Patellar subluxation, with no articular lesion
	B)	Patellar subluxation with grade 1–2 chondromalacia
	C)	Patellar subluxation with grade 3–4 arthrosis
	D)	Patellar subluxation with a history of dislocation and minimal or no chondromalacia
	E)	Patellar subluxation with a history of dislocation, with grade 3–4 arthrosis
Type II	A)	Patellar tilt and subluxation with no articular lesion
	B)	Patellar tilt and subluxation with grade 1–2 chondromalacia
	C)	Patellar tilt and subluxation with grade 3–4 arthrosis
Type III	A)	Patellar tilt with no articular lesion
	B)	Patellar tilt with grade 1–2 chondromalacia
	C)	Patellar tilt with grade 3–4 arthrosis
Type IV	A)	No malalignment and no articular lesion
	B)	No malalignment and grade 1–2 chondromalacia
	C)	No malalignment and grade 3–4 arthrosis

SOURCE: Fulkerson J, Hungerford D: *Disorders of the Patellofemoral Joint.* Baltimore, Williams & Wilkins, 1990.

45 PATIENTS

Type 1 - Sublux without tilt

18 Patients, 21 Knees

Type 2 - Sublux with tilt

14 Patients, 19 Knees

Type 3 - Tilt without sublux

19 Patients, 25 Knees

FIGURE 8-1
Patterns of patellar malalignment. *(Reproduced from Reference 7.)*

TABLE 8-2
Classification of Patellofemoral Disorders

I. Trauma (conditions caused by trauma in the otherwise normal knee)
   A. Acute trauma
      1. Contusion
      2. Fracture
         a. Patella
         b. Femoral trochlea
         c. Proximal tibial epiphysis (tubercle)
      3. Dislocation (rare in the normal knee)
      4. Rupture
         a. Quadriceps tendon
         b. Patellar tendon
   B. Repetitive trauma (overuse syndromes)
      1. Patellar tendinitis ("jumper's knee")
      2. Quadriceps tendinitis
      3. Peripatellar tendinitis (e.g., anterior knee pain of the adolescent due to hamstring contracture)
      4. Prepatellar bursitis ("housemaid's knee")
      5. Apophysitis
         a. Osgood-Schlatter disease
         b. Sinding-Larsen-Johanssen disease
   C. Late effects of trauma
      1. Posttraumatic chondromalacia patellae
      2. Posttraumatic patellofemoral arthritis
      3. Anterior fat pad syndrome (posttraumatic fibrosis)
      4. Reflex sympathetic dystrophy of the patella
      5. Patellar osseous dystrophy (11)
      6. Acquired patella infera
      7. Acquired quadriceps fibrosis

II. Patellofemoral dysplasia
   A. Lateral patellar compression syndrome
      1. Secondary chondromalacia patellae
      2. Secondary patellofemoral arthritis
   B. Chronic subluxation of the patella
      1. Secondary chondromalacia patellae
      2. Secondary patellofemoral arthritis
   C. Recurrent dislocation of the patella
      1. Associated fractures
         a. Osteochondral (intraarticular)
         b. Avulsion (extraarticular)
      2. Secondary chondromalacia patellae
      3. Secondary patellofemoral arthritis
   D. Chronic dislocation of the patella
      1. Congenital
      2. Acquired

III. Idiopathic chondromalacia patellae

IV. Osteochondritis dissecans
   A. Patella
   B. Femoral trochlea

V. Synovial plicae (anatomic variant made symptomatic by acute or repetitive trauma)
   A. Medial patellar ("shelf")
   B. Suprapatellar
   C. Lateral patellar

SOURCE: Merchant AC: The classification of patellofemoral disorders. *Arthroscopy* 4:235, 1988.

Lateral Patellar Subluxation

When the patella is chronically displaced out of the femoral trochlea, it usually leads to feelings of patellar instability and apprehension. Frequently, patellar *subluxation* is associated with patellar *tilt* (type II, Fig. 8-2). Occasionally, subluxation is not associated with tilt (type I malalignment). Subluxation without tilt (type I, Fig. 8-3) is most common in patients who have generalized ligamentous laxity. Subluxation without tilt may also occur after isolated lateral retinacular release in a patient with type II malalignment (in this instance tilt may be relieved without correcting subluxation). The differentiation of tilt from subluxation has been too frequently overlooked, sometimes leading to inappropriate treatment of patients. Understanding that subluxation represents only abnormal placement of the patella in the medial/lateral plane as opposed to tilt (Fig. 8-4) will enable the clinician to better understand patients with extensor mechanism instability.

One should understand, at this point, the difference between *subluxation* and *subluxability*. A patella, which is *chronically* aligned such that it rides up on the lateral trochlea, out of its central position in the trochlea, exhibits subluxation. When a patella, under most activities, tracks centrally in the trochlea but is abnormally prone to displacement out of the trochlea with extreme rotation or position of the leg, it is *subluxable*.[2] One way to differentiate these is with an external rotation radiographic view, such as that described by Malghem and Maldague.[3] Such patients may have absolutely normal tangential radiographs and tomographic studies of the patellofemoral joint and normal static alignment as well as normal functional alignment until extremes of rotation are created. Those authors who recommend "quadrant displacement" of the patella are evaluating subluxability but *not* subluxation.

Most commonly, lateral subluxation of the patella is accompanied by tilt. For purposes of under-

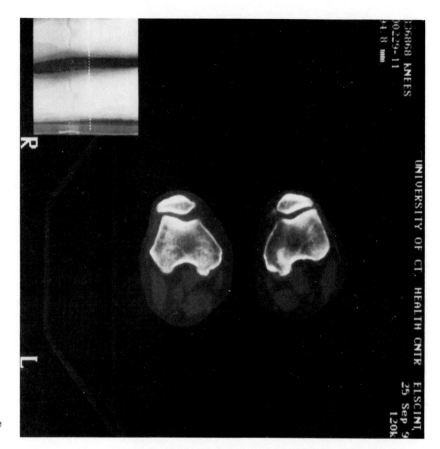

FIGURE 8-2
Computerized tomographic (CT) image of type
II malalignment, subluxation with tilt.

standing these malalignment problems, however, it
is important to recognize that the subluxation component and the tilt component of malalignment are separate (see Table 8-1).

Medial Subluxation

Occasionally a patient complains of medial displacement of the patella out of the trochlea. Most commonly, this occurs as a result of excessive lateral
retinacular release (sometimes including complete
detachment of the main vastus lateralis tendon) or
lateral retinacular release in a patient who had no
preexisting malalignment. Hughston and Deese[4] have
described the entity of medial patellar subluxation
and this has been further elaborated by Shellock,
Mink, and Fox.[5] It is our opinion that true medial
subluxation occurs extremely rarely *except* as a result
of surgery.

We have noted also that the central ridge of the
patella tends to rotate in a medial direction in association with patellar tilt. It is extremely important to
recognize this entity (see Fig. 8-4) of *medial rotation
of the central patellar ridge*, because it may be caused
by tightness of the lateral retinaculum and will be
best treated by *lateral* release if it is associated with
tilt and chronic patellofemoral pain.

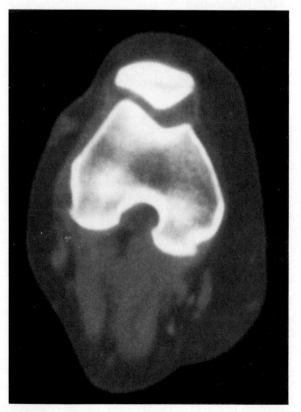

FIGURE 8-3
Computerized tomographic (CT) image of type I malalignment,
subluxation without tilt.

137

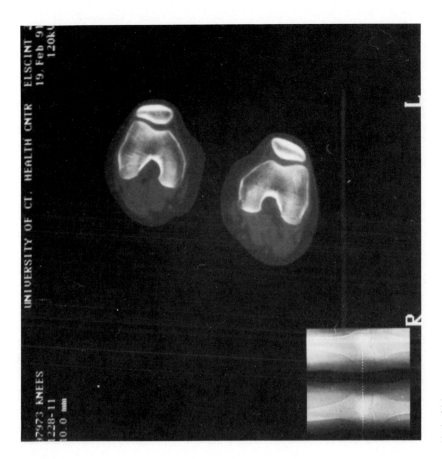

FIGURE 8-4
Tilted patellae with rotation of the central patellar ridge caused by a tight *lateral* retinaculum.

Patellar Dislocation

Most patients who have experienced patellar dislocation (Fig. 8-5) give a history of the patella going out of place and then having to push it back into place. Sometimes, however, the patella will relocate spontaneously. It is worth noting that such patients sometimes think they have had a *medial* patellar dislocation. This is most often because the prominent medial femoral condyle after lateral dislocation of the patella is striking to the patient and gives the false impression that it *is* the patella. To understand problems of

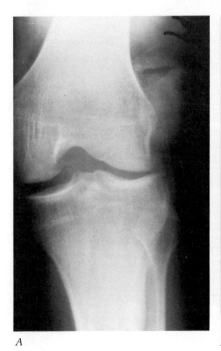

A

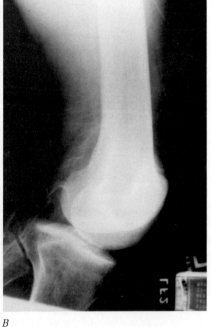

B

FIGURE 8-5
The dislocated patella. *A.* Anteroposterior view *B.* Lateral view.

patellar dislocation, one should differentiate those patients who have chronic malalignment leading to dislocation from those who have a strictly traumatic dislocation with no preexisting malalignment. Many of the studies published on patellar dislocation have failed to recognize this differentiation, making the analysis of treatment results questionable. One might expect that a patient who has surgery aimed at correcting alignment will be much more likely to achieve improved function if there has been preexisting malalignment. If one sustains a traumatic patellar dislocation, never having had malalignment, and then has lateral release, it is less likely that the surgical procedure will bring benefit. Finally, one should differentiate those patients who have *permanent* patellar dislocation (a patella that is always outside of the femoral trochlea) from those having a transient dislocation, or recurrent dislocations.

CLINICAL EVALUATION

The history is helpful in patients with a patellar instability problem. The patient may relate a history of chronic pain in the anterior knee with no subjective experience of patellar instability. On the contrary, the patient may relate a history of apprehension and patellar instability with little or no history of anterior knee pain except as it relates to acute episodes of patellar displacement. The astute clinician will note this difference in the history. As stated earlier, the clinician should also differentiate the patient with patellar dislocation and a *preexisting* history of patellar pain/instability from the patient with a history of preexisting patellar trauma and dislocation without a history of the anterior knee pain.

The clinician should not be fooled by a history of medial patellar dislocation. Often, as noted earlier, the patient feels the *medial* femoral condyle and assumes it is the patella when, in fact, the patella has gone lateral.

Subtleties in the history are helpful. Pain associated with a grating sensation may forebode a true articular breakdown, whereas aching pain along with medial or lateral *border* of the patella is more often associated with peripatellar retinacular pain, plica, or osteophyte. It is easy to be fooled, but most patients, given enough time to tell their story, will give signals as to the nature and location of their problem.

The physical examination will, of course, include a full examination of the back, hips, knees, and lower extremity alignment. The Lesegue test (straight leg raising) may indicate a radicular form of anterior knee pain. Pain on rotation of the hip or a lack of

normal hip motion may forebode anterior knee pain referred from the hip. Tightness of hamstrings or quads should be noted because specific nonoperative treatment may help to relieve such problems. Observing the patient in normal stance and gait will elucidate functional disorders such as excessive hip anteversion and resulting internal rotation of the femoral trochlea *away* from the patella, excessive knee valgus and associated increase of the functional quadriceps (Q) angle, external tibial torsion, pronation, or antalgia.

Examining the patient supine is helpful. After the hip and back are examined, the clinician should seek evidence of a meniscus, cruciate ligament, articular, or rheumatologic condition in the knee. The presence or absence of effusion, however slight, should be noted. The crux of doing a good examination of the anterior knee is *differentiation of peripatellar retinacular pain and tightness from articular pain and irregularity.* Patients with patellar instability often have components of both.

On examining the knee, it is best to start with a slow and careful palpation of every component of the peripatellar retinaculum (Fig. 8-6). Starting proxi-

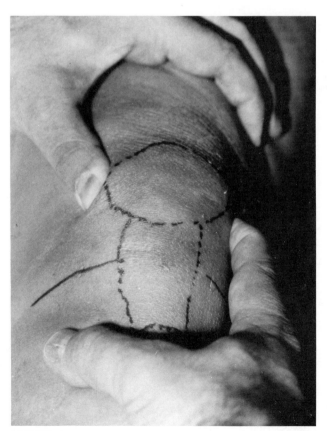

FIGURE 8-6
Palpation of the peripatellar retinaculum.

mally, *palpate for tenderness* in the distal quadriceps and then progress distally along the lateral retinaculum and then to the patellar tendon. Palpate the medial retinaculum for tenderness. Subsequently, the clinician should *look for evidence of retinacular laxity or tightness.* The patella *should be displaced laterally* to see if this causes apprehension and to quantitate the amount of lateral patella displacement possible. *Evaluate medial displacement of the patella*, particularly in patients who have had lateral retinacular release. In general, though, we have found this less helpful than observing patellar tracking actively and passively.

Next, the clinician should *evaluate patellar tilt.* By raising the lateral facet of the patella away from the lateral trochlea (Fig. 8-7), the clinician can gain an appreciation of lateral retinacular tightness and tethering of the patella on the lateral side.[6] This clinical evaluation should give an impression of whether the patella is tilted, and whether this tilt can be easily corrected by elevating the lateral patella away from the trochlea. Normally the examiner should be able to raise the lateral patella to the horizontal plane or slightly beyond.

Next, *observe the tracking* of the patella to see how it engages the trochlea on flexion and extension of the knee. The patient is encouraged to flex the knee actively from a position of full extension, and subsequently the examiner observes patellar tracking while passively flexing the knee.

Finally, the examiner should carefully evaluate old scars around the anterior knee for evidence of a painful retinacular nodule or neuroma. This is an extremely important, and often overlooked, part of the examination.

RADIOGRAPHIC EXAMINATION

The anteroposterior (AP) and lateral radiographs may reveal evidence of *patella alta* or *baja,* degenerative changes, bipartite patella, osteoporosis, loose body, or other conditions contributing to anterior knee pain or instability. The axial view should be examined for both *congruence* (centering of the patella in the trochlea) and *tilt* (alteration of patellar balance in the trochlea such that the medial facet of the patella rotates away from the medial facet of the trochlea and the lateral patella facet is tethered against the lateral trochlea), although tilt is particularly difficult to evaluate. On the routine axial radiograph, there is not a reliable reference plane for determining tilt (the anterior trochlea line is too unreliable because of its anatomic variability).

It is important to use a standard axial view, preferably at a relatively low knee flexion angle (45 degrees knee flexion or less) in addition to standard AP and lateral radiographs. The Merchant (Fig. 8-8) axial view (or the Laurin 20 degrees knee flexion axial view) are most helpful. Second, patellar alignment should be studied in a position of normal, functional lower extremity alignment. There is no place for arbitrary or sloppy patient positioning in the evaluation of patellar alignment, and the physician should insist on careful control of patient position for these studies. Third, one must realize that there is image overlap on traditional axial radiographs such that error or misinterpretation may occur.

Nonetheless, axial radiographs of the patella are all that the clinician will need in the majority of patients with patellofemoral pain and malalignment. The axial x-ray may reveal subluxation, tilt, or dislo-

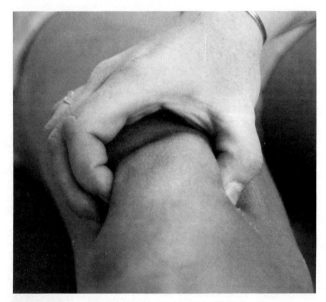

FIGURE 8-7
Elevation of the lateral patellar facet away from the trochlea will give an indication of lateral retinacular tightness and tilt.

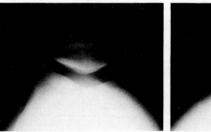
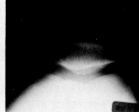

FIGURE 8-8
Merchant axial view of the patella.

cation. Additional expensive studies, such as computed tomography (CT) and magnetic resonance imaging (MRI), are not needed in most cases. In addition to a standard axial radiograph, one may wish to evaluate "subluxability" with the external rotation view of Malghem and Maldague.[3] This study by itself, however, is not reliable for understanding patellar alignment and is best used only as a "window" to functional displacement of the patella.

When axial radiographs do not provide enough information to make a decision about patellar alignment, particularly when surgery is likely, one may obtain tomographic images of the patellofemoral joint (PFJ). CT provides the needed information but MRI may be used also for this purpose, although it may be more expensive. To obtain useful CT images of the PFJ, the patient must be placed in a scanner gantry in normal standing alignment, and tomographic images must be taken at 10 to 20 degrees knee flexion where the patella has normally become engaged and centered in the femoral trochlea.[1,7] Also, it is **imperative** that the images be taken at the **precise** midpatella transverse plane. If this is not done, results may be misinterpreted. The *midpatella transverse plane* is the articulating plane of the patella and images distal to this may show the nonarticular distal pole of the patella (Fig. 8-9). Using bolsters to carefully position the patient in the scanner gantry will usually allow a satisfactory tomographic study. The technician should not take any films until the midpatella transverse plane has been accurately identified, perhaps with the help of a radiologist. Normally, both knees are imaged at the same time, taking care to obtain the tomographic images *through both posterior femoral condyles* (Fig. 8-10). The posterior condyles, while providing an excellent reference plane for evaluating tilt, also may be used in the evaluation of subluxation. A perpendicular line drawn from the posterior con-

dyle line through the center of the trochlea will provide an accurate plane for medial/lateral displacement of the patella.

Three-dimensional CT (Fig. 8-11) is even more helpful because serial images of the PFJ are possible, and the interpreting physician can choose the appropriate images to interpret. To fully evaluate patellar alignment in the patient with suspected chronic subluxation or dislocation, we recommend midpatellar transverse tomographic images at 15, 30, and 45 degrees knee flexion. Proper interpretation of these studies, then, will follow the protocol of Fulkerson and Hungerford.[1] Normally, the patellar tilt angle (lateral patella facet relative to the posterior femoral condyle line) should be greater than 12 degrees, and the congruence angle should be zero (patella centered in the trochlea). These criteria of normal alignment have been established in 20 normal knees and have been reported previously.[1,2,7]

ARTHROSCOPIC EVALUATION AND TREATMENT OF PATIENTS WITH CHRONIC PATELLAR INSTABILITY

Arthroscopy will not be needed in the majority of patients with mild patellar instability. Such patients can be managed readily with bracing, taping, exercises, strengthening, modification of activity, and reassurance in many cases. Patients with recurrent episodes of significant instability that limits normal activities, however, may require surgical intervention (usually including arthroscopy) at some point.

It is imperative that the clinician understand the difference between radiographic determination of appropriate patellar alignment and arthroscopic criteria of normal patellar alignment. Radiographic studies have shown that the normal patella engages the troch-

FIGURE 8-9
Tomographic images taken through the nonarticular distal pole of the patella may given an erroneous impression of articular malalignment. Apparent medial subluxation due to a distal cut *(A)*, well centered midpatella cut *(B)*, of the same knee.

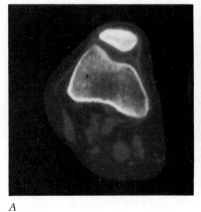 *A*

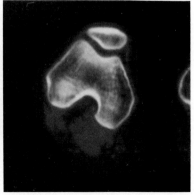 *B*

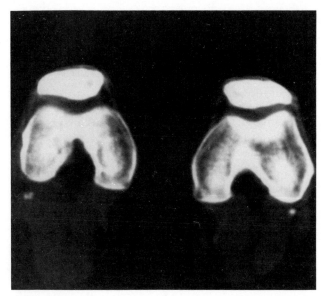

FIGURE 8-10
Quality tomographic studies of the patellofemoral joint must transect the midpatella transverse plane and both posterior femoral condyles.

Nonetheless, one may use the arthroscope to confirm an opinion about patellar tracking that has been based on careful clinical examination and precise radiographs, preferably including precise tomographic images. In the author's opinion, arthroscopic assessment of patellar alignment should be reserved primarily for this type of confirmation and not so much for definitive assessment of patellar alignment.

Arthroscopy is most appropriate as an adjunct to definitive surgery for patellar instability. In the decision-making process, the clinical examination and radiographs will usually enable a clinician to make a definitive decision regarding appropriate surgery for those individuals who have failed nonoperative treatment. Arthroscopy is most useful, nonetheless, in evaluating articular lesions immediately before performing definitive surgery.[1]

In general, the approach is to tailor the surgical treatment to correct the specific mechanical disorder and, hopefully, to unload any significant articular lesions. Localization and quantification of articular lesions, then, becomes extremely important in the final decision-making regarding definitive surgery. The arthroscope permits evaluation in this regard. In particular, it is important to note if any specific articular lesions will be made worse or subjected to increased stress by surgery. In particular, one should look for lesions at the proximal and medial aspect of the patella when surgery is performed to shift contact stresses to these areas. Since tibial tubercle anteriorization will shift the patellar contact area proximally on the patella, the surgeon should know if there is a distal medial facet or lateral facet articular lesion (Fig. 8-13) that will benefit from the shift of contact onto the more proximal medial facet at the time of surgery. Likewise, any large articular lesion on the proximal medial facet may preclude surgery, which will add increased load to this area. Localization of such lesions is difficult without direct visualization, and the

lea early in flexion, usually by 10 to 15 degrees knee flexion in asymptomatic individuals. Arthroscopic evaluation, on the other hand, has shown a different picture. Using the arthroscope, one will note that a normal patella does not always engage the trochlea until 30 to 40 degrees knee flexion or more (Fig. 8-12). One must consider that the knee is distended with fluid, the quadriceps are usually paralyzed, a leg holder may be in place, there is sometimes a tourniquet in place, and instruments are in the knee joint. Consequently, the criteria for normal alignment are vastly different using the arthroscope from those criteria using radiographic images. In the author's opinion, radiographs, particularly tomographic images, will give a better appraisal of patellar alignment and a more valid picture of patellar tracking.

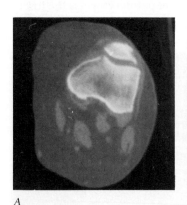

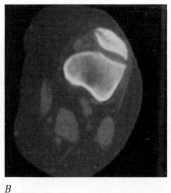

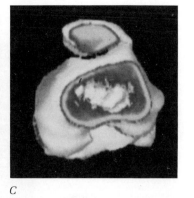

A   *B*   *C*

FIGURE 8-11
Three-dimensional CT images of the patellofemoral joint allow selective sectioning of the joint at any level using the computer. Proximal *(A)* and distal *(B)* cuts are demonstrated in the same knee. A series of these images will permit three-dimensional reconstruction *(C)*.

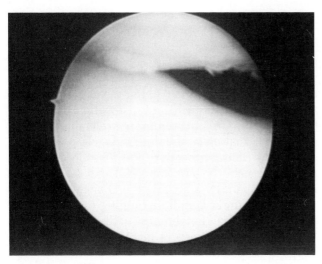

FIGURE 8-12
Arthroscopic view of the patella shows tilting of a normally aligned patella (by clinical examination and radiographs) with the knee flexed 30 degrees. This tilt may be created by fluid, quadriceps paralysis, and instruments and should not be considered pathologic unless it is confirmed by clinical and radiographic studies.

arthroscope is the best tool available for this process of articular lesion localization and quantification, short of direct observation of the patella at the time of open surgery.

Occasionally, the arthroscopic surgeon will find unsuspected lesions in the knee at the time of patellar alignment surgery. Loose bodies may be noted and occasionally meniscus tears, which may contribute to pain, will be found at the time of definitive patellofemoral surgery. The arthroscope also permits evaluation of articular surfaces in the medial and lateral compartments.

Definitive surgical treatment may be possible using the arthroscope. Arthroscopic lateral release and realignment will be covered elsewhere in this text-

book. For the patient, it makes little or no difference whether lateral release is done arthroscopically or through a short $1\frac{1}{2}$- to 2-inch lateral incision using direct visualization and retractors. In the author's experience, lateral release using this mini-incision technique with direct visualization permits optimal release, the best possible access to hemostasis, and direct release of the inferolateral retinaculum, which is difficult or impossible to visualize at the time of arthroscopic lateral release. It is important not to leave a residual band that may become painful in some patients, and therefore, when lateral release is performed either arthroscopically or open, it should be complete, paying thorough attention to hemostasis.

At the time of performing lateral release, whether arthroscopic or open, the surgeon may wish to place a nerve stimulator over the femoral nerve (Fig. 8-14). Anesthesiology can usually do this. This technique permits a good quadriceps contraction under anesthesia such that the operating surgeon may note if there has been adequate release. This is a helpful and simple technique at the time of arthroscopic (or open) surgery to confirm appropriate dynamic patellar

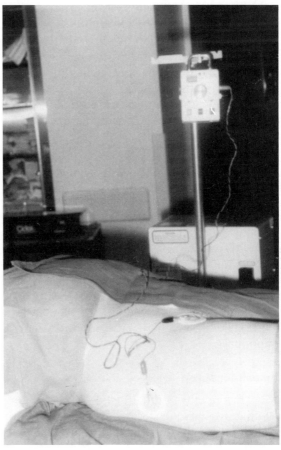

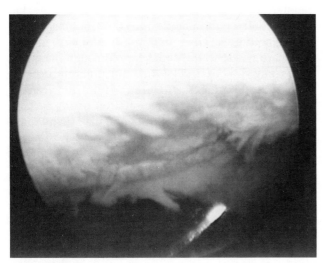

FIGURE 8-13
Arthroscopic view of lateral facet patellar articular breakdown.

FIGURE 8-14
Femoral nerve stimulation at the time of surgery will permit quadriceps contraction and its effects on patellar alignment.

alignment, and to test patellar centralization throughout a range of motion.

Arthroscopic patellar shaving is most appropriate in conjunction with definitive surgery to unload a deficient area of patellar articular cartilage. Isolated arthroscopic patellar shaving offers little advantage to the majority of patients, and, in the author's opinion, should be used only to debride loose fragments of cartilage when more definitive treatment of the patellar articular lesion is undertaken. Occasionally, there may be an appropriate indication to do isolated arthroscopic patellar shaving in the posttraumatic patellar arthrosis patient in whom direct patellar articular cartilage injury has given rise to fibrillation and articular cartilage flaps which are, in themselves, symptomatic. This may be true either on the patellar or trochlear side of the joint. On the other hand, shaving a patellar articular lesion that is under constant stress from malalignment may bring little or no benefit unless the malalignment problem itself is corrected.

In the author's opinion, isolated arthroscopic (or open) lateral release for patellar subluxation is questionable except when subluxation is mild. Lateral release is helpful in relieving tilt but is inconsistent in controlling subluxation.[1] Consequently, isolated arthroscopic lateral release for the patient with significant subluxation (type I or II malalignment) must be considered with skepticism, and the possibility of a tibial tubercle transfer or a cautious medial retinacular imbrication must be considered to control significant lateral patellar displacement.

OPEN SURGICAL TREATMENT

In certain instances nonoperative and arthroscopic treatment will be insufficient in the treatment of patients with patellar instability. As previously noted, lateral retinacular release is insufficient for control of significant patellar instability (as opposed to tilt). The key to success, then, is to correct the *vector* of patellar alignment, by placing the patella in the femoral trochlea so that it will stay there through a functional range of motion.

Trillat Procedure

Jay Cox has reviewed the Elmslie–Trillat procedure for realigning the extensor mechanism.[8] This procedure, which involves medialization of the tibial tubercle by using a flat osteotomy deep in the tibial tubercle, will diminish the Q angle and will effectively place the lateralized extensor mechanism in an

alignment that will permit correct tracking of the patella. The Trillat procedure is appropriate for patients who have chronic patellar instability, particularly when there is recurrent dislocation. In the author's opinion, this procedure is preferable to those procedures that place the tibial tubercle posteriorly, such as the Hauser procedure. Furthermore, handling patellar instability and abnormal extensor mechanism alignment by adjusting the Q angle, using the Trillat procedure, avoids tightening the medial aspect of the PFJ. Such tightening of the medial PFJ can lead to increased pressure medially in the effort to support the patella in a medial direction.

The technique for performing a Trillat procedure is well described.[8] Basically, the surgeon creates a flat osteotomy deep to the tibial tubercle with a short pedicle of anterior tibial bone permitting shift of the tibial tubercle in a medial direction. The author prefers to place two screws in the transferred tibial tubercle lagging the transferred pedicle to the posterior cortex with cortical screws to ensure firm fixation. A lateral retinacular release is always done at the time of the Trillat procedure and degenerated cartilage on the patella is debrided arthroscopically or through the lateral release incision.

Medial Imbrication

Tibial tubercle transfer is not feasible in the skeletally immature patient. Therefore, in such patients with chronic patellar instability (either recurrent subluxation or dislocation), a careful medial reefing (imbrication) of the medial patellar retinaculum may be needed, in addition to lateral release, to control instability of the patella. Using soft tissue imbrication, the concept is similar to that of medial tibial tubercle transfer, namely: realignment of the extensor mechanism to deliver the patella into the trochlea during normal activities. The inherent problem with medial imbrication is that the force vector through the quadriceps may still be laterally directed, potentially causing ultimate stretching and failure of the imbrication. Excessive hip anteversion, pronation of the feet, or an excessively lateral tibial tubercle may lead to failure of the imbrication. The risks are excessive medial tightness causing posteriorly directed force on the patella and resultant aggravation of impending or incipient patellar arthrosis, medial scar pain, or eventual stretching of the medial imbrication resulting in recurrent instability.

The author prefers to keep medial imbrication as benign as possible when it is necessary. A short $1\frac{1}{2}$- to 2-inch medial peripatellar incision in the region of the vastus medialis obliquus (VMO) will permit the surgeon to advance the VMO and some of the medial retinaculum down to the level of the junction of the distal and middle thirds of the patella. The medial retinaculum and tendinous portion of the VMO are advanced in a lateral direction to hold the patella more medially. Usually this retinacular/VMO imbrication is advanced no more than 1 cm. Multiple sutures, preferably nonabsorbable, are placed to maintain the retinacular/VMO imbrication. The surgeon should look carefully at the alignment of the patella following placement of the initial sutures to ensure that the patella has not been tilted medially or drawn too far in a medial direction.

Another variant of soft tissue medial imbrication is the Galeazzi procedure[9] in which the semitendinosus tendon is left at its insertion distally and detached at the musculotendinous junction, bringing the semitendinosus tendon back to the patella through a drill hole to hold the patella in a medial direction (Fig. 8-15). This procedure is usually appropriate for the skeletally immature patient and may be used in preference to medial imbrication. The Galeazzi procedure has the advantage of avoiding posteriorly directed forces on the patella as are likely to occur with a medial imbrication.

Following medial imbrication or Galeazzi procedure, a period of immobilization has been traditional, usually 5 to 6 weeks. To avoid lateral scarring, atrophy, and disuse, the author prefers to start early, limited range of motion and partial weight bearing. This requires secure fixation of the repair with multiple nonabsorbable sutures.

Anteromedial Tibial Tubercle Transfer (AMTTT)

Many patients with patellar instability have some degree of patellar arthrosis related to the chronic imbalance of pressures on patellar articular cartilage. The patient with true excessive lateral pressure syndrome (ELPS) as described by Ficat[10] will benefit from unloading the lateral facet at the time of improving the extensor mechanism vector by medial transfer of the tibial tubercle. Similarly, many patients have distal medial facet patellar arthrosis, related to chronic instability, with a lesion at the "critical zone"[1] of the patella. Such patients will benefit from anterior and medial transfer of the tibial tubercle. This may be accomplished through the anteromedial tibial tubercle originally described in 1983.[11]

It is important to recognize the *medial* transfer will be limited to some extent when one does an AMTTT. This is because the oblique osteotomy shifts the tibial tubercle anteriorly in exchange for less medialization. If considerable medialization of the tubercle is necessary (as in the case of severe patellar lateralization and some patients with patellofemoral dysplasia), one should use a standard Trillat procedure to titrate the medialization, and rely on bone graft, as described by Maquet,[12] to achieve tibial tubercle anteriorization.

Nonetheless, in most patients, one can achieve the needed medialization and concomitant decompression of the distal and lateral patella facets using AMTTT (Fig. 8-16). AMTTT also distracts the released lateral retinaculum, thereby minimizing any risk of retinacular scar contracture.

TECHNIQUE

After arthroscopy to quantitate and localize the patellar articular lesions, the surgeon will make a lateral peripatellar longitudinal incision extending from the midproximal patella to a point about 5 cm distal to the tibial tubercle.[1,11,13] A lateral release is done, and care taken to preserve the main vastus lateralis tendon. The patella can be examined then and debrided as necessary.

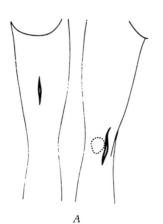 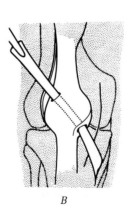 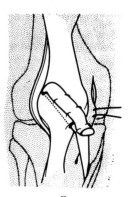

FIGURE 8-15
Galeazzi procedure. *(Reproduced from Reference 9.)*

A   *B*   *C*

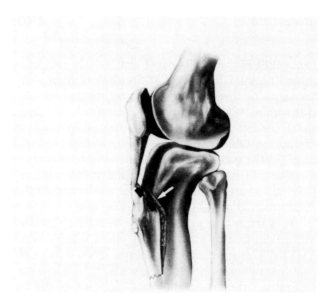

FIGURE 8-16
Anteromedial tibial tubercle transfer. *(Reproduced from References 1 and 13.)*

At this point, the anterior compartment is identified and the proximal anterior tibialis muscle released directly off bone only at its most proximal extent, leaving the anterolateral tibial exposed for a distance of about 7 to 10 cm below the tibial tubercle. The whole lateral side of the tibia should be exposed at this level, such that the junction of the lateral and posterior tibia can be seen.

Starting just at the medial aspect of the patellar tendon insertion, and using the Hoffman drill guide, several long drill bits are directed from anteromedial to posterolateral such that an osteotomy plane is defined. These drill bits must not penetrate out of the posterior cortex of the tibia, or into the tibialis anterior muscle at any time, so excellent retraction and control are imperative. The deep peroneal nerve and the anterior tibial artery are just behind the junction of the lateral and posterior aspects of the tibia at this

level (Fig. 8-17). The osteotomy should be fashioned to *taper* anteriorly as the osteotomy goes distal.

Once the osteotomy plane is defined, an oscillating saw or broad osteotomes may be used to make the osteotomy cut, but a cut proximally at the anterolateral aspect of the osteotomy must be made from a point just proximal to the patellar tendon insertion to the tip of the most proximal drill bit deep to the tibial tubercle.

After creating the osteotomy, the tibial tubercle is shifted in an anterior and medial direction and locked in the corrected position using two cortical screws placed through the transferred bone pedicle and fixed using a slight lag effect in to the posterior tibial cortex (Fig. 8-18). After achieving meticulous hemostasis, a large hemovac is left in the wound (usually for 24 h) and the wound is closed in layers.

Patients are started on immediate active and passive flexion to 90 degrees and kept on crutches partial weight bearing for 4 to 6 weeks. Results with this technique were reviewed in 1990.[1, 13]

Open Surgical Treatment Summary

In the surgical treatment of patients with patellar instability, the clinician should design the surgical plan to treat tilt when present (lateral release), the abnormal alignment vector, and arthrosis. The Trillat procedure is most appropriate for correcting the extensor mechanism vector, and a medial imbrication will occasionally be indicated when tibial tubercle transfer is not possible (as in the skeletally immature patient). When arthrosis is a problem, the surgeon may want to combine a distal realignment procedure with anterior shift of the tibial tubercle. This can be accomplished using an anteromedial tibial tubercle transfer.[1, 13]

ACKNOWLEDGEMENTS

The authors wish to acknowledge Susan Philo for dedicated secretarial support.

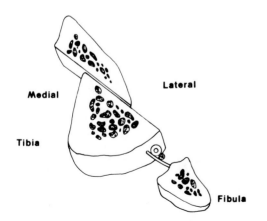

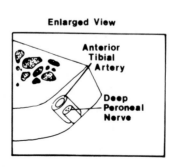

FIGURE 8-17
The proximity of the anterior tibial artery and deep peroneal nerve to osteotomy. *(Reproduced from References 1 and 13.)*

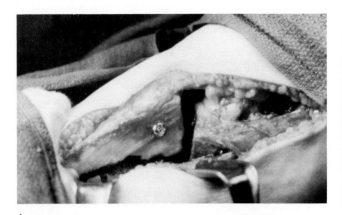

A

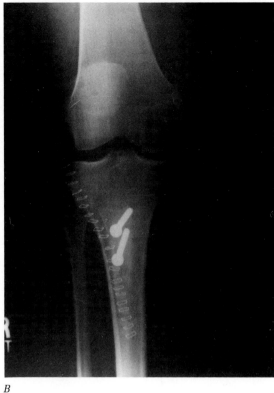

B

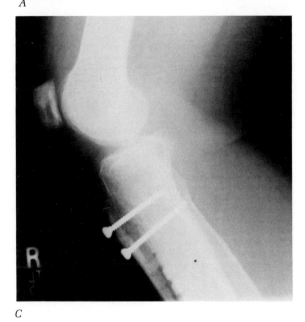

C

FIGURE 8-18
Anteromedial tibial tubercle transfer in shifted position *(A)*, and postoperative AP radiograph *(B)*, and lateral radiograph *(C)*.

REFERENCES

1. Fulkerson J, Hungerford D: *Disorders of the Patellofemoral Joint.* Baltimore, Williams & Wilkins, 1990.
2. Fulkerson J, Shea K: Current concepts: Disorders of patellar alignment. *J Bone Joint Surg* 72-A:1424, 1990.
3. Malghem J, Maldague B: Patellofemoral joint 30° axial radiograph with lateral rotation of the leg. *Radiology* 170:566, 1989.
4. Hughston J, Deese M: Medial subluxation of the patella as a complication of lateral retinacular release. *Am J Sports Med* 16:383, 1988.
5. Shellock F, Mink J, Fox J: Patellofemoral joint: Kinematic MR imaging. *Radiology* 168:551, 1988.
6. Fulkerson J: Awareness of the retinaculum in evaluating patellofemoral pain. *Am J Sports Med* 10:147, 1982.
7. Schutzer S, Ramsby G, Fulkerson J: Computed tomographic classification of patellofemoral pain patients. *Orthop Clin North Am* 17:235, 1986.
8. Cox J: Evaluation of the Roux–Elmslie–Trillat procedure for knee extensor realignment. *Am J Sports Med* 10:303, 1982.
9. Baker R, Carroll N, Dewar P, Haugh J: Semitendinosus tenodesis for recurrent dislocation of the patella. *J Bone Joint Surg* 54B:103, 1972.
10. Ficat C, Bailleux A: Syndrome d'hyperpression externe de la routle. *Rev Chir Orthop* 61:39, 1975.
11. Fulkerson J: Anteromedialization of the tibial tuberosity for patellofemoral malalignment. *Clin Orthop* 177:176, 1983.
12. Maquet P: Advancement of the tibial tuberosity. *Clin Orthop* 115:225, 1976.
13. Fulkerson J, Becker G, Meaney J, Miranda M, Folcik M: Anteromedial tibial tubercle transfer without bone graft. *Am J Sports Med* 18:490, 1990.

147

CHAPTER 9

Medial Patellar Subluxation

Robert A. Eppley

INTRODUCTION

Idiopathic medial patellar subluxation has only recently been recognized as a distinct clinical entity. Merchant, in fact, in a recent extensive classification of patellofemoral disorders,[1] doesn't even list it (refer to Chap. 10 and Table 10-1). Medial instability, however, has long been known as a potential complication of surgeries directed at medializing the distal extensor mechanism.[2–8] More recently, it has been shown to be a relatively common complication of lateral retinacular release.[9–12] Failure has, in turn, led to the recognition of idiopathic medial patellar subluxation.

New methods of studying dynamic patellar tracking, taking into account lower extremity rotational malalignment and patellar translation, tilt, and rotation, have offered new insights into patellar motion.[13–19] Kinematic magnetic resonance imaging (MRI) has been particularly sensitive as a diagnostic tool in the recognition of medial subluxation.[11] The actual incidence and significance of medial subluxation is currently debated and is not completely understood. We have coined the term "patella adentro," in recognition of the terms patella alta and baja, to describe this entity.

IATROGENIC MEDIAL SUBLUXATION

Medial patellar subluxation or dislocation after extensor mechanism surgery occurs more commonly than previously recognized.[2,4,5,6,9,11] It was first reported after distal realignment procedures described by Hauser or Roux-Goldthwait[5] and is now recognized as a relatively common complication of lateral retinacular release surgery.[7,9,10,11]

MEDIAL SUBLUXATION FOLLOWING EXTENSOR REALIGNMENT

Distal Realignment

Southwick described a patient who developed medial dislocation following medialization of the tibial tubercle using the dovetail technique.[8] "Slight lateral repositioning of the patellar tendon" was required for correction. Blazina reported a 12 percent incidence of medial instability following the Hauser procedure, particularly in patients "with a shallow femoral sulcus or dysplastic patella where an exact balance of muscle pull is necessary to prevent the patella from moving lateral or medially." Lateralization of the lateral portion of the patellar tendon was suggested as treatment for this complication.[2]

Chrisman reported data on 3 of 47 patients who required reoperation for medial dislocation following Hauser procedures,[4] and Templeman and McBeath presented case reports of 2 patients with medial subluxation complicating Roux-Goldthwait procedures.[5] The latter authors emphasize the importance of dynamic intraoperative evaluation of patellofemoral mechanics, using local anesthesia and having the patient extend the knee during surgery.

Lanier described a case of "stuck medial patella" following the Hauser-Hughston procedure, an operation which involved tibial tubercle realignment, advancement of the vastus medialis, and patellar shaving.[3] The patient developed patellar fusion to the medial femoral condyle, requiring reoperation.

Medial Retinacular Advancement

Larson cautioned against advancing the medial quadriceps too distally beyond the midline of the patella, or too laterally, for fear of causing patellar rotation and "undue pressure on the medial facet," causing either discomfort or limitation of flexion.[20] Hughston similarly cautioned that "misplacement of the VMO advancement by as little as one or two mm can impart abnormal rotary forces to the patella; or in the case of the patient with loose retinacular type of subluxation, actually cause medial displacement to occur."[21]

Hughston noted the presence of medial femoral condylar defects[22] and Nicholas described medial subluxation and "stuck patella" as a result of "vastus medialis or medial capsular or meniscal patellofemoral ligament adhesions which take the patella to the medial side."[23]

Teitge found medial patellar tilting in 25 of 47 patients who had undergone iliotibial band lateral extra-articular tenodesis for anterolateral rotatory instability.[6] He notes the importance of balancing the medial and lateral retinaculum when stabilizing the patella in general.

We have identified nine patients with medial subluxation following distal realignment procedures.[24] These patients all had either an inappropriate or overly aggressive medialization of the tibial tubercle, resulting in medial subluxation (Fig. 9-1). They tended to subluxate medially during the initial degrees of knee flexion. One patient continued to dislocate laterally in flexion despite marked medial subluxation in extension (Figs. 9-2 and 9-3).

MEDIAL PATELLAR SUBLUXATION FOLLOWING LATERAL RETINACULAR RELEASE

Betz first described one case of medial subluxation following lateral release.[10] Deese and Hughston's recognition of medial subluxation in 30 knees following lateral release was particularly influential in increasing our awareness of this entity.[11] These patients all developed markedly increased pain following lateral release surgery and, on examination, the patella could be easily subluxated medially by the examiner. Many patients had undergone lateral release for nonspecific symptoms and signs such as anterior knee pain, patellar apprehension, and popping and catching sensations. None of the patients demonstrated lateral patellar subluxation in the normal knee. Three patients who underwent CT scanning showed marked atrophy of the vastus lateralis. No other preoperative clinical or radiographic abnormalities could be identified.

Similarly, Shellock, et al.,[9] reported a 63 percent incidence of medial subluxation in 40 patients with persistent pain following lateral release. Kinematic MRI was diagnostic for medial subluxation during the initial 30 degrees of knee flexion (Fig. 9-4). Seventeen of 43 patients showed medial subluxation of the contralateral, unoperated knee as well.

The recognition of medial subluxation following lateral release has led to increased selectivity when advocating this procedure and to greater vigilance in assessing preoperative patellar tracking abnormalities. Lateral release has been performed for a variety of patellofemoral symptoms in the past, including "pain of otherwise unclear etiology."[25] Unfortunately, results have been varied accordingly, with reported "success" rates ranging from 14 percent to 100 percent.[10,26,27,28,29,30,31,32] More recently, a consensus seems to be arising that lateral release has predictable results in patients with significant lateral patellar tilt, a tight lateral retinaculum and a normal Q angle.[13,33]

Chondromalacia and anterior knee pain are not indications for lateral release in the absence of these criteria, particularly in patients with hypermobility or rotational malalignment.[33] By performing a lateral release, the delicate patellar balance may be disrupted, potentially causing medial subluxation and exacerbation of symptoms. Obviously, patients who track medially or both medially and laterally prior to

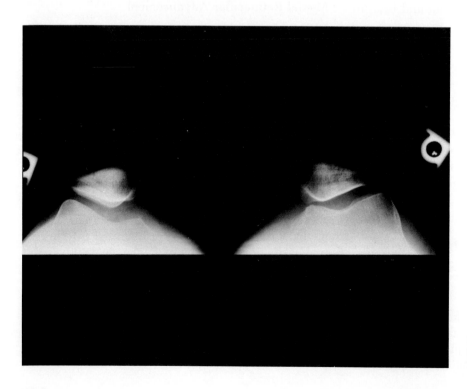

FIGURE 9-1
Medial patellar subluxation following tibial tubercle realignment surgery.

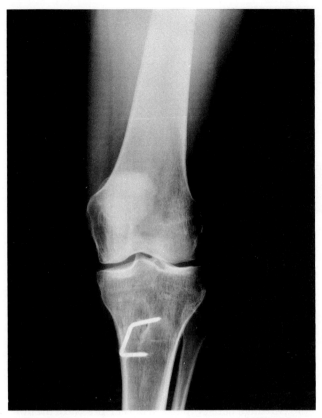

FIGURE 9-2
Patient in Fig. 9-1 with medial patellar subluxation in extension and *lateral* dislocations in flexion; status postdistal realignment.

lateral release will have poor postoperative results. The "failures" of lateral release point out the need to carefully examine all aspects of patellofemoral mechanics preoperatively and observe for medial subluxation.

IDIOPATHIC MEDIAL PATELLAR SUBLUXATION

Idiopathic medial subluxation is a distinct entity which has only recently been described.[9] Using kinematic MRI, which is very sensitive in detecting small degrees of patellar subluxation during the initial 30 degrees of knee flexion, Shellock et al. found a 40 percent incidence of medial subluxation in the unoperated knee of patients who had failed lateral release surgery on the opposite knee[9] (Fig. 9-5). Considering that patellar malalignment is often bilateral,[20,34] it is likely that medial subluxation existed before the lateral retinacular release in certain patients, but was not detected by conventional techniques.[9] Shellock et al.[9] and others[11] suspect that many of the lateral retinacular release procedures performed on patients who develop medial patellar subluxation postoperatively were done for nonspecific patellar symptoms,

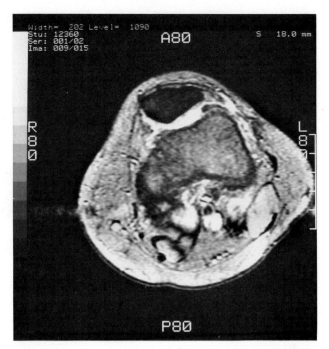

FIGURE 9-3
Medial patellar subluxation following distal realignment.

without careful attention to determine the presence of lateral subluxation or tilt. It is possible that some of the patients who developed medial subluxation after lateral release may have had a degree of medial instability prior to the procedure.

Prior to the advent of kinematic MRI, idiopathic medial patellar subluxation was only alluded to.

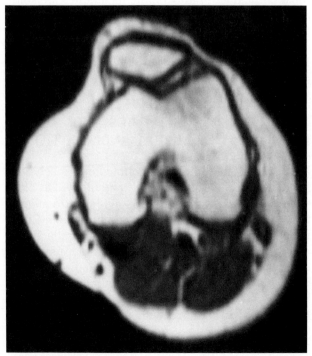

FIGURE 9-4
Kinematic MRI showing idiopathic medial patellar subluxation.

151

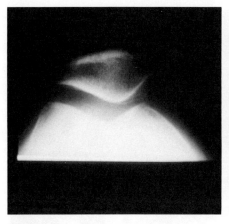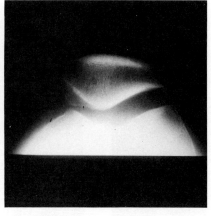

FIGURE 9-5
Bilateral idiopathic medial patellar subluxation. *Courtesy of James Fox, M.D.*

Nicholas[35] stated: "the patella can also move medialward and is influenced by internal tibial rotation during knee extension." He found that the tighter lateral attachments, along with the prominent larger medial condyle prevent medial dislocation, but that "internal femoral torsion combined with external tibial rotation causes a marked side to side or oblique movement of the patella in response to the weight bearing axes at the ankles and hips."[35]

We believe that this "side to side" patella translation and tilt may result in medial subluxation in certain patients. This subluxation is less obvious because of the anatomic confines medially and because it occurs only during the dynamic, multidirectional patellar motion which occurs during the gait cycle. Most clinical and radiographic techniques are static and will not detect the patellar motion. Kinematic MRI, particularly when dynamic, can detect subtle degrees of idiopathic medial patellar subluxation. Further study is ongoing to determine the clinical relevance of these findings and theories.

THE EXTENSOR MECHANICS AND PATHOLOGY OF MEDIAL SUBLUXATION

Most scientific studies of patellofemoral mechanics have concentrated on "lateral" pathology. On close examination, however, there is evidence to suggest that medial pathology may be present as well. Chondromalacia of the medial femur and patella facet[36] and fibrillation of the medial facet cartilage have been observed intraoperatively and attributed to disuse.[37] Chondromalacic changes of the medial facet suggesting excessive medial compression have been identified on MRI in patients with medial subluxation.[16] Outerbridge[38] described medial facet chondromalacia resulting from excessive pressure between the medial facet and the medial femoral condyle during the initial 30 degrees of flexion.

Fulkerson[39] described a subset of patients with pain solely in the medial patellofemoral joint. Ten percent had pain which was "more ill-defined and less clearly retinacular, raising the possibility of true medial facet pain in these patients."

Insall[40] stated that most young patients with patellofemoral pain have malalignment, and Ficat and Hungerford[35] showed that pressure on chondromalacic cartilage caused pain, whereas pressure on normal cartilage did not. If these hypotheses are true, then medial subluxation in conjunction with medial facet chondromalacia suggests that incongruent medial compression may be present and symptomatic.

PATELLOFEMORAL CONTACT ZONES

Studies of patellofemoral contact zones show medial contact at certain degrees of flexion and rotation in some patients. Ahmed[41] found that as the knee flexed from 10 degrees to 20 degrees, the contact pressure zone was medial, lateral, or both, showing wide variation in cadavers tested. Others have shown that the patella moves side to side during flexion.[34,37,42] Sikorski[43] found that patients with chondromalacia demonstrate abnormal femoral rotation when taking weight on the flexed knee and that the medial femoral condyle rises instead of dropping. "It is possible that it may then abut on the medial facet of the patella," a hypothesis which would explain the findings that the pathologic changes of chondromalacia tend to start on the medial patellar facet.[38,43,44]

Patellofemoral mechanics are complicated and variable among individuals. Rotation, tilt, and shift all contribute to the resultant contact areas. Van Kampen and Huiskes[15] found medial tilting and rotation of the patella, which was strongly influenced by tibial rotation. Others have documented this three-dimensional tracking pattern which is influenced by dynamic, axial, and rotational forces during knee mo-

152

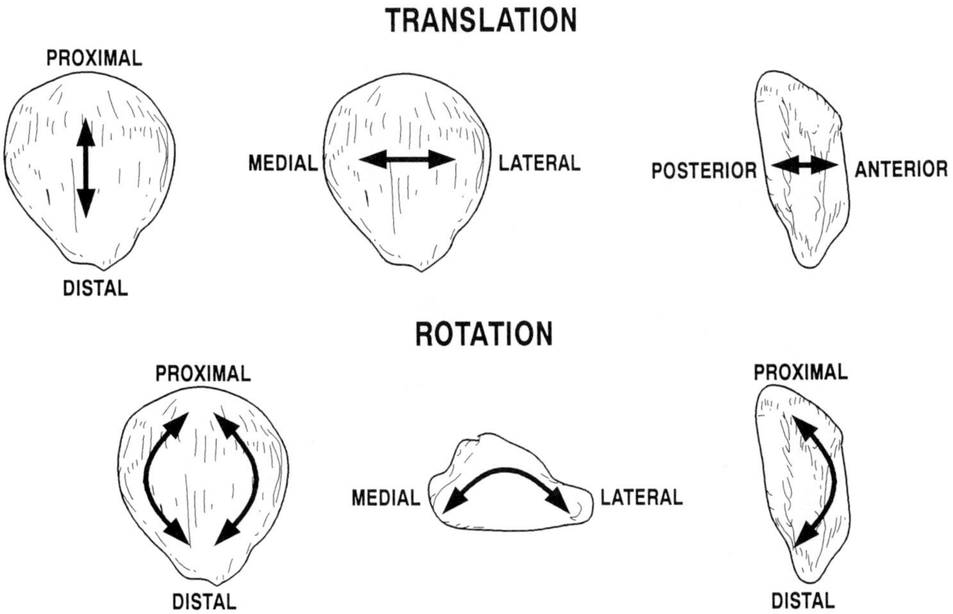

TRANSLATION

PROXIMAL

DISTAL

MEDIAL — LATERAL

POSTERIOR — ANTERIOR

ROTATION

PROXIMAL

DISTAL

MEDIAL — LATERAL

PROXIMAL

DISTAL

FIGURE 9-6
Three-dimensional patellar motion.

tion [12,15,35,45] (Fig. 9-6). Medial shift up to 4 mm and medial rotation to 20 degrees has been described. Nicholas[35] stated that "internal tibial rotation and internal femoral rotation causes the patella to face medially in walking, with side to side movement and a characteristic gait." James[46] noted the difficulties involved in treating patients with "squinting patellae" and so-called "miserable malalignment."

THE DIAGNOSIS OF MEDIAL PATELLAR SUBLUXATION

We are currently attempting to identify the distinct clinical characteristics of over 100 patients who have idiopathic medial subluxation on kinematic MRI (see Fig. 9-4). These patients have had persistent patellofemoral complaints, refractory to traditional rehabilitation aimed at strengthening the medial quadriceps. None had undergone prior surgery. They, in general, have excessive femoral anteversion, external tibial rotation, squinting patellae, and patellae which are easily subluxated medially on clinical exam (Figs. 9-7 through 9-10). A subluxation suppression test, observing for a decrease in symptoms when the patella is held laterally during knee motion, is performed (Fig. 9-11).

When assessing a patient for medial patellar subluxation, the gait is observed for rotational malalignment and medial, lateral or medial-to-lateral translation, rotation or tilt of the patella (see Fig. 9-6). Videotaping the gait cycle on a treadmill may be useful (Fig. 9-12). Rarely, arthroscopic evaluation is performed using local or selective epidural anesthesia to allow direct viewing of active patella motion. This technique allows for assessment of the true dy-

namic patellar tracking during active knee motion, showing the effects of quadriceps pull in conjunction with tibiofemoral rotation.

Most patients with medial patellar subluxation on kinematic MRI have normal Q angles and normal

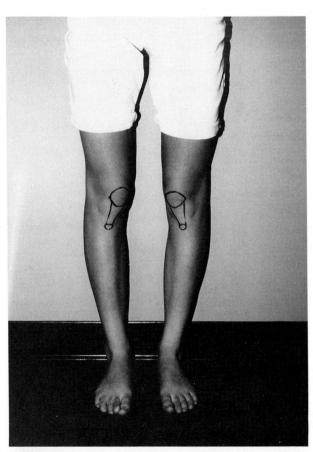

FIGURE 9-7
Medial patellar subluxation with "squinting patella" and typical excessive femoral anteversion.

153

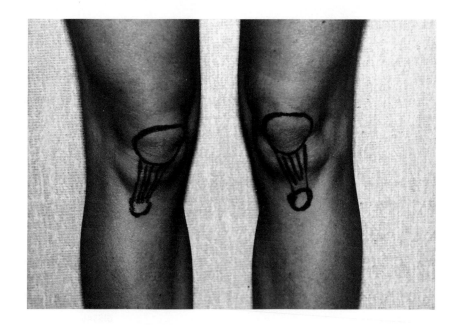

FIGURE 9-8
Medial patellar subluxation.

x-rays. We are attempting to better define the clinical characteristics of this patient population who are presently diagnosed by kinematic MRI.

SUMMARY

Inconsistent success rates in the treatment of patello-femoral disorders imply an incomplete understand-ing of the relevant pathology. Medial patellar sublux-ation is a newly described entity which is currently being defined. It can follow ill-advised or overaggres-sive lateral retinacular release or tibial tubercle re-alignment surgeries. Medial patellar subluxation also exists as an isolated, idiopathic entity in presently unknown frequency.

At present, there is little consistent scientific data to fully define the pathomechanics of this disor-

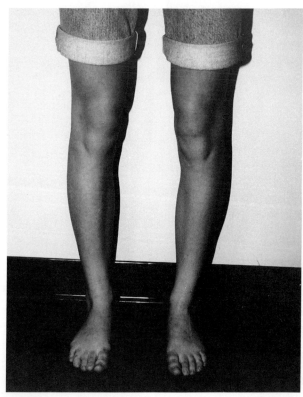

FIGURE 9-9
"Squinting patellae."

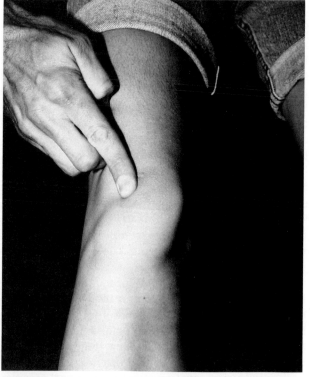

FIGURE 9-10
"Preoperative" examination demonstrating lack of lateral retinacu-lar tightness.

154

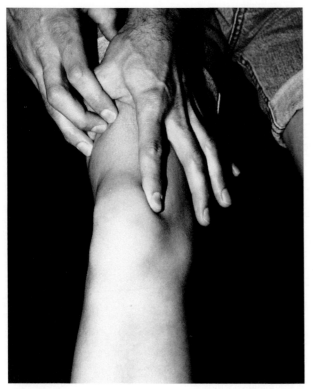

FIGURE 9-11
The subluxation-suppression test for medial subluxation.

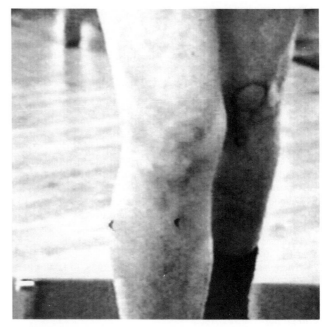

FIGURE 9-12
Treadmill testing showing marked medialization of the left patella.

der. Dynamic analysis of the patellofemoral joint with studies such as kinematic MRI may offer clearer insights into the complicated and variable mechanics of patellar tracking.

Increased awareness of medial patellar subluxa-tion will hopefully prevent the unnecessary or even harmful complications of inappropriate lateral re-lease or other extensor realignment procedures. We stress the importance of dynamic clinical radiologic and intraoperative methods of observing patellofem-oral mechanics on an individual basis. Through these techniques we can hope to better recognize and fur-ther define medial patellar subluxation as a distinct clinical entity.

REFERENCES

1. Merchant AC: Classification of patellofemoral disorders. *Arthroscopy* 4:235, 1988.
2. Blazina ME: Complications of the Hauser Procedure, in *The Injured Adolescent Knee*, edited by JC Kennedy. Baltimore, Williams & Wilkins, 1979, p. 198.
3. Lanier BE: Stuck medial patella. *NY State J Med*, Oct. 1977, p. 1955.
4. Chrisman OD, Snook GA, Wilson TC: A long-term prospective study of the Hauser and Roux-Goldthwait procedure for recurrent patellar dislocation. *Clin Orthop* 144:27, 1979.
5. Templemen D, McBeath A: Iatrogenic patellar malalignment following Roux-Goldthwait proce-dure, corrected by dynamic intraoperative realignment. *J Bone Joint Surg* 68A:1096, 1986.
6. Teitge RA, Indelicato PA, Kerlan RK, et al: Iliotibial band transfer for anterolateral rotatory instability of the knee. *Am J Sports Med* 8:223, 1980.
7. Teitge RA: Recurrent medial subluxation and dislocation. Unpublished manuscript, 1989.
8. Southwick WO, Becker GE, Albright JA: Dovetail patellar tendon transfer for recurrent dislocating patella. *JAMA* 204:117, 1968.
9. Shellock FG, Mink JH, Deutsch A, et al: Evaluation of patients with persistent symptoms follow-ing lateral retinacular release by kinematic MRI of the patellofemoral joint. *Arthroscopy* 6:226, 1990.
10. Betz RR, Magill JT, Longergan RP: The percutaneous lateral retinacular release. *Am J Sports Med* 15:477, 1987.
11. Hughston JC, Deese M: Medial subluxation of the patella as a complication of lateral retinacular release. *Am J Sports Med* 16:383, 1988.
12. Daniel DM, Teitge RA, Grana WA, et al: Knee and leg: Soft tissue trauma, in *Orthopaedic Knowledge Upgrade 3*, American Academy of Orthopaedic Surgeons, pp 563–567.
13. Fulkerson JP, Schutzer SF, Ramsby GR, Bernstein RA: Computerized tomography of the patello-femoral joint before and after lateral release or realignment. *Arthroscopy* 3:19, 1987.
14. Huberti HH, Hayes WC: Patellofemoral contact pressures. *J Bone Joint Surg* 66A:715, 1984.

155

15. Van Kampen A, Huiskes R: The three dimensional tracking pattern of the human patella. *J Orthop Res* 8:372, 1991.

16. Shellock FG, Mink JH, Fox JM: Patellofemoral joint kinematic MR imaging to assess tracking abnormalities. *Radiology* 168:551, 1988.

17. Shellock FG, Mink JH, Deutsch AL, et al: Patellar tracking abnormalities: Clinical experience with kinematic MR imaging in 130 patients. *Radiology* 172:799, 1989.

18. Ahmed AM, Burke DL, Yu A: In-vitro measurement of static pressure distribution in synovial joints. Part II. Retropatellar surface. *Transactions of the ASME* 105:226, 1983.

19. Inoue M. Shino K, Hitoshi H, et al: Subluxation of the patella: Computed tomography analysis of patellofemoral congruence. *J Bone Joint Surg* 70A:1331, 1988.

20. Larson RL: Subluxation-dislocation of the patella, in *The Injured Adolescent Knee*, edited by JC Kennedy. Baltimore, Williams & Wilkins, 1979, p. 199.

21. Hughston JC, Walsh WM: Proximal and distal reconstruction of the extensor mechanism for patellar subluxation. *Clin Orthop* 144:36, 1979.

22. Hughston JC: Reconstruction of the extensor mechanism for subluxation patella. *Am J Sports Med* 1:6, 1972.

23. Nicholas JA: Correspondence, April 15, 1975, in Lanier BE: *Stuck Medial Patella. NY State J of Med*, Oct. 1977, p. 1955.

24. Fox JM, Eppley RA: Patella adentro: Medial patellar subluxation. Unpublished data, 1990.

25. Krompinger WJ, Fulkerson JP: Lateral retinacular release for intractable lateral retinacular pain. *Clin Orthop* 179:191, 1983.

26. Dzioba RB: Diagnostic arthoscopy and longitudinal open lateral release. *Am J Sports Med* 18:343, 1990.

27. Strand, T, Alho A, Rangstad TS, et al: Patellofemoral disorders treated by operations. *Acta Orthop Scan* 54:914, 1983.

28. Schonholtz GJ, Zahn MG, Magee CM: Lateral retinacular release of the patella. *Arthoscopy* 3:269, 1987.

29. Bigos SJ, McBride CG: The isolated lateral retinacular release in the treatment of patellofemoral disorders. *Clin Orthop* 186:75, 1984.

30. Merchant AC, Mercer RL: Lateral release of the patella. A preliminary report. *Clin Orthop* 103:40, 1974.

31. Ogilvie-Harris DJ, Jackson RW: The arthroscopic treatment of chondromalacia patellae. *J Bone Joint Surg* 66B:660, 1984.

32. Cerullo G, Puddu G, Conteduca F, et al: Evaluation of the results of extensor mechanism reconstruction. *Am J Sports Med* 16:93, 1988.

33. Kolowich PA, Paulos LE, Rosenberg RD, Farnsworth S: Lateral release of the patella: Indications and contraindications. *Am J Sports Med*, 18:359, 1990.

34. Ficat RP, Hungerford DS: *Disorders of the Patellofemoral Joint*. Paris, Masson, 1977.

35. Nicholas JA: Dynamic causes of patellar pain. *Orthop Review* 2(3), March 1973.

36. McGinty JB, McCarthy JC: Endoscopic lateral retinacular release. *Clin Orthop* 158:120, 1981.

37. Goodfellow J, Hungerford DS, Woods C: Patellofemoral joint mechanics and pathology. Chondromalacia patellae. *J Bone Joint Surg* 58B:291, 1976.

38. Outerbridge RE, Dunlop JAY: The problem of chondromalacia patellae. *Clin Orthop* 110:177, 1975.

39. Fulkerson JP: The etiology of patellofemoral pain in young active patients: A prospective study. *Clin Orthop* 179:129, 1983.

40. Insall J, Falvo KA, Wise DW: Chondromalacia patellae. *J Bone Joint Surg* 58A:1, 1976.

41. Ahmed AM, Burke DL, Hyder A: Force analysis of the patellar mechanism. *J Orthop Res* 5:69, 1987.

42. Wang CJ: A study of patellofemoral contact in human knees. *J Med Soc NJ* 75(5), 1978.

43. Sikorski JM, Peters J, Watt I: The importance of femoral rotation in chondromalacic patellae as shown by serial radiography. *J Bone Joint Surg* 61B:435, 1979.

44. Abernethy PJ, Townsend PR, Rose RM, Radin EL: Chondromalacia patellae as a separate clinical entity. *J Bone Joint Surg* 60B:205, 1978.

45. Takai S, et al: Rotational alignment of the lower limb in osteoarthritis of the knee. *Int Orthop* 9:209, 1985.

46. James SL: Chondromalacia of the patella in the adolescent, in *The Injured Adolescent Knee*, edited by JC Kennedy. Baltimore, Williams & Wilkins, 1979, p. 205.

CHAPTER 10

The Lateral Patellar Compression Syndrome

Alan C. Merchant

HISTORICAL PERSPECTIVE

The concept of diagnosis of a lateral patellar compression syndrome (LPCS) was first described and defined by Ficat and colleagues in 1975 in an original article entitled "Syndrome d'Hyperpression Externe de la Rotule."[1] The delightful and almost whimsical illustrations from that article deserve republication (Fig. 10-1).

The idea of an LPCS was developed further by Ficat and Hungerford 2 years later in their classic textbook, *Disorders of the Patello-Femoral Joint.*[2] Unfortunately, in this textbook Ficat's original designation for this syndrome was inaccurately translated from French to English as *excessive lateral pressure syndrome* (ELPS), omitting his reference to the patella entirely. A literal translation is syndrome of hyperpressure laterally of the patella. Reworded into English idiom this becomes lateral patellar compression syndrome, a more accurate translation of Ficat's original terminology, which maintains the reference to the patella for clarity. This might seem to be a small

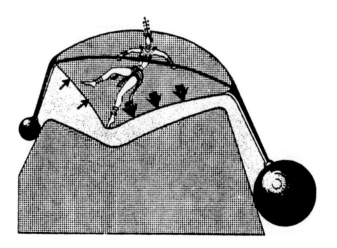

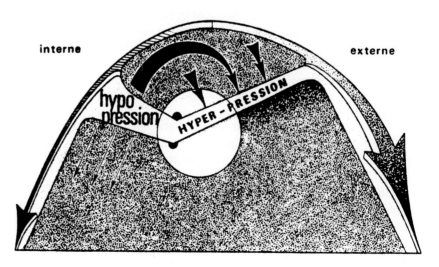

FIGURE 10-1
Illustrations from the original article defining the lateral patellar compression syndrome. *(Reproduced with permission from Ficat P, Ficat C, Bailleaux: Syndrome d'hyperpression externe de la rotule (S.H.P.E.). Rev Chir Orthop 61:39, 1975.)*

point of contention for those who have not struggled to review the literature on patellofemoral disorders. This literature contains a profusion of vague and ill-defined terms that makes accurate comparison of treatment protocols and outcome studies impossible.

This text was the first monograph in English devoted entirely to the subject. As stated in the preface to this volume, the authors' purpose was "to fill a significant gap in the literature" concerning what was then "the forgotten compartment of the knee." In truth, the patellofemoral joint was indeed the "forgotten compartment" at that time. For example, the initial designs for knee replacement arthroplasties completely ignored the patellofemoral joint by replacing only the femorotibial compartments, yet mistakenly called them "total" knee replacements. Before the 1970s only two diagnoses were commonly used relating to anterior knee pain or instability: chondromalacia patellae and recurrent dislocation of the patella. Chondromalacia patellae was considered a final and primary diagnosis with little attention given to the pathomechanics of these lesions. In the United States, the usual surgical treatment for chondromalacia was arthrotomy and shaving, and for recurrent dislocations it was the ill-conceived Hauser procedure. If the arthrosis became too disabling, all too often the patella was considered dispensable and was discarded entirely by patellectomy.

The term *chondromalacia patellae* was first used to designate lesions of the articular cartilage arising from trauma. Aleman is credited with being the first to use this term as early as 1917 and published his classic paper "Chondromalacia Post-Traumatica Patellae" in 1928.[3] Until 1936, the association between a traumatically induced lesion of the patellar articular cartilage found at surgery and the persistent anterior knee symptoms was accepted and understood. In that year Owre published a paper studying chondromalacia found at autopsy.[4] The incidence of these lesions increased with age, but a significant proportion occurred in the teenage years. This use of the same terminology to describe both a condition found at autopsy as well as a clinical syndrome led to an era of increasing confusion. As the years passed, chondromalacia patellae began to be used as a diagnosis by many authors and clinicians without any direct knowledge of the condition of the articular cartilage, finally becoming almost synonymous with anterior knee pain.

The 1970s saw the development of clinically practical radiographic techniques which gave accurate, consistent, and reproducible axial views of the patellofemoral joints[5-7] (Fig. 10-2). The routine use of these axial views in all new patients with knee complaints led Ficat to the concept of LPCS. It had long been understood that recurrent dislocation of the patella could lead to damage of the articular cartilage as the patella slipped over the lateral condyle and reduced back again. But now an accurate axial view demonstrated chronic subluxation (malalignment) of the patella (CSP) in a group of patients who had never experienced episodic dislocations but who presented with anterior knee pain and subpatellar crepitation. This explained their secondary chondromalacia as a result of a chronic localized overload of the articular cartilage. Still a significant number of patients complained of anterior knee pain whose axial view radiographs revealed no patellar subluxation. By correlating a careful physical examination of the extensor mechanism with subtle findings on the axial radiographs, Ficat was able to define this new syndrome.

DEFINITION AND DIAGNOSIS

The original definition for LPCS from Ficat and Hungerford's text[2] remains the best. "It is, then, a syndrome in which the patella is well centered in the trochlear sulcus and stable, but in which there is a functional lateralization onto a physiologically and often anatomically predominant lateral facet."

In the second edition of *Disorders of the Patellofemoral Joint* by Fulkerson and Hungerford,[8] the original terminology is supplemented by a new term *Patellar tilt/compression* and redefined as a syndrome "characterized clinically by pain and radiologically by patellar tilt as evidenced on the axial patellofemoral radiograph, computerized tomography (CT) scan, or magnetic resonance imaging (MRI)." This new terminology not only adds to the confusion of patellofemoral disorders, but also the new definition shifts the focus away from the idea of "functional lateralization" and its implied increased quadriceps angle and onto a radiologic finding (tilt), which most of the time must be discovered by CT scan or MRI. The original terminology and definition appear preferable.

One must remember that the existence of excessive lateral pressure alone does not establish the diagnosis of the LPCS; the patella must be centered and stable in the trochlea as well. In the next more severe form of patellofemoral dysplasia, CSP, excessive lateral pressure is frequently present, but in this case the patella is subluxed and incongruent in the trochlea as well.

History

The presenting complaint of the patient with LPCS is anterior knee pain that can arise quite spontaneously, follow repetitive overuse, or persist after direct or indirect trauma. The precipitating trauma can be deceptively minor. Because anterior knee pain has so many other causes, for example, patellar tendinitis ("jumper's knee") or prepatellar bursitis ("house-

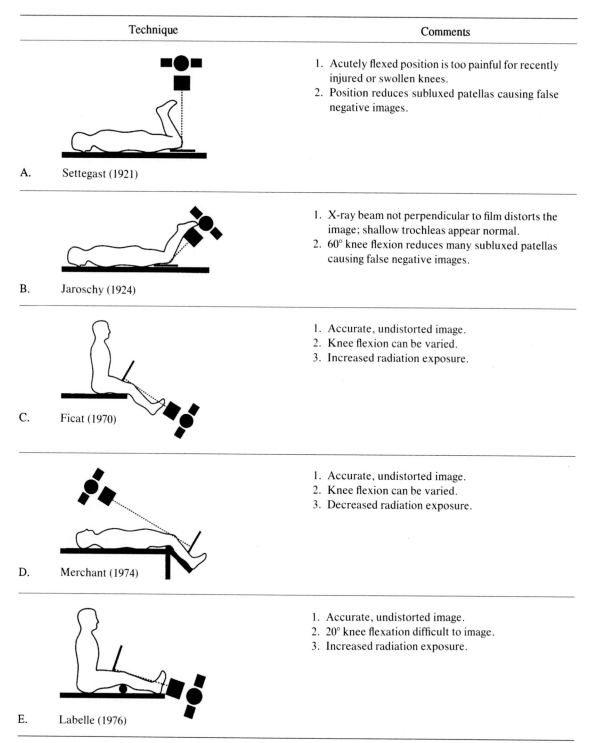

Technique	Comments
A. Settegast (1921)	1. Acutely flexed position is too painful for recently injured or swollen knees. 2. Position reduces subluxed patellas causing false negative images.
B. Jaroschy (1924)	1. X-ray beam not perpendicular to film distorts the image; shallow trochleas appear normal. 2. 60° knee flexion reduces many subluxed patellas causing false negative images.
C. Ficat (1970)	1. Accurate, undistorted image. 2. Knee flexion can be varied. 3. Increased radiation exposure.
D. Merchant (1974)	1. Accurate, undistorted image. 2. Knee flexion can be varied. 3. Decreased radiation exposure.
E. Labelle (1976)	1. Accurate, undistorted image. 2. 20° knee flexation difficult to image. 3. Increased radiation exposure.

FIGURE 10-2
Axial patellofemoral radiographic techniques.

maid's knee"), these other causes must be ruled out by a careful clinical evaluation.

The patient frequently admits to the knee giving way or "going out," leading the unwary clinician toward a diagnosis of recurrent dislocation of the patella. But one must be careful and persistent in extracting the history to discover exactly what the patient means by these terms. Patients frequently refer to a knee (or back, for that matter) "going out" and mean that it suddenly became painful, not that it physically collapsed. Furthermore, during a particular activity, they might feel a sudden stab of anterior knee pain that causes a momentary reflex inhibition of the quadriceps to unload the patellofemoral joint. This certainly feels as if the knee gives way, but almost never results in a fall nor is there any subsequent effusion so characteristic of a recurrent patellar dislocation.

The typical pain is anterior and almost anywhere in the patellofemoral, extensor mechanism. It is aggravated by flexed knee activities such as hiking, climbing, or descending stairs, squatting, kneeling, running, and the like. Anterior knee pain associated with prolonged sitting (a "theater ache") is common. Because the location, character, and features of the pain are nearly identical to other patellofemoral disorders, one must look to the physical examination and radiographs to make the diagnosis.

Physical Examination

If we remember that the definition of LPCS requires the existence of a "functional lateralization" of the patella, then the physical examination should focus on a search for the features known to cause it. For simplicity these features can be grouped into three areas: those causing an increased anatomic quadriceps (Q) angle, those that weaken the medial forces on the patella, and those that increase the lateral pull. Of course, these features can occur in various degrees of severity and in various combinations in any given patient. For instance, a patient with a mild increased Q angle, a mild vastus medialis obliquus (VMO) deficiency, and a mild lateral retinacular tightness can suffer just as much as one with a normal Q angle, a normal VMO, but a severe hypertrophy of the lateral retinaculum. Both patients would have LPCS, but their prognosis and ultimate treatment would differ because of the different etiologies.

To avoid confusion when discussing the Q angle, we must differentiate between the true Q angle and the anatomic Q angle. The *true Q angle* is defined as the complimentary angle of a line representing the resultant line of force of the quadriceps and a line along the patellar tendon. In the normal knee, a line from the anterior superior iliac spine to the center of the patella approximates that resultant line of force, but in actuality this line really measures only the *anatomic Q angle*. For example, a patient may have a significant deficiency of the vastus medialis obliquus along with a normal anatomic Q angle when measured from the anterior superior iliac spine. The medial muscular deficiency causes the resultant line of force of the quadriceps to swing lateral to the anterior superior iliac spine increasing the true angle.

Because the true Q angle is a functional and dynamic measurement of the lateralizing forces on the extensor mechanism and the LPCS is defined as "functional lateralization" of the patella, the two become inseparable. In fact, LPCS could be thought of as a true Q angle syndrome.

However, we cannot measure the true Q angle by physical examination, so in this discussion as in other clinical studies the term Q angle refers to the anatomic Q angle, which we can measure. Measurement of the Q angle is important not only to help establish an accurate diagnosis but also to record where the anatomic abnormalities are within the extensor mechanism so that a logical nonoperative and surgical treatment program can be developed. Measurement and documentation of the Q angle is of such prime importance in LPCS and other patellofemoral dysplasias that a detailed discussion about it is appropriate.

If the physical examination begins with the patient sitting on the edge of the examination table, the first assessment of the Q angle can be made with the knee flexed at 90 degrees. Normally in this position a line through the center of the patellar tendon will line up exactly with the center axis of the leg, giving a value of zero degrees. Any displacement of the tibial tubercle laterally will increase this angle and is considered abnormal (Fig. 10-3). Because the patella is centered in the trochlea at 90 degrees flexion, this measurement has been termed the *tubercle-sulcus angle*.[9] However, this method of measurement only measures the distal limb of the Q angle. Therefore, the Q angle should be more accurately measured and recorded with the patient supine and the knee fully extended. One limb of the goniometer should point to the anterior superior iliac spine and the other to the tibial tubercle (Fig. 10-4). The normal value for men is about 10 degrees and for women about 15 degrees.[10]

There is disagreement about whether or not to have the quadriceps contracted at the time of measurement. I believe it should be relaxed for the following reasons. The Q angle as measured is part of an anatomic approximation of the dynamic equilibrium of the forces at work on the patella during active use. Most patellofemoral symptoms are generated by vigorous flexed knee activities with the knee flexed between 30 and 60 degrees and the patella centered within the trochlea. If the patient has a J sign with the patella shifting laterally in terminal active extension as it leaves the trochlea, then the Q angle is falsely straightened toward normal. Instead, the quadriceps should remain relaxed and the examiner should be sure the patella is centered in the trochlea for measurement. If the patient has a significant patella alta so that the patella does not engage the sulcus in full extension, then the examiner should slowly lift the relaxed knee with one hand while the other feels the patella center in the trochlea. Then the examiner should hold the patella centered in that position as the knee is allowed to extend onto the table and the Q angle should be measured there. We all recognize that the tibia externally rotates in terminal extension with the "screw home" mechanism, which increases the Q angle, but if all knees are measured in this same manner, than the comparisons are meaningful.

Anatomic variants that increase the Q angle include valgus deformity of the knee, lateral displacement of the tibial tubercle, and rotational malalignment of the femur, tibia, or both. The anterior knee pain from the combination of internal femoral torsion and compensatory external tibial torsion (the "miserable malalignment" of James)[11] is, in final analysis, an LPCS.

The most common abnormality that weakens the medial force on the patella is a congenital deficiency of the VMO in which the distal fibers insert much too high and not into the upper third of the patella where they should. This leaves a characteristic hollow adjacent to the patella medially as the patient actively holds the leg suspended and the knee flexed 30 to 45 degrees. This hollow is easily seen in most patients but can be impossible to spot in the obese.

Other causes of medial weakness can be quadriceps atrophy, chronic effusion with distension of the weaker medial retinaculum, disruption of the medial retinaculum or VMO from previous dislocation of the patella, and prior surgery through a medial parapatellar incision.

Finally, during the physical examination a search needs to be made for factors exerting an increased lateral force on the patella. The most common of these is hypertrophy and excessive tightness of the lateral retinaculum. It is simple to evaluate by

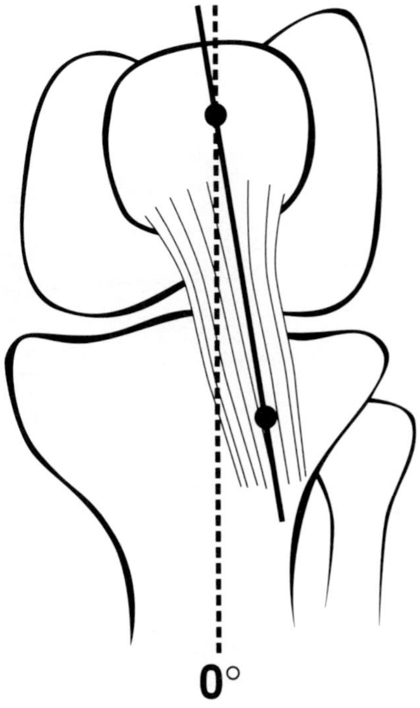

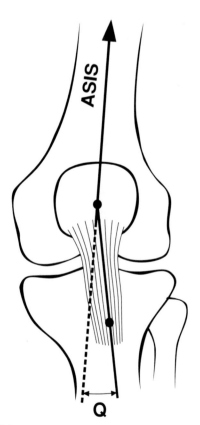

FIGURE 10-3
With the knee flexed 90 degrees the tubercle-sulcus angle should be 0 degrees. This one is abnormal.

FIGURE 10-4
Measurement of the anatomic Q angle with the knee in extension. ASIS, anterior superior iliac spine. Q, Q angle.

assessing the passive medial excursion or "glide" of the patella. Just as one checks for excessive passive lateral motion of the patella and the production of apprehension as the patella glides too far laterally, the medial glide should be checked at the same time as well. With the knee flexed to 30 degrees and the quadriceps relaxed, the normal patella can be moved about one finger breadth medially. Again, the most common cause for lateral retinacular tightness is congenital and thought to be part of the patellofemoral dysplasias. Other causes are posttraumatic scaring, postsurgical fibrosis, and reflex sympathetic dystrophy.

Radiologic Evaluation

After obtaining a history of anterior knee pain and finding the physical features of increased functional lateralization of the patella, the axial view radiograph is the third examination necessary to establish the diagnosis of LPCS. An accurate axial view is needed to establish the fact that the patella is indeed "centered in the trochlear sulcus." In fact, if the patella is shown to be subluxed laterally, then the diagnosis changes to CSP.

As was mentioned earlier, it was the careful study of axial view radiographs obtained on every patient with knee complaints that led to the description of this syndrome. The most direct finding of excessive lateral pressure is narrowing of the joint space compared to the asymptomatic side. Because the contact areas on the patella change with the degree of flexion, Ficat insisted on axial views at 30, 45, and 60 degrees to study almost all of the articular surface. For joint space narrowing to occur, there must be some degree of softening of the articular cartilage (chondromalacia). If an arthrogram is to be done, an axial view with the contrast media will demonstrate the diminution, and if the damage has progressed to breakdown and fissuring, the dye will be seen to invade the articular cartilage. However, chondromalacia is not a *sine qua non* for the diagnosis of LPCS; it is considered a secondary change. Ficat and Hungerford[2] reported that 20 percent of their cases of LPCS did not demonstrate any evidence of narrowing on any of the three axial views. Obviously the occurrence and frequency of secondary changes of chondromalacia are a function of how far the condition has progressed before the patients are studied. Fortunately several indirect signs of excessive lateral pressure can be found on the axial view before chondromalacia is present.

The most common indirect evidence of increased lateral compression found on the axial view is thickening or sclerosis of the subchondral bone of the lateral patellar facet (Fig. 10-5). At the same time there is a relative osteopenia of the medial portion of the patella. In addition, the trabeculae of the patella, which are usually oriented perpendicular to a line drawn transversely across the patella, become oriented perpendicular to the lateral facet. All these findings are an expression of Wolff's law of bone's adaptation to applied forces.

Other less common findings are traction osteophytes on the lateral patellar margin, thickening or calcification of the soft tissues of the lateral retinaculum, hypoplasia of the lateral femoral condyle, and bipartite patella (Fig. 10-6).

Before leaving the subjects of the definition and diagnosis of LPCS, it should be noted that excellent clinicians have not confirmed the existence of this syndrome despite a diligent clinical and radiographic search. Perhaps this discrepancy is caused by the failure to use accurate, undistorted axial radiographs taken at 30 to 45 degrees of knee flexion, or perhaps it is merely a confusion of terminology.

CLASSIFICATION

It is evident that LPCS shares many common features with CSP and recurrent dislocation of the patella (RDP). Therefore, these three diagnoses are placed as subgroups within the larger division of patellofemoral dysplasia. They can be thought of as a continuum with LPCS representing the most common and mild form of patellofemoral dysplasia and RDP the most

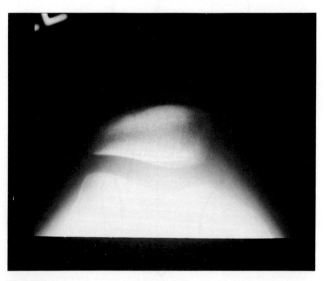

FIGURE 10-5
Axial view radiograph of the knee shows osseous changes secondary to excessive lateral pressure. See text and Fig. 10-6*A*.

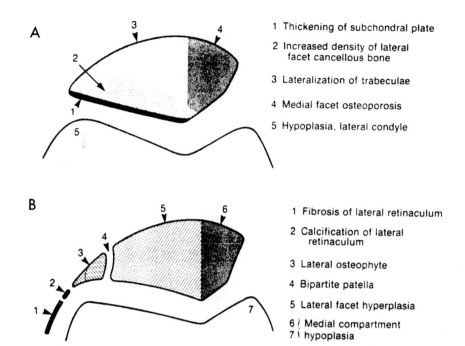

FIGURE 10-6
A. Radiologic signs of excessive lateral pressure. *B.* Radiologic signs of excessive lateral retinacular tension. *(Reproduced with permission from Ficat P, Hungerford DS: Disorders of the Patellofemoral Joint. Baltimore, Williams & Wilkins, 1977.)*

1 Thickening of subchondral plate
2 Increased density of lateral facet cancellous bone
3 Lateralization of trabeculae
4 Medial facet osteoporosis
5 Hypoplasia, lateral condyle

1 Fibrosis of lateral retinaculum
2 Calcification of lateral retinaculum
3 Lateral osteophyte
4 Bipartite patella
5 Lateral facet hyperplasia
6 } Medial compartment
7 } hypoplasia

uncommon and more severe expression. Table 10-1 demonstrates how these patellofemoral dysplasias fit into the overall classification of patellofemoral disorders.

The other major attribute of this classification of patellofemoral disorders is that the term *chondromalacia patellae* is eliminated as a diagnosis used by itself. It is returned to its original and proper usage as a descriptive term for a pathologic condition of articular cartilage. Using the terms *secondary chondromalacia patellae* and *idiopathic chondromalacia patellae* focuses the clinician's attention on a search for the cause for the chondromalacia.

TREATMENT

Nonoperative Treatment

The initial treatment of LPCS depends on the mode of onset. If the onset is traumatic, usually the patient is not seen initially because the effects of the trauma are expected to be transient. It is only when the anterior knee pain persists longer than anticipated, the patient comes in or is referred. Only then is the underlying dynamic imbalance discovered. Frequently, symptoms are from overuse, especially related to flexed knee activities. The first advice should be to place the knee at relative rest by avoiding the physical activities that cause the symptoms. If inflammation is part of the presentation, then the usual measures of ice and anti-inflammatory medications are added.

The most important part of the treatment, however, is focused on regaining the functional balance of the patella and the extensor mechanism by exercise. If the quadriceps or hamstring muscles are contracted, stretching exercises are prescribed. Contracture of these antagonistic thigh muscles is a frequent finding and a common cause for anterior knee pain in the adolescent patient.

Because the quadriceps muscle plays such an important role in the dynamic balance of the patella, its strengthening becomes the major rehabilitative effort from beginning to end. Earlier we discussed the different lateralizing forces on the patella: a deficient VMO, an increased Q angle, and tightness of the lateral retinaculum. Of these three, only the effect of the VMO can be materially improved by exercise; the other two require surgical correction, if necessary. In most patellofemoral disorders, the quadriceps will be weakened in proportion to the severity of the problem. This will occur naturally by disuse as the patient avoids the flexed knee activities that cause the pain. Therefore, the initial goal is to restore them to normal strength, but beyond that, the final goal is to build greater strength to compensate for the imbalance that caused the functional lateralization in the first place.

If the muscle is extremely weak, quadriceps setting then straight leg raising exercises can be started. Recumbent straight leg weight lifting follows, but the limit here is about 8 to 10 lb because more weight will strain the hip and lower back. It is at this juncture, in the commendable desire to gain more strength, that most patellofemoral rehabilitation programs fail. Too often these patients are placed on either short arc (30 degree) isotonic progressive resistive exercises or an isokinetic resistive machine, which are both nonphysiologic for the patellofemoral joint. During normal physiologic activities such as climbing or jump-

TABLE 10-1
Classification of Patellofemoral Disorders

I. Trauma (conditions caused by trauma in the otherwise normal knee)

    A. Acute trauma
1. Contusion
2. Fracture
    a. Patella
    b. Femoral trochlea
    c. Proximal tibial epiphysis (tubercle)
3. Dislocation (rare in the normal knee)
4. Rupture
    a. Quadriceps tendon
    b. Patellar tendon

    B. Repetitive trauma (overuse syndromes)
1. Patellar tendinitis ("jumper's knee")
2. Quadriceps tendinitis
3. Peri-patellar tendinitis (e.g., Anterior knee pain of the adolescent due to hamstring contracture)
4. Pre-patellar bursitis ("housemaid's knee")
5. Apophysitis
    a. Osgood-Schlatter disease
    b. Sinding-Larsen-Johanssen's disease

    C. Late effects of trauma
1. Post-traumatic chondromalacia patellae
2. Post-traumatic patellofemoral arthritis
3. Anterior fat pad syndrome (post-traumatic fibrosis)
4. Reflex sympathetic dystrophy of the patella
5. Patellar osseous dystrophy
6. Acquired patella infera
7. Acquired quadriceps fibrosis

II. Patellofemoral Dysplasia

    A. Lateral patellar compression syndr. (LPCS)
1. Secondary chondromalacia patellae
2. Secondary patellofemoral arthritis

    B. Chronic subluxation of the patella (CSP)
1. Secondary chondromalacia patellae
2. Secondary patellofemoral arthritis

    C. Recurrent dislocation of the patella (RDP)
1. Associated fractures
    a. Osteochondral (intra-articular)
    b. Avulsion (extra-articular)
2. Secondary chondromalacia patellae
3. Secondary patellofemoral arthritis

    D. Chronic dislocation of the patella
1. Congenital
2. Acquired

III. Idiopathic Chondromalacia Patellae

IV. Osteochondritis dissecans
    A. Patella
    B. Femoral trochlea

V. Synovial plicae (anatomic variant made symptomatic by acute or repetitive trauma)
    A. Medial patellar ("shelf")
    B. Suprapatellar
    C. Infrapatellar
    D. Lateral patellar

Adapted from Merchant AC: Classification of patellofemoral disorders. *Arthroscopy* 4:235, 1988.

ing, the increased load on the patellofemoral joint as the knee is flexed is mediated by an increase in the contact surface area.[12] In contrast, if the knee is extended against an isokinetic machine or a free weight, the patellofemoral joint reaction force increases as the contact surface area shrinks, thus exceeding the physiologic unit load on the patellar articular cartilage. In a knee already compromised by a patellofemoral imbalance or actual subluxation, the result is further damage to the hyaline cartilage. **Never use resistive extension exercises in patellofemoral disorders!**

There are two alternative methods to gain additional quadriceps strength while still avoiding the nonphysiologic and damaging techniques of resistive knee extensions. Both use progressive resistive isometric quadriceps exercises with the knee in full extension. The method described by DeHaven and colleagues[13] requires the use of a so-called double action weight bench (Fig. 10-7). We have used another technique[14] as a simple home exercise quite successfully for years (Fig. 10-8). Resistance levels of 20 to 40 lb can be achieved depending on the patient's size, general strength, and vigor. The use of the weight bench technique provides a mechanical advantage and much higher levels can be obtained. These two methods cannot damage the articular cartilage of the patellofemoral joint because the patella rests above the trochlea during the exercise.

Once the symptoms have subsided, physiologic closed-end exercises such as cycling, climbing, running, and leg presses can be judiciously added. If the patient wishes to return to sports, a patellar brace is advisable. Many are on the market and for LPCS it should have a hole for the patella to avoid additional compression and a lateral buttress pad to apply a medially directed force.

Success for the nonoperative treatment program in patients with LPCS approximates 90 percent. But to be successful the program must be persistent and monitored. Just telling a patient to do the exercises is frequently not enough; follow-up evaluations are necessary. Furthermore, I am amazed how often a written physical therapy prescription is ignored, and the patient is placed on a resistive knee extension, usually on an isokinetic machine.

Operative Treatment

Surgery should be considered only after a proper, prolonged, and monitored nonoperative treatment program has failed. Having said that, not even all patients who remain symptomatic after such a program should have an operation. Two factors become paramount in counseling patients about surgery: the degree of disability caused by the LPCS and the physical cause or causes of its functional lateralization. As an example, if a high school student has made a *bona fide* effort at a proper nonoperative program and the only limitation remains long distance running, then I believe a frank discussion with the parents and the student encouraging other alternative sports would be preferable to surgery. Regarding the causative factors, we frequently encounter patients whose LPCS is secondary to bilateral internal femoral torsion with compensatory external tibial torsion ("miserable malalignment") who remain symptomatic in almost all flexed knee activities. Surgical correction with bilateral femoral and tibial derotation osteotomies presents too many risks to be considered.

For these reasons when finally considering surgery, it becomes vitally important to reexamine the patient to confirm the physical causes of the functional lateralization. These are the abnormalities that need to be corrected if possible. The most simple realignment surgery is the lateral retinacular release. If the patient has a tight lateral retinaculum, release it; if it is not tight, leave it alone.

Arthroscopy provides an excellent opportunity to inspect and document the secondary chondromalacia patellae. If there is only softening or early crevicing, no shaving is indicated. Only loose, fragmented,

and unstable cartilage should be conservatively debrided. Arthroscopy also can reveal an unsuspected intra-articular cause for anterior knee pain, such as a pathologic synovial plica.

When an isolated lateral release is properly performed on a tight retinaculum for the correct indications and the knee intelligently rehabilitated, it is a relatively safe outpatient procedure with low morbidity. However, correction of an abnormally large anatomic Q angle will require a medial tibial tubercle transfer, which raises the levels of risk, length of hospitalization, morbidity, and temporary disability significantly. For these reasons, the surgeon must try to estimate to what degree each abnormality found on the physical examination is affecting the functional lateralization of the patella.

Starting with the deficient VMO, its anatomic appearance can vary from mild to severe. Its effect on functional lateralization certainly can be increased by quadriceps deconditioning or atrophy, thus precipitating the symptoms of LPCS. On the other hand, it is the only physical abnormality that can be improved by proper isometric quadriceps exercises discussed previously. If the surgeon is honestly con-

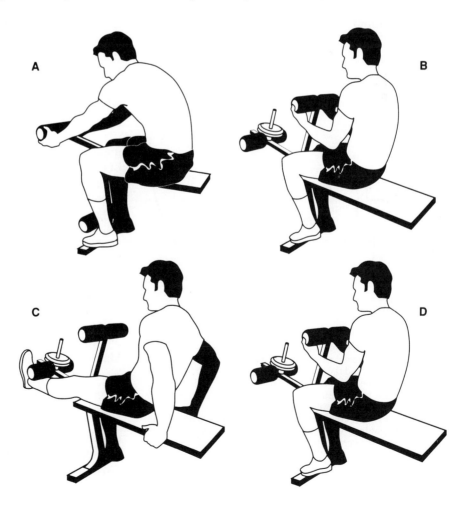

FIGURE 10-7
Isometric progressive resistive quadriceps exercises using a weight bench. *A.* The patient uses the hamstring pads to lift the weights with his arms not the leg *(B). C.* One knee is then extended without any resistance, held straight, and the weights are placed onto the ankle for 5 s. The quadriceps maintains the resistance isometrically until the weights are lifted again by the arms so the knee can be relaxed to 90 degrees without resistance *(D).* The exercise can be repeated with the same knee, or the opposite knee can be extended to accept the weights while the first one rests.

vinced that the patient has achieved the goals of the nonoperative program and remains symptomatic, then the focus shifts to a surgical correction of the tight lateral retinaculum or the increased Q angle. Furthermore, because the medial stabilizers of the patella in LPCS have never been stretched or torn by recurrent dislocations, their surgical imbrication and advancement are almost never necessary.

Evaluating the effect of a tight lateral retinaculum is somewhat easier. With the patient's knee flexed about 30 degrees and the quadriceps relaxed, the examiner should be able to push the patella medially about one finger breadth or 15 mm normally. Therefore, an excursion of 0 to 5 mm represents a severe tightness, 5 to 10 mm moderate, and 10 to 15 mm mild. Armed with this information and an accurate measurement of the anatomic Q angle, the surgeon can begin to establish a reasonable prognosis for the different surgical options. In general, the tighter the lateral retinaculum, the better the prognosis for an isolated lateral release; and the greater the anatomic Q angle, the worse the prognosis for an isolated lateral release.

Discussion of a few clinical scenarios will be helpful. As usual, decision-making at the extremes is easy. The patient with a severely tight lateral retinac-

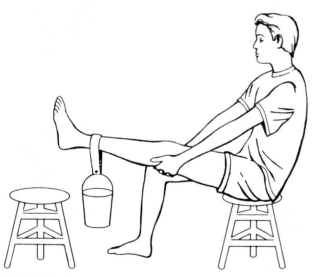

FIGURE 10-8
Safe isometric progressive resistive quadriceps exercises. The patient starts with the heel resting on the opposite seat, the weight resting on the floor, and the quadriceps relaxed. For each repetition the patient contracts the quadriceps, lifts the weight with the arms, holding the knee fully extended, and holds the weight off the floor a few inches for 5 s before returning to the resting position. Use of the arms while seated allows much greater weight to be lifted than in supine straight leg weight lifting. *(Reproduced with permission from Merchant AC: Patellofemoral disorders, in Operative Orthopaedics, vol 3, edited by MW Chapman. Philadelphia, Lippincott, 1988, 1699–1707.)*

ulum and a Q angle at or near normal has an excellent prognosis after a lateral release alone. Conversely, the patient with only mild tightness of the lateral retinaculum and a Q angle of 25 degrees or more should not be considered for an isolated lateral release. In the middle, I would strongly advise that the patient or patient and parents help make the decision. If the patient demonstrates moderate tightness of the lateral retinaculum as well as a moderate increase in the Q angle measuring 20 to 25 degrees, then the prognosis for an isolated lateral release falls to the 50 percent to 70 percent successful range in my experience. After a frank discussion of the risks involved and the benefits expected, I have no disagreement with attempting the more simple lateral release first, with the full understanding that a medial tibial tubercle transfer might well be necessary in the future. The danger with this approach is that patients quickly forget this discussion[15] and need to be reminded of it frequently throughout the course of treatment to avoid disappointment or, worse yet, anger at the need for additional surgery. In the same context, the surgeon should not consider the need for a subsequent medial tibial tubercle plasty a failure of the lateral release but rather an inaccurate patient selection. Given the relatively large difference in risk and morbidity between these two surgical options, in a patient with a relatively low sports and activity level, I frequently opt for a more conservative lateral retinacular release and have not been disappointed, even when the occasional patient requires further realignment surgery.

When the tibial tubercle needs to be transferred medially to correct the abnormally large Q angle in LPCS, the same principles relating to surgical realignment in recurrent dislocation of the patella should be followed. The surgeon must be sure that the lateral tether of the retinaculum has been released as well. The tibial tubercle should never be moved posteriorly on the sloping medial face of the tibia as in the ill-fated Hauser procedure. This posterior shift will decrease the mechanical advantage of the extensor mechanism and increase the patellofemoral joint reaction force leading to iatrogenic chondromalacia patellae. This has just the opposite effect on the extensor biomechanics as elevation of the tibial tubercle in the Maquet procedure.

When moving the tibial tubercle medially for LPCS, the surgeon has the opportunity to move it anteriorly as well. The amount of anterior displacement in extensor mechanism realignment surgery usually depends on the degree of articular cartilage damage found in the patellofemoral joint. The greater the patellofemoral osteoarthrosis, the higher the ante-

Epidemiology

Most frequently jumper's knee is found in volleyball, basketball and soccer players; but many authors reported also track-and-field athletes (high and long jumpers, sprinters, throwers), dancers, cyclers, fencers and several other sport players among their patients.[1,4,9–12] In his series Martens[13] reported 90 cases of jumper's knee: volleyball (31) and soccer (29) prevailed over other sports (7), basketball (4), and cycling (4). According to Stanish,[5] volleyball and basketball players represent 75 percent of the jumper's knee population. In De Paulis' series,[14] volleyball players represent 45 percent, other athletes 24 percent, and basketball players 7 percent. Finally, in our practice, jumper's knee represents 4.5 percent of the whole knee pathology; among 391 cases, we found 32 soccer players, 22 volleyball players, 22 track-and-field athletes, 21 skiers, 13 tennis players, and only 7 basketball players; 370 patients have been treated conservatively and 21 surgically.

Etiopathogenesis

According to many authors,[5,10,12,15–18] the main cause of jumper's knee is the repetitive loading on the extensor mechanism that occurs during the repeated impacts of the limb on the ground with the knee in semiflexion (volleyball, basketball, soccer), or in the moment in which the foot leaves the ground (sprinters, jumpers), or in acceleration, deceleration, stopping, or cutting (rugby, football, soccer, basketball, throwing).

That sudden and repeated overload can originate a traction lesion of the quadriceps or patellar tendon, consisting in microtearing and fraying of the fibers, followed by focal degeneration and, sometimes, calcification.

Usually it involves the deep central fibers near the insertion, because they are less elastic and subjected to a higher rate of elongation when the knee is bent.

According to an epidemiology study done in 1984,[15] the high frequency of playing (four to five times a week) and the hard floor surfaces are more causative than age, sex, years of playing, and type of training.

The same study shows that no statistically significant relationship can be found between patellar tendinitis and morphologic factors, as high-riding patella.

In adolescents the same factors can be the reason for Osgood-Schlatter disease or, less frequently, Sinding-Larsen-Johansson disease.[7]

These must be considered as traction tendinitis (better than epiphysitis), which occur at the distal or proximal insertion of the infrapatellar tendon, in such a poorly vascularized area, and cause a partial avulsion of the tendon attachment, followed by calcification.

The onset of a chronic adhesive peritendinitis, with or without tendinosis, can be brought back to a prolonged exertion, as occurs in long distance runners; in fact these athletes can be afflicted with patellar peritendinitis (and Achilles tendinitis) more often than sprinters.

Gross and Microscopic Pathologic Anatomy

In the *insertional tendinopathies* (jumper's knee) the bone–tendon junction generally has a normal macroscopic appearance, without any gross degeneration of the tendon or chondromalacia of the patella.

On the contrary, in all cases there are always several microscopic abnormalities at the bone–tendon junction, consisting in pseudocystic cavities filled up by necrotic and fragmented tissue or loose areola tissue with capillaries, which in some areas take the shape of mucoid degeneration or fibrinoid necrosis[19] (Figs. 12-2 and 12-3).

In the fibrocartilaginous area usually the "blue line" is missing and the fibrocartilage itself is thicker than normal with some areas consisting of myxomatous tissue or classifications.

As previously reported, usually those lesions involve the deep central fibers at the insertion of the tendon.

In *pure peritendinitis* the peritenon shows marked signs of inflammation with infiltration of plasma cells.

In *peritendinitis with a tendinosis* the tendon belly is wider, thicker, yellowish, and adherent to the peritenon. Some cavities or calcified areas can be found in the context of the tendon, in which it is impossible to point out focal infiltration of plasma cells and proliferating capillaries disarranging the collagen fibers bundles (Fig. 12-4*A–E*).

In *pure tendinosis* the peritenon is intact and the inflammatory or degenerative process involves only the tendon belly. Tendinosis is a frequent finding in spontaneous ruptures of the patellar tendon.[1]

History and Clinical Examination

Pain localized at the patellar apex (or base) is the prevailing symptom of jumper's knee; usually sport players complain of pain arising at the beginning or at the end of the game or training and disappearing with warm-up or rest.

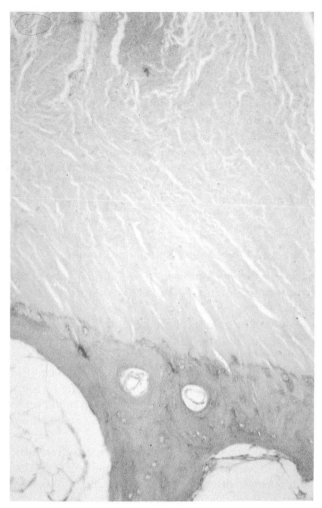

FIGURE 12-2
Normal proximal osteotendinous junction of the patellar tendon in 24-year-old man. From above to below it is possible to distinguish: tendon tissue, fibrocartilage, mineralized fibrocartilage, bone; between fibrocartilage and mineralized fibrocartilage it is possible to point out the "blue line." H&E, ×110.

Blazina[4] and Roels[20] classified these symptoms as stage 1 and 2 of the disease.

When pain does not disappear with warm-up or rest it can severely limit the participation in sports: this is stage 3 according to Blazina (Table 12-1). Stanish and Curwin[5] proposed a more complete classification in six levels (Table 12-2).

In the worst stages, pain and stiffness can arise during daily life activities, such as going upstairs or downstairs, or keeping the knee in a bent position for a long time (sitting at the movies, driving a car). Tenderness is always evoked by palpation, more often at the lower pole of the patella (patellar tendinitis) and especially pushing the kneecap downward with the knee in full extension so that the apex can arise (Fig. 12-5).

Sometimes the pain is localized at the upper pole (quadriceps tendinitis) or at the tibial tuberosity.[12]

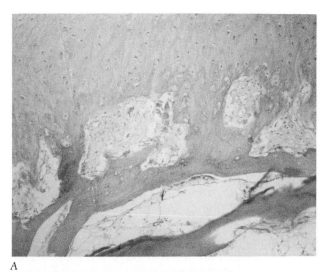

A

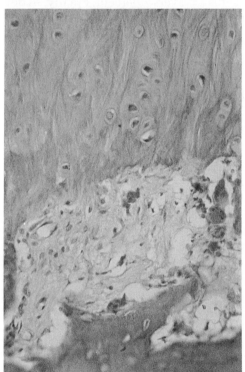

B

FIGURE 12-3
A. Proximal osteotendinous junction of the patellar tendon in jumper's knee: the "blue line" is missing, the fibrocartilage is thicker than normal; pseudocysts are present and filled with loose fibrous tissue, capillaries and chondroclasts H&E, ×110. B. The same area at higher magnification, ×350.

Pain can be exacerbated by squatting or applying a sudden pressure downward on the leg while the patient is straightening his knee.[3] Usually there is no radiation of the pain, which disappears in full extension of the knee. Sometimes it is possible to appreciate a mild swelling of the tendon belly, which is painful to palpation (peritendinitis), or a "popping" sensation at the proximal insertion of the infrapatellar tendon.

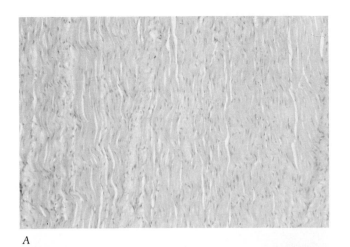

A

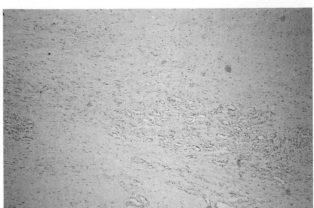

B

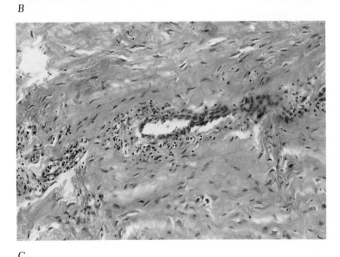

C

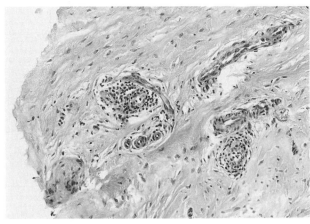

D

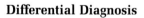

E

FIGURE 12-4

A. Normal appearance of patellar tendon. H&E, ×110. *B–E.* Pathologic appearance of patellar tendon with focal infiltration of capillaries disarranging the bundles of fibers. H&E; *B*, ×90; *C*, ×110; *D*, ×110; *E*, ×170.

Differential Diagnosis

The differential diagnosis includes[5]:

1. *Synovial infrapatellar plica*—can provoke locking sensations in extension and pain in superomedial or superolateral quadrant of the knee.
2. *Meniscopathies*—can cause real locking episodes, sharp pain localized at the joint line and joint effusion.

TABLE 12-1
Blazina's Classification

Stage 1	Pain after sports activity
Stage 2	Pain at the beginning of sports activity disappearing with warm-up and sometimes reappearing with fatigue
Stage 3	Pain at rest and during activity; inability to participate in sports
Stage 4	Rupture of the patellar tendon

181

TABLE 12-2
Stanish's Classification

Level 1	No pain
Level 2	Pain with extreme exertion only
Level 3	Pain with exertion and 1–2 h after
Level 4	Pain during any athletic activity and 4–6 h after; performance level decreased
Level 5	Pain immediately after the beginning of sports activity; withdrawal from activity
Level 6	Pain during daily activities; inability to participate in any sports

3. *Patellofemoral arthrosis and chondromalacia*—possible to find anterior knee pain in squatting or jumping, without point tenderness; the "grinding" sign is often present.

4. *Bursitis*—among the four bursae around the knee joint (suprapatellar, prepatellar, subcutaneous, and deep infrapatellar) especially the deep infrapatellar bursitis can mimic jumper's knee; but it must be remembered that pain localized at the tibial tubercle (as in deep infrapatellar bursitis) is uncommon in tendinitis occurring beyond adolescence.

5. *Fat pad inflammation (Hoffa's disease)*—distinguished by swelling and pain occurring when the fat pad is squeezed.

6. *Osgood-Schlatter and Sinding-Larsen-Johansson diseases*—considered as peculiar types of traction tendinitis in adolescents; they are characterized by pain localized at the tibial tubercle or at the lower pole of the patella (very rarely at the upper pole) and by radiographic findings (see below).

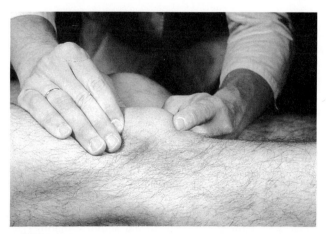

FIGURE 12-5
Clinical examination. Tenderness at the lower pole of the patella (Puddu's sign).

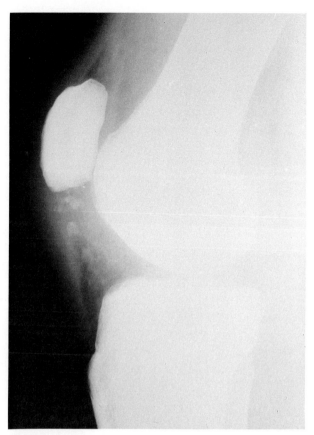

FIGURE 12-6
Radiography shows calcifications in the tendon in jumper's knee.

Instrumental Diagnosis

RADIOGRAPHY

The lateral radiogram is sufficient to show the presence of calcification at the lower (Fig. 12-6) or upper pole of the kneecap or in the tendon belly; when ossicles are localized near the tibial tuberosity, they are generally a result of Osgood-Schlatter disease (Fig. 12-7).

In adolescents, the lateral radiogram is an unavoidable test to confirm the presence of a traction epiphysitis such as Osgood-Schlatter or Sinding-Larsen-Johansson disease and to follow their evolution.

Some other bony conditions related to patellar tendinitis such as patella baja or high-riding patella are pointed out by radiography.

COMPUTED TOMOGRAPHY (CT)

A CT scan is a computerized test that allows the examiner to obtain transverse images of the knee so that the tendon width and the patellar height can be measured at different levels.[21]

The axial tomogram of tendon and peritenon is the best view to evaluate the presence of swelling and

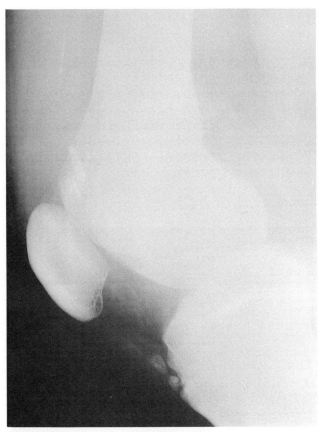

FIGURE 12-7
Ossicles as result of Osgood-Schlatter disease in a 20-year-old man.

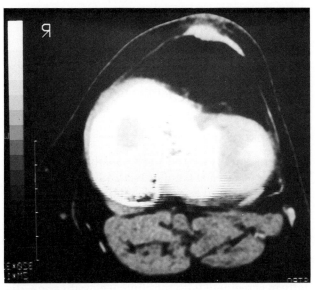

FIGURE 12-8
CT scan. Peritendinitis of the patellar tendon, which appears thicker and larger than normal.

inflammation (Fig. 12-8): the tendon appears thicker, enlarged, and less homogeneous than normal.

The disadvantages of this technique are the high exposure to radiation and the high cost of the examination.

MAGNETIC RESONANCE IMAGING (MRI)

Although MRI is expensive too, it is a noninvasive examination and allows the physician to obtain multiplanar images (coronal, axial, and especially sagittal view).

Quadriceps and patellar tendons appear dark in T1 weighted images and they contrast sharply with subcutaneous, prefemoral, and infrapatellar fat.

Reicher[22] classified MRI appearances of the extensor mechanism into three categories:

1. Complete interruption or avulsion of the tendon. The tendon appears totally discontinued; hemorrhage and edema surround the tendon.

2. Focal increased signal without complete disruption; it means a severe tendinitis or a partial tear and is frequent in older patients with degenerated tendon.

3. Masslike area (Fig. 12-9) posterior to the distal part of the patellar tendon, moderately significant

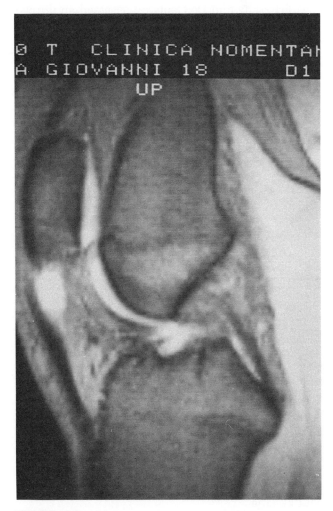

FIGURE 12-9
MRI. Image of a patellar tendinitis with a cyst in the context of the proximal third of the tendon.

183

on T1 images, but extremely bright on T2 images. It indicates an infrapatellar bursitis; the same image in an anterior position means a prepatellar bursitis.

ULTRASONOGRAPHY

Ultrasonography is the most sensible and specific instrument test for patellar tendinitis.

It is a noninvasive and relatively cheap procedure, useful to study the intimate structure of tendon and peritenon, even during quadriceps contraction (dynamic test), and proper to monitor the progressive changes occurring during and after treatment.

Monetti's ultrasonographic classification[23] is totally in agreement with the clinical classification, distinguishing the insertional tendinopathies (jumper's knee) from the peritendinitis with or without tendinosis, in which even ruptures can be included (Figs. 12-10 through 12-12).

Fritzschy and De Gautard[24] assessed an ultrasonographic classification in three stages:

1. *Pure inflammatory stage*—characterized by edema of tendon fibers.
2. *Stage with irreversible anatomic lesions*—the tendon has a heterogenous appearance, with hyperechoic and hypoechoic areas together with edema.

3. *Final stage of lesion*—the tendon sheath is irregularly thickened, tendon fibers appear heterogenous, and swelling is no longer present.

Therefore, ultrasonography provides complete anatomic information; the only disadvantage is that its execution, interpretation, and reproducibility are strictly related to the examiner.

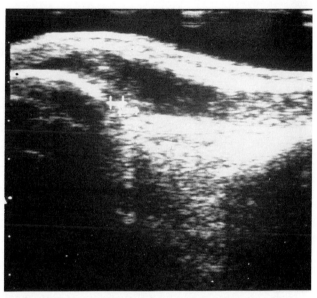

FIGURE 12-11
Ultrasonography. Infrapatellar tendon rupture (longitudinal scan) with presence of microcalcifications at the patellar insertion.

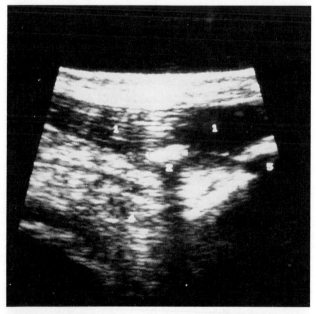

FIGURE 12-10
Ultrasonography. Infrapatellar tendinitis with calcifications (longitudinal scan): *1.* patellar tendon; *2.* calcification; *3.* skin; *4.* Hoffa's fat pad; *5.* tibia.

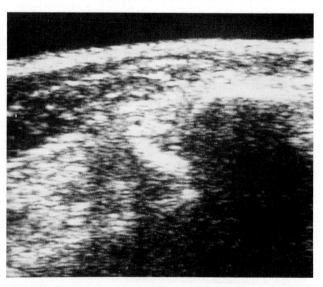

FIGURE 12-12
Ultrasonography. Quadriceps tendinitis with calcification at distal insertion (longitudinal scan).

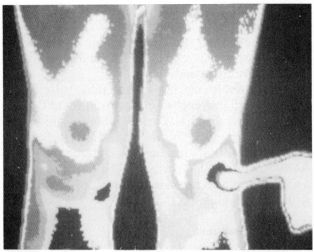

FIGURE 12-13
Telethermography shows a "red spot" at the lower pole of the patella in bilateral jumper's knee.

TELETHERMOGRAPHY

Telethermography[23] (Fig. 12-13) is another noninvasive technique, rapidly and easily feasible, and suitable to assess and follow the evolution of inflammatory processes of the patellar (and quadriceps) tendon; its peculiarity consists in the possibility of grading the inflammation on a specific color scale.

Conservative Treatment

Conservative treatment is recommended in the first two stages according to Blazina's classification and in the second to fifth stages of Stanish's classification, but it is the first choice even in the worst stages.[5,6]

First of all, to prevent the onset of pain, all physicians recommend an adequate warming-up (5 to 10 min) with stretching and eccentric exercises before the activity (see below), ice packs after the activity, and elastic knee supports or brace (Fig. 12-14) to be worn during training and games. The mechanism of the brace compresses the tendon insertions on the kneecap and stabilizes the patella; during flexion of the knee the compression increases, thus decreasing the tensile strength and contributing to relief of pain and swelling.

Medical therapy consists of nonsteroidal anti-inflammatory drugs (NSAIDs) for several weeks and local anti-inflammatory ointments.

A prolonged period of rest is sometimes required to allow the recovery of the tendon; cast or immobilization is less popular now than in the past.

The most important item of conservative treatment is the rehabilitative schedule, including the eccentric program, as established by Stanish and Curwin.[12] It consists of four phases:

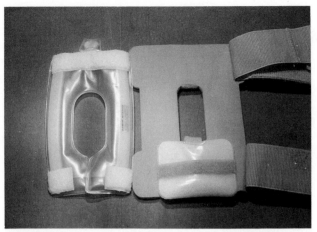

A

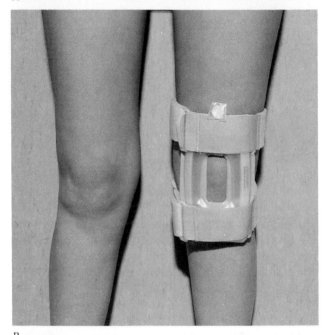

B

FIGURE 12-14 *A,B*
Brace Aircast for jumper's knee: the inflatable device compresses the tendinous insertions on the kneecap; the compression increases during the knee flexion.

1. Static stretching of hamstrings (Fig. 12-15)
2. Static stretching of quadriceps (Fig. 12-16)
3. Eccentric exercises (semisquatting movements)
4. Ice packs after stretching again

Stretching is recommended to resolve the quadriceps tightness, which is an etiologic factor.

The eccentric exercises include semisquatting and slow movements followed by return to an upright position at the same speed. When discomfort disappears, speed is increased gradually, until the patient can rapidly "drop and stop" without any pain.

The importance of the eccentric program depends on the increase of the elasticity of the muscle–

185

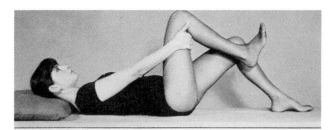

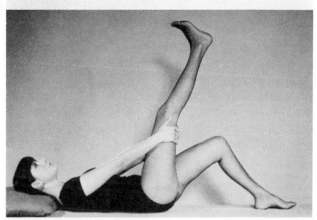

FIGURE 12-15
Stretching of the hamstrings.

Ultrasonography and telethermography, together with clinical examination and patient complaints, are helpful parameters to monitor the evolution of quadriceps and patellar tendinitis during conservative treatment.

Local steroid injection in the tendon belly should be avoided to prevent secondary ruptures of the tendon. Instead, mesotherapy could be the right way to inject a small quantity of anti-inflammatory drugs together with local anesthetic, directly in the derma so that medications can reach the tendon and the peritenon through the surrounding capillary plexus, without damaging the tissue.

Surgical Treatment

Surgery is recommended in the most severe stages of quadriceps and patellar tendinitis when conservative treatment has failed (Blazina's third stage, Stanish's sixth level).

First of all, we recommend an arthroscopy to evaluate and treat any intra-articular pathology (i.e., chondromalacia of the patella, loose bodies, plicae); then a longitudinal lateral paratendinous incision is performed and the peritenon is opened.

In the insertional tendinopathies, the tendon near the insertion usually appears normal (or just a little bit thicker than normal); a few longitudinal scarifications are carried out in the tendon belly (Fig. 12-17) and the distal (or proximal) pole of the kneecap is drilled (Fig. 12-18).

Otherwise, in lower pole involvement, in accordance with Fritschy[24] we suggest removing a triangular-shaped osteotendinous "flap" from the apex to the medium third of the tendon and then suturing the remaining tendon with Vicryl (or catgut) interrupted sutures (as to take the central third of the patellar tendon to replace the anterior cruciate ligament

tendon unit and of the tensile strength of the tendon.

The load on the tendon can be increased with "plyometric exercises" (or "depth jumping"). The athlete drops from a height; the load increases with the drop height. This movement resembles the jump of volleyball or basketball and is followed by concentric contraction and vertical jumping (Kovalev, 1981, cited in Ref. 5).

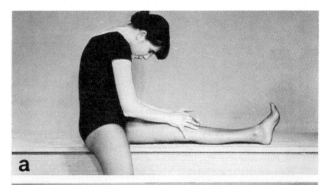

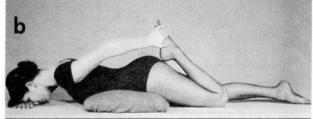

FIGURE 12-16
A. Stretching of the hamstrings. *B.* Stretching of the quadriceps.

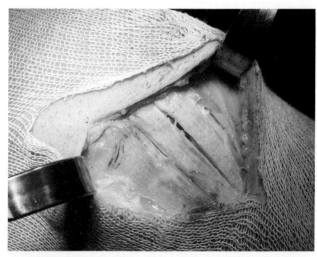

FIGURE 12-17
Surgical technique 1: Multiple scarifications of the patellar tendon.

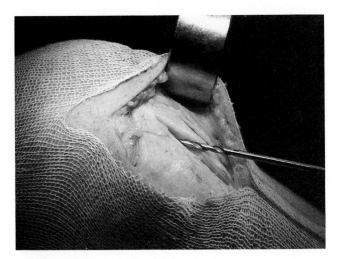

FIGURE 12-18
Surgical technique 1: Drilling of the patellar apex.

[ACL], without detaching its distal insertion) (Fig. 12-19). In these cases, drilling is not required. After surgery, a walking splint in full extension of the knee is applied for 4 weeks.

Isometric exercises are started from the first day after the operation; gentle passive range of motion exercises are allowed using the continuous passive motion machine from 2 weeks after surgery, but the splint has to be reapplied to walk with weight bearing.

If malalignment of the extensor mechanism with chondromalacia of the patella is associated with patellar tendinitis, the realignment has to be performed at the same time, together with shaving of the cartilage or chondrectomy.

In the rare distal patellar tendinopathies, a skin incision is carried out on the tibial tubercle; in adult patients who suffered from Osgood-Schlatter disease during adolescence, the remaining ossicles (if any) have to be removed from the context of the tendon (Fig. 12-20); the tendon itself has to be opened and scarified and the tubercle drilled.

In peritendinitis with tendinosis resistant to conservative treatment, surgery consists of opening the peritenon (generally thicker than normal) and the tendon belly (generally thin and sclerotic) and then scarifying the tendon longitudinally (as in Achilles peritendinitis).[8] The sheath is left open and its central third removed.

Postoperative management is the same as in the insertional tendinopathies.

IATROGENIC TENDINITIS

An iatrogenic peritendinitis can be found in those patients who had an arthroscopy performed using the central transpatellar tendon portal and confirmed by

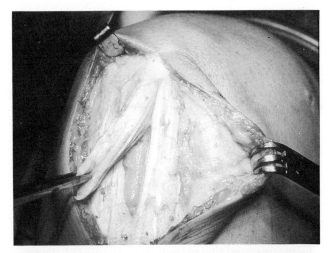

A

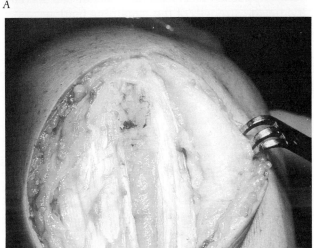

B
FIGURE 12-19
Surgical technique 2: Removal of an osteotendinous flap from the apex to the intermediate third of the tendon.

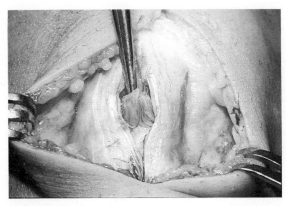

FIGURE 12-20
Removal of Osgood-Schlatter's ossicles from the tibial tubercle.

CT scan (Fig. 12-21) or MRI; however, no tendon weakness or rupture is reported by the authors who use this portal routinely.[12]

According to our experience, a small percentage (5 percent) of patients who had an ACL reconstruction using the central third of the patellar tendon complain of an insertional proximal patellar tendinitis, sometimes associated with a peritendinitis; CT scan, MRI, and ultrasonography demonstrated satisfactorily that the central longitudinal defect of the tendon has completely healed at 8 to 16 months after the operation[14] and experimental studies[25] have proved that at the fourth month after surgery no loss of tensile strength is found.

In 1984 Bonamo and colleagues[26] reported, however, the first two cases of rupture of the patellar tendon after using its central third to replace the ACL. They supposed that at least three factors can decrease the tensile strength of the remaining tendon:

1. An excessive tension during closure of the longitudinal defect that can cause a focal necrosis followed by fibrosis and tertiary calcification within the tendon;

2. The reduction in mass of the tendon;

3. The interruption of the normal vascular supply to the proximal third and the disruption of the infrapatellar fat pad due to manipulation during surgery (trans-defect portal, therefore, has to be avoided).

RUPTURES

Ruptures represent the ultimate stage of patellar tendinitis (Blazina's fourth stage). They occur in four different ways:

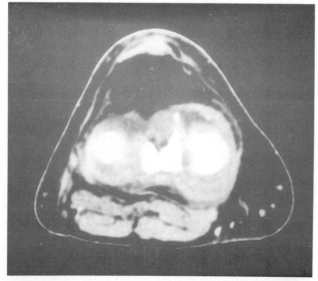

FIGURE 12-21
Infrapatellar tendinopathy as a consequence of transpatellar tendon arthroscopic portal. The tendon appears wider; peritendinitis is present.

1. In patients afflicted with systemic diseases weakening the tendon and osseous strength (i.e., systemic lupus erythematosus, rheumatoid arthritis, renal failure, hyperparathyroidism) after a mild injury of the extensor mechanism of the knee.[27,28]

2. In patients with severe degrees of patellar-quadriceps tendinitis or degeneration in which a direct shot or a sudden heavy weight bearing on the flexed knee can produce either a disruption of the quadriceps patellar tendon or an avulsion ("decalottement") of the tendon from the patellar pole.[9,20,29,30]

3. In the literature about 10 cases of bilateral infrapatellar tendon spontaneous and concurrent rupture have been reported in healthy patients after a sudden loading on the extensor mechanism.[31]

4. A severe direct injury on the proximal tibial epiphysis can produce a traumatic disruption of the patellar tendon, usually together with tears of the other ligamentous structures of the knee (ACL, posterior cruciate ligament [PCL], menisci, collateral ligaments).

Clinical examination shows tenderness and swelling over the anterior aspect of the knee and total inability to extend the knee despite active contraction of the quadriceps.

Radiographs can show a high-riding patella (Fig. 12-22) when the infrapatellar tendon is disrupted, and an inferior displacement of the kneecap when the quadriceps is involved.

In the avulsion of the tendon from the patellar pole, some osseous fragments in the distal portion of quadriceps tendon (Fig. 12-23) or in the proximal end of the patellar tendon can be revealed.[29]

Hemarthrosis is present in quadriceps disruption and absent in infrapatellar rupture, because only the former is deeply covered with synovial membrane in contiguity with the knee joint.

Ultrasonography (see Fig. 12-11), CT scan, and MRI (Fig. 12-24) can confirm the rupture of the tendon and the associated injuries, if any.

Treatment of Ruptures

In *quadriceps tendon rupture* (Fig. 12-25*A*), the surgical approach is vertical median. An end-to-end suture is performed using resorbable suture (Vicryl). Sometimes it is necessary to freshen the free borders of rupture and to reinforce the suture with long-term resorbable materials [PDS-band (Ethicon)] (Fig. 12-25*B*) or aponeuroses flaps from vastus medialis and lateralis.

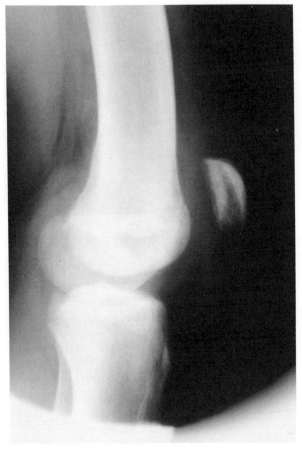

FIGURE 12-22
Radiography shows a high-riding patella in infrapatellar tendon disruption.

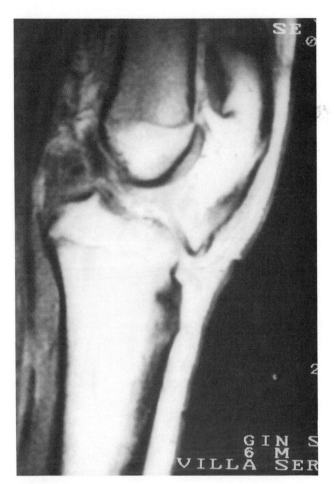

FIGURE 12-24
MRI: Patellar tendon disruption associated with ACL and PCL tears in a posterior traumatic knee dislocation.

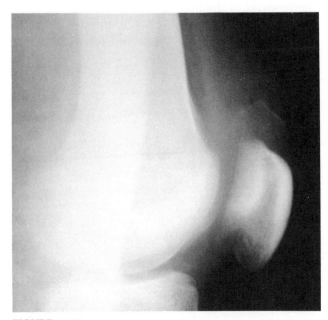

FIGURE 12-23
Radiography shows an avulsion of the quadriceps tendon from the patellar base.

In quadriceps avulsions, it is necessary to perform an osteotendinous suture by drilling transosseous tunnels on the proximal pole of the patella. A metal wire cerclage can be required to ensure the suture.

In *patellar tendon rupture* (Fig. 12-26*A*) an end-to-end suture can be performed with good results. Reinforcement is performed with PDS band (Fig. 12-26*B*) or a flap of quadriceps tendon, when necessary; tendinosis, in fact, is often present in spontaneous ruptures of the patellar tendon.

In *avulsions from the lower pole of the patella* (Fig. 12-27), it is necessary to use an osteotendinous suture after the removal of bony chips detached from the patella; a metal wire reinforcement can be added to ensure the reinsertion in the comminuted avulsions.

In the rare *distal avulsions*[30] from the tibial tubercle after the removal of bone fragments, it is better to drill two holes in the tibia to pass the suture coming from the tendon. When the bone fragment detached from the tibial tuberosity is large enough, it is preferable to fix it with a staple.

189

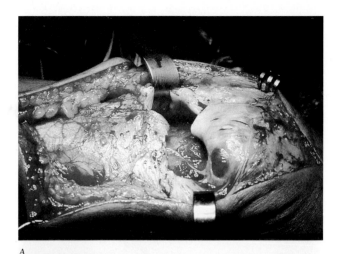

A

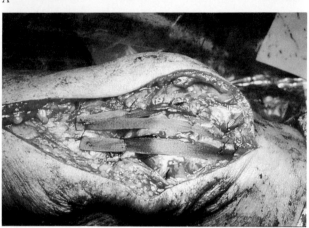

B

FIGURE 12-25
A. Neglected rupture of the quadriceps tendon. *B.* Its repair with PDS-band (Ethicon) augmentation.

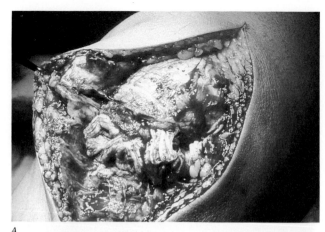

A

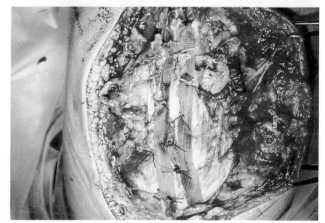

B

FIGURE 12-26
A. Patellar tendon rupture. *B.* Its repair with PDS-band (Ethicon) augmentation.

With every suture, the postoperative treatment consists of 4 to 6 weeks of immobilization in a cylinder cast or splint in full extension of the knee. Partial weight bearing with splint and gentle range of motion passive exercises with continuous passive motion are started 2 or 3 weeks after surgery; the recovery is complete in about 2 months.

The neglected tears of the extensor mechanism tendons generally heal with a pathologic elongation; clinical examination reveals a dramatic weakness of the extension of the knee.

Radiography show a high-riding patella in infrapatellar tendon tears or a patella baja in quadriceps tears, and gross calcification (Fig. 12-28) at the lower or upper pole of the patella.

Sometimes after an avulsion or repeated tears at the level of the bone–tendon junction, it is possible to point out a double patella (Fig. 12-29).

The neglected tears of the patellar tendon require a Z shortening and suture of the patellar ligament and, sometimes, a Z lengthening of the quadriceps tendon.[17]

The neglected avulsions of the lower pole require the removal of the bone fragments from the context of the tendon, freshening and shortening of the proximal part of the tendon itself, and reinsertion with transbone suture or cerclage.

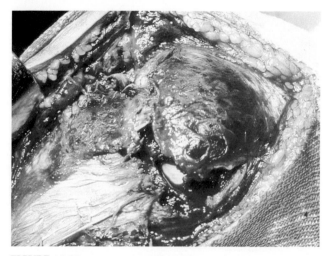

FIGURE 12-27
Avulsion of the patellar tendon from the lower pole of the patella.

190

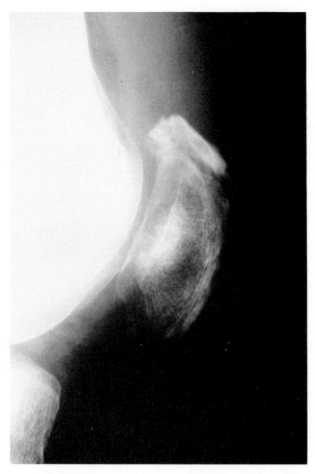

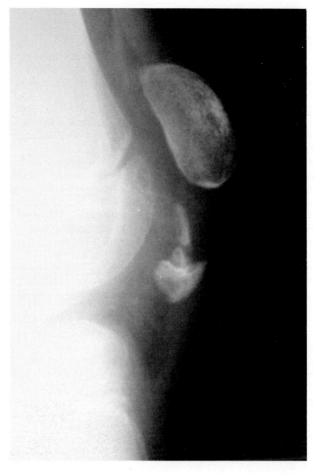

FIGURE 12-28
Radiography shows calcification at the distal insertion of the quadriceps tendon (neglected avulsion).

FIGURE 12-29
Gross calcifications of the infrapatellar tendon (double patella) in a neglected avulsion.

ACKNOWLEDGEMENTS

The authors thank G. Monetti, MD, Radiologist at the S. Maria Nuova Arcispedale in Reggio Emilia (Italy) for providing the ultrasonographic images; F. Nardi, MD, Professor in the Pathologic Anatomy Institute of the University "La Sapienza" of Rome (Italy) for the histologic assistance; and Mario Spinelli, MD, Associate Professor at the Orthopaedic Clinic of the University of Pisa (Italy), for providing the slides on neuroreceptors.

REFERENCES

1. Perugia L, Ippolito E, Postacchini F: *I tendini. Biologia, patologia, clinica.* Milano, Masson, 1981.
2. Scapinelli R: Blood supply of the human patella. *J Bone Joint Surg* 49B:563, 1967.
3. Scapinelli R: Studies on the vasculature of the human knee joint. *Acta Anat (Basel)* 70:305, 1968.
4. Blazina ME, Kerlan RK, Jobe FW: Jumper's knee. *Orthop Clin North Am* 4:665, 1973.
5. Stanish WD, Curwin KS: *Tendinitis. Its Etiology and Treatment.* Toronto, Collamore Press, 1984.
6. Stanish WD, Curwin KS, Lamb H: The biomechanical analysis of chronic patellar tendinitis and treatment with eccentric loading, in *Surgery and Arthroscopy of the Knee: 2d Congress of the European Society.* Berlin-Heidelberg, Springer-Verlag, 1988.
7. Medlar RC, Lyne DE: Sinding-Larsen-Johansson disease. *J Bone Joint Surg* 60A:1113, 1978.
8. Puddu G, Ippolito E, Postacchini F: A classification of Achilles tendon disease. *Am J Sports Med* 4:145, 1976.

9. Bassett FH III, Panayotis NS, Carr WA: Jumper's knee: Patella tendinitis and patellar tendon rupture. *AAOS Symposium on the Athlete's Knee* 8:96, 1980.

10. Ferretti A, Neri M, Mariani P, Puddu G: Considerazioni eziopatogenetiche sul ginocchio del saltatore. *Ital J Sports Traumatol* 5:101, 1983.

11. Insall J: *Surgery of the Knee*. New York, Churchill-Livingstone, 1983.

12. Smillie IS: *Injuries of the Knee Joint*. Edinburgh, Churchill-Livingstone, 1976.

13. Martens M, Wouters P, Burssens A, Mulier JC: Patellar tendinitis: Pathology and results of treatment. *Acta Orthop Scand* 53:445, 1982.

14. De Paulis F: Ruolo della TC e della RM, in Trattato di medicina dello sport applicata al calcio, edited by Vecchiet L, Calligaris A, Montanari G, Resina A. Firenze, Menarini, 1990, pp 345–364.

15. Ferretti A, Puddu G, Mariani P, Neri M: Jumper's knee: An epidemiological study of volleyball players. *Physician and Sport Med* 12:97, 1984.

16. Kujala UM, Aalto T, Osterman K, Dahlstrom S: The effect of volleyball playing on the knee extensor mechanism. *Am J Sports Med* 17:766, 1989.

17. Mandelbaum BR, Bartolozzi A, Carney B: A systematic approach to reconstruction of neglected tears of the patellar tendon. *Clin Orthop* 235:268, 1988.

18. Mariani P, Puddu G, Ferretti A: Il ginocchio del saltatore. *Giorn Ital Ort Traumatol* 4:85, 1978.

19. Ferretti A, Ippolito E, Mariani P, Puddu G: Jumper's knee. *Am J Sports Med* 11:58, 1983.

20. Roels J, Martens M, Mulier JC, Burssens A: Patellar tendinitis (jumper's knee). *Am J Sports Med* 6:362, 1978.

21. Passariello R, Trecco F, De Paulis F, et al: Computed tomography of the knee joint: Technique of study and normal anatomy. *J Comput Assist Tomogr* 9:1035, 1983.

22. Mink JH, Reicher MA, Crues JV III: *MRI of the Knee*. New York, Raven Press, 1988.

23. Monetti G: *Ecografia muscolo-tendinea e dei tessuti molli*. Milano, Solei, 1989.

24. Fritschy D, De Gautard R: Jumper's knee and ultrasonography. *Am J Sports Med* 16:637, 1988.

25. Cabaud HE, Feagin JA, Rodkey WG: Acute ACL injury and augmented repair. Experimental studies. *Am J Sports Med* 8:395, 1980.

26. Bonamo JJ, Krinick RM, Sporn AA: Rupture of the patellar ligament after use of its central third for ACL reconstruction. *J Bone Joint Surg* 66A:1294, 1984.

27. Cirincione RJ, Baker BE: Tendon ruptures with secondary hyperparathyroidism. *J Bone Joint Surg* 57A:852, 1975.

28. Maddox PA, Garth WP: Tendinitis of the patellar ligament and quadriceps (jumper's knee) as an initial presentation of hyperparathyroidism. *J Bone Joint Surg* 68A:228, 1986.

29. Dejour H, Walch M: *La pathologie femoro-patellaire*. Lyon, 1987.

30. Douglas Bowers K: Patellar tendon avulsion as a complication of Osgood-Schlatter's disease. *Am J Sports Med* 9:356, 1980.

31. Sherlock DA, Phil D, Hughes A: Bilateral spontaneous concurrent rupture of the patellar tendon in the absence of associated local or systemic disease. *Clin Orthop* 237:179, 1988.

CHAPTER 13

Synovial Folds—Plicae

Dinesh Patel
Cato T. Laurencin
Akihiro Tsuchiya
Mary Dutka

INTRODUCTION

The presence of synovial folds (Figs. 13-1 and 13-2) in the knee is a common observation by arthroscopists. Anatomists,[1–5] embryologists, and surgeons[6–9] have studied synovial folds and reported extensively in the literature. The advent of arthroscopy further delineated and classified synovial folds into separate easily identifiable entities (Fig. 13-3). Four plicae of the knee exist: suprapatellar, infrapatellar, medial, and (rare) lateral.[9] This chapter reviews salient features of knee plica anatomy and pathophysiology and presents methods for treatment.

PLICA EMBRYOLOGY

Ogata and Uhthoff[10] studied the embryologic development of synovial plicae through dissections of 116 knees of embryos and fetuses. The joint space of the

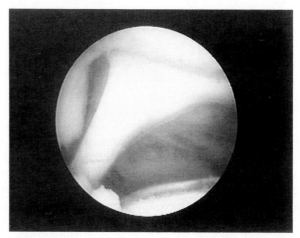

FIGURE 13-2
Thickened synovial fold—plica.

knee was found to form at 8 weeks' gestation, as multiple small cavitations about the distal femur. At 12 weeks' gestation, a single synovial cavity was formed at the knee joint with remaining strands of mesenchymal tissue that could form plica. At 11 to 20 weeks' gestation, a suprapatellar plica was found in 33 percent of fetuses, a mediopatellar plica was found in 37 percent of fetuses, and an infrapatellar plica was found in 50 percent of fetuses.

SUPRAPATELLAR PLICA

The suprapatellar plica (Fig. 13-4) arises from the undersurface of the quadriceps tendon and attaches on the superomedial and lateral walls of the knee joint. This plica can take many forms, from domed to crescent shape, and has smooth, sharp, thick, or translucent edges. Joyce and Harty[4] found the suprapatellar plica to be present in varying sizes in 89 percent of their cadaver dissections. An imperforate septum was found in 7 percent and a small central resorption termed a *porta* (see Fig. 13-4) was found in 9 percent.

Any conditions resulting in scarring, thickening (Fig. 13-5), or inflammation of this plica can result

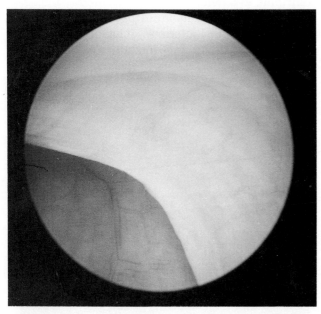

FIGURE 13-1
Classical arthroscopic appearance of plica (duplication of synovial fold).

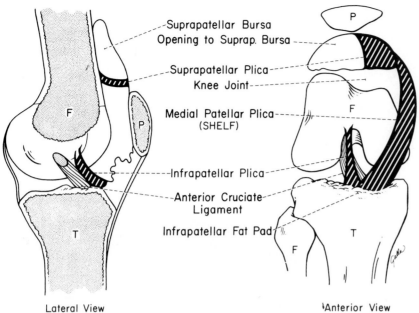

Lateral View

Anterior View

FIGURE 13-3
Anatomy of plicae.

Labels in figure:
Suprapatellar Bursa
Opening to Suprap. Bursa
Suprapatellar Plica
Knee Joint
Medial Patellar Plica (SHELF)
Infrapatellar Plica
Anterior Cruciate Ligament
Infrapatellar Fat Pad

in symptoms of a pathologic suprapatellar plica. A catching or popping sensation can occur as the thickened plica travels across the patella or femoral condyles with flexion and extension of the knee. When suprapatellar plicae have small openings for communication between the suprapatellar pouch and the knee joint proper, loose bodies may sometimes be found hidden in the suprapatellar pouch.

Importance

1. If thicker—compression changes in femur and patella
2. If thicker—may restrict total flexion because of pain
3. Common hiding place for debris or loose bodies when the opening is small

4. Occasionally soft tissue neoplasms seen behind suprapatellar plicae

INFRAPATELLAR PLICA

This plica is commonly called the ligamentum mucosum (Fig. 13-6) and extends from the infrapatellar fat pad at its midportion to the tip of the intercondylar notch. It is a synovial fold that runs parallel to and above the anterior cruciate ligament and may lie in continuity with the ligament, be partially separated by a fenestration, or be completely separate. A small artery may lie in association with this plica and may contribute to a hemarthrosis if ruptured.

If large, the ligamentum mucosum may make visualization of the anterior cruciate ligament, infrapatellar fat pad, and anterior horns of the menisci

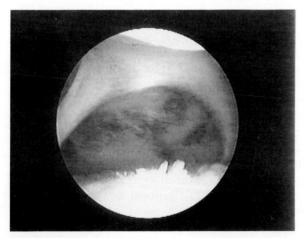

FIGURE 13-4
Suprapatellar plica porta—arthroscopic view.

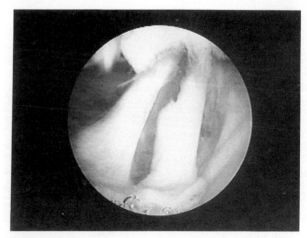

FIGURE 13-5
Thickened duplicated suprapatellar plica—arthroscopic view.

194

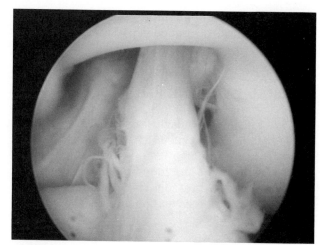

FIGURE 13-6
Infrapatellar plica—ligamentum mucosum.

difficult. Additionally, a large ligamentum mucosum can make manipulation of arthroscopic instruments in the knee difficult.

MEDIAL PATELLAR PLICA

This plica (Fig. 13-7) has been described as plica synovialis mediopatellaris, medial shelf, wedge, cleat, plica alaris elongata, medial interarticular band, and Iino's band and originates on the superomedial wall of the knee joint and extends obliquely to insert on the medial portion of the infrapatellar fat pad (see Fig. 13-7). It can arise in continuity with the suprapatellar plica, have a separate attachment, or occur in the absence of the suprapatellar plica. The incidence of this structure has varied between 18.5 percent and 55 percent, largely depending on the interpretation of the individual investigators (Table 13-1). Practically speaking, every knee has a plica of some kind.

Pathogenesis

Chronic swelling from internal derangement of a knee or direct injury, like a dash board, to the anteromedial femoral condyle can cause thickening (Fig. 13-8) and fibrosis. When the knee is flexed and extended this thickened band can compress the patella and the femoral condyle causing chondromalacia changes (Figs. 13-9 and 13-10) and pain. This band can also cause subluxation in flexion and extension causing clicking, mimicking a patellofemoral or meniscal problem.

Symptoms

A painful knee with or without clicking or swelling, which may mimic patellar pain, is a common presentation of patients. Joggers and swimmers (breast strokers) commonly have symptoms from this.

Physical Examination

A palpable painful cord, one finger breadth medial to the medial border of the patella is noted; stimulat-

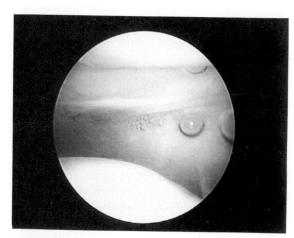

FIGURE 13-7
Medial plica—arthroscopic view.

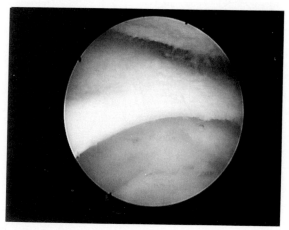

FIGURE 13-8
Thickened medial plica—arthroscopic view.

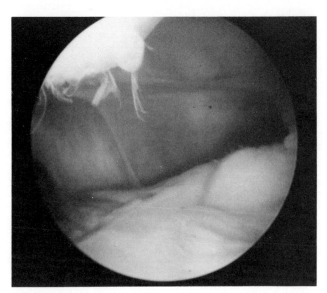

FIGURE 13-9
Medial plica with patella chondromalacia.

ing the same symptoms could be an indicator that medial plica is the cause of problems. Occasionally, lack of terminal flexion or extension may be found. Valgus knee, patella laxity, increase in Q angle, swelling or decrease in motion may or may not be present.

Studies

Radiography is of no value, but an arthrogram or a magnetic resonance imaging scan (MRI) can diagnose the suprapatellar and medial plicae easily. Medial patellar plica diagnosis by radiologic (arthrogram and MRI) criteria requires special knowledge.

Significance

A large medial plica can prevent the movement of the arthroscope from the superior compartment to

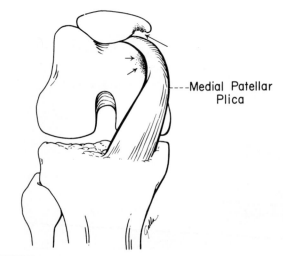

FIGURE 13-10
The medial plica with chondromalacia.

the medial compartment unless the knee is hyperextended and the arthroscope is passed under the medial plica.

LATERAL PATELLAR PLICA

This is a rare entity transversing the lateral fat pad to the lateral wall of the knee.[9] There is no significance, unless it is large. Large lateral plicae, by virtue of their priority to the popliteus tunnel, may make it difficult to pass arthroscopic instruments for visualization of the popliteus tendon and associated structures.

PSEUDOPLICA

Patients who have had previous open surgery for any condition, including infection, may form pseudoplicae in the suprapatellar pouch, lateral gutters, and ligamentous mucosum region. Scar tissue in the intercondylar notch region following anterior cruciate reconstruction is commonly seen to prevent extension or terminal flexion of the knee because of pain or tension.

TREATMENT

Conservative

Initial treatment for pain and disability from pathologic plicae should be conservative. Localized ice and elastic support with a hole for the patella should be used in conjunction with a physical therapy program emphasizing stretching exercises and strength building. Amatuzzi[11] examined 136 cases of pathologic synovial plica treated conservatively and found results to be good in 40 percent of cases and average in 20 percent of cases. They believed these results underscored the need for initial conservative therapy before surgical correction is considered. In a prospective study of 30 athletes with pathologic plicae, Rovere[12] injected a long-acting anesthetic agent and a steroid into the medial patellar plica region. He found that 73 percent of these patients had full relief and were able to return to full activity.

Arthroscopic Surgery

Plicae refractory to conservative measures should undergo arthroscopic surgical treatment.[7,13–15]

The arthroscopic evaluation is performed in a standard operating room environment with local, regional, or general anesthesia. Local anesthesia (5 mL 0.5% Marcaine with 1:200,000 epinephrine) is used to infiltrate the arthroscopic portals. The 30-degree, 5-mm arthroscope is inserted either through a superolateral patellar or midlateral patellar portal, while an inferolateral patellar portal is used for insertion of instruments (punch, scissors, shaver). Plica should be excised only if there is no associated pathology such as a torn meniscus or torn anterior cruciate ligament. If the patient has been placed under local anesthesia, pulling the medial plica during arthroscopy with reproduction of symptoms is diagnostic for plica as the cause of pain. The plica is then infiltrated with 15 mL 0.5% Marcaine with 1:200,000 (to prevent bleeding and for postoperative pain relief) and excised. Complete excision (as opposed to simple incising or sectioning) is recommended to ensure that further mechanical irritation from the plicae does not take place. One should avoid cutting the capsule, otherwise the patella may sublux laterally.

SUMMARY

The indications for arthroscopic surgery include:

1. A clinically painful palpable cord
2. A thickened, subluxating plica with or without associated cartilage changes (fibrillation or groove formation) on the patella or femur
3. Reproduction of the patient's symptoms on stretching the plica with a probe (if arthroscopy is performed under local anesthesia)
4. No evidence of other clinical or arthroscopic abnormalities (meniscal or ligamentous pathology)

A number of studies have examined the results of arthroscopic surgery for the treatment of pathologic plicae and have found efficacy in its use. For example, Hansen and Boe[16] reported data on 53 consecutive patients who underwent treatment for symptomatic medial patellar plica. They found 80 percent of patients obtaining good to excellent results (according to the Lysholm score) and 59 percent of patients were completely symptom free. The senior author[8,14,17] has had similarly positive results in the use of arthroscopy for pathologic plica.

It should be emphasized that overdiagnosis of plica[14] as a cause of pain and disability should be avoided. Although pathologic plicae do occur, they are rarely a cause of pain.

REFERENCES

1. Gray DJ, Gardner W: Prenatal development of the human knee and superior tibiofibular joints. *Med J Anat* 86:234, 1950.
2. Hohlbaum J: Die bursa suprapatellaris und ibre Beziehungen zum Kniegelenke. Ein Beitrag zur Entwicklung der angeborenen Schleimbeutel. *Beitr Z Klin Chir* 128:412, 1923.
3. Iino S: Normal arthroscopic findings of the knee joint in adult cadavers. *J Jap Orthop Assoc* 14, 1939.
4. Joyce JJ, Harty M: Surgery of the synovial fold, in *Arthroscopy: Diagnosis and Surgical Practice*, edited by W Cassells. Philadelphia, Lea & Febiger, 1984, pp 201–209.
5. Pipkin G: Knee injuries: The role of the suprapatellar plica and suprapatellar bursa in simulating internal derangements. *Clin Orthop* 74:161, 1971.
6. Hughston JC, Stone M, Andrews JR: The suprapatellar plica: Its role in internal derangement of the knee (abstract). *J Bone Joint Surg* 55A:1318, 1973.
7. Jackson RW, Marshall DJ, Fujisawa Y: The pathologic medial shelf. *Orthop Clin North Am* 13:307, 1982.
8. Patel D: Arthroscopy of the plicae-synovial folds and their significance. *Am J Sports Med* 6:217, 1978.
9. Schonholtz GJ, Magee CM: The synovial plicae of the knee joint. *Contemp Orthop* 12:31, 1986.
10. Ogata S, Uhthoff HK: The development of synovial plica in human knee joints: An embryotic study. *Arthroscopy* 6:315, 1990.
11. Amatuzzi M, Fazzi A, Varella M: Pathologic synovial plica of the knee: Results of conservative treatment. *Am J Sports Med* 18:466, 1990.
12. Rovere GD, Adair DM: Medial synovial shelf plica syndrome. Treatment by intraplical steroid injection. *Am J Sports Med* 13:382, 1985.
13. Koshino T, Okamoto R: Resection of painful shelf (plica synovialis mediopatellaris) under arthroscopy. *Arthroscopy* 1:136, 1985.
14. Patel D: Synovial lesions: Plicae, in *Operative Arthroscopy*, edited by JB McGinty. New York, Raven Press, 1991, pp 361–372.
15. Rosenberg TD, Paulos LE, Parker RD, Abbott PJ: Arthroscopic surgery of the knee, *Operative Orthopaedics*, edited by MW Chapman. Philadelphia, Lippincott, 1987, pp 1585–1604.
16. Hansen H, Boe S: The pathological plica in the knee. Results after arthroscopic resection. *Arch Orthop Trauma Surg* 108:282, 1989.
17. Patel D: Plica as a cause of anterior knee pain. *Orthop Clin North Am* 17:273, 1986.

18. Aoki T, Takano Y, Kishimoto C: A case of internal derangement of the knee to the so-called shelf. *J Jap Orthop Assoc* 39:922, 1965.

19. Blackburn TA, Eiland G, Bandy C: An introduction to the plica. *J Orthop Sports Phys Ther* 3:171, 1982.

20. Broom MJ, Fulkerson JP: The plica syndrome. A new perspective. *Orthop Clin North Am* 17:279, 1986.

21. Caffinire JY, Bruch JM: Pli synovial interne et chondropathie rotulienne. A propos de 13 cas opérés. *Rev Chir Orthop* 67:4799, 1981.

22. Hardaker WT, Whipple TL, Bassett FH: Diagnosis and treatment of the plica syndrome of the knee. *J Bone Joint Surg* 62A:221, 1980.

23. Kinnard P, Levesque RY: The plica syndrome. A syndrome of controversy. *Clin Orthop* 183:141, 1984.

24. Klein W: The medial shelf of the knee. A follow-up study. *Arch Orthop Trauma Surg* 102:67, 1983.

25. Munzinger U, Ruckstuhl J, Scherrer H, et al: Internal derangement of the knee joint due to pathologic synovial folds: The mediopatellar plica syndrome. *Clin Orthop* 155:59, 1981.

26. Nottage WM, Sprague NF, Auerbach BJ, Shaihiaree H: The medial patellar plica syndrome. *Am J Sports Med* 11:211, 1983.

27. O'Connor RL: *Arthroscopy.* Philadelphia, Lippincott, 1977.

28. O'Dwyer KJ, Peace PK: The plica syndrome. *Injury* 19:350, 1988.

29. Richmond JC, McGinty JB: Segmental arthroscopic resection of the hypertrophic mediopatellar plica. *Clin Orthop* 178:185, 1983.

30. Vilpeau C, Beguin J, Aubriot JH, et al: Place du repli mediopatellaire dans la pathologie du genou. *Am Chir* 35:325, 1981.

CHAPTER 14

Bursae of the Knee

Dinesh Patel
Cato T. Laurencin
Akihiro Tsuchiya

INTRODUCTION

Bursae are thin sacs that can lie along skin, tendon, ligament, or bone.[1] They allow surrounding surfaces to glide on each other with less friction and thereby preserve the integrity of important structures. True bursae are lined with synovium and may or may not communicate with a joint. Normally, bursae are in the form of enclosed clefts and may be hardly noticeable.[1] However, when affected by trauma, inflammation, or frank infection they may become prominent.

ANATOMY

Figures 14-1, 14-2, and 14-3 show the bursae of the knee. Superficially, a prepatellar bursa is present sub-

cutaneously at the level of the lower pole of the patella. A superficial infrapatellar bursa lies subcutaneously to the upper portion of the infrapatellar tendon, and over the region of the tibial tuberosity lies a subcutaneous bursa.

At the next layer, a subfascial prepatellar bursa can be present, invested by the connective tissue of the lower portion of the patella.

The deep bursae are numerous and mainly protect tendon and ligaments from bony prominences. A subtendinous prepatellar bursa can be found under the quadriceps tendon, lying between it and the upper portion of the patella.[2] A large suprapatellar bursa can be found between the quadriceps tendon and the anterior surface of the femur. Because in most

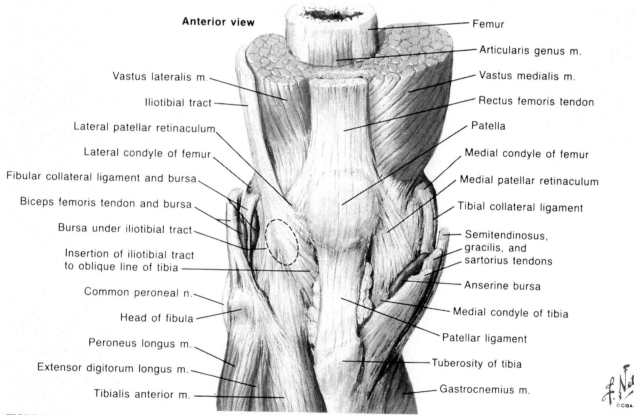

Anterior view

Femur
Articularis genus m.
Vastus medialis m.
Rectus femoris tendon
Patella
Medial condyle of femur
Medial patellar retinaculum
Tibial collateral ligament
Semitendinosus, gracilis, and sartorius tendons
Anserine bursa
Medial condyle of tibia
Patellar ligament
Tuberosity of tibia
Gastrocnemius m.

Vastus lateralis m.
Iliotibial tract
Lateral patellar retinaculum
Lateral condyle of femur
Fibular collateral ligament and bursa
Biceps femoris tendon and bursa
Bursa under iliotibial tract
Insertion of iliotibial tract to oblique line of tibia
Common peroneal n.
Head of fibula
Peroneus longus m.
Extensor digitorum longus m.
Tibialis anterior m.

FIGURE 14-1
Anatomy of bursae of the knee, anterior view.

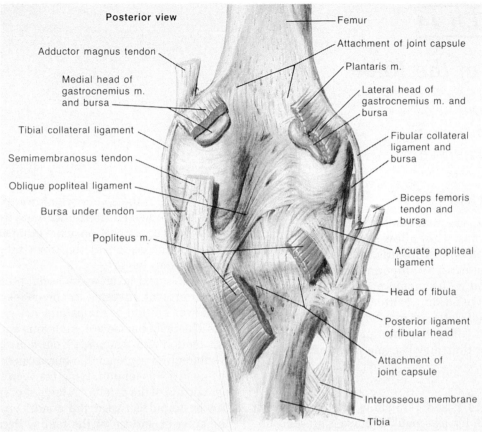

Posterior view

Adductor magnus tendon

Medial head of gastrocnemius m. and bursa

Tibial collateral ligament

Semimembranosus tendon

Oblique popliteal ligament

Bursa under tendon

Popliteus m.

Femur

Attachment of joint capsule

Plantaris m.

Lateral head of gastrocnemius m. and bursa

Fibular collateral ligament and bursa

Biceps femoris tendon and bursa

Arcuate popliteal ligament

Head of fibula

Posterior ligament of fibular head

Attachment of joint capsule

Interosseous membrane

Tibia

FIGURE 14-2
Anatomy of bursae of the knee, posterior view.

patients the suprapatellar bursa freely communicates with the knee joint, the suprapatellar bursa is more commonly termed a suprapatellar pouch or recess. Inferiorly, the deep infrapatellar bursa can be found between the patellar tendon and the tibia.

Voshell and Brantigan[3] have identified lateral bursae in association with the tibial collateral ligament (TCL). They noted five locations under the TCL that these bursae can be found and have seen as many as three bursae under the TCL in the same knee. In addition, a bursa associated with the iliotibial tract can be found at the level of the superior pole of the patella.

A number of bursae can be found on the medial side of the knee. Bursae in association with the fibular collateral ligament have been identified by Hendryson.[4] Subtendinous bursae in association with the sartorius muscle have been found deep to its tendon, between the tendons of the gracilis and semitendinosus. These bursae often communicate with the pes anserine bursa, a large bursa located between the tendons of the sartorius, gracilis, and semitendinosus, and the tibia.

Posteriorly, a bursa exists under the tendon of the lateral gastrocnemius muscle and acts as a buffer between it and the posterior capsule of the knee.

Likewise, a similar bursa exists under the tendon of the medial gastrocnemius muscle, lying between the tendon and posteromedial capsule. Finally, a bursa can be found in association with the semimembranosus tendon, lying between the semimembranosus and medial head of the gastrocnemius. This bursa can communicate in many cases with the bursa of the medial gastrocnemius, which can then communicate with the knee.

PATHOLOGIC STATES

Prepatellar Bursitis

MECHANISM

Inflammation of the prepatellar bursae can be caused by acute trauma or by repetitive irritation, resulting in the commonly termed housemaid's knee. Direct blows to the knee through collisions between athletes,[5] falls directly onto turf,[6] or in some sports[7] such as wrestling[8] can produce prepatellar bursitis. In addition, Janecki and Hechtman have reported a case of acute prepatellar bursitis resulting from a lost meniscal fragment after arthroscopic meniscectomy.[9]

200

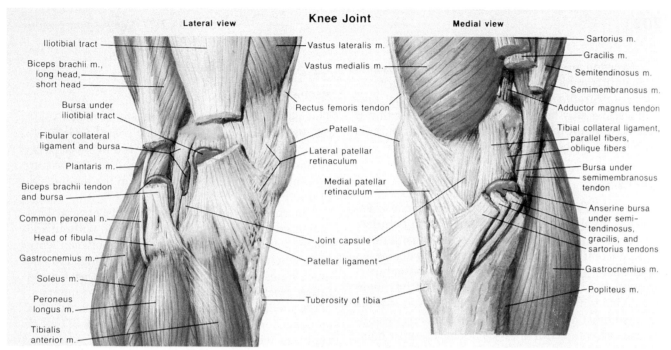

Knee Joint

Lateral view

Iliotibial tract

Biceps brachii m., long head, short head

Bursa under iliotibial tract

Fibular collateral ligament and bursa

Plantaris m.

Biceps brachii tendon and bursa

Common peroneal n.

Head of fibula

Gastrocnemius m.

Soleus m.

Peroneus longus m.

Tibialis anterior m.

Vastus lateralis m.

Vastus medialis m.

Rectus femoris tendon

Patella

Lateral patellar retinaculum

Medial patellar retinaculum

Joint capsule

Patellar ligament

Tuberosity of tibia

Medial view

Sartorius m.

Gracilis m.

Semitendinosus m.

Semimembranosus m.

Adductor magnus tendon

Tibial collateral ligament, parallel fibers, oblique fibers

Bursa under semimembranosus tendon

Anserine bursa under semi-tendinosus, gracilis, and sartorius tendons

Gastrocnemius m.

Popliteus m.

FIGURE 14-3A
Anatomy of bursae of the knee, lateral views.

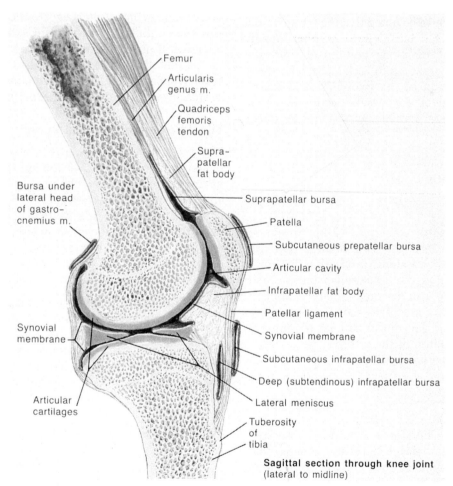

Femur

Articularis genus m.

Quadriceps femoris tendon

Supra-patellar fat body

Bursa under lateral head of gastro-cnemius m.

Suprapatellar bursa

Patella

Subcutaneous prepatellar bursa

Articular cavity

Infrapatellar fat body

Patellar ligament

Synovial membrane

Subcutaneous infrapatellar bursa

Deep (subtendinous) infrapatellar bursa

Lateral meniscus

Tuberosity of tibia

Synovial membrane

Articular cartilages

Sagittal section through knee joint
(lateral to midline)

FIGURE 14-3B
Anatomy of bursae of the knee, lateral sagittal view.

Pyogenic prepatellar bursitis can occur in association with trauma[8] and is usually caused by *Staphylococcus* or *Streptococcus* species.[10,11] Prepatellar bursal swelling may be so great in these settings that it may be difficult to distinguish a prepatellar bursitis from a frank knee joint infection.

TREATMENT

Treatment of acute prepatellar bursitis is conservative and involves ice, compression, and immobilization of the knee. Aspiration should be considered if bursal distention causes significant pain or decreased range of motion. Treatment of acute prepatellar bursitis with intrabursal injections of steroid has been associated with significant rates of infection[10] and is not recommended. Chronic swelling causing disability can be treated with drainage but may require complete excision. Arthroscopic excision of chronic bursitis tissue has been possible in rare cases.[12]

The treatment of pyogenic prepatellar bursitis involves aspiration of the bursa for drainage and for fluid culture and the initiation of an antistaphylococcal antibiotic. It should be noted that the white blood cell count in infected bursal fluid may be low in comparison to joint infections, and bursal fluid cultures routinely may take up to 72 h to become positive.[13] Immobilization of the extremity and warm soaks should be used. If the bursal infection is refractory to this treatment, formal incision and drainage may be necessary.

Infrapatellar Bursitis

MECHANISM

Inflammation of the subcutaneous or deep infrapatellar bursa results in localized swelling and obliteration of the normal depression surrounding the infrapatellar tendon. Like the prepatellar bursae, the infrapatellar bursae can become inflamed due to trauma, inflammatory processes such as gout, or infection.[14] The use of the central patellar tendon approach for introduction of the arthroscope or other instruments into the knee can potentially cause an infrapatellar bursitis.[12]

TREATMENT

The treatment of this bursitis is as outlined for prepatellar bursitis and includes rest, ice, and nonsteroidal anti-inflammatory medications. For pyogenic forms and infrapatellar bursitis, aspiration and initiation of antibiotics is required.

Pes Anserine Bursitis

MECHANISM

The pes anserine bursitis is an injury that usually results from overuse activities. It occurs specifically in runners but has also been observed in breast stroke swimmers.[13,15–17] Pain, swelling, and tenderness are present 6 cm below the joint line on the medial side of the tibia.[18]

In runners, pes anserine bursitis occurs when increased mileage routines are initiated without adequate intervals for rest and stretching between workouts, when running includes hill climbing, and adequate hamstring stretching has not been performed. Stress fractures, benign and malignant tumors of bone, medial meniscus tears, hamstring tendinitis, and degenerative joint disease of the knee all may be confused with pes anserine bursitis.[13]

TREATMENT

The inflammation usually responds to a regimen of rest, ice, nonsteroidal anti-inflammatory medications, hamstring stretching exercises, ultrasound, and knee taping to help prevent external rotation of the knee. If pes anserine bursitis occurs in a runner, the patient should be counseled to reduce mileage, shorten the running stride, and continue hamstring stretching and strengthening exercises.

Tibial Collateral Ligament Bursitis

The diagnosis of TCL bursitis is based on findings of tenderness over the TCL at the joint line in a patient having no history of mechanical symptoms.[3] Kerlan and Glousman[19] reported data on 91 patients diagnosed with TCL bursitis. With a conservative treatment program, 62 percent showed improvement and required no operative intervention.

Fibular Collateral Ligament Bursitis

Fibular collateral ligament bursitis presents with localized tenderness and swelling at the lateral joint line. The bursa itself may be from 0.6 to 2.5 cm in diameter[20] and can lie anterior or posterior to the fibular collateral ligament. Treatment of this lesion is nonsurgical; the use of a steroid injection into the bursa may rarely be necessary.

Popliteal Cyst (Baker's Cyst)

MECHANISM

The popliteal cyst, otherwise termed Baker's cyst after W. M. Baker who described the entity in 1877,[21] represents a distended bursa located in the region of the semimembranosus muscle. In most cases, the bursa involved in the cyst is the medial gastrocnemius bursa (located under the medial head of the gastrocnemius), the semimembranosus bursa (located between the semimembranosus and the medial tibial condyle), or the gastrocnemius-semimembranosus bursa described by Rauschning[22] (located between the semimembranosus tendon and the medial head of the gastrocnemius).

Many investigators have pointed out the differences in pathophysiology of popliteal cysts in children and adults.[23–25] In adult patients, popliteal cysts are frequently associated with intra-articular pathology, whereas in the pediatric population, this is not the case. Tears of the medial meniscus have been the most frequent intra-articular pathology associated with popliteal cysts.[26]

It is important to recognize that the popliteal cyst must be differentiated from other possible causes of masses in the posterior knee. These include popliteal artery aneurysm, thrombophlebitis, pyogenic abscess, and tumors such as lipoma, xanthoma, and fibrosarcoma.

TREATMENT

Although some investigators have found that excision of popliteal cysts in children, with and without postoperative immobilization, provides excellent results with little if any recurrence,[25] others such as Gristina and Wilson[24] have suggested that with observation, popliteal cysts in children gradually disappear.

For adults, meniscal or other intra-articular pathology should be sought and rectified. This will usually result in the disappearance of the cyst.[8] If the popliteal cyst continues to be present, excision may be considered.

REFERENCES

1. *Gray's Anatomy*, 36th ed. Philadelphia, Saunders, 1980.
2. Hollingshead WH: *Anatomy for Surgeons*. Philadelphia, Harper and Row, 1982.
3. Voshell AF, Brantigan OC: Bursitis in the region of the tibial collateral ligament. *J Bone Joint Surg* 26:793, 1944.
4. Hendryson IE: Bursitis in the region of the fibular collateral ligament. *J Bone Joint Surg* 28:446, 1946.
5. Smillie I: *Injuries to the Knee Joint*, 4th ed. Edinburgh, E & S Livingstone, 1970.
6. Larson RL, Osternig LR: Traumatic bursitis and artificial turf. *Am J Sports Med* 2:183, 1974.
7. Gecha SR, Torg E: Knee injuries in tennis. *Clin Sports Med* 7:435, 1988.
8. Mysnyk MD, Wroble RR, Foster DT, et al: Prepatellar bursitis in wrestlers. *Am J Sports Med* 14:46, 1986.
9. Janecki CJ, Hechtman KS: Prepatellar bursitis: A complication of arthroscopic surgery of the knee due to a lost meniscal fragment. *Arthroscopy* 5:343, 1989.
10. Canoso JJ, Sheckman PR: Septic subcutaneous bursitis: Report of 16 cases. *J Rheumatol* 6:196, 1979.
11. Canoso JJ, Yood RD: Reaction of superficial bursae in response to specific disease stimuli. *Arthritis Rheum* 22:1361, 1979.
12. Patel D: Personal communication.
13. Boland A: Soft tissue injuries of the knee, in *The Lower Extremity and Spine in Sports Medicine*, edited by JA Nicholas, EB Hershman. St. Louis, Mosby, 1986.
14. Taylor PW: Inflammation of the deep infrapatellar bursa of the knee. *Arthritis Rheum* 32:1063, 1989.
15. D'Ambrosia R, Drez D: *Prevention and Treatment of Running Injuries*. Thorofare, NJ, CB Slack, 1982, pp 77–84.
16. Helfet AJ: *Disorders of the Knee*, 2d ed. Philadelphia, Lippincott, 1982.
17. James SL, Bates BT, Osternig LR: Injuries to runner. *Am J Sports Med* 6:40, 1978.
18. Fitzgerald RH (ed): *Orthopaedic Knowledge Update 2*. Park Ridge, IL, American Academy of Orthopaedic Surgeons, 1987.
19. Kerlan RK, Glousman RE: Tibial collateral ligament bursitis. *Am J Sports Med* 16:346, 1988.
20. Justis EJ: Nontraumatic disorders, in *Campbell's Operative Orthopaedics*, 7th ed, edited by AH Crenshaw. St. Louis, Mosby, 1987, pp 2247–2261.
21. Baker WM: On the formation of synovial cysts in the leg in connection with disease in the joint. *St. Bartholomew Hosp Rep* 13:245, 1877.
22. Rauschning W: Popliteal cysts and their reaction to the gastocnemico-semimembranosus bursa. Studies on the surgical and functional anatomy. *Acta Orthop Scand Suppl* 179, 1979.

23. Childress HM: Popliteal cysts in association with undiagnosed posterior lesions of the medial meniscus. The significance of age in diagnosis and treatment. *J Bone Joint Surg* 52A:1487, 1970.

24. Gristina AG, Wilson PD: Popliteal cysts in adults and children. A review of 90 cases. *Arch Surg* 88:357, 1964.

25. Touloukian RJ: Popliteal cyst in childhood. *Surgery* 60:629, 1971.

26. Wolfe RD, Coloff B: Popliteal cysts. An arthrographic study and reivew of the literature. *J Bone Joint Surg* 52A:1057, 1972.

CHAPTER 15

Patella Infera

Lonnie E. Paulos
John L. Pinkowski

INTRODUCTION

Although other overuse and traumatic injuries of the patellofemoral joint are more common, no discussion of nonosseous lesions of the patella would be complete without addressing patella baja or infera. These terms refer to an inferior vertical position of the patella in relation to the femorotibial articulation. Although the term *patella infera* has been used in the descriptions of postoperative syndromes, the terms *baja* and *infera* can be used interchangeably, referring only to patellar location. In this chapter, the term infera will be used for consistency.

Patella infera has been known to occur developmentally, but it is more often a complication or direct result of patellofemoral or knee surgery. In this chapter, we will present a framework of classification, diagnosis, prevention, and treatment of complications.

CLASSIFICATION AND ETIOLOGY

Anterior knee pain is a common complaint among patients with knee symptoms. A large differential diagnosis exists, consisting of multiple etiologic factors. Careful clinical correlation is necessary in evaluating patients with a patella infera because the mere existence of patella infera may not account for all or any of the patient's complaints.

Patella infera is rarely seen as an independent entity, but it does exist as a normal variant. It has been reported to occur in achondroplastic dwarfs and in children with poliomyelitis without causing any functional problems.[14] Cameron and Jung have also noted osteoarthritis as a rare cause of infera in their total knee arthroplasty recipients.[9] Osgood–Schlatter's disease has also been associated with this entity,[25] but whether the infera causes the disease, or the disease causes the infera, could not be established. Patients with a tight extensor mechanism may increase stress on the developing tibial tubercle causing apophysitis. Alternatively, the inflammation from the apophysitis may cause scarring and contracture, leading to patella infera.

Secondary causes such as surgical procedures about the knee and traumatic insults account for almost all cases seen. Since little information has been tabulated on this subject to date, we propose a classification system based on etiology (Table 15-1).

DIAGNOSIS

Methods

HISTORY

All problem solving in medicine begins with a careful history. Most patients presenting to the office with symptoms secondary to patella infera will have had previous surgery or a lower extremity condition causing immobilization of the knee. It is important to inquire about the exact date of the surgery, immobilization, or onset of pain. Information regarding the type and duration of immobilization; the degree of pain in the postoperative or postinjury state; the type, duration, and intensity of physical rehabilitation; and the mode of subsequent treatment intervention must also be obtained. Patients with this syndrome will complain of knee stiffness, pain, altered gait,

TABLE 15-1
Etiologic Classification of Patella Infera

I. Genetic
    A. Achondroplasia

II. Developmental
    A. Normal variant

III. Infectious
    A. Poliomyelitis

IV. Degenerative
    A. Osteoarthritis

V. Traumatic
    A. Patellar tendon rupture
    B. Fracture of the tibial tubercle

VI. Iatrogenic
    A. Tibial tubercle surgery
    B. The postoperative knee
        1. Arthroscopy
        2. Total knee arthroplasty
        3. Cruciate ligament reconstruction
        4. Tibial osteotomy

crepitation, and perhaps weakness. The current and past history of medications prescribed (nonsteroidal anti-inflammatory drugs, corticosteroids, or narcotics) is helpful in determining the patient's response to treatment and also in defining the patient's pain tolerance.

PHYSICAL EXAMINATION

Following a careful history, the physical examination can alert the physician to the syndrome of patella infera. In 1899, Schulthess reported his observation that with the knee flexed at 90 degrees, the patella normally sinks in between the femoral condyles and this produces a rounded contour of the knee.[31] Those patients with profound patella infera lose this contour and the knee takes the appearance of the distal femoral condyles. However, if a large amount of swelling occurs this may not be obvious.

Palpation of the patella or patellar tendon may reveal a significant amount of tenderness depending on the degree of inflammation present at examination. Patellofemoral crepitation often accompanies the postoperative patella infera syndrome. Other qualitative clues defining the amount of inflammation present include swelling, erythema, and warmth.

When assessing patellar mobility, the medial, lateral, superior, and inferior gliding motion should be determined. Often, the patella becomes entrapped and loses its usual mobility. Comparison to the contralateral patella is helpful in unilateral traumatic or postoperative cases.

RADIOGRAPHIC

Several reported radiographic methods are used to determine the height relationship of the patella to the femorotibial joint.[10] Most are based on the lateral radiograph by using an index or ratio. These measurements depend on osseous anatomy and are therefore less accurate in the immature skeleton. These measurements are important because they define the normal range of patellar height. With guidelines of this type, corrective surgery to restore normal patellar biomechanics is possible. When using any of these methods, serial radiography is helpful. Preoperative radiographs or radiographs of the unaffected opposite knee increase the accuracy of these measurements by reducing individual variability. Noyes and colleagues[28] showed that there is no significant difference between the right and left knees in the same individual using three different radiographic methods. Statistically, a difference of > 15 percent was considered significant. The measurement of choice

should achieve certain goals. The method should be quick and easy to use, accurate, reproducible, and independent of knee position, joint size, and magnification.

Anteroposterior Radiographs

The outline of the patella is visible on the anteroposterior projection of the knee. The relationship of the inferior pole to the joint line gives the clinician only a rough estimate of the vertical height of the patella. The tip of the inferior pole of the patella is normally located at the level of the femorotibial joint line[7] (Fig. 15-1). Because the inferior nonarticular extension of the patella has a great normal variation, this particular method is not extremely accurate.

Lateral Radiographs

Boon-Itt Method In 1930, Boon-Itt developed a complex method of measuring patellar height based on geometric calculations.[6] This has been found to be too difficult to use[20] in the clinical setting and therefore has never gained widespread acceptance.

Blumensaat Method Blumensaat[5] developed a method of measurement based on a 30 degree flexed knee lateral radiograph. At this position, a direct extension of the roof of the intercondylar notch (*Blumensaat's line*) should touch the inferior pole of the patella (Fig. 15-2).

Even though this measurement is simple, it is not without its flaws. A criticism of this technique is that the 30 degree radiograph is difficult to reproduce, and others have reported that it is inaccurate.[7,19,20,21,22]

Jacobsen and Bertheussen[22] examined 100 knees in 50 patients using this method. The average distance from the inferior pole to Blumensaat's line was 17 mm with the knee flexed at 30 degrees. The range between the 2.5 and 97.5 percentile was 7 mm and 29 mm, respectively, thereby refuting Blumensaat's observations. This study also emphasized the need to correct the absolute measurement for physical proportions of the patient. This eliminates the difference seen between male and female populations based on size, and also between extremes of size in the same sex.[22]

Brattström Method In 1970, Brattström searched for an alternative to Blumensaat's method of measuring patellar height.[7] His prime concern was to identify patella alta and its association to symptomatic knees without a history of dislocations. Brattström examined 100 knees and found Blumensaat's measurement method inaccurate. To test Blumensaat's method, the variability of Blumensaat's line in rela-

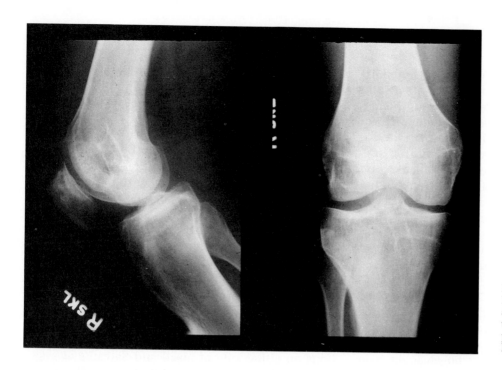

FIGURE 15-1
Patella infera after anterior cruciate ligament reconstruction. Notice that the inferior pole of the patella is located below the joint line on the AP radiograph.

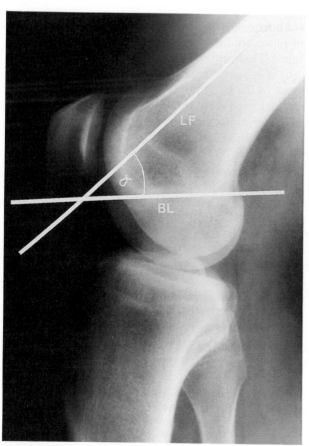

FIGURE 15-2
Blumensaat's line (*BL*) is located at the roof of the intercondylar notch and classically is tangential to the inferior pole of the patella. The axis of the femur (*LF*) intersects Blumensaat's line to form the angle alpha (α), as determined by Brattström.[¹]

tion to the long axis of the femur was determined. Using a lateral radiograph, a line is drawn along the long axis of the femur, which intersects Blumensaat's line. The angle of intersection, alpha (see Fig. 15-2), varied between 27 degrees and 60 degrees (average 45 degrees), suggesting that Blumensaat's method has a wide range of variability, affecting its accuracy. Jacobsen and Bertheussen also measured this angle in 100 knees and found a slightly narrower range (26 degrees to 40 degrees) of variability. Brattström found that an alteration of ±10 degrees in the angle (α) (average 45 degrees) would alter the intersection of Blumensaat's line with the patella by ±10 mm. A "false" infera would be seen at 35 degrees and a "false" alta at 55 degrees.[7] Correcting for this variability in the angle α, Brattström arbitrarily defined patella alta as any patella 10 mm above Blumensaat's line but set no measure for patella infera.

Ninety Degree Flexion Lateral   Labelle and Laurin found a method of measurement using the 90 degree flexed knee radiograph.[24] A line drawn down the anterior aspect of the femur passes over the top of the superior pole of the patella in 97 percent of normal knees. The superior pole of the patella lies above this line in those patients with patella alta and below this line in those with patella infera.

Insall–Salvati Method   In 1971, Insall and Salvati published their method of measuring patellar height in an effort to assist with the surgical planning of distal and medial transfer of the tibial tubercle.[20] They

207

examined 44 lateral radiographs of knees flexed exactly 30 degrees, and did not find a single knee in which the lower pole of the patella touched Blumensaat's line. All 44 patients had their patellae positioned above this line. In fact, in 41 patients the patella was located $\geq$ 10 mm above Blumensaat's line. Based on the principles that the infrapatellar tendon is not elastic and that the point of insertion into the tibia is constant, Insall and Salvati established a measurement relating the patellar length (LP) to the patellar tendon length (LT) (Fig. 15-3).

The LP is determined by measuring its greatest diagonal length. LT is determined by measuring along its posterior surface from the origin on the inferior pole of the patella to its insertion into the tibia. The tibial attachment site can be measured by finding a rather constant notch located at the tibial tubercle. In their initial article, the ratio was defined as LT:LP; in a later article published in 1972, however, the ratio used was LP:LT. In his book, published in 1984, Insall used his initial LT:LP ratio.[21]

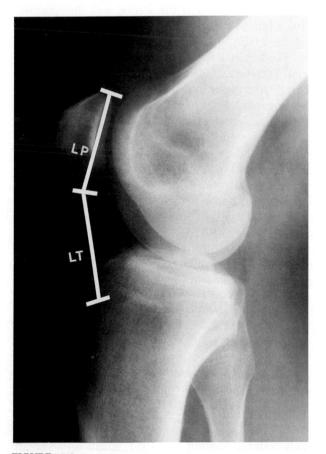

FIGURE 15-3
The Insall–Salvati ratio is derived by determining the greatest length of the patella (*LP*), and the length of the patellar tendon (*LT*). The LT:LP ratio is approximately 1.0.

Insall and Salvati also examined two ratios in the knee to verify that the physical proportions were consistent. First, they examined the relationship between the location (height) of the patellar tendon insertion from the tibial plateau (HI) to the length of the patellar tendon (LT:HI). The ratio, LT:HI, was felt to be quite constant. The second ratio compared the width of the femoral condyles at the intercondylar line (Blumensaat's line) to the length of the patellar tendon. This ratio, LP:WCBL, also was found to be consistent, reflecting this method's usefulness in joints of all sizes. If there was a great variation in either of these two ratios, it would have invalidated the LP:LT measurements.[20] After reviewing 114 knee radiographs showing meniscal pathology but otherwise considered normal, Insall and Salvati determined that an average LT:LP ratio is 1.02, with a standard deviation of 0.13. Using two standard deviations on either side of Insall and Salvati's average, the normal range would be 1.28 to 0.76. This range encompasses 96 percent of the normal population (Fig. 15-4).

Blackburne–Peel Method In 1977, Blackburne and Peel reported another method of measuring patellar height.[3] Their ratio is obtained by comparing the height of the patellar articular surface above the tibial plateau to the length of the patellar articular surface, with the knee flexed >30 degrees (PA:TA; Fig. 15-5).

The drawbacks of the Insall–Salvati method according to Blackburne and Peel are: (1) the measurement depends on the tibial tubercle being a standard distance below the tibial plateau, (2) the exact point of distal patellar tendon attachment to the tibia may be difficult to determine if it is not prominent or if there is calcification from Sinding–Larsen–Johannsen disease or Osgood–Schlatter disease, and (3) the length of the nonarticular portion of the inferior pole of the patella is too variable.

The mean ratio for 121 normal knees in men was 0.805 (SD of 0.14) and for 50 normal knees in women, 0.806 (SD of 0.13). They defined normal as 0.8 and patella alta as 1.0 but gave no value for patella infera. We suggest that the normal range, consisting of two standard deviations above and below the mean, is 0.54 to 1.06.

Because this method has the least amount of variability, we feel this is the measurement of choice.

BIOMECHANICS AND PATHOPHYSIOLOGY

Diagnosing the presence of patella infera is meaningful, but perhaps a more important issue is deter-

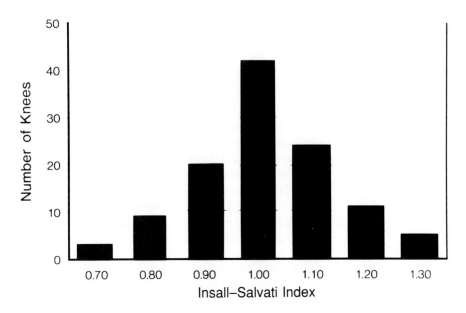

FIGURE 15-4
The normal Insall–Salvati Index (LT:LP) distribution of the 114 knees initially reported.

mining how infera interferes with normal knee kinematics. In an elaborate study by Hehne,[16] experimental distal tibial tubercle transfers were performed on cadavers to evaluate contact area and pressure at different flexion angles of the knee. He found that the

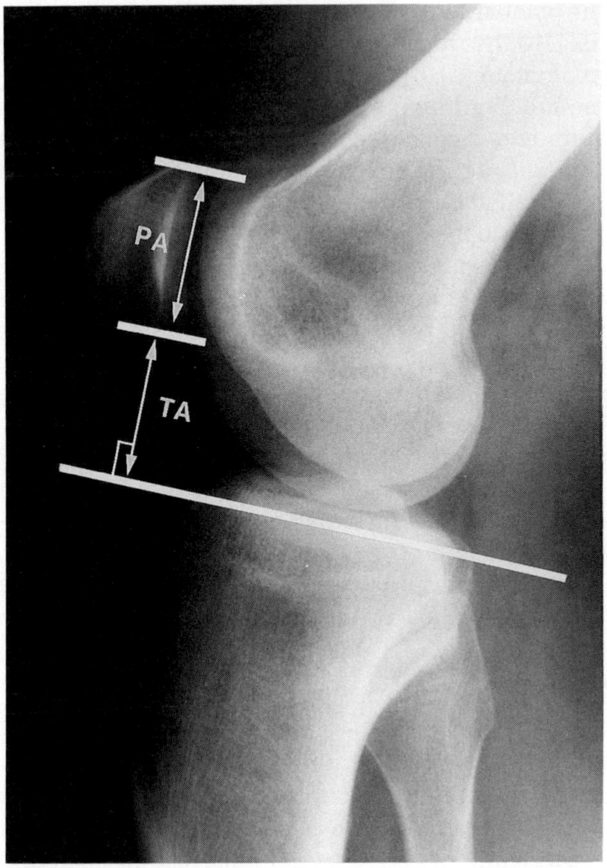

FIGURE 15-5
The Blackburne and Peel ratio is determined by measuring the length of the articular surface of the patella (*PA*) to the height of the articular cartilage above the tibial plateau (*TA*). The normal ratio, PA:TA, is approximately equal to 0.8.

contact areas on the articular surface of the patella are reduced and exhibit higher pressures. This same effect was postulated to explain the high rate of postoperative osteoarthritis in long-term studies of patients with infera. Since Hehne's study was performed on normal cadaver knees, a follow-up study showing how contact areas and pressures are affected in knees with patella alta or infera is needed.

The functional effect of patella infera is to tighten the extensor mechanism. This is thought to lead to increased patellar articular pressures and restrict knee flexion.[2,18,23,27]

CLINICAL APPLICATIONS

Patella infera exists in several clinical situations. Patella infera is most commonly found secondary to a traumatic or surgical event, but despite the etiology there are common features in the pathophysiology and treatment. The most extensive description of patella infera and its treatment is found in an article published by Paulos and colleagues[29] describing the infrapatellar contracture syndrome.

Infrapatellar Contracture Syndrome

The patella may become entrapped in the knee (patellar entrapment syndrome or PES) as a direct result of surgery or injury. A specific subset of PES, as elaborated by Paulos and colleagues,[29] is the complication of infrapatellar contracture syndrome (IPCS). It was initially recognized in patients who had a unique combination of loss of both flexion and extension range of motion.

The classification of this entity has been recognized as primary or secondary. In the primary group, an exaggerated fibrohyperplasia of the anterior soft tissues of the knee is present. These individuals have

209

an intensified healing response. In the secondary group, a surgical procedure combined with prolonged immobilization typically leads to a lack of extension. Other causes of secondary IPCS include nonisometric ligament surgery, infection, reflex sympathetic dystrophy, entrapped meniscus, quadriceps insufficiency, and neuromuscular disorders.

There are three important stages of IPCS and each has a recommended method of treatment and ultimate prognosis.

STAGES

Stage I—Prodromal Stage—(2 to 8 weeks)
This stage is recognized by induration of the synovial, fat pad, and retinacular tissues. Physical examination reveals a painful range of motion, restricted patellar mobility, tenderness along the patellar tendon, and a quadriceps lag. A *quadriceps lag* is defined as a greater passive than active range of motion. A clue, in many of these patients, is a difficult and painful rehabilitation progression.

Stage II—Active Stage—(6 to 20 weeks)
The indurated tissues have now formed a "shelf" beneath the patella (Fig. 15-6). The patellar motion becomes more limited with restriction of glides and tilts; superior glide is restricted the most. Patellar crepitus is now found (see Fig. 15-6).

At this stage many of the patients have had vigorous, forceful physical therapy or manipulations, which have intensified this condition. Passive and active range of motion are now the same and the quadriceps has a large amount of atrophy. Both intra-

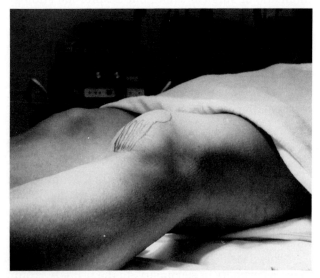

FIGURE 15-6
The "shelf" sign caused by induration and fibrosis is demonstrated in this clinical photograph.

articular and extra-articular involvement are present. The patient cannot achieve full extension and walks with a "short leg" gait.

Stage III—Burned Out Stage—(8 months to years)
Inflammation and induration have now subsided with the result of developmental patella infera. Patellar mobility, therefore, is not as restricted as in stage II. Significant loss of flexion and extension are still presented combined with marked quadriceps atrophy. Patellofemoral arthrosis is noted by severe crepitus and a diminished joint space on Merchant radiographs. Some patients who are at the end of this stage have patella infera and patellofemoral arthrosis as their only remaining physical signs.

RADIOGRAPHIC FINDINGS

An early finding in these patients is osteopenia of the knee; later findings include patella infera and associated patellofemoral arthrosis.

BIOMECHANICS

The patellar tendon normally has a discrete insertion distal to the tibial plateau on the tibial tubercle. The inflammatory response seen with infrapatellar contracture syndrome results in a fibrous proliferation behind the patellar tendon. This scarification process secondary to the inflammation causes adherence of the patellar tendon proximal to the tibial tubercle insertion, up to the level of the tibial plateau.

Biomechanically, the patellofemoral joint contact force is composed of the force from the quadriceps muscle proximally and the patellar tendon attachment distally. In IPCS, as the insertion of the patellar tendon becomes more proximal, the effective force from the patellar tendon becomes more posteriorly directed. The posterior redirection of the patellar tendon force increases the patellofemoral joint contact force, as it contributes a greater component toward the femoral trochlea in knee flexion (Fig. 15-7). Occasionally, a proximal slide of the tibial tubercle is necessary to correct the biomechanics (Fig. 15-8).

PATHOLOGY

Those patients requiring surgery gave Paulos and colleagues[29] an opportunity to define the gross and microscopic pathology from this disease. The findings at surgery are quite consistent. Cadaver dissections by these authors were used to suggest an anatomic basis for the pathophysiology seen.

Between 3 and 6 months after the onset, severe induration and fibrosis of the capsular, fat pad, and synovial tissues are seen. The amount of this tissue

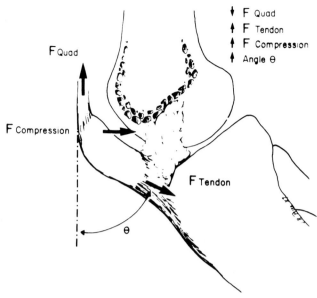

FIGURE 15-7
The scarification process effectively moves the patellar tendon force vector more proximal and posterior than its usual location. This increases the force of compression on the patellofemoral joint. F Quad, force of the quadriceps tendon; F Compression, force of patellar compression; F Tendon, force of the patellar tendon; Θ, the angle between F Tendon and F Quad.

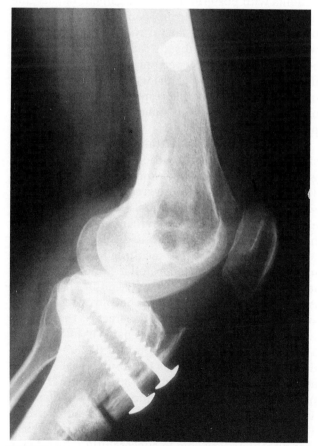

FIGURE 15-8
To establish normal patellar biomechanics, a proximal slide of the tibial tubercle is occasionally performed.

present may prevent entrance to the joint arthroscopically without endangering the hyaline cartilage. Biopsy of this tissue reveals a dense, disorganized collagen connective tissue. The patella becomes adherent to the fibrotic fat pad, which occupies the entire anterior space from the intercondylar notch to both joint lines. The histology of the fat pad shows that the fatty tissue is replaced with a dense fibrotic tissue associated with inflammation (Fig. 15-9). Fibrous tissue is abundant anteriorly and in the medial and lateral gutters.

Patients with long-standing disease may develop a fibrotic pannus that impinges into the joint and damages the hyaline cartilage in three ways. The pannus causes mechanical injury to the joint, which is made worse by range of motion in forceful physical therapy. Secondly, the pannus interferes with hyaline nutrition. Thirdly, although not proven, there may be an increase in enzyme formation in the pannus, which could lead to further chemical degradation of the hyaline cartilage. Biopsies in these areas illustrate a loss of glycosaminoglycans accompanied by subchondral bone atrophy.

The anatomic dissections allowed the authors to define the fascial and fibrofascial tissues that become involved in this entity. All these structures have the potential to contribute to the fibrous hyperplasia: fibrous tissue surrounding the patellar tendon, the fibrofatty fat pad and its extensions beneath the patellar tendon and into the medial and lateral joint, the patellofemoral ligaments (Kaplan's ligaments) that attach to the anterior horns of both menisci, and the ligamentum mucosa.

TREATMENT RECOMMENDATIONS

Ideally, prevention is the best treatment for IPCS. Early identification and treatment is the key to a satisfactory prognosis. Those patients treated extensively in the initial stage will do better than those seen in stage III, when the damage to the joint has already occurred.

Avoidance of this complication is best achieved by the same measures used to treat stage I disease. The physician should use early range of motion, manual patellar mobilization by the therapist and patient, judicious use of anti-inflammatory medication including, at times, corticosteroids and electrical muscle stimulation. Those patients with an unusual amount of pain and failure to progress with physical therapy should be identified for addition of other therapeutic measures. These could include analgesics, corticosteroid dose packs, or use of a transcutaneous electrical nerve stimulation unit. All postoperative patients, and most of those in stage I of IPCS, should respond to this program of treatment.

The timing of operative intervention is critical.

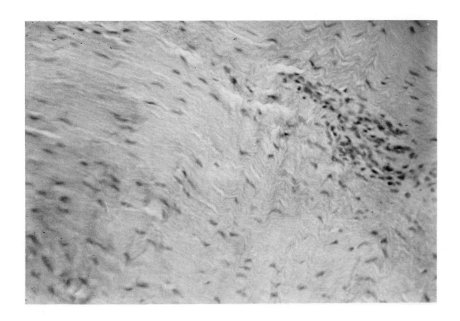

FIGURE 15-9
Photomicrograph demonstrates the dense, disorganized collagen tissue, associated with inflammation that replaces the fat pad.

Usually, a patient who has failed to progress in physical therapy and who has PES should have surgery postponed for 4 to 12 weeks. During this period, the patient should continue to gain quadriceps strength, while the surgeon waits for the pain, swelling, and inflammation to decrease.

When the patient has reached stage II or III, the best treatment is by anterior, medial, and lateral intra-articular and extra-articular capsular debridement and release, followed by physical therapy. The best circumstances for operative intervention are at a time of decreased inflammation and when the patient has good quadriceps strength. Open debridement includes lateral retinacular release, anterior debridement, and partial fat pad resection. The intra-articular and extra-articular freeing of the patellar tendon and patella should be performed medially, superiorly, and inferiorly. Often a medial arthrotomy is needed to effectively accomplish this. If a ligament procedure was performed, evaluation for notch impingement, overtensioning, or a nonisometric placement of the ligament should be assessed. It is sometimes helpful to perform this procedure under an epidural anesthetic to allow the patient to visualize the range of motion attained at surgery. The epidural can then be kept in place postoperatively to allow effective continuous passive range of motion without pain.

Paulos and colleagues[29] reviewed data on 28 cases of IPCS, 19 of which were in the primary IPCS category. These patients were followed for at least 1 year (average 18 months); the 16 females and 12 males were aged 11 to 52. IPCS followed a surgical procedure in all except for 2 patients in whom entrapment occurred after minor anterior knee trauma. The most common surgical procedure leading to IPCS was an-

terior cruciate ligament reconstruction (19 patients). In these patients, there were no differences in the type of graft, timing of surgery, or combined extra-articular, meniscal, or medial collateral ligament repair. The remaining surgical cases consisted of 2 patients with posterior cruciate ligament reconstructions, 4 patients with arthroscopy alone or with partial meniscectomy or lateral release, and 1 patient with a proximal and distal realignment. Paulos and coworkers[29] estimate 5 percent of patients having an injury or surgery of the knee will develop this abnormal fibrosclerotic healing response. The distribution of the surgical procedures may reflect their surgical practice.

In their experience, patients had a loss of extension (range 7 degrees to 35 degrees, average 17 degrees) and loss of knee flexion (range 60 degrees to 139 degrees, average 98 degrees), and moderate to severe quadriceps atrophy that was associated with an antalgic gait. Over 75 percent of their patients had patellofemoral crepitus and diffuse synovitis and peripatellar inflammation resulting in a shelf sign in most patients. Restricted patellar mobility, particularly in the superior glide, was seen in all patients. After treatment, the 28 patients had an average extension loss of 5 degrees (range 0 degrees to 10 degrees), with an average increase in extension at follow-up of 12 degrees. The average amount of flexion was 133 degrees (range 115 degrees to 145 degrees), with an average increase in flexion of 35 degrees. Over 90 percent of patients had symptoms of patellofemoral arthrosis and 16 percent demonstrated patella infera. The most distressing outcome in these patients is that no athlete was able to successfully return to the preinjury level of sports and patients who were laborers had not returned to their former employment.

212

Treatment recommendations in the past have advised various posterior releases to relieve loss of extension. The procedures were used primarily in pediatric and neuromuscular disorders and were designed to release the contracted posterior capsule and hamstring tendons to gain extension.

Sprague[33] and Payr[30] both advocate release of the suprapatellar pouch and the peripatellar gutters; however, Sprague suggests that patients who do not improve after arthroscopic debridement of these areas have extra-articular involvement.

In light of the past treatment of flexion and extension contractures, Paulos was able to achieve correction using anterior intra-articular and extra-articular debridement combined with manipulation without resorting to posterior surgical release. Posterior release should only be considered if a previous posterior surgical approach has been used and accounts for the contracture.

Proximal Tibial Osteotomy

Valgus-producing proximal tibial osteotomies are routinely performed in adults to unload an arthritic medial compartment. In the standard technique for adults, the osteotomy is executed above the tibial tubercle. The closing wedge osteotomy then moves the tibial tubercle slightly proximal to its previous location and can result in patella infera. Perhaps a more common pathophysiologic explanation for infera after tibial osteotomy is that long immobilization time after surgery allows fibrohyperplasia to occur about the infrapatellar tendon.

Using the Insall–Salvati method, Staeheli and colleagues[34] noted that in patients undergoing condylar total knee arthroplasty, patella infera was present in 4 of 32 patients (12.5 percent). All 4 patients have Insall–Salvati ratios between 0.83 and 0.90.

Windsor[35] analyzed 45 knees that had undergone proximal tibial osteotomy that needed subsequent revision to total knee arthroplasty. He noted that 38 patients (84 percent) had patella infera as determined by the Insall–Salvati method, using a ratio of less than 0.8.

Scuderi and colleagues[32] analyzed data on 60 patients to see if any alteration in patellar height was present after proximal tibial osteotomy. Postoperative radiographs were measured using the Insall–Salvati (ratio <0.8) and Blackburne and Peel (ratio <0.54) methods. Eighty-nine percent of patients had a lower patella using the former method and 76 percent using the latter method. Actual patella infera was noted in 16.7 percent and 7.6 percent, respectively. However, they did not find any correlation between the postoperative height of the patella and the need for subsequent revision to a total knee replacement or the success of the tibial osteotomy. There appears to be a wide variance in the incidence of patella infera after proximal tibial osteotomy and the true incidence lies between a large range from 7.6 percent to 84 percent.

Total Knee Arthroplasty

Patella infera can exist in the preoperative state or it can be created by altering the joint during arthroplasty; it can also occur postoperatively in the healing phase.

Preoperative patella infera, as already mentioned, is unusual. Rare cases of patella infera have been seen in osteoarthritic patients undergoing total knee arthroplasty,[8] but joint replacement itself can alter the joint line causing patella infera. The principles of knee surface replacement demand the maintenance of the naturally occurring joint line. This is accomplished by avoiding excessive bone cuts on the tibia and femur, as well as paying attention to deficient bone stock. In those few patients where patella infera is seen secondary to osteoarthritis, maintenance of the joint space may then leave a patellar component that fails to contact the femoral component. Instead, the proximal quadriceps mechanism is forced to articulate in the prosthetic trochlea. It may therefore be necessary in these instances to perform a proximal slide of the tibial tubercle by osteotomy and internal fixation.

Alternatively, poor technique in total knee arthroplasty may yield a joint line that is too far proximal, creating patella baja. Often this will require revision of the arthroplasty. Revision of the total knee arthroplasty for treatment of patella infera has not consistently yielded satisfactory results.[15]

Bryan[8] reported on two cases of postoperative patella infera which were felt to cause anterior knee pain after total knee arthroplasty. His findings at revision surgery are remarkably similar to the IPCS as described by Paulos and colleagues[29] and surgical correction of the soft tissues follows the same principles. The only aspect that seemed to differ was that in Bryan's revision total knees, the posterior capsular sulci had to be reestablished by elevating the posterior capsule off of the femur. Facilitation of soft tissue resection was obtained by removal of the tibial tray. His results for pain relief and increase in functional range of motion were gratifying. The good results seemed to have lasted in most patients and the incidence of recurrence has been reported as rare. Bryan felt that inadequate mobilization secondary to pain inhibition may have attributed to the formation of fibrous adhesions in the fat pad, suprapatellar pouch, and posterior sulci. He describes fibrous hypertrophy of the fat pad in the infrapatellar area combined with capsular adhesions.

Based on the premise that pain created by tight anterior structures will limit flexion, Bryan suggests three technical errors that could increase the possibility of development of patella infera: (1) increasing the overall thickness of the patella by using a patellar component that is too thick or a bone cut that is not thick enough, (2) using a thick tibial component or an insufficient bone cut on the tibia, and (3) performing an excessively tight closure of the capsule to the patellar tendon anteromedially.

Distal Patellar Realignment and Hauser Procedures

Patellar subluxation and dislocation have been associated with patella alta.[1,7,11,14,17,19,25,26] Those patients resistant to rehabilitation continue to have instability. The distal realignment procedures consider the abnormal amount of lateral and superior positioning of the tibial tubercle and its associated biomechanical alteration. Realizing that patella infera can occur not only from improper surgical repositioning but also from alterations in normal healing, one must be cognizant of what can be done to prevent this complication. Understanding the normal patellar height rela-

tionships aids in the repositioning of the tibial tubercle and early mobilization with proper physical therapy after surgery provide benefit.

Blazina and colleagues[4] recognized that patella infera occurred as a complication in 10 of 40 (25 percent) Hauser procedures. Their patient's symptoms included retropatellar pain, crepitus, limitation of motion, and disability; physical examination and radiography revealed evidence of distal displacement of the tibial tubercle.

Others have reported the incidence of patella infera in tibial tubercle surgery. Fielding[13] only found it in 3 of 377 (0.8 percent) patients undergoing Hauser procedures. Chrisman[11] mentioned in his evaluation of Hauser procedures that 4 of 47 (8.5 percent) tibial tubercles were transferred too far distally or medially leading to severe arthritis.

Reviewing a series of patients treated by conservative or surgical methods with a diagnosis of recurrent patellar dislocation, Crosby and Insall[12] found no relationship of patellar height to the incidence of osteoarthritis. They felt that the medial and not the distal transfer was responsible for a high incidence of osteoarthritis. Unfortunately, in the series the patients examined were not randomly assigned to treatment groups; therefore, those undergoing surgery may not only have had greater symptoms but also existing chondrosis. It is also unclear what kind of immobilization, bracing, and rehabilitation were used in the treatment groups.

REFERENCES

1. Bentley G: Surgical treatment of chondromalacia patellae. *J Bone Joint Surg* 60B:74, 1900.
2. Bessette GC, Hunter RE: The Maquet procedure. A retrospective review. *Clin Orthop* 232:159, 1988.
3. Blackburne J, Peel T: A new method of measuring patellar height. *J Bone Joint Surg* 58B:241, 1977.
4. Blazina ME, Fox JM, Carlson GJ, Jurgutis JJ: Patella baja. A technical consideration in evaluating results of tibial tubercle transplantation. *J Bone Joint Surg* 58A:1027, 1975.
5. Blumensaat C: Die Lageabweichungen und Verrenkungen der Kneischeibe. *Ergen Chir Orthop* 31:149, 1938.
6. Boon-Itt, SB: The normal position of the patella. *J Roentgen Soc* 24:389, 1930.
7. Brattström H: Patella alta in nondislocating knee joints. *Acta Orthop Scand* 41:578, 1970.
8. Bryan RS: Patella infera and fat-pad hypertrophy after total knee arthroplasty. *Tech Orthop* 3:29, 1988.
9. Cameron HU, Jung YB: Patella baja complicating total knee arthroplasty: A report of two cases. *J Arthroplasty* 3:177, 1988.
10. Carson WG, James SL, Larson RL, et al: Patellofemoral disorders: Physical and radiographic evaluation. Part II. Radiographic examination. *Clin Orthop* 185:178, 1984.
11. Chrisman OD, Snook GA, Wilson TC: A long-term prospective study of the Hauser and Roux–Goldthwaite procedures for recurrent patellar dislocation. Clin Orthop 144:27, 1979.
12. Crosby EB, Insall J: Recurrent dislocation of the patella. Relation of treatment to osteoarthritis. *J Bone Joint Surg* 58A:9, 1976.
13. Fielding JW, Liebler WA, Krishne-Urs ND, et al: Tibial tubercle transfer: A long-range follow-up study. *Clin Orthop* 144:43, 1979.

14. Fulkerson JP, Hungerford DS: *Disorders of the Patellofemoral Joint*, 2d ed. Baltimore, Williams & Wilkins, 1990.

15. Goldberg VM, Figgie EF III, Figgie MP: Technical considerations in total knee surgery: Management of patella problems. *Orthop Clin North Am* 20:189, 1989.

16. Hehne HJ: Biomechanics of the patellofemoral joint and its clinical relevance. *Clin Orthop* 258:73, 1990.

17. Hughston JC, Walsh WM: Proximal and distal reconstruction of the extensor mechanism for patellar subluxation. *Clin Orthop* 144:36, 1979.

18. Hungerford DS, Barry M: Biomechanics of the patellofemoral joint. *Clin Orthop* 144:9, 1979.

19. Insall J, Goldberg V, Salvati E: Recurrent dislocation and the high riding patella. *Clin Orthop* 88:67, 1972.

20. Insall J, Salvati E: Patella position in the normal knee joint. *Radiology* 101:101, 1971.

21. Insall J: *Surgery of the Knee*. New York, Churchill-Livingstone, 1984.

22. Jacobsen K, Berthensen K: The vertical location of the patella. *Acta Orthop Scand* 45:436, 1974.

23. Karrison J, Bunkertorp O, Lansinger O, et al: Lowering of the patella secondary to anterior advancement of the tibial tubercle for the patellofemoral pain syndrome. *Arch Orthop Trauma Surg* 105:40, 1986.

24. Labelle H, Laurin CA: Radiologic investigation of normal and abnormal patellae. *J Bone Joint Surg* 57B:530, 1976.

25. Lancourt JE, Cristini JA: Patella alta and patella infera. Their etiologic role in patellar dislocation, chondromalacia, and apophysitis of the tibial tubercle. *J Bone Joint Surg* 57A:1112, 1975.

26. Marks KE, Bentley G: Patella alta and chondromalacia. *J Bone Joint Surg* 60B:71, 1978.

27. Mendes DG, Soudery M, Iusim M: Clinical assessment of Maquet tibial tuberosity advancement. *Clin Orthop* 222:228, 1987.

28. Noyes FR, Wojtys EM, Marshall MT: The early diagnosis and treatment of developmental patella infera syndrome. *Clin Orthop* 265:241, 1991.

29. Paulos LE, Rosenberg TD, Drawbert J, et al: Infrapatellar contracture syndrome: An unrecognized cause of knee stiffness with patella entrapment and patella infera. *Am J Sports Med* 15:331, 1987.

30. Payr E: Zür operativen behandlung der kniegelensteife. *Zentralbl Chir* 44:809, 1917.

31. Schulthess W: Zür pathologie und therapie der spastischen gliederstarre. *Z Orthop Chir* 6:1, 1899.

32. Scuderi G, Cuomo F, Scott WN: Lateral release and proximal realignment for patellar subluxation and dislocation. A long term follow-up. *J Bone Joint Surg* 70A:856, 1988.

33. Sprague N, O'Conner R, Fox J: Arthroscopic treatment of postoperative knee fibroarthrosis. *Clin Orthop* 166:165, 1982.

34. Staeheli JW, Cass JR, Morrey BF: Condylar total knee arthroplasty after failed proximal tibial osteotomy. *J Bone Joint Surg* 69A:19, 1987.

35. Windsor RE, Insall JN, Vince KG: Technical considerations after total knee arthroplasty after proximal tibial osteotomy. *J Bone Joint Surg* 70A:547, 1988.

SECTION V

Fractures

CHAPTER 16

Fractures (Including Traumatic, Stress, and Bipartite Patella)

Neal L. Thomson

INTRODUCTION

The patella is vulnerable to injury because of its relatively unprotected position in the anterior aspect of the knee joint. A blow to the front of the knee joint, directly striking the patella, is more likely to cause significant damage in the flexed knee than the extended knee.[1] The patella, being an integral part of the extensor mechanism of the knee joint, and the surrounding soft tissues must be considered when assessing damage to the front of the knee. Management of patella fractures requires an exact knowledge of the anatomy of the extensor mechanism.

Although vulnerable to direct trauma, the bony structure of the patella may also be damaged in ballistic activities such as high jumping, skiing, and violent rotating sports. Longitudinal stress with the knee flexed can cause a transverse fracture, whereas direct trauma commonly results in either a transverse or a comminuted fracture. Lateral dislocation of the patella may be associated with fractures at the lower pole or osteochondral fractures. Comminuted fractures or osteochondral fractures may be complicated by the occurrence of loose bodies in the knee joint and radiographs do not always reveal their presence.

Management of fractured patellae must consider damage to the extensor mechanism and involvement of the articular surface of the patella. The adolescent and the young adult should have particular attention paid to repair of the quadriceps mechanism and restoration of the articular surface of the patella. Failure to achieve these aims will lead to a loss of normal function and power of knee extension. In the older age group, and with undisplaced fractures, more conservative measures are applicable to management regimes. Excellent results can be expected without surgical interference.

The patella should be preserved if at all possible. The goal of management of the displaced patella fracture is to restore accurately the articular surface and achieve early mobilization with fixation to prevent fracture displacement, achieve union, and regain full range of movement and power of knee extension.[2] Failure to manage displaced patella fractures adequately will result in irregularity of the articular surface and probable later patellofemoral arthrosis.

MECHANISM OF INJURY

The position of the patella makes it vulnerable to direct trauma. Industrial, domestic, and motor vehicle accidents account for the majority of patella fractures. The most common fracture seen up until the advent of seat belts, now compulsory in many countries, was "the dashboard injury"[3]—direct impingement of the patella onto the metallic dashboard with the knee in a flexed position, resulting in either a transverse[1] (Fig. 16-1) or comminuted fracture[4] (Fig. 16-2). The comminuted fracture is often referred to as a stellate fracture. The force, transmitted through the patella, either produces a transverse split or a crush fracture of the body of the patella with extensive disruption of the articular surface of the patella. Chondral damage to the trochlear articular surface of the femur may also occur.

The transverse fracture[5,6] is more commonly seen at the midposition of the patella or below the midline, following a direct blow or during violent athletic activity, such as jumping and gymnastics[7] (see Fig. 16-1C). This type of fracture has been reported as an indirect fracture occurring in childhood.[8]

A crush injury or stellate fracture is commonly produced in older people by falling forward, landing

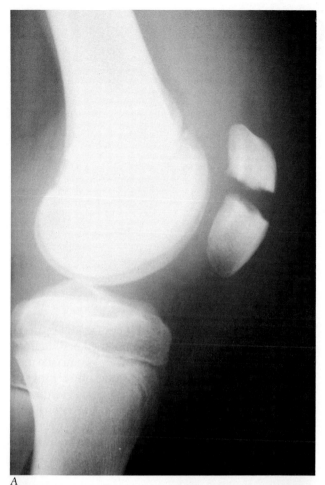

A

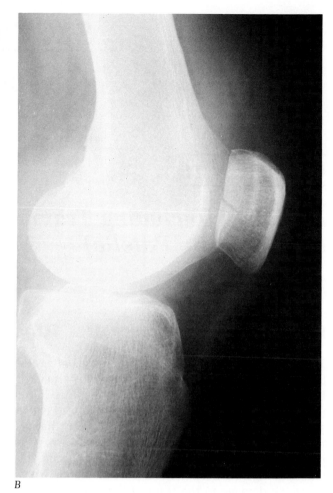

B

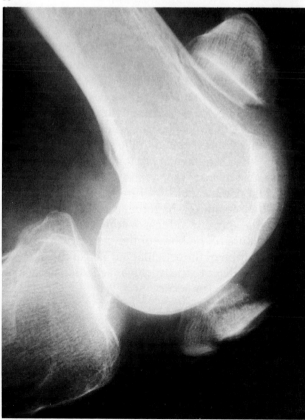

C

FIGURE 16-1
A. Transverse fracture, following direct blow to the knee or during
violent athletic activity.   *B.* Undisplaced transverse fracture. *C.*
Widely displaced transverse fracture with retinacular disruption.

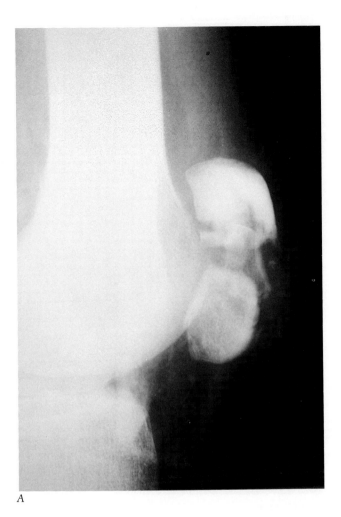

A

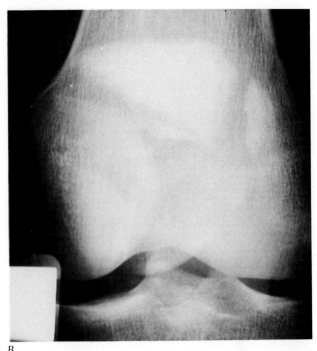

B

FIGURE 16-2
A. Comminuted fracture. Lateral radiograph tends to mask the comminution. *B.* Anteroposterior radiograph shows degree of comminution.

directly on the front of the knee. This injury is the second most common cause of patella fracture.

There is often involvement of the soft tissues of the extensor mechanism at the time of patella fracture. The retinaculum on the medial and lateral sides of the patella may be torn. Quite extensive involvement of the retinaculum may be encountered if there is violent flexion of the knee at the time of injury. The tear in the retinaculum may extend for 5 to 6 cm around the medial and lateral aspects of the knee.

Lesser degrees of comminution are encountered depending on the force at impact. Lower pole fractures[9] or vertical fractures[10–12] (Fig. 16-3) are observed depending on the angle and the direction of force at the time of impact. A not unusual fracture is comminution of the lower pole of the patella without involvement of the articular surface (Fig. 16-4). In this instance, it is important to determine that the patella tendon is still intact at the tendon insertion because management will depend on this finding. Less commonly, with a direct blow to the front of the knee joint the finding will be a vertical fracture of the patella. The vertical fracture is more common on the lateral aspect of the patella due to impingement of the

lateral facet as it climbs the lateral femoral condyle. Accurate restoration of the articular surface should be the aim of treatment of this fracture if the fragment is large and involves a significant portion of the lateral facet of the patella.

During violent exertional activity, avulsion fractures of the upper or lower poles of the patella may be seen.[13,14] The more common injury is quadriceps avulsion without bony damage or disruption of the patella tendon. Avulsion of either the quadriceps muscle or the patella tendon should always be looked for when there is interference with the function of the extensor mechanism. Loss of active extension of the knee or extensor lag should make one think of this diagnosis.

The sleeve fracture,[7,15,16] commonly seen in children, is a small bony fragment with a large cartilaginous articular component not visible on x-rays. Its occurrence and its association with patella dislocation should be recognized. This fracture is commonly overlooked.

Major osteochondral fractures[17,18] (Fig. 16-5) may occur during episodes of patella dislocation during cutting and turning maneuvers under load. With ex-

219

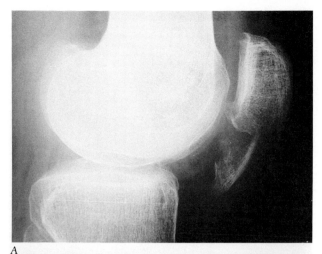

A

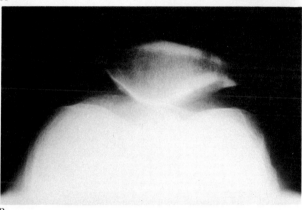

B

FIGURE 16-3
A. Comminuted fracture of lower pole.   B. Vertical fracture lateral margin.

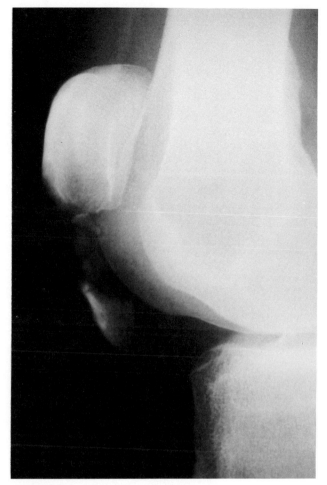

FIGURE 16-4
Fracture of the lower pole with avulsion of the patella tendon.

ternal tibial rotation on the extended knee or in instances of violent body contact, the patella may dislocate and then relocate with such force that a shear fracture of the inferior portion of the medial facet of the articular surface is produced. A fragment may fracture from the lateral femoral condyle during the relocation phase. This shear fracture of the inferomedial surface of the patella or the femoral fracture may, on occasion, be of such a size that necessitates open reduction and internal fixation.

Avulsion fractures can occur on the medial side of the patella during episodes of dislocation (Fig. 16-6). They occur due to violent contraction of the vastus medialis obliquus causing a vertical avulsion fracture at the site of insertion of the vastus medialis obliquus muscle into the patella. They are not intra-articular and do not occur in conjunction with the shear fracture of the articular surface.

Overuse or repetitive activity may, at times, produce a stress fracture[6,19,20] of the patella without a significant history of injury, although this is not a common site for stress fracture.

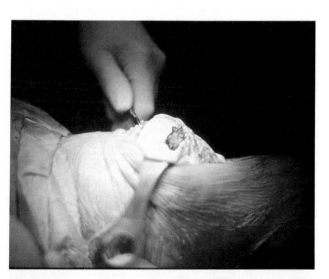

FIGURE 16-5
Site of major osteochondral fracture of medial facet of patella following patella dislocation.

220

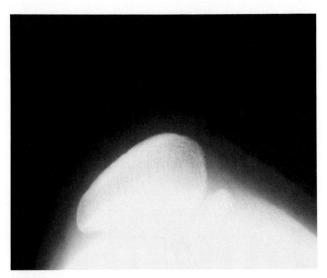

FIGURE 16-6
Avulsion fracture from the medial border of the patella in adolescent with recurrent patella dislocation.

The presence of a bipartite patella may be the site of a stress injury.[21] The bipartite patella can become symptomatic on occasions following a fall on to the knee resulting in damage to the fibrous area between the bony fragments.[22] At other times, overuse leads to a stress area of the fibrous junction, which becomes painful. Painful bipartite patella should not be confused with a definite traumatic fracture of the superolateral pole of the patella.[23]

CLASSIFICATION (see Table 16-1)

INCIDENCE

Fractures of the patella (Fig. 16-7) are said to account for 10 percent of all fractures.[5] Fractures of the patella

TABLE 16-1
Classification

1.	Transverse fracture	Displaced Undisplaced
2.	Comminuted fracture (stellate)	
3.	Vertical fracture (longitudinal) (lateral marginal)	Displaced Undisplaced
4.	Avulsion fracture	Superior pole Inferior pole Medial
5.	Sleeve fracture	
6.	Sheer fracture (osteochondral)	Major Minor
7.	Stress fracture	Body of patella Bipartite

are seen in all age groups but are less frequent in childhood and adolescence. Below the age of 16 years, the incidence varies from 1.34 percent[24] to 3 percent.[25] The mean age is reported as 40 years by Thomson[26] and 41.9 by Nummi.[27] Males tend to predominate in most of the series reported, ranging from 63.8 percent to 89 percent. Bilateral fractures occur infrequently. Refracture has been reported but is again infrequent.

The most common fracture in sporting individuals is the transverse fracture, occurring in some 50 percent to 80 percent of all cases. Taken overall, before the advent of seat belts, the most common injury was the comminuted or stellate fracture. This fracture accounts for well over 50 percent of cases seen and approximately 30 percent in the sporting individual. The vertical fractures occur in 12 percent to 25 percent and avulsion fractures in 5 percent. The other types of fractures tend to be less common and even relatively infrequent.

DIAGNOSIS

Patella fracture will usually be diagnosed on the history and physical examination. A history of a direct blow to the patella region with subsequent severe pain, giving way of the knee, and inability to walk suggest patella fracture. Sudden severe pain about the anterior aspect of the knee during ballistic activity and inability to weight bear or straight leg raise, will indicate possible damage in the region of the extensor mechanism. Physical examination commonly reveals a defect in the bony structure of the patella and tenderness at the site of the fracture. A tense hemarthrosis is often present although this may dissipate rapidly if the retinaculum is torn. In absence of a tense hemarthrosis, an extensor lag is suggestive of disruption of the extensor mechanism.

Confirmation of the fracture by x-ray diagnosis is not always possible on standard anteroposterior and lateral views. Special patella views with the beam parallel to the patella and the knee in as much flexion as possible will show some longitudinal and vertical avulsion fractures that cannot be seen on standard anteroposterior and lateral films. The use of oblique films may reveal otherwise undiagnosed small patella fractures. Special views may prove helpful.

Arthroscopy has proved helpful in the diagnosis of chondral and bony damage to the articular surface of the patella following patella dislocation. In a personal series of 27 knees suffering patella dislocation, two large shear type osteochondral fractures were diagnosed by arthroscopy that failed to be detected by radiographic measures.

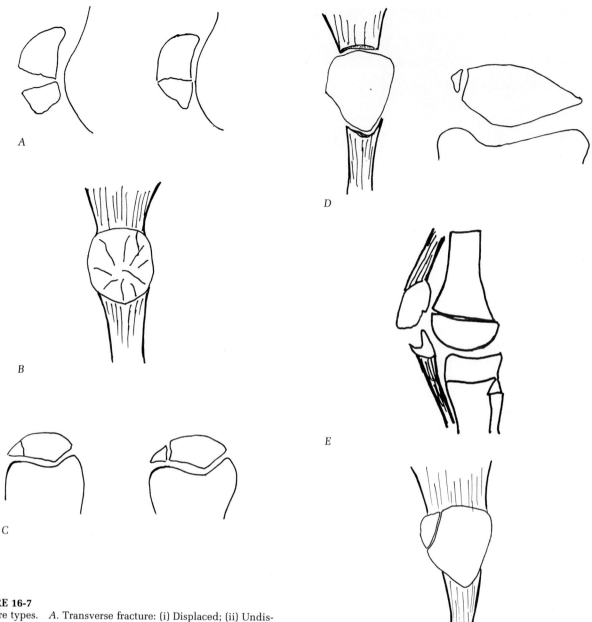

FIGURE 16-7
Fracture types. *A.* Transverse fracture: (i) Displaced; (ii) Undisplaced. *B.* Comminuted fracture. *C.* Longitudinal fracture: (i) Undisplaced; (ii) Displaced. *D.* Marginal fractures: superior, inferior, medial. *E.* Sleeve fracture; the avulsed lower pole is mainly cartilaginous. *F.* Bipartite patella.

A bone scan should be performed in sports participants suffering anterior knee pain to exclude the possibility of stress fracture to the patella following overuse or overactivity of the extensor mechanism if the diagnosis is uncertain. The occurrence of stress fractures in the body of the patella has been most infrequent. This is probably explained by the fact that the bony portion of the patella is well invested by the aponeurosis of the medial and lateral retinacular and the expansion of the quadriceps insertion into the upper pole of the patella, which tends to support the bony architecture and no doubt reinforces the bone, protecting it from stress injury.

MANAGEMENT OF PATELLA FRACTURE

In the early 1880s, methods of treatment for patella fracture were conservative, using splinting, elevation, immobilization in hyperextension with hip flexion, and elastic bandages with early massage.

Early methods of reduction of fracture fragments included Malgaigne's hook, subcutaneous suture, or wire suture. Percutaneous cerclage wire was also used.

Cameron of Glasgow reported the use of a silver wire to internally fix fracture fragments of the patella.[28] This was the first operation to fix patella fracture fragments. The procedure was advocated by Lister.[29]

In 1909, Heineck recommended the following surgical procedures[30]:

1. The fracture must be reduced.
2. The bony fragments must be maintained in intimate apposition until organic union has been effected.
3. The continuity of denuded soft tissues must be reestablished.
4. The functional integrity of the knee joint must be restored.

The Aims of Management

1. *Preserve the Patella.* Patellectomy leads to weakening of knee extension, loss of protective function of the patella, quadriceps weakness, and occasional painful ossification of the reconstructed ligamentous structures.

2. *Restore the Anatomy.* Restoration of anatomic alignment and position is important. Undisplaced fractures may be treated conservatively. The accurate apposition of articular surface of the patella is more likely to give better functional results.

3. *Open Reduction.* Displaced fractures should be openly reduced and rigidly fixed if possible. On occasion, simple fractures will be found to be more comminuted than expected. Rigid fixation may not be possible due to comminution of fragments or porosity of the bone. In these instances cerclage wires or suture fixation may be the only means of approximating the fragments.

4. *Mobilization.* Early mobilization of fractures should be considered following adequate fixation. It is not uncommon to see shortening of the patella ligament, patella baja, or fibroarthrosis following immobilization of fractures. Mobilization is also recommended to prevent the complications of knee stiffness, quadriceps weakness, and patella tendon shortening. Fractures with 1 mm to 2 mm separation without a step can be treated by immobilization but are more likely to displace if early motion is instituted.

5. *Extensor Mechanism.* Preservation and repair of the adjacent medial and lateral retinaculum of the extensor mechanism is as important as reduction of the fracture to prevent weakness of quadriceps function, loss of knee extension, and weakness of knee extension.

6. *Loose Bony Fragments.* Exploration of the joint should be undertaken at the time of surgery.

Lavage of the joint will remove loose bony fragments, which are common with complex crush fractures and may be present in simple fractures.

7. *Rehabilitation.* Early rehabilitation should help shorten postoperative morbidity. The use of continuous passive motion may be helpful. Early return of quadriceps function will lessen the occurrence of complications associated with these fractures and will enhance quadriceps rehabilitation.

Conservative Management

INDICATIONS

1. Undisplaced fracture
2. Intact extensor mechanism
3. Separation of 2 mm to 3 mm may be considered acceptable[31]
4. Comminuted fracture in the elderly with intact extensor mechanism

The undisplaced fracture with an intact extensor mechanism should be treated conservatively. A tense hemarthrosis producing distention of the joint with excessive pain should be aspirated. Immobilization by plaster cylinder or knee immobilizer will allow early introduction of static quadriceps exercises and later straight leg raising. Early protected partial weight bearing is allowed with the use of crutches. Knee flexion without strain is possible at 4 weeks. At this time the fracture should be relatively stable. The use of continuous passive motion will enhance rehabilitation at this stage.

The severely comminuted fracture in the older patient is often treated conservatively if the patient is able to straight leg raise at initial examination, indicating an intact extensor mechanism and probably stability of the fracture. Immobilization is not usually required and early mobilization is advised. The patient is made to use crutches to protect the patella during weight bearing.

Operative Management

PATELLECTOMY

Patellectomy[32–35] is often the treatment of choice where there is severe comminution or in instances where there are no large fragments. If the articular surface cannot be reconstituted without a step, patellectomy will often be necessary. Restoration of the articular surface must be achieved without a step in the articular surface or separation of fragments. Bone union with a step or deformity is more likely to lead to later osteoarthritis.

Some authors have recommended patellectomy in all instances[36] except for minor fracture. Others have stated that patellectomy is never the method of choice.[3, 37, 38] It should be remembered that the results of patellectomy are not uniformly successful.[39] Early reports indicated that patellectomy did not compromise knee function[40] and that the patella played little part in knee function.[35] Later investigations have repudiated these statements, indicating the important function of the patella in enhancing quadriceps function.[41–43]

Indications

1. Severely comminuted patella fracture with disruption of the articular surface, which cannot be restored in the younger and middle age group.

2. Displaced fracture where the articular surface cannot be reconstituted and there are no large fragments.

3. Major trauma where the articular surface of distal femur is significantly damaged.

Procedure

If patellectomy is performed, all bony fragments should be removed with particular attention being paid to preserving the fascia overlying the patella and the retinacular structures on the medial and lateral sides of the patella.

Repair of the soft tissues and reconstitution of the extensor mechanism requires special attention to anatomic details. Anatomic studies[44,45] on the effects of excision of the patella and division of the medial and lateral retinacular should be noted. Patella excision alone with intact retinacular structures allows knee extension with reduced power. Sectioning of the retinacular structures with the patella still in place also reduces the power of knee extension. Satisfactory return of function without loss of flexion and the return of adequate power of knee extension requires attention to special surgical repair of the soft tissue. The ruptures in the medial and lateral retinacular must be traced to their limits and repaired. Double breasting of the retinacular structures longitudinally can then be achieved to close the defect remaining after patella excision; the fascia overlying the anterior aspect of the excised patella can be used to reinforce this double-breasted repair. Approximation of the quadriceps tendon to the patella tendon has not been found to be necessary as excellent return of knee extension can be achieved if the method of double breasting the retinacular is used (Fig. 16-8). The return of knee flexion during rehabilitation is more rapid with this type of reconstruction. Extension lag can occur initially but is not a late problem once quadriceps power develops. In the author's hands, this has proved an excellent method for exten-

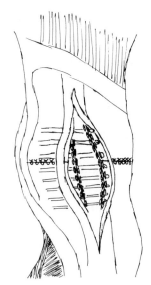

FIGURE 16-8
Reconstruction of the extensor mechanism after patellectomy for fracture of the patella. Longitudinal repair of the defect.

sor mechanism reconstruction after patellectomy. Early mobilization can be achieved and splintage can usually be discarded after 4 to 6 weeks.

The Soto–Hall technique of patellectomy is described in Campbell's *Operative Orthopaedics*.[45]

PARTIAL PATELLECTOMY

Partial patellectomy has been advocated by a number of authors because of the difficulty in approximating the articular surface accurately and the possibility of nonunion. The procedure commonly used is to excise the lower fragment, usually the smaller fragment in a transverse fracture, and reattach the patella tendon to the raw surface of the remaining bone using two modified mattress sutures. This operation is also extremely applicable to comminuted fractures of the lower pole of the patella. The technique was originally reported by Thomson.[26]

Other fractures suitable for partial patellectomy are vertical fractures close to the periphery of the bone involving little of the articular cartilage or osteochondral fractures of the medial facet, which are not suitable for replacement.

Vertical avulsion fractures from the medial side of the patella are usually extra-articular and operative treatment for their removal is not usually considered necessary. If there is wide detachment of the fragment with avulsion of the vastus medialis obliquus, then more appropriate treatment would be to reattach the muscle to the medial side of the patella.

Bostman and colleagues,[4] in a series of 64 comminuted displaced fractures, used tension band wiring in 21, partial patellectomy in 33, and total patellectomy in 10 patients. They reported that partial exci-

224

sion showed satisfactory results provided that at least three-fifths of the patella could be preserved.

Indications

1. Transverse fracture where there is difficulty in achieving a smooth articular surface
2. Transverse fractures with one large and one small fragment
3. Comminuted fractures where a large fragment can be preserved

Procedure

In the situation where there is a comminuted lower pole of the patella and a large remaining portion, operative treatment by excision of the lower pole and reattachment of the patella tendon to the raw bony surface can give excellent results. Particular attention should be given to reattaching the tendon. The method described by Andrews and Hughston[46] (Fig. 16-9) using mattress-type sutures passed through drill holes in the patella and approximating the patella tendon have given satisfactory results. Protected early motion is possible.

Chiroff[47] has reported a technique whereby the patella ligament is inserted into a transverse groove created in the proximal patella fragment following partial patellectomy of a comminuted lower pole and this anastomosis is protected by a tension band. The author has no experience with this technique. It is stated that a large surface area for more satisfactory tendon-to-bone healing is provided and relatively early motion of the knee can be initiated.

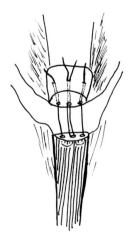

FIGURE 16-9
Partial patellectomy after Andrews and Hughston. The distal fragment is excised and the tendon reattached to the raw surface of the larger fragment. Sutures are passed through drill holes in the bone. The retinaculum is repaired.

INTERNAL FIXATION OF PATELLA FRACTURES

Many types of wiring techniques have been used[48-51] (Fig. 16-10). An encircling wire is one of the oldest methods used for patella fractures. Wiring through longitudinal drill holes has been used (Fig. 16-11). The technique of tension band wiring has been described on many occasions with good results reported.[4,51-53]

Lotke[49] advocated to preserve the bony fragments and enhance union of the fracture by better forms of internal fixation.

Indications

1. Transverse fractures or fractures with more than two fragments where rigid fixation and a smooth articular surface is achieved.

Methods

Experimental studies by Weber and colleagues,[54] to determine whether any of the commonly used wiring techniques are rigid enough to allow early motion in the treatment of transverse fractures of the patella, indicated that separation of the fracture fragments was much less with the Magnusson wiring and modified tension ban wiring than with circumferential wiring or standard tension band wiring (Fig. 16-12).

It was concluded that if early motion was to be used in treatment techniques that used anchorage of the wire directly into bone and repair of the retinaculum, adequate fixation was required.

These experiments showed that tension band wiring did not prevent separation of the fragments at the articular surface. The experiment showed in simulated transverse fracture that the articular surfaces of the fragments separated widely and with knee flexion and extension the anatomic alignment was further disturbed.

Circumferential wiring was also ineffective with the articular surfaces clearly separated with full active extension.

Magnusson wiring (see Fig. 16-12A) was found to have movement from 10 degrees to full extension, whereas with modified tension band wiring with the wire loop anchored to Kirschner wires, there was no separation of fragments throughout the entire range of zero to 90 degrees.

Lotke and Ecker have also cast doubt on the use of circumferential wiring, AO tension band wiring, and longitudinal wiring. They have recommended the use of a technique named LAB/C[49] (Fig. 16-13). This technique uses longitudinal anterior bands with cerclage wire. The use of the cerclage wire is recommended with severe comminution. They report data

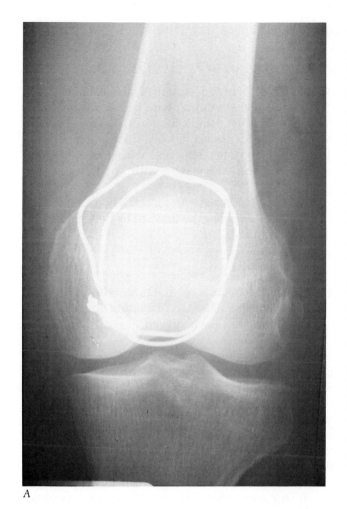

A

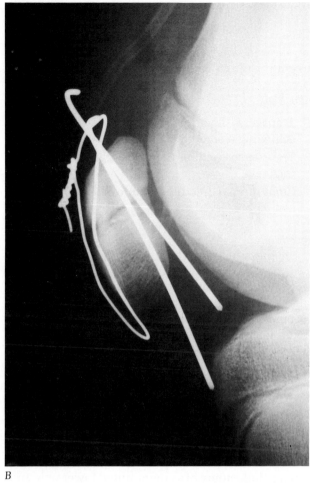

B

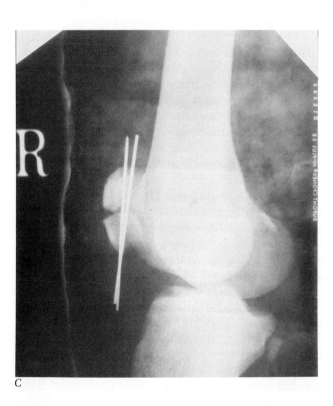

C

FIGURE 16-10
A. Cerclage wiring of patella.   *B.* Tension band wiring.   *C.* Inadequate wiring technique using longitudinal wires.

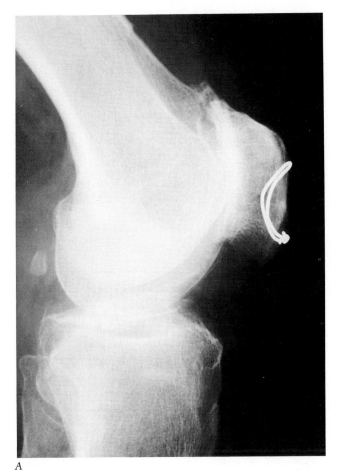

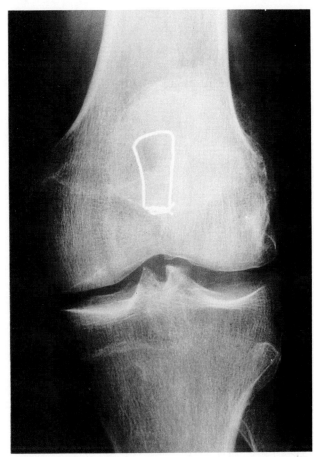

A   B

FIGURE 16-11
Wire inserted into a fractured patella 28 years before patient presented with symptoms of
patellofemoral arthritis.

on 16 patients with follow-up of 6 months to 6 years. Most patients were asymptomatic with only three noting some discomfort on stairs or after prolonged activity.

Cadaveric studies carried out by Curtis[9] showed that a combination of cerclage and tension band wiring proved to be significantly stronger than a simple tension band technique (Fig. 16-14).

OPEN REDUCTION AND INTERNAL FIXATION USING WIRES OR SCREWS

Kirschner wires with a bent tip or screws have been used to internally fix transverse and longitudinal fractures. Certain operative difficulties are encountered with these procedures as it is almost impossible to ensure accurate reduction of the articular surfaces. The failure of anatomic reduction with an articular step or gap of > 2 mm is more likely to lead to later development of patellofemoral osteoarthritis followed by pain and reduced function.

Large osteochondral fragments separated from the medial facet of the patella at the time of patella dislocation can be adequately managed by open re-duction and internal fixation using a Herbert compression screw.[55] The screws can be buried deep to the articular cartilage and do not need to be removed at a second operation.

OPEN REDUCTION AND EXTERNAL COMPRESSIVE SKELETAL FIXATION

An unusual form of treatment is reported by Liang and Wu.[56] Twenty-seven patients with separated fractures of the patella were treated by open reduction combined with external compressive skeletal fixation.

If it was impossible to reduce some of the fragments, they were removed. At an average of 3.1 years of follow-up, 24 of 27 patients were reported to have excellent results.

PERCUTANEOUS TENSION BAND WIRING

Leung and colleagues[48] have reported data on five cases with excellent results using this technique. The fractures were mildly displaced or undisplaced with intact retinacular fibers.

227

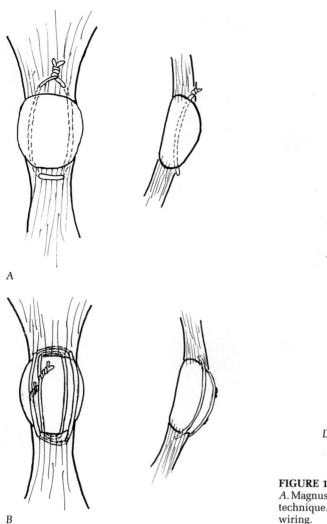

A

B

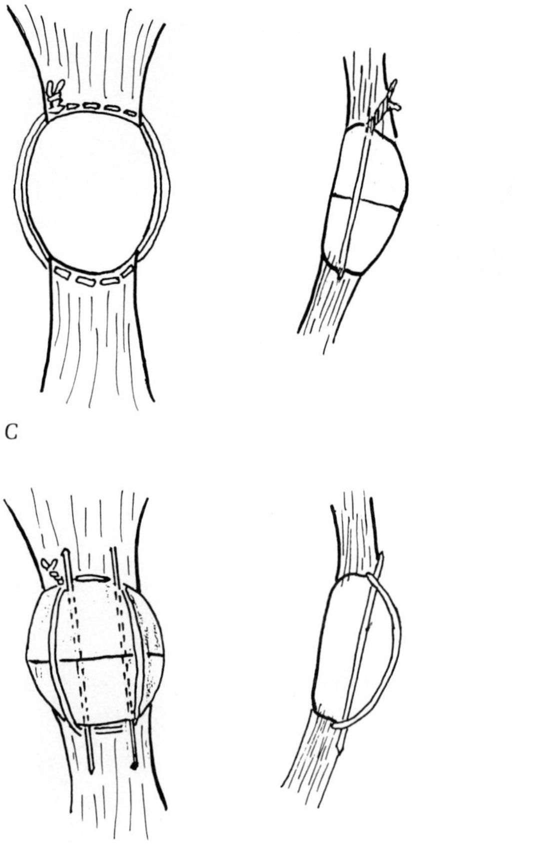

C

D

FIGURE 16-12
A. Magnusson wiring technique.   B. Modified tension band wiring technique.   C. Circumferential wiring.   D. Standard tension band wiring.

Summary of Management

The final decision on the course of management will sometimes be difficult. At one end of the spectrum are undisplaced fractures with intact extensor mechanism, which are suitable for conservative manage- ment with early mobilization. The end result is very satisfactory.

Some fractures are so severely comminuted that the articular surface cannot be reconstructed and pat- ellectomy is the only choice. In the middle ground,

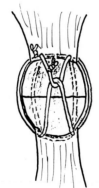

FIGURE 16-13
Lotke LAB/C wiring technique.

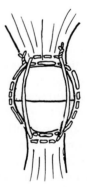

FIGURE 16-14
Curtis combination cerclage and tension band wiring.

internal fixation and partial patellectomy must be used to reconstruct the patella articular surface and to preserve as much of the patella as possible to enhance extensor mechanism function.

The correct operative procedure will be determined by the experience and ability of the surgeon to reconstitute the articular surface. This is especially applicable in younger individuals who are more likely to develop patellofemoral symptoms from degenerative arthrosis if reduction is adequate.

COMPLICATIONS

Inadequate reduction of displaced patella fractures is likely to lead to degenerative changes in the patellofemoral articulation. The occurrence of a gap of 2 mm to 3 mm or step in the articular surface is associated with an increased incidence of narrowing of the patellofemoral articulation (10 to 15 years after the injury) particularly in association with the lateral facet. Lateral patellofemoral arthrosis may develop. Femorotibial arthrosis has not been found to be a common association with patella fracture.[57]

Nonunion of patella fracture is rare. Refracture of the patella after treatment is uncommon.[58] Refracture may occur following prolonged immobilization leading to osteoporosis. Patella magna may result from crush injuries to the patella. Prolonged immobilization may lead to an increased incidence of patella baja, shortened patella ligament, and arthrofibrosis with later increase in the incidence of patellofemoral arthritis.

Loose bodies in the knee joint following patella fracture can lead to functional disability associated with locking. This often requires removal of a loose fragment.

Although original reports stated that patellectomy was compatible with normal quadriceps function, it is now well recognized that patellectomy is associated with quadriceps weakness, knee pain, and reduced functional ability.[59] There may also be calcification in the reconstructed extensor mechanism. Smaller fragments are compatible with pain-free function, but larger areas of new bone formation can lead to residual knee pain and functional impairment.

Failure to adequately repair the retinacular structures will lead to quadriceps weakness and weakness of knee extension. Knee stiffness and extensor lag are noted after inadequate reconstruction of the extensor mechanism and poor rehabilitation.

The most common complication following patella fracture is patient complaint of disturbance in normal function of the knee joint. The patient will complain of aching, pain with activity, giving way, occasional swelling, and weakness of knee extension.

RESULTS OF TREATMENT

It is important to recognize that the reports on the long-term morbidity following fractured patellae vary. Excellent results have been reported for management by total excision. Other authors have not reported such successful results.

Long-term studies have been carried out by a number of authors.[2,4,27,57,60] Assessment of these results would indicate that total excision of the patella did not result in a normal knee in the majority of instances. Sixty to 90 percent of the patients had residual complaints of ache, weakness, and giving way. Wilkinson reported on 31 cases followed 4-1/2 to 13 years, with the following results: excellent 22 percent, good 39 percent, and poor 39 percent.[39] Sanderson stated 63 percent were considered satisfactory at follow-up.[60]

Levack stated that patellectomy had better results than internal fixation. He reported 60 percent good, 20 percent fair, and 20 percent poor results for patellectomy.[2]

Partial patellectomy would appear to give superior results with 50 percent of patients stating they have normal function. But the reason may be that the initial injury was less severe. Full recovery can be achieved when the fragment removed at partial patellectomy is only small without significant involvement of the articular surface or interference with the extensor mechanism. Sanderson reported 65 percent were considered satisfactory.[60]

Excellent results are achieved with anatomic replacement of fragments especially when the fracture has occurred due to traction and not compression; the latter resulting in damage to the articular surface of the patella or the underlying femur. Full functional recovery can be expected after anatomic reduction and internal fixation when the fracture is produced by traction. Sanderson reported 55 percent excellent results for the internally fixed group.[60] Hung reported on results of the tension band principles with 81 percent excellent and good results.[52] Levack reported on 30 patients treated with internal fixation with 31 percent good, 33 percent fair, and 36 percent poor results.[2]

Bostrom in his review of 422 patella fractures, of which 135 were treated mainly by osteosynthesis, reported that of those available for follow-up 79 percent were excellent or good.[5]

Conservative treatment in the correctly selected patient can give excellent results. Sanderson reports 83 percent excellent results. Bostrom states 99 percent excellent or good.

Patient expectations for full recovery of function should be modified in the presence of extensive damage to articular surface, severe damage to the extensor mechanism, and with total or partial patellectomy.

Edwards[61] reports in a 30-year follow-up of 40 patients that two-thirds of the patients who had more than 2 mm diastasis or 1 mm incongruity had complaints and reduced quadriceps strength. All patients had a reduction in the lateral patellofemoral distance. The patella length was increased and the patella tendon length shortened in patients with an original diastasis.

SUMMARY

It is important to assess the fracture adequately, to remove only those portions of the patella that are absolutely necessary, and to obtain adequate reduction with excellent internal fixation to maximize the outcome of fractures of the patella.

REFERENCES

1. Belman DAJ, Neviaber RT: Transverse fracture of the patella in a child. *Trauma* 13:917, 1973.
2. Levack B, Flannagan JP, Hobbs S: Results of surgical treatment of patella fractures. *J Bone Joint Surg* 67B: 416, 1985.
3. Smillie IS: Dashboard fractures of the patella. *Br Med J* 2:203, 1954.
4. Bostman O, Kivilusto O, Nirhamo J: Comminuted displaced fractures of the patella. *Injury* 13:196, 1982.
5. Bostrom A: Fractures of the patella. *Acta Orthop Scand* 143 (suppl) :1, 1972.
6. Dickason JM, Fox JM: Fracture of the patella due to overuse syndrome in a child. *Am J Sports Med* 10:248, 1982.
7. Hughes AW: Avulsion fracture involving the body of the patella. *Br J Surg* 19:119, 1985.
8. Hanel DP, Burdge RE: Consecutive indirect patella fractures in an adolescent basketball player. *Am J Sports Med* 9:5, 1981.
9. Curtis MJ: Internal fixation of fractures of the patella. *J Bone Joint Surg* 72B:2, 1990.
10. Dowd GSE: Marginal fractures of the patella. *Injury* 14(3):287.
11. Kleinberg S: Vertical fracture of the articular surface of the patella. *JAMA* LXXXI:1205, 1928.
12. Lapidus PW: Longitudinal fractures of the patella. *J Bone Joint Surg* 14:351, 1932.
13. Suguira Y, Kaneko F: Rupture of the patella ligament with avulsion of lower pole of patella—A case report. *Ortho Surgery (Tokyo)* 23:384, 1972.
14. Tibone JE, Stephan JL: Bilateral fractures of the inferior poles of the patellae in a basketball player. *Am J Sports Med* 9:215, 1981.
15. Heckman JD, Alkire CC: Distal patellar pole fractures. *Am J Sports Med* 12:6, 1984.
16. Hougton GR, Ackroyd CE: Sleeve fractures of the patella in children—A report of three cases. *J Bone Joint Surg* 61B:165, 1979.
17. Milgram JE: Tangential osteochondral fracture of the patella. *J Bone Joint Surg* 25:271, 1943.
18. Vainionpaa S, Laasonen E, Silvennoinen T, et al: Acute dislocation of the patella. *J Bone Joint Surg* 72B:366, 1990.
19. Devas MB: Stress fractures of the patella. *J Bone Joint Surg* 42B:71, 1960.
20. Jerosch JG, Castro WHM, Jantea C: Stress fracture of the patella. *Am J Sports Med* 17:579, 1989.
21. Weaver JK: Bipartite patellae is a cause of disability in the athlete. *Am J Sports Med* 5:137, 1977.
22. Green LT Jr: Painful bipartite patellae—A report of three case. *Clin Orthop* 110:197, 1975.
23. Echeverria TS, Bersani FA: Acute fracture stimulating a symptomatic bipartite patella. *Am J Sports Med* 8:48, 1980.
24. Diebold O: Uber Kniescheibenbrache in Kindesafter Langenbecks. *Arch Klin Chur* 147:664, 1927.
25. Jarvinen A: Uber die kniescheibenbruche und ihre behandlung unter besonderer berucksichtigung der dauerresultate im licht der nachantersurhaurgen. *Acta Soc Med Deudeum* 32:80, 1942.
26. Thomson JEM: Comminuted fractures of the patella. Treatment of cases presenting one large fragment and several small fragments. *J Bone Joint Surg* 17:431, 1935.
27. Nummi J: Fracture of the patella. A clinical study of 707 patellar fractures. *Ann Chir Gyn Fenn* 60(suppl):179, 1971.
28. Cameron HC: Transverse fracture of the patella. *Glasgow Med J* 10:289, 1878.
29. Lister Lord J: A new operation for fracture of the patella. *Br Med J* 2:850, 1877.
30. Heineck AP: The modern operative treatment of fractures of the patella. 1. Based on the study of other pathological states of this bone. 2. An analytical review of over 100 cases treated during the last ten years by the open operative method. *Surg Gynecol Obstets* 9:177, 1909.

31. Bohler L: *Treatment of Fractures,* 2d ed. Vienna, Wm Maudrick, 1929.

32. Cohn BNE: Total and partial patellectomy. An experimental study. *Surg Gynecol Obstet* 79:526, 1944.

33. Hey Groves EW: A note on the extension apparatus of the knee joint. *Br J Surg* 24:747, 1937.

34. Watson-Jones R: Excision of patella. *Br Med J* II:195, 1945.

35. Brooke R: Treatment of fracture of the patella by excision. A study of morphology and function. *Br J Surg* 24:733, 1956.

36. O'Donoghue DH: Treatment of fractures of the patella. *North W Med (Seattle)* 57:1592, 1958.

37. Baumgartl F: *Das Keniegetenk,* Berlin, Springer-Verlag, 1964.

38. De Palma AF, Flynn JJ: Joint changes following experimental partial and total patellectomy. *J Bone Joint Surg* 40A:395, 1958.

39. Wilkinson J: Fracture of the patella treated by total excision. A long term follow up. *J Bone Joint Surg* 59B:352, 1977.

40. Brooke L: Fracture of the patella. Analysis of 54 cases treated by excision. *Br Med J* 1:231, 1946.

41. Haxton HA: The function of the patella and effects of its excision. *Surg Gynecol Obstet* 80:389, 1945.

42. Jensenius H: On the result of excision of the fractured patella. *Acta Chir Scand* 102:275, 1951.

43. Maquet PGJ: *Biomechanics of the Knee.* 2d ed. Berlin, Springer-Verlag, 1984.

44. Bruce J, Walmsley R: Excision of patella. Some experimental and anatomical observations. *J Bone Joint Surg* 24:311, 1942.

45. Crenshaw AH (ed): *Campbell's Operative Orthopaedics* 5th ed. St. Louis, Mosby, p 178, 1971.

46. Andrews JR, Hughston JC: Treatment of patella fractures of partial patellectomy. *South Med J* 70:809, 1977.

47. Chiroff RT: A new technique for the treatment of comminuted transverse fractures of the patella. *Surg Gynecol Obstet* 145:909, 1977.

48. Leung PC, Mak KH, Lee SY: Percutaneous tension band wiring—A new method of internal fixation for mildly displaced patellar fractures. *Trauma* 23:62, 1983.

49. Lotke PA, Ecker ML: Transverse fractures of the patella. *Clin Orthop* 158:180, 1981.

50. Ma Y-Z, Zhand Y-F, Qu K-F, Yeh Y-C: Treatment of fractures of the patella with percutaneous suture. *Clin Orthop* 191:235, 1984.

51. Muller ME, Allgower M, Willenegger H: *Manual of Internal Fixation.* New York, Springer-Verlag, 1979.

52. Hung LK, Chan KM, Chow YW, Leung PC: Fractured patella. Operative treatment using the tension band principle. *Injury* 16:343, 1985.

53. Moschinski D, Kleinschmid F: *Results of Operative Management of Patella Fractures.* Unfall-heilkunde, 81:14, 1978.

54. Weber MJ, Janecki CJ, McLeod P, et al: Efficacy of various forms of fixation of transverse fractures of the patella. *J Bone Joint Surg* 62A:215, 1980.

55. Rae PS, Khasawneu ZM: Herbert screw fixation of osteochondral fractures of the patella. *Injury* 19:116, 1988.

56. Liang Q-Y, Wu J-W: Fracture of the patella treated by open reduction and external compressive skeletal fixation. *J Bone Joint Surg* 69A:83, 1987.

57. Cargill AO'R: The long term effect on the tibiofemoral compartment of the knee joint of comminuted fractures of the patella. *Injury* 6:309, 1975.

58. Rees D, Thompson SK: Refracture of the patella. *Injury* 16:559, 1985.

59. Wass SH, Davies ER: Excision of the patella for fracture with remarks on ossification in the quadriceps tendon following the operation. *Guy's Hosp Rep* 91:35, 1942.

60. Sanderson MC: The fractured patella. A long term follow up study. *Aust NZ J Surg* 45:49, 1975.

61. Edwards B: ᴰatella Fractures. *Acta Orthop Scand* 60:712, 1989.

SECTION VI
Pain Dysfunction Syndrome

CHAPTER 17

Reflex Sympathetic Dystrophy of the Knee

F. Edward Pollock, Jr.
Gary G. Poehling
L. Andrew Koman

INTRODUCTION

Reflex sympathetic dystrophy (RSD) is a perplexing pathologic entity manifested by persistent pain and loss of function in the affected area. Until recently, however, the syndrome was not well described in the knee, and persistent knee pain was traditionally thought to be due to various posttraumatic or postoperative conditions.[1] Now with the publication of several series of patients with RSD of the knee,[2-8] the syndrome must be regarded as a significant potential complication following a traumatic or a surgical insult to the knee.

The historical reluctance to describe RSD in the knee may be due to several factors. First, the pathogenesis and natural history of dystrophy is not well defined for any area of the body, even though initial descriptions of the symptoms date from 1864.[3,9] Second, recognition of the syndrome is often delayed by repeated diagnostic and therapeutic interventions that inadequately address the underlying disease process. Third, no treatment for RSD has proven consistently effective,[8] perhaps because of the dynamic evolution of the disease over time. Finally, the prolongation of symptoms often results in increasing frustration for both patient and physician, culminating in delayed diagnosis, randomly selected therapeutic interventions, and frequent permanent partial disability judgments.

DEFINITION

Schutzer and Gossling have defined RSD as an exaggerated response of an extremity to an injury.[10] This response is manifested by four characteristics: (1) intense or unduly prolonged pain, (2) vasomotor disturbances, (3) delayed functional recovery, and (4) trophic changes in the soft tissues.[10] We believe that dystrophy must be suspected whenever recovery from a traumatic or surgical insult is delayed for longer than would be expected given the magnitude of the injury.[11]

RSD appears to be an abnormal expression of the normal physiologic response to injury.[11] Most persons who sustain an injury to the knee will experience transient symptoms of hyperpathia (increased pain), allodynia (sensation of pain following a nonpainful stimulus), burning discomfort, vasomotor abnormalities, and functional deficit. These symptoms generally subside as recovery progresses. However, the RSD patient's symptoms do not subside, and they often escalate, leading to unremitting pain, vasospasm, edema, and immobility. If these conditions are allowed to persist, amelioration will be extremely difficult and perhaps impossible.

PATHOGENESIS

Numerous investigators have suggested various theories regarding the pathophysiology of RSD; many of these have been summarized in reviews by Bonica,[12] Wall,[13] Payne,[14] and Schwartzman and McLellan.[15] Three main areas have been suggested as possible sources leading to the perception of the chronic pain and disability of RSD—the central nervous system (CNS), the peripheral nerves, and nutritional blood flow in the affected area (Fig. 17-1).

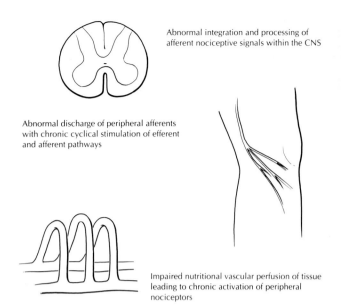

Abnormal integration and processing of afferent nociceptive signals within the CNS

Abnormal discharge of peripheral afferents with chronic cyclical stimulation of efferent and afferent pathways

Impaired nutritional vascular perfusion of tissue leading to chronic activation of peripheral nociceptors

FIGURE 17-1
Theories of pathogenesis of RSD.

Melzak and Wall were among the first to suggest that awareness of pain is subject to modulation within the substantia gelatinosa of the CNS.[16] Their "gate control system" proposed that stimulation of small, unmyelinated peripheral fibers caused the opening of gates and the subsequent sensation of pain. Wall has refined this theory and emphasized the difference between acute and chronic pain.[13] Roberts has proposed the presence of wide-dynamic-range neurons in the CNS, which are sensitized by peripheral afferent mechanoreceptors.[17] Schott has reviewed a number of proposed mechanisms and has concluded that fibers in both the CNS and the sympathetic system play a critical role in the development of RSD.[18,19]

Others have emphasized lesions in the peripheral nervous system. Devor has proposed the presence of "ectopic pacemaker" capability, which develops at the site of peripheral nerve injury and is sensitive to α-adrenergic stimulation.[20] Abnormal afferent discharge is produced whenever these areas are depolarized by nearby sympathetic efferents. Blumberg and Janig have postulated similar continuous activities in myelinated and nonmyelinated peripheral neurons,[21] and Cline and colleagues have noted that sensitization of peripheral C nociceptive fibers produces hyperalgesia.[22] We have also noted the association between sensory nerve damage and RSD in the knee.[7]

RSD secondary to microvascular abnormalities has also been suggested. Stolte and colleagues[23] and Fulkerson and Hungerford[24] have suggested that abnormalities of local blood flow might be associated with RSD; Rosen has shown that capillary blood flow is reduced in the dystrophic hand and has postulated

that decreased vasomotor activity may be the cause.[25] Gross has postulated that damage to innervated vessels produces "irritation centers" which produce pain in regions associated with the vascular nerve supply.[26] Cooke and Ward have recently suggested that locally acting neuroactive and vasoactive peptides mediate loss of thermoregulatory control in the vasculature and account for the persistent pain.[27] The true pathogenesis of RSD probably involves both peripheral and central mechanisms interacting to produce pain with unusual topography and chronicity.

As for RSD in the knee, several investigators have observed that the syndrome is often associated with symptoms about the patellofemoral joint[5,6,8] and Lagier[28] and Lequesne and colleagues[29] have described roentgenographic and bone scan evidence of patellofemoral involvement. Despite these observations, the pathogenesis of knee RSD remains obscure.

DIAGNOSIS

The diagnosis of RSD must be considered in any patient with unexplained pain about the knee, especially if the patellofemoral joint appears to be involved. Because no sensitive or specific test for RSD is currently available, the diagnosis must depend on careful scrutiny of presenting symptoms, interpretation of objective tests against the background of the clinical presentation, and a high index of suspicion for the syndrome.

Most patients will have a history of either traumatic or surgical injury to the knee.[1,7] The pain associated with RSD is characteristic; burning sensations predominate, but complaints of aching or shooting pains are also common.[30] Limited range of motion and stiffness are invariably noted on physical examination,[3,6] along with difficulty in bearing weight on the extremity. Palpation of the knee often reveals pain localized to the patella, the femoral condyles, or the patellofemoral articulation; the tibia is less often involved.[28,29,31]

Laboratory studies are helpful only in differentiating RSD from infection, arthritis, and malignant neoplasms. The complete blood cell count, chemistry profile, erythrocyte sedimentation rate, and rheumatoid tests will all be normal if dystrophy alone is the cause of the pain.

A variety of objective tests are available to further define the disease process. These include: plain radiographs (anteroposterior and lateral view of the knee, and a skyline view of the patella), a three-phase technetium bone scan (TcBS), isolated cold stress testing/laser–Doppler fluxmetry (ICST/LDF), thermography, pharmacologic neural blockade, and endurance testing.

Radiologic Evaluation

Radiographs of the knee made early in the course of RSD are uniformly normal.[3] Lesquesne and colleagues have described a diffuse and generalized osteoporosis about the knee occurring a few weeks after the onset of symptoms (Fig. 17-2); the articular margins are not affected, and once symptoms have improved, the osteoporosis resolves.[29] This finding has been associated histologically with active bone remodeling,[24,28,32] and has been noted in conditions other than RSD.[33] Tietjen has stressed the importance of obtaining a skyline view of the patella because of its frequent involvement in the disease process.[3]

Three-Phase Bone Scanning

Increased periarticular uptake on TcBS is often present in multiple joints of the affected extremity in patients with RSD of the knee.[1,29,34] The increased uptake is thought to reflect increased blood flow to bone resulting in hyperemia and increased bone metabolism. The test has been repeatedly shown to have excellent *specificity* in the presence of RSD,[34,35] but recent studies of TcBS in both upper and lower extremities have suggested that the *sensitivity* of the

test ranges from 44 percent to 60 percent.[34,36] The test is more likely to be positive in the later stages of RSD of the lower extremity.[34] Tietjen noted that two-thirds of the patients in this study had a positive TcBS.[3]

Isolated Cold Stress Testing/Laser–Doppler Fluxmetry

ICST/LDF assesses the dynamic sympathetic response of an extremity to changes in environmental temperature.[37,38] The test is performed using a modified refrigeration unit, thermistors attached to each digit of both feet, and laser–Doppler probes secured to the pulp of each great toe (Fig. 17-3). A 20-min period of cooling in an ambient temperature of 6°C (45°F) to 10°C (50°F) is used as a provocative thermal stress for maximal stimulation of the sympathetic efferents of the extremity. The 20-min period of rewarming at room temperature that follows estimates sympathetic withdrawal. We have recently described normal patterns of temperature and LDF response to the test.[37,38] The two normal response curves are shown in Fig. 17-4. The temperature of both feet should be similar and LDF will fluctuate symmetrically with the temperature curves.

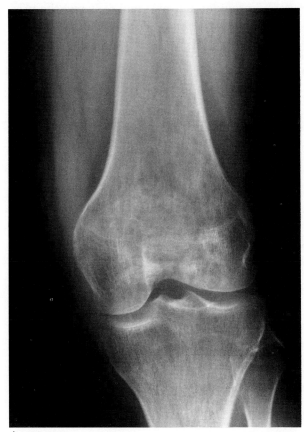

A

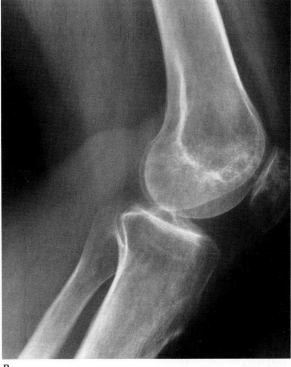

B

FIGURE 17-2
Radiographs of a 32-year-old woman with RSD of the knee. There is generalized periarticular osteopenia, especially in the distal femur and patella. *A.* AP. *B.* Lateral.

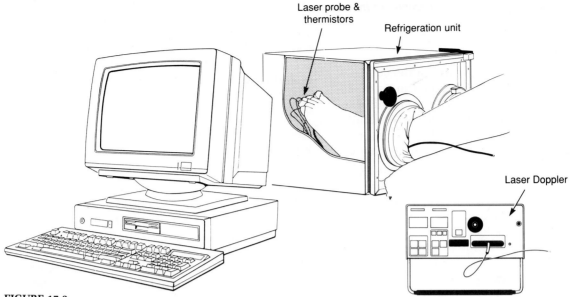

FIGURE 17-3
Equipment required to perform ICST/LDF.

Patients with RSD of the knee will demonstrate asymmetric responses in both temperature curves and LDF (Fig. 17-5). The test appears to be sensitive to vasomotor disturbance, which occurs in 80 percent to 90 percent of RSD patients.[7,11] However, the specificity of the test for RSD is poor and its diagnostic value has not been examined prospectively.

Thermography

Little is known about the application of thermography to RSD of the knee. Fulkerson and Hungerford have stated that thermography is a reliable and practical means of documenting the surface vascular changes that occur in RSD.[24] Uematsu and colleagues retrospectively reviewed 24 patients with RSD of the lower extremity and found abnormal thermograms in 94 percent of patients; 32 percent of these studies showed the painful area to be warmer and 62 percent showed it to be colder.[39] They concluded that thermography provided a useful tool to detect the presence of sympathetic dysfunction. Despite this promising report, however, much of the information about thermography is anecdotal and needs confirmation by prospective evaluation.

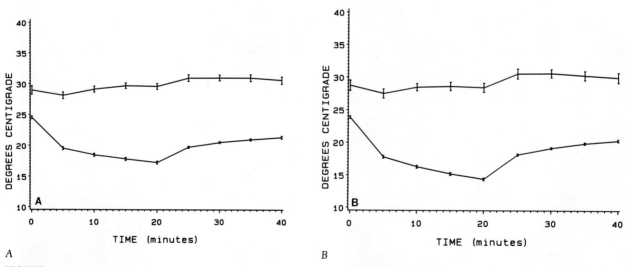

A   *B*

FIGURE 17-4
Temperature response curves for ICST of the foot performed on 72 subjects with normal lower extremities. The surface skin temperatures of each foot behave similarly and show two distinct normal patterns of response. Warm and cold responses are represented by mean temperature ± standard error of the mean.   *A.* Left foot.   *B.* Right foot. *(Reproduced with permission from Pollock FE Jr, Koman LA, Neal MB, et al: Foot Ankle 10:229, 1990.)*

236

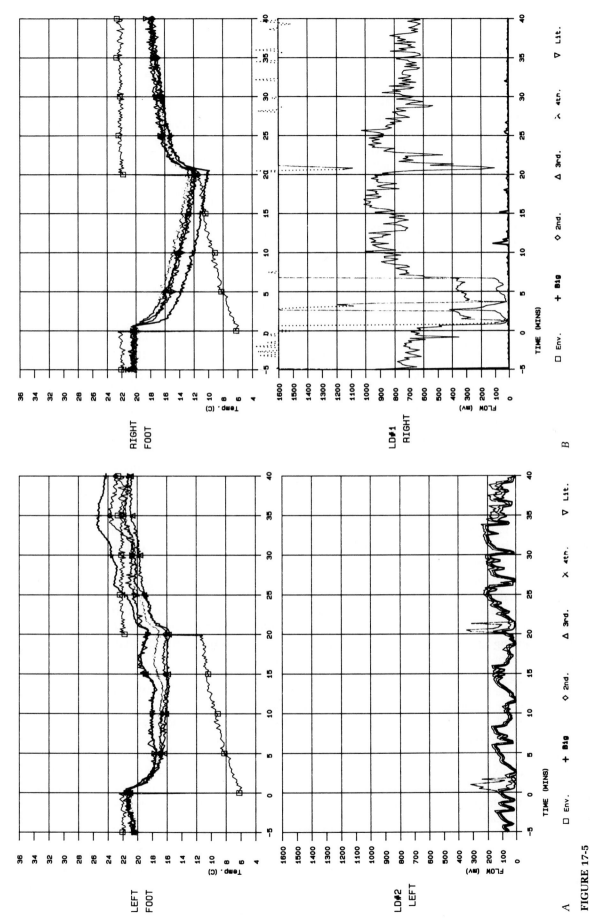

FIGURE 17-5

ICST and LDF of 38-year-old man with RSD of the left knee. The temperature response of the left foot shows several abnormalities, including low average baseline temperature, asymmetric responses of the left toes during both cooling and rewarming phases of the test, and asymmetric responses between feet. LDF demonstrates unusual variation in blood flow suggesting abnormal control of microvascular blood flow in the left lower extremity. *A.* Left foot. *B.* Right foot.

237

Pharmacologic Neural Blockade

Several investigators have suggested that lumbar sympathetic blockade should be used to establish the diagnosis of RSD, and Patman and colleagues consider that the relief of pain following sympathetic blockade is the most important diagnostic criterion in the evaluation of RSD.[40] Others have emphasized that failure to relieve pain with a sympathetic block suggests that the patient does not have RSD.[5,6] The study also has prognostic value: the amount of pain produced by the block has been reported to correlate with improvement following sympathectomy.[6,41]

Endurance Testing

Endurance testing is extremely effective means of documenting functional deficits.[5,11] Patients are tested with the Cybex II isokinetic dynameter and evaluated for strength, power, and endurance in both the affected and the normal extremity, and comparisons between the two sides are then made. Ogilvie-Harris and Roscoe have reported that deficits in endurance testing are more apparent than strength and power testing.[5] The test is difficult to falsify, and it provides quantitative information about functional impairment in the knee, but is not specific for RSD.

TREATMENT

Effective treatment of RSD of the knee requires diligence and patience on the part of both the patient and the physician. No treatment has proved to be consistently effective in alleviating pain and restoring function, and multiple therapeutic modalities are often required to promote improvement.

Early treatment has been shown to be the most important factor influencing clinical improvement. Numerous studies have shown that patients treated within 6 to 12 months after the onset of dystrophic symptoms have much better pain relief and functional improvement than those whose symptoms are of longer duration.[5,6–8] This is true also for dystrophy affecting other areas of the body.[15]

Most treatments are directed toward decreasing the sympathetic hyperactivity that characterizes RSD. Therapeutic modalities that have proved to be effective include physical therapy, various oral medications, pharmacologic sympathetic blockade, surgical or chemical sympathectomy, and various adjuvant therapies.

Physical Therapy

Active and active-assisted range of motion exercises are begun immediately after the diagnosis of RSD has been made to deter atrophy and stiffness in the knee. Tietjen has emphasized that extreme gentleness and patient cooperation are necessary to effect improvement by this method.[3]

Patients unable to tolerate physical therapy are asked to perform standing stress therapy.[11] The patient bears small amounts of weight on the affected extremity for short periods during the day, and keeps a log of the amount of time tolerated and the amount of pain experienced. Progress is often slow, but it allows the achievement of limited goals while applying some physiologic loading to the knee.

Oral Medications

Amitriptyline is a tricyclic antidepressant that is useful in treating the "burning" pain associated with RSD. The drug decreases sympathetic outflow by blocking reuptake of norepinephrine. A dose of 25 to 50 mg taken at bedtime is usually effective but may be adjusted as necessary. Amitriptyline may be used in conjunction with other agents, except guanethidine, which displaces norepinephrine in presynaptic vesicles (see below).[11]

Nifedipine has been shown to improve nutritional blood flow[42,43] and has been used to treat lower extremity dystrophy with good success.[44,45] The drug may be taken in 10- to 20-mg increments three times daily or once daily in a 30-mg sustained-release preparation.

Anticonvulsants suppress ectopic discharge in peripheral and CNS neurons[14] and have been effective in reducing the "shooting" or "stabbing" pain characteristic of patients with posttraumatic neuralgia.[46] These drugs include phenytoin, carbamazepine, clonazepam, and sodium valproate.

α-Receptor blockade produces arterial vasodilation and may facilitate more normal modulation of afferent signals to the CNS.[14,47] These drugs have been reported to be effective in the treatment of patients with causalgia; their efficacy in patients with RSD of the knee is unknown.

Corticosteroids have been used successfully to treat RSD by a number of investigators.[35,48] Typical dosages range from 60 to 80 mg daily for 2 weeks, followed by a tapering dosage over another 2-week period. The regimen may be repeated if symptoms recur and reported side effects are rare.[35]

Pharmacologic Sympathetic Blockade

Three types of sympathetic blockade are available to reduce the elevated sympathetic tone associated with RSD: intravenous regional blockade, lumbar sympathetic ganglia blockade, and continuous blockade using epidural anesthesia.

Hannington-Kiff has described excellent results using intravenous guanethidine administered under conditions similar to Bier block anesthesia.[49,50] Guanethidine displaces norepinephrine in presynaptic vesicles and, therefore, should not be used with amitriptyline, which would inhibit uptake of the drug into the terminal neuron.[11] Pain relief typically lasts 12 to 36 h but may last as long as 6 months.[51] The test may serve both diagnostically and therapeutically in the evaluation of RSD.[14]

Blockade of lumbar sympathetic ganglia is the most widely recognized treatment for patients with refractory RSD. Blocks are generally performed with small volumes of long-acting anesthetic agents and are usually well tolerated.[14] Katz and Hungerford reported good relief of pain in 58 percent of patients who underwent lumbar sympathetic blockade; the remaining 42 percent had fair relief.[6] However, 89 percent of the patients had recurrence of their symptoms. The duration of pain decrease has been reported to outlast the duration of action of the anesthetic agent, especially if the block is performed shortly after symptoms become manifest.[2,14]

Cooper and colleagues have recently reported data on 14 patients with RSD of the knee treated with epidural block anesthesia followed by epidural narcotics.[8] All patients underwent physical therapy and continuous passive motion of the knee during hospitalization, and all had been treated shortly after the onset of symptoms. With over 2 years of follow-up, 11 of the 14 patients were cured with no functional deficit; 2 patients had intermittent "aching"; and 1 patient had no relief of symptoms. This therapeutic technique holds promise for the total alleviation of symptoms in patients with RSD that is recognized and treated promptly.

Surgical or Chemical Sympathectomy

Surgical or chemical ablation of the lumbar sympathetic ganglion is generally reserved for patients who have experienced only transient relief from intravenous or sympathetic ganglion blockade. Many patients have good pain relief initially, but the pain may recur in as many as one-third.[14] Katz and Hungerford noted that in their patients who had sympathectomies, the amount of pain relief provided by the surgery could be predicted by the amount obtained transiently with a sympathetic block.[6]

Adjuvant Therapies

Numerous other forms of treatment have been suggested in the treatment of RSD. Temperature-contrast baths and nonsteroidal anti-inflammatory agents have been used with good success during courses of physical therapy.[3] The benefits of electrical nerve stimulation in patients with causalgia[16,52] have been described. Biofeedback, occupational therapy, and psychiatric testing may aid in pain relief, as well as provide emotional and psychological support.[11] Many of these treatments may be used in conjunction with other treatments the patient is receiving.

Tietjen has stressed that the most important therapy that can be offered the patient with RSD of the knee is the establishment of a good doctor–patient relationship.[3] Patients will be frustrated by the chronic pain and functional loss associated with RSD and will require patience, understanding, and encouragement from physicians, nurses, and therapists if they are to become and remain motivated to work toward improvement.

SUMMARY

Reflex sympathetic dystrophy of the knee is a complication that often follows traumatic or surgical insult to the knee. The syndrome is defined as an exaggerated physiologic response to an injury, and may be characterized by (1) intense or unduly prolonged pain, (2) vasomotor disturbances, (3) delayed functional recovery, and (4) trophic changes in the soft tissues. The pain often involves the patellofemoral articulation and produces limited range of motion and stiffness of the knee. No currently available objective testing technique allows sensitive and specific identification of dystrophic patients. However, plain x-ray films, TcBS, and ICST/LDF all aid in the diagnostic evaluation of the patient with chronic knee pain. Effective treatment of RSD requires prompt recognition of the syndrome, followed by a combination of treatments designed to maintain strength and range of motion while decreasing symptoms of sympathetic hyperactivity in the extremity.

REFERENCES

1. Kim HJ, Kozin F, Johnson RP, Hines R: Reflex sympathetic dystrophy syndrome of the knee following meniscectomy. Report of three cases. *Arthritis Rheum* 22:177, 1979.
2. Lagier R, Boussina, I, Mathies B: Algodystrophy of the knee. *Clin Rheumatol* 2:71, 1983.
3. Tietjen R: Reflex sympathetic dystrophy of the knee. *Clin Orthop* 209:235, 1986.
4. Doury P, Pattin S, Eulry F, et al: L'Algodystrophie du genou. A propos d'une sereis de 125 observations. *Rev Rhumat* 54:655, 1987.

5. Ogilvie-Harris DJ, Roscoe M: Reflex sympathetic dystrophy of the knee. *J Bone Joint Surg* 69B:804, 1987.

6. Katz MM, Hungerford DS: Reflex sympathetic dystrophy affecting the knee. *J Bone Joint Surg* 69B:797, 1987.

7. Poehling GG, Pollock FE Jr, Koman LA: Reflex sympathetic dystrophy of the knee after sensory nerve injury. *Arthroscopy* 4:31, 1988.

8. Cooper DE, DeLee JC, Ramamurthy S: Reflex sympathetic dystrophy of the knee. Treatment using continuous epidural anesthesia. *J Bone Joint Surg* 71A:365, 1989.

9. Shelton RM, Lewis CW: Reflex sympathetic dystrophy: A review. *J Am Acad Dermatol* 22:513, 1990.

10. Schutze SF, Gossling HR: The treatment of reflex sympathetic dystrophy. *J Bone Joint Surg* 66A:625, 1984.

11. Poehling GG, Koman LA, Pollack FE Jr: Reflex sympathetic dystrophy of the knee, in *Complications in Arthroscopy,* edited by NF Sprague III. New York, Raven Press, 1989, pp 53–72.

12. Bonica JJ: Causalgia and other reflex sympathetic dystrophies. *Adv Pain Res Ther* 3:41, 1979.

13. Wall PD: Mechanisms of acute and chronic pain. *Adv Pain Res Ther* 6:95, 1984.

14. Payne R: Neuropathic pain syndromes, with special reference to causalgia and reflex sympathetic dystrophy. *Clin J Pain* 2:59, 1986.

15. Schwartzman RJ, McLellan TL: Reflex sympathetic dystrophy. A review. *Arch Neurol* 44:555, 1987.

16. Melzak R, Wall PD: Pain mechanisms: A new theory. *Science* 150:971, 1965.

17. Roberts WJ: A hypothesis on the physiologic basis for causalgia and related pains. *Pain* 24:297, 1986.

18. Schott GD: Mechanisms of causalgia and related clinical conditions. The role of the central and of the sympathetic nervous system. *Brain* 109:717, 1986.

19. Schott G: Clinical features of algodystrophy: Is the sympathetic nervous system involved? *Funct Neurol* 4:131, 1989.

20. Devor M: Nerve pathophysiology and mechanisms of pain in causalgia. *J Auton Nerv Syst* 7:371, 1983.

21. Blumberg H, Janig W: Reflex patterns in the postganglionic vasoconstrictor neurons following chronic nerve lesions. *J Auton Nerv Syst* 14:157, 1985.

22. Cline MA, Ochoa J, Torebjork HE: Chronic hyperalgesia and skin warming caused by sensitized C nociceptors. *Brain* 112:621, 1989.

23. Stolte BH, Stolte JB, Leyten JF: De Pathofysiologie von ist Schoulder-Hand Syndroom. *Ned Tijdschr Genesskd* 114:1208, 1970.

24. Fulkerson JP, Hungerford DW: Reflex sympathetic dystrophy and chronic pain, in *Disorders of the Patellofemoral Joint,* 2d ed. Baltimore, Williams & Wilkins, 1990, pp 247–264.

25. Rosen L: Videophotometric skin capillaroscopy for assessment of microvascular disturbances. *J Oslo City Hosp* 39:107, 1989.

26. Gross D: Pain and autonomic nervous system. *Adv Neurol* 4:93, 1974.

27. Cooke ED, Ward C: Vicious circles in reflex sympathetic dystrophy—a hypothesis: Discussion paper. *J R Soc Med* 83:96, 1990.

28. Lagier R: Partial algodystrophy of the knee. An anatomico-radiological study of one case. *J Rheumatol* 10:255, 1983.

29. Lequesne M, Kerboull M, Bensasson M, et al: Partial transient osteoporosis. *Skeletal Radiol* 2:1, 1977.

30. Nathan PW: Pain and the sympathetic system, in *Autonomic Failure: A Textbook of Clinical Disorders of the Autonomic Nervous System,* 2d ed, edited by R Bannister. Oxford, Oxford University Press, 1988, pp 733–747.

31. Hungerford DS: Dystrophie sympathique reflexe et chondromalacie de la rotule. *Rev Chir Orthop* 66:259, 1980.

32. Arlet J, Ficat P, Durroux R, et al: Histopathologie des lesions osseuses et cartilagineuses dan l'algodystrophie sympathique reflexe du genou: A propos de 16 observations. *Rev Rhum Mal Osteoartic* 48:325, 1981.

33. Kozin F, Genant HK, Bekerman C, McCarty DJ: The reflex sympathetic dystrophy syndrome. II. Roentgenographic and scintigraphic evidence of bilaterality and of periarticular accentuation. *Am J Med* 60:332, 1976.

34. Intenzo C, Kim S, Millin J, Park C: Scintigraphic patterns of the reflex sympathetic syndrome of the lower extremities. *Clin Nucl Med* 14:657, 1989.

35. Kozin F, Ryan LM, Carrerra GF, et al: The reflex sympathetic dystrophy syndrome (RSDS). III. Scintigraphic studies, further evidence for the therapeutic efficacy of systemic corticosteroids, and proposed diagnostic criteria. *Am J Med* 70:23, 1981.

36. Werner R, Davidoff G, Jackson MD, et al: Factors affecting the sensitivity and specificity of the three-phase technitium bone scan in the diagnosis of reflex sympathetic dystrophy syndrome in the upper extremity. *J Hand Surg,* 14A:520, 1989.

37. Pollock FE Jr, Koman LA, Neal MB, et al: Use of isolated cold stress testing in determining normal lower extremity thermoregulation. *Foot Ankle* 10:229, 1990.

38. Pollock FE Jr, Koman LA, Smith BP, et al: Assessment of normal lower extremity thermoregulation by isolated cold stress testing and laser Doppler fluxmetry. Transactions of the 36th Annual Meeting of Orthopaedic Research Society 15:590, 1990.

39. Uematsu S, Hendler N, Hungerford D, et al: Thermography and electromyography in the differential diagnosis of chronic pain syndromes and reflex sympathetic dystrophy. *Electromyogr Clin Neurophsiol* 21:165, 1981.

40. Patman RD, Thompson JE, Persson AV: management of post-traumatic pain syndromes: Report of 113 cases. *Ann Surg* 177:780, 1973.

41. Toumey JW: Occurrence and management of reflex sympathetic dystrophy (causalgia of the extremities). *J Bone Joint Surg* 30A:883, 1948.

42. Ostergren J, Fagrell B: Videophotometric capillaroscopy for evaluating drug effects on skin microcirculation—A double-blind study with nifedipine. *Clin Physiol* 4:169, 1984.

43. Fagrell B: The relationship between macro- and microcirculation. Clinical aspects. *Acta Pharmacol Toxicol (Copenh)* 58:67, 1986.

44. Prough DS, McLeskey CH, Poehling GG, et al: Efficacy of oral nifedipine in the treatment of reflex sympathetic dystrophy. *Anesthesiology* 62:796, 1985.

45. Paulson RR: Reflex sympathetic dystrophy in a teenaged girl. *Postgrad Med* 81:66, 1987.

46. Swerdlow M: Anticonvulsant drugs and chronic pain. *Clin Neuropharmacol* 7:51, 1984.

47. Ghostine SY, Comair YG, Turner DM, et al: Phenoxybenzamine in the treatment of causalgia. Report of 40 cases. *J Neurosurg* 60:1263, 1984.

48. Kozin F, McCarty DJ, Sims J, Genant H: The reflex sympathetic dystrophy syndrome. I. Clinical and histologic studies: Evidence for bilaterality, response to corticosteroids and articular involvement. *Am J Med* 60:321, 1976.

49. Hannington-Kiff JG: Intravenous regional sympathetic block with guanethidine. *Lancet* 1:1019, 1974.

50. Hannington-Kiff JG: Hyperadrenergic-effected limb causalgia: Relief by IV pharmacologic norepinephrine blockade (Letter). *Am Heart J* 103:152, 1982.

51. Loh L, Nathan PW, Schott GD, Wilson PG: Effects of guanethidine infusion in certain painful states. *J Neurol Neurosurg Psychiatry* 43:446, 1980.

52. Meyer GA, Fields HL: Causalgia treated by selective large fibre stimulation of peripheral nerve. *Brain* 95:163, 1972.

SECTION VII
Degenerative Lesions

CHAPTER 18

Patellofemoral Arthritis—General Considerations

Ronald P. Karzel
Wilson Del Pizzo

INTRODUCTION

Degeneration of the articular cartilage of the patellofemoral joint is one of the most common problems encountered by knee surgeons. Despite the common occurrence of the problem, however, significant controversy exists about the causes of the articular cartilage degeneration, as well as the optimal treatment. Chondromalacia of the patella was first described by Aleman in 1928.[1] Chondromalacia is the pathologic finding of softened cartilage on the articular surface of the patella. This is often noted incidentally at the time of surgical evaluation of the knee for other problems and is often asymptomatic. Chondromalacia is a problem that is apparently more common in the younger age groups. One long-term follow-up study has shown that most individuals with a clinical diagnosis of chondromalacia treated nonoperatively did not ultimately develop clinically significant patellofemoral arthritis.[2] It appears that in young individuals, the capacity for repairing damage to the cartilage matrix is much greater, and therefore most of these patients will respond favorably to conservative treatment. Likewise, degenerative changes to the patellofemoral joint are common in middle-aged and elderly patients. Studies have shown degenerative changes of the patellar cartilage in from 40 percent to 60 percent of patients at autopsy, and from 20 percent to 50 percent of patients at the time of knee arthrotomy for other diagnoses.[3] Despite the relatively high incidence of degenerative changes of the patellofemoral joint with aging, most patients are not significantly symptomatic. However, when the patients in this older age group develop patellofemoral symptoms, they have less capacity for cartilage repair and are less likely to respond to conservative treatment. In these patients, operative intervention is more likely to be required for relief of symptoms.

Patients with symptomatic patellofemoral arthritis are begun initially on a conservative treatment regimen. This will usually be successful for younger patients with chondromalacia and will sometimes be successful for older patients with less severe patellofemoral involvement. Although patients often continue to have a mild to moderate level of symptoms after conservative treatment, surgical intervention may be avoided. In general, at least several months of conservative treatment will be attempted before considering operative intervention. We believe that most surgical procedures for patellofemoral arthritis should be considered salvage procedures, with the goal of surgical intervention being a decrease in disabling pain, sufficient to allow the patient to return to many activities of daily living. We consider these procedures to be "salvage-type" procedures, in that it is unlikely that the patient will have an asymptomatic, fully functional, normal knee after surgery. An important part of surgical intervention, therefore, is preoperative counseling of the patient about realistic expectations following the surgery, and of the probable need for continued activity modification postoperatively. Operative options range from arthroscopy and debridement of the chondral lesion to total patellectomy. In between these two procedures of the patellofemoral joint are the Maquet tibial tubercle elevation and patellofemoral modular prosthetic replacement.

NONOPERATIVE TREATMENT PROGRAM

Initial management of patellofemoral disorders is generally with a nonoperative treatment program.

243

This is most likely to be successful in the younger patient population with patellofemoral symptoms, but no significant radiologic changes of joint space narrowing or malalignment. Initial rehabilitation is directed at decreasing pain and inflammation. Generally, the patient will be treated with a trial of anti-inflammatory medication, intermittent icing, and rest. Many patients have already learned through experience which activities place forces across the patellofemoral joint and exacerbate their pain. These include activities that require flexion of the knee with quadriceps loading, such as climbing stairs or inclines, squatting, kneeling, or crawling. Patients are often symptomatic as well when sitting for long periods of time with the knee in a flexed position, such as while driving a car or sitting in a theater. Education of the patient about activities that cause patellofemoral pain, and of ways to modify activities to avoid placing stress across the patellofemoral joint, can be helpful in reducing symptoms. Also important is a program of strengthening and stretching. Generally, in the early stages, strengthening exercises consist primarily of quadriceps isometric exercises, as well as strengthening of the adductor muscles of the thigh and the hamstrings. Hamstring, quadriceps, and Achilles stretching are also important. Electrical stimulation of the vastus medialis obliquus and sometimes the use of biofeedback or patellar taping techniques may also be beneficial. A brace designed for increased patella support without pressure over the patella is often used.

Additional strengthening exercises can be added for those patients who respond well to the initial phases with decreased patellofemoral pain. Exercises are used that build strength, power, and endurance in the involved extremity without aggravating patellofemoral problems. Exercise is also beneficial in helping patients to lose weight. In particular, nonimpact activities, such as swimming (avoiding the breaststroke kick), stationary biking with the seat height properly adjusted for minimal resistance, and the use of a Nordic-type ski track exercise can be tolerated by many of these patients. Activities should be done in moderation and not at a level that causes pain. Icing should be continued after activity. At this point, short arc quadriceps as well as hamstring curl strengthening may be added. In the younger age group, isokinetic strengthening and eccentric quadriceps exercises may also be used. Weight loss is generally desirable in these patients because activities such as stair climbing may result in three to five times the body weight across the patellofemoral joint and squatting may result in forces of up to seven times body weight across the patellofemoral joint.[4] Losing

and maintaining large amounts of weight loss are often difficult, particularly in patients who have difficulty exercising because of patellofemoral pain. However, it should be emphasized that even weight loss in the 10- to 20-lb range may significantly benefit the patellofemoral joint and improve the overall patellofemoral mechanics. As previously mentioned, most patients with chondromalacia of the patella and some patients with degenerative arthritis of the patellofemoral joint will respond favorably to these nonoperative measures. For patients who fail to respond and continue to be significantly disabled by their patellofemoral pain, a surgical procedure may subsequently become necessary. These procedures are considered further in the remainder of this chapter.

SURGICAL PROCEDURES

The most common surgical procedures for isolated patellofemoral arthritis include arthroscopic debridement, Maquet elevation of the tibial tubercle, patellofemoral replacement, and patellectomy. In this chapter, factors influencing the decision to perform each of these procedures are discussed. The remaining chapters in the section present the individual procedures and techniques in greater detail.

Arthroscopic Debridement

Given the lesser magnitude of arthroscopic procedures than of open surgical procedures, arthroscopic treatment of patellofemoral arthritis is often the first step. An overall decreased morbidity, faster recovery time, and faster speed of rehabilitation are generally ascribed to arthroscopic techniques. For patients in whom surgery is contemplated for patellofemoral arthritis, arthroscopy is usually offered as the initial procedure. Arthroscopy should include diagnostic evaluation of the patient's knee, allowing evaluation of the extent of patellofemoral arthritis, the extent of arthritis in the other compartments, and other associated pathology such as meniscal tears. Arthroscopy should also evaluate patellofemoral tracking as the knee is moved through a range of motion. It should be emphasized to the patient preoperatively that arthroscopic patellar shaving is not a cure for the problem. Many authors have found the removal of fibrillated and damaged cartilage can improve the patient's pain and function.[5–7] However, in our experience, arthroscopy is more likely to be a temporizing procedure that will not completely cure the patient. Patients should continue to expect symptoms in their knee following arthroscopy, particularly if they overuse the knee.

At the time of surgery, patellar alignment is assessed. For patients with appropriate alignment of the extensor mechanism, arthroscopic patellar shaving is done alone. This is most appropriate for the patient with grade 3 chondromalacia, in which extensive flap formation and fissuring are present. Fibrillated cartilage that appears to be loosening is removed. No attempt is made to remove articular cartilage down to the level of subchondral bone. Theoretically, removing fibrillated cartilage prevents eventual loosening and release of the cartilage into the joint, a process thought to lead to enzymatic reaction and synovitis, which aggravates the underlying arthritic process. In patients who have patellar malalignment at the time of arthroscopy, arthroscopically assisted lateral release using electrosurgical technique has been used for a number of years. Theoretically, lateral release will help to allow some realignment of the patellofemoral mechanism, and hopefully will also allow some mechanical decompression of the arthritic patella.[8–11] Many patients' patellae will remain malaligned following such a procedure. When these patients are recreationally active and young, a small medial incision to allow plication of the medial retinaculum is then performed concomitantly with lateral release in an attempt to further realign the patella. No advancement of the vastus medialis obliquus is performed because it is felt that this will weaken the quadriceps mechanism, slowing the rehabilitation program and increasing the patient's postoperative pain and morbidity. In addition to providing a therapeutic modality, arthroscopy also allows determination of the overall level of arthritic involvement of the patellofemoral compartment. This allows postoperative discussion with the patient of the potential clinical outcome following this procedure. In our clinical experience, patients who have significant involvement of a grade 3 to 4 level chondromalacia of the patella and trochlear groove have no more than a 50 percent chance of being helped by an arthroscopic approach to their problem. Even when successful in giving pain relief, significant activity modification will often be necessary, and future progression of the problem may still occur.

Maquet Tibial Tubercle Elevation

For the patient with severe patellofemoral arthritis who has failed conservative management and subsequent arthroscopic intervention, our procedure of choice is generally the Maquet tibial tubercle elevation. We consider this to be an end-stage salvage type of procedure. It is a procedure done for patients who are generally quite incapacitated because of their pa-

tellofemoral symptoms. First introduced by Maquet in 1963, he has since reported further on the results of this procedure.[12,13] Maquet calculated biomechanically joint reaction forces occurring across the patellofemoral joint. He reasoned that by increasing the lever arm of the quadriceps muscle, and increasing the angle formed by the pull of the quadriceps muscle of the patellar tendon, joint reaction force could be significantly lowered.[13] The elevation is most effective in reducing joint reactive force when the knee is almost fully extended. He recommended a 2.0- to 2.5-cm advancement of the tibial tubercle to achieve the calculated reduction of 50 percent in compressive forces across the patellofemoral joint.[12] Using this technique, Maquet reported 36 good or excellent results out of 37 cases, at a mean follow-up period of 4.7 years.[12] The patient who failed in his series developed skin necrosis over the elevated tubercle.

Ferguson and coworkers tested Maquet's mathematical model in the laboratory.[14] They found that after an elevation of 1.25 cm, most of the decrease in patellofemoral contact stress had occurred. Further elevation gave relatively little improvement in patellofemoral contact stress, but appeared to markedly increase the incidence of complications such as skin necrosis and cosmetic deformity. Ferguson reported 85 percent satisfactory results in his patients, with a satisfactory result defined as pain relief sufficient to allow resumption of lost functions and activities.[15] Other authors have documented satisfactory results in from 63 percent to 97 percent of patients, with the latter number being the results of Maquet.[12,16–18] In our own series of 51 patients, 73 percent had improvement in their pain and 57 percent had improvement in their limitations in activity following the anterior tubercle elevation.[19] Despite the improvement in pain, however, the majority of these patients still did not have pain-free knees. Their pain was more tolerable and their activities somewhat increased, but pain was still present.[19] Complication rates in the various series have ranged from 18 percent to 40 percent, with the most significant complications including wound infections, skin necrosis, and stress fractures of the proximal tibial tubercle.[18]

Because of the relatively low percentage of patients who gain complete pain relief and because of the high complication rate, the Maquet procedure must be considered a salvage procedure. Clearly not all patients undergoing the Maquet procedure will be significantly improved, and some may suffer complications that make them worse. We offer this procedure to young or middle-aged patients who have disabling patellofemoral symptoms and who have exhausted other forms of treatment. These patients must be fully informed preoperatively about the significance of the Maquet procedure, including the potential morbidity, the prolonged healing time, and realistic expectation of results. All of our patients undergoing the Maquet tibial tubercle elevation have failed nonoperative protocol, most have had previous arthroscopic procedures including patellar shaving and, in some, arthroscopic lateral release. These patients are generally middle-aged and have pain that affects their work, activities of daily living, and recreational life-style. Patients are counseled not to expect a significant improvement or significant change in their work capability, with the goal being instead, a tolerable level of daily pain and ability to perform more of their activities of daily living. Despite the Maquet operation, the patient will still have an arthritic patellofemoral joint that can be overloaded with vigorous activities and overuse. Even in those patients who are improved by the procedure, it is unlikely that complete relief of patellofemoral pain with activities such as kneeling, squatting, crawling, or other activities requiring deep knee flexion will occur. We consider the Maquet procedure to be an end-stage procedure and not a temporizing procedure prior to performing other patellofemoral surgery. It continues to be our most often used salvage procedure for certain groups of patients with disabling patellofemoral arthritis.

Patellectomy

Although patellectomy was previously a commonly performed procedure for degenerative arthritis of the patellofemoral joint with satisfactory results in up to 85 percent of patients,[20,21] the procedure is rarely used at present. Ivey and coworkers reported a failure rate of 39 percent in 51 patients undergoing patellectomy.[22] Failure required reoperation, most commonly for continued extensor mechanism malalignment, or for continued degeneration of the groove or tibial femoral joint. Several biomechanical studies have documented the significant loss of extensor torque that occurs following this procedure.[23-25] Maquet[13] has also raised questions about the possibility of increasing tibial femoral contact stresses and subsequent arthritis due to alteration of the normal patellofemoral biomechanics by patellectomy. Finally, patellectomy creates problems for subsequent total knee arthroplasty in those patients who later go on to develop tibial femoral arthritis. For these reasons, patellectomy is infrequently used except in cases of severe comminution of the patella following patellar fracture.

Patellofemoral Replacement

Modular patellofemoral replacement is rarely used in our practice. Most of the patients in the past who would have been candidates for patellofemoral replacement are now the patients who are surgical candidates for the Maquet tibial tubercle elevation. These are the middle-aged patients with isolated patellofemoral arthritis with intact medial and lateral tibial-femoral compartments. Elderly patients with patellofemoral arthritis will usually have arthritic changes in the other knee compartments, and therefore are candidates for total knee arthroplasty. Likewise, younger and more active patients who undergo patellofemoral replacement will be committed to further knee arthroplasties if the procedure fails. Given the concerns about long-term results of implants in younger patients, patellofemoral replacement is not recommended in the younger age groups. Although noncemented press fit components may increase the longevity of the prosthesis in younger patients, the concerns for future failures in this group should still be considered. Initial reports have shown improvement in symptoms in approximately 75 percent of patients. The procedure has significant morbidity as well as a prolonged recovery time, and most of the patients still retain some symptoms.[26,27] Resurfacing of the patella alone produced satisfactory results in only 55 percent of patients at short-term follow-up, and this procedure has been abandoned.[28]

CONCLUSIONS

We recommend initial nonoperative treatment for most patients with patellofemoral arthritis. Most patients will respond satisfactorily to nonoperative treatment. For those patients failing nonoperative treatment, initial arthroscopic evaluation with debridement of articular cartilage flaps and possible lateral retinacular release is the next step. Patients failing this procedure may then be offered the option of anterior tibial tubercle elevation. We consider the Maquet elevation to be an end-stage salvage procedure. No additional surgery is advised if the Maquet procedure is unsuccessful in certain groups of patients. We rarely use patellectomy or patellofemoral replacement procedures at present because they are used in only very specific cases. Total knee arthroplasty is used in elderly patients with patellofemoral arthritis because they have concomitant arthritic changes in the tibial femoral compartments. Specific indications and techniques of each of these procedures are discussed more fully in the following chapters in this section.

REFERENCES

1. Aleman O: Chondromalacia post-traumatic patellae. *Acta Chir Scand* 63:149, 1928.
2. Karlson S. Chondromalacia patella. *Acta Chir Scand* 83:349, 1939.
3. Vuorinen O, Paakkala T, Tuuturii T, et al: Chondromalacia patellae: Results of operative treatments. *Arch Orthop Trauma Surg* 104:175, 1985.
4. Scott RP: Prosthetic replacement of the patellofemoral joint. *Orthop Clin North Am* 10:129, 1979.
5. Insall J: Patellar pain: Current concept review. *J Bone Joint Surg* 64A:147, 1983.
6. Ogilvie-Harris DS, Jackson RW: Arthroscopic treatment of chondromalacia patella. *J Bone Joint Surg* 66B:660, 1984.
7. Schonholtz GJ, Ling B: Arthroscopic chondroplasty of the patella. *Arthroscopy* 1:92, 1985.
8. Fox JM, Ferkel RD: Use of electrosurgery and arthroscopic surgery, in *Arthroscopic Surgery*, edited by J Parisien. New York, McGraw-Hill, 1988, pp. 313–330.
9. Miller GK, Dickason JM, Fox JM, et al: The use of electrosurgery for arthroscopic subcutaneous lateral release. *Orthopedics* 5:309, 1982.
10. Schonholtz GJ, Zahn MG, Magee CM, et al: Lateral retinacular release of the patella. *Arthroscopy* 3:269, 1987.
11. Sherman OH, Fox JM, Sperling H, et al: Patellar instability. Treatment by arthroscopic electrosurgical lateral release. *Arthroscopy* 3:152, 1987.
12. Maquet P: Advancement of the tibial tuberosity. *Clin Orthop* 115:225, 1976.
13. Maquet P: Mechanics and osteoarthritis of the patellofemoral joint. *Clin Orthop* 144:70, 1979.
14. Ferguson AB, Brown TD, Fu FH, Ruthouski R: Relief of patellofemoral contact stress by anterior displacement of the tibial tubercle. *J Bone Joint Surg* 61A:159, 1979.
15. Ferguson AB: Elevation of the insertion of the patellar ligament for patellofemoral pain. *J Bone Joint Surg* 64A:776, 1982.
16. Rorbruch JD, Campbell RD, Insall J: Tibial tubercle elevation (the Maquet operation): A clinical study of 31 cases. *Orthop Trans* 3:291, 1979.
17. Radin EL: The Maquet procedure: Anterior displacement of the tibial tubercle. *Clin Orthop* 213:241, 1986.
18. Bessette GC, Hunter RE: The Maquet procedure: A retrospective review. *Clin Orthop* 232:159, 1988.
19. Friedman MJ, Pachelli AF, Fox JM, et al: Modified Maquet tibial tubercle elevation: A retrospective review. *J Knee Surg* 3:114, 1990.
20. Bentley G: The surgical treatment of chondromalacia patella. *J Bone Joint Surg* 60B:74, 1978.
21. West FE: End results of patellectomy. *J Bone Joint Surg* 44A:1089, 1962.
22. Ivey FM, Blazina ME, Fox JM, Del Pizzo W: Reoperation following patellectomy for chondromalacia. *Orthopedics* 2:134, 1979.
23. Kaufer H: Mechanical function of the patella. *J Bone Joint Surg* 53A:1551, 1971.
24. Watkins MP, Harris BA, Wender S, et al: Effect of patellectomy on the function of the quadriceps and hamstrings. *J Bone Joint Surg* 65A:390, 1983.
25. Wendt PP, Johnson RP: A study of quadriceps excursion, torque, and the effect of patellectomy on cadaver knees. *J Bone Joint Surg* 67A:726, 1985.
26. Blazina ME, Fox JM, Del Pizzo W, et al: Patellofemoral replacement. *Clin Orthop* 144:98, 1979.
27. Lubinus HH: Patella guide bearing total replacement. *Orthopedics* 2:120, 1979.
28. Insall J, Tria AJ, Aglietti P: Resurfacing of the patella. *J Bone Joint Surg* 62A:933, 1980.

CHAPTER 19

Tibial Tubercle Elevation

Mary Isham
Kenneth M. Singer
Thomas Helpenstell

INTRODUCTION

Patellofemoral arthralgia is a common cause of knee pain that often responds to conservative treatment. In some instances, however, the pain is refractory to nonoperative treatment and becomes disabling. For these patients, surgical options are available. Before deciding on a specific procedure, it is helpful to try to determine as precisely as possible the etiology of the pain (i.e., instability, osteoarthritis, malalignment). Failure to do so may result in a poor outcome regardless of the procedure.

Tibial tubercle elevation has been described to relieve the pain for patients with specific patellofemoral disorders. Evaluation of published results, however, reveals significant inconsistency and it is sometimes difficult to determine who will do well following tibial tubercle elevations.

This chapter summarizes the current knowledge available and combines that with the authors' recommendations regarding the place of tibial tubercle elevation in the treatment of patients with patellofemoral disorders.

BIOMECHANICS

Anterior displacement of the tibial tubercle was first described in 1963 by Paul Maquet of Liège, Belgium.[1,2] In search of an alternative to patellectomy, he based the procedure on the premise that patellofemoral joint degeneration was caused by stress overload of the tissues, both cartilaginous and osseous. He proposed an eloquent mechanical model to reduce the compressive forces across the patellofemoral joint.

The anterior displacement of the tibial tubercle alters the joint mechanics in three ways.

1. Anterior displacement lengthens the lever arm, thereby reducing the force that the quadriceps must generate to perform the same work.

2. Anterior displacement opens or increases the angle (beta) between the quadriceps vector and patellar tendon vector, which markedly decreases the patellofemoral compressive forces.

3. Tibial tubercle elevation rotates the patella and shifts the forces on the patella superiorly, increasing the patellar contact area, decreasing the stress per unit of area, and off-loading some of the force onto the quadriceps tendon.

By using knee models, Maquet estimated that elevating the tibial tubercle 2 cm would reduce the patellofemoral force by 50 percent during normal gait.[1] However, subsequent to his initial publication, others have studied the biomechanics of tibial tubercle elevation in detail and have come to varying conclusions.

In 1972, Bandi placed stress transducers beneath cadaveric patellae and demonstrated reduced forces after tibial tubercle elevation.[3]

Ferguson and colleagues used implanted pressure transducers and found significant reductions in pressure with a 1.25-cm elevation, but minimal additional reduction with further elevation.[4] Burke and Ahmed did a similar study, but found progressive unloading of the patellofemoral joint with elevations of 2 to 3 cm.[5] Since these studies were all done on cadaveric patellae with relatively normal articular cartilage, it is unclear whether the effects are the same on knees with underlying patellofemoral disease.

A geometric analysis of forces in areas of contact of the patellofemoral joint was published by Nakamora and coworkers in 1985.[6] Their analyses showed a diminution of patellofemoral compressive forces with increasing tubercle elevation; however, there was an alarming increase in tibiofemoral shear forces and a significant decrease in the contact area of the patella, which ultimately would result in increased pressure. This study substantiates Ferguson's proposal that the optimal alteration of patellofemoral biomechanics occurs at about 1 cm of elevation.

More recently, Lewallen and colleagues studied cadaveric knees with varying degrees of degenerative changes and tested them at 1.25 cm and 2.5 cm of tibial tubercle elevation.[7] They found a progressive decrease in contact force and contact area, but no significant change in contact pressure.

At present, the changes that occur at the patellofemoral joint following tibial tubercle elevation are not yet fully understood.

CLINICAL RESULTS

In 1976, Maquet reported data on 39 patients who had undergone isolated anterior tibial tubercle elevations with a follow-up period ranging from 1 to 10 years with a 4.7-year average.[2] The patients ranged in age from 19 to 81 years (average, 50 years). Indication for surgery had been patellofemoral osteoarthritis, chondromalacia of the patella, and generalized osteoarthritis of the knee. Thirty-seven of 39 patients had good to excellent results by Dr. Maquet's grading system, which implies relief of pain and a functional knee. One failure occurred in a patient who underwent high tibial osteotomy and the other in a patient who, with multiple scars from previous surgeries, developed necrotic flaps and required removal of the graft. However, no study to date has been able to reproduce these results.

Subsequent studies have reported variable results. Hirsch reported on nine knees in eight patients, aged 20 to 32 years, who underwent 2 to 2.5 cm of tibial tubercle elevation.[8] At an average of 29 months' follow-up, results showed six excellent, one good, and one fair, with three complications (skin necrosis, muscle herniation, and scar formation).

A larger and prospective series by Sudmann was reported in 1980.[9] Thirty-two knees in 28 patients with the diagnosis of chondromalacia patella who had been symptomatic for a range of 6 months to 4 years underwent 10 to 23 mm of tibial tubercle elevation. At 8 to 34 months' follow-up, 30 of 32 patients achieved satisfactory results and were able to return to work. There were two infections, three deep venous thromboses (DVT), and one loss of tubercle elevation for a serious complication rate of 18 percent.

Ferguson[7] can be credited with one of the largest series and with stratifying the results based on pathologic diagnosis. In 1982, he reported data on 184 patients who underwent a 1.25-cm advancement of the tibial tubercle. The patients were evaluated at a minimum of 2-years of follow-up with an overall success rate of 85 percent using the "all or none" rating system. The group with the highest success rate (92 percent) included patients with patellofemoral arthritis who, coincidentally, had the lowest average number of previous surgical procedures. Patients with a history of patellar dislocation or posttraumatic problems had success rates of 83 percent and 84 percent, respectively.

When patellofemoral pain with severe malalignment was used as an indication for tubercle elevation, Fulkerson achieved good relief of symptoms in 8 patients using 9 mm of anterior translation of the tubercle along with medialization.[10] He found mild to moderate chondromalacia patellae in 40 patients.

In the young adult, Radin reported an overall success rate of 90 percent in 36 patients; the highest success rate was 94 percent in the posttraumatic group of 14 knees.[11] Those who had arthrosis secondary to subluxation achieved an 88 percent success rate, and the postpatellectomy group of 6 patients had a success rate of only 66 percent. He advocated 2 to 2.5 cm of elevation and the avoidance of internal fixation if possible. Along with his success rate was a 5 percent incidence of serious complications and 19 percent minor complications. He felt perioperative problems were minimized by using an incision that begins lateral to the patella, crossing medially over the tubercle and extending down the leg. He elevated entirely from the medial side, leaving the lateral soft tissue attachments, and pie-crusted the skin to relieve tension.

In 1986, Heatley reported a prospective study in which he followed 27 patients an average of over 7 years.[12] He used a qualitative rating system and found a significant deterioration in success rates between 3- and 6-year follow-up intervals. At 3 years the rates were 65.5 percent good, 13.8 percent fair, and 20.7 percent poor. By 6 years, the percentages were 53.6 percent, 14.3 percent, and 32.1 percent, respectively. At 6 years, when the results were stratified according to pathologic diagnosis, the highest success rate was achieved in patients with chondromalacia patellae in whom 5 of 6 (83 percent) had good results. The group with patellofemoral osteoarthritis achieved 43 percent good, 21 percent fair, and 35 percent poor results. In 4 patients who had previous patellar dislocation, 1 (25 percent) was good, 2 (50 percent) were fair, and 1 (25 percent) was a failure. Of those who had undergone previous surgery, 4 (80 percent) had good results and 1 (20 percent) poor. Four of 27 patients (13 percent) experienced complications, including one deep infection and three fractures of the tibial crest.

Radin reported in 1986 that the results were better in his patients who had 2 to 2.5 cm of elevation (94 percent success) than in those who only had 1.25 cm (67 percent success).[13] He felt that patellofemoral arthrosis was a major indication and also reported a fairly high complication rate.

CHAPTER 20

Patellofemoral Arthroplasty

Ronald P. Grelsamer
Philippe Cartier

INTRODUCTION

Patellofemoral arthroplasty, otherwise known as patellofemoral replacement surgery, is a prosthetic resurfacing of both the patella and the trochlea. As with any other implant surgery, patellofemoral arthroplasty is a salvage procedure designed to bring symptomatic and functional improvements to arthritic patellae for which no simpler soft tissue or bone procedure will do. Patellofemoral arthroplasties are therefore not competing with lateral releases, medial plications, or Trillat-type procedures. Patellofemoral arthroplasty is in a league with patellectomies, Maquet-type procedures, spongialization, and total knee replacement (TKR) surgery.

Patellectomy

Removal of the patella has been reported on repeatedly since the early part of the twentieth century. It is a resection arthroplasty of the patellofemoral joint, the premise being that the knee can function adequately without a patella. Issues surrounding this procedure include short-term function, cosmesis, and long-term effects on the femorotibial articulations. Numerous publications support both sides of these issues (see Chap. 21).

Maquet-type Procedures

Elevating the tibial tubercle can decrease the intraarticular pressure of the patellofemoral joint. However, this decrease is unpredictable, as it is a complex function of changes in load and contact areas.[1] Maquet-type procedures are insufficient for adequate pain relief when the arthritic process is advanced. The exact arthritic threshold above which a Maquet-type procedure will not work remains to be determined and is probably quite patient dependent. Overall, we have been disappointed with these procedures and are resorting to them with decreasing frequency (see Chap. 19).

Spongialization

This operation is an extension of Pridie's localized subchondral perforations and was described by Ficat in 1979.[1a] It consists of removing subchondral bone down to cancellous (spongy) bone over the entire diseased area. The theories behind both the Pridie and Ficat operations "rest on the same principle of regeneration of tissue from the marrow of the underlying cancellous bone" as Ficat felt that the subchondral bone itself is a significant source of pain. It also seems to us that by thinning the patella the surgeon might be decreasing the patellofemoral stresses during knee flexion. However, despite these theoretical possibilities and some encouraging early reports in the literature, we have not had much success with this operation.

Total Knee Replacement

This operation will provide pain relief for any knee ailment. The issues are: (1) is the sacrifice of two healthy compartments justified? (2) is this the most cost-effective procedure? and (3) is the function afforded the patient as good as that provided by other procedures (such as a patellofemoral replacement)?

Patellofemoral Replacement

The first arthroplasties dating back to 1955 resurfaced the patella only and did so with a metallic implant.[2] Such replacements were reported on in the 1970s,[3,4] but we are aware of just one study[5] reporting reasonable long-term results with this approach. Although the patella is more prone to degeneration than the trochlea—perhaps secondary to a difference in the properties of their articular cartilage[6]—candidates for a patellar arthroplasty usually have enough degeneration on both sides of the articulation to warrant resurfacing of both. Lubinus reported on a patellofemoral replacement in 1979[7] as did Blazina and colleagues.[8] Both featured a polyethylene patellar button and a metallic trochlear component. Other implants have since been described (see Choice of Implant). Bechtol and Blazina deserve the greatest credit for introducing the concept of patellofemoral arthroplasty as we know it today.

PREOPERATIVE EVALUATION

The surgeon must confirm that the patient's symptoms are essentially from the patellofemoral joint and that this compartment is "significantly" arthritic (see Maquet section above).

Clinical Evaluation

In addition to asking the patient to point to the area(s) of pain, we perform the "stair test": the patient goes up a large step with the affected leg first. As the patient rises up to the step he or she is asked to point with one finger to the painful area. The same is repeated with the patient going down the step with the unaffected leg first. If the patient points only to the front or sides of the patella this is a good (though imperfect) sign of isolated patellofemoral involvement. If the patient also points to one of the joint lines, this is worrisome with respect to the possibility of more diffuse arthritis.

The clinical evaluation also involves assessing the overall alignment of the extensor mechanism. Only patients with posttraumatic arthritis are likely to have a normal alignment. The quadriceps (Q) angle may be abnormal and may contribute to an excessive lateral pull on the patella. The patella may be tilted and subluxed as a result of a tight lateral retinaculum and of a dysplastic vastus medialis obliquus. These pathologic factors will need to be addressed at surgery.

Roentgenographic Evaluation

The axial (Fig. 20-1) and lateral views will have presumably demonstrated patellofemoral arthritis. Standing and standing flexion views are needed to assess the femorotibial compartments.

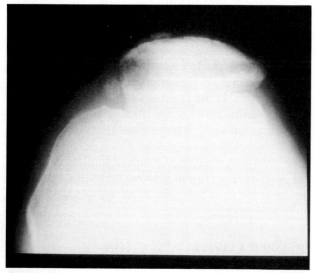

FIGURE 20-1
End-stage arthritis of patellofemoral joint.

Magnetic Resonance Imaging (MRI)/Arthroscopy

These modalities can be more sensitive to the presence of arthritis than radiographs or a clinical examination, but they may be overly sensitive. It has already been shown in one study that (femorotibial) unicompartmental replacements can function well with a less than perfect contralateral side.[9] The same can be true with patellofemoral replacements. No firm pronouncement can be made with respect to the use of MRI or arthroscopy except to say that they can be useful in borderline cases (more so arthroscopy as of this writing).

CHOICE OF IMPLANTS

The success of total knee arthroplasty has made the choice of a polyethylene patellar button and of a metallic trochlear component standard among current manufacturers of such implants. Differences between implants center around the depth, length, and method of fixation of the trochlear component.

Patients with severe, isolated patellofemoral arthritis often have a dysplastic trochlea that contributes to patellar instability. Other components of patellar malalignment are usually also present (weak vastus medialis obliquus, increased Q angle, among others). Accordingly, we have favored an implant that features a deep, "non-anatomic" trochlea and a correspondingly V-shaped patellar button. The combination provides a measure of geometric constraint to dislocation. This geometric constraint cannot be entirely counted on to prevent dislocation (see Surgical Technique). When the trochlea has a normal topography, consideration can be given to a custom implant. The fixation of the trochlear component can be provided by a central peg (Blazina-Richards, Lotus) or by a few small pegs (Cartier-Richards, Grammont[10]). The large central peg can be advantageous in osteoporotic bone.

SURGICAL TECHNIQUE

The Trochlea

Regardless of the implant used certain principles apply[11]: osteophytes must be removed from the notch because they can impinge against the spines and they can lead to poor placement of the trochlear implant. The tip of the trochlear component should not overhang the notch lest it impinge against the spines (Fig. 20-2). As noted earlier, the trochlea (and therefore the condyles) will often be dysplastic. The component should not be tilted medially or laterally in an attempt to have the implant rest perfectly on both condyles. This can lead to dislocation. The surgeon should accept the possibility of cement buildup on one side. A custom implant can be an alternative assuming the trochlear dysplasia is sufficiently mild.

The Patella

The technique is similar to that used in total knee surgery. The thickness of patella resected must result in a patella of normal thickness once the implant is positioned. If an implant with a steep trochlea is used, the ridge on the trochlea must line up with the trochlear groove (Fig. 20-3). This can be less straightforward than it appears as the patella is operated on in a rotated and everted position.

Extensor Realignment

This is a critical yet sometimes overlooked aspect of the procedure. Patients who undergo a patellofem-

oral replacement often have a severe malalignment that caused the arthritis in the first place. If the malalignment is not sufficiently corrected the patella will continue to sublux or dislocate, and the patient will be dissatisfied. Blazina and coworkers and Arciero and colleagues have made similar observations.[8,12] In our review of 72 patellofemoral arthroplasties we found that 61 had a concomitant realignment procedure including 34 tibial tuberosity transfers: 18 medially, 13 cephalad, 1 laterally, and 2 posteriorly (reversal of Maquet). Patients whose patella "catches" as the knee goes from flexion to extension often have patella baja, itself a complication of previous surgery. Even when the tibial tuberosity is transferred cephalad, the baja condition can recur making it one of the more frustrating orthopaedic conditions.[11,13] Accordingly, the preoperative detection of patella baja is a contraindication to patellofemoral arthroplasty.

Medial/Lateral Compartment Pathology

Presumably the preoperative work-up will have ruled out significant arthritis of the other compartments. There are two possible approaches to the knee with bicompartmental arthritis (with one of the compartments being the patellofemoral joint): (1) placement of a total knee prosthesis or (2) placement of a femorotibial unicompartmental implant along with the patellofemoral replacement. The latter approach has the advantage of leaving both cruciates and an entire compartment intact. If a resurfacing implant is used for the femorotibial compartment, bone stock may be maintained. This approach is clearly more indicated in the younger patient whose surgeon is comfortable with unicompartmental arthroplasty.

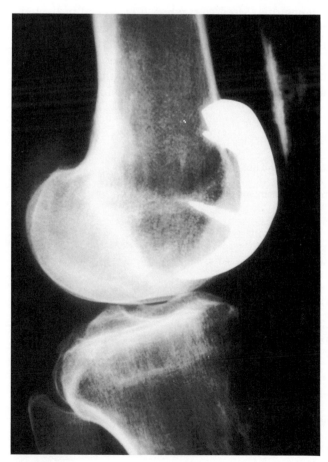

FIGURE 20-2
Patellofemoral replacement (lateral view). The distal tip of the trochlear implant is flush with the true trochlear groove. It does not rest on osteophytes and does not impinge on the tibial spines.

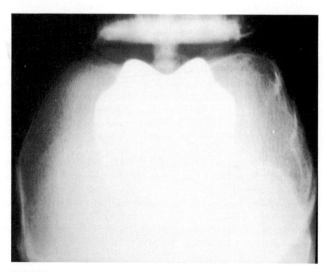

FIGURE 20-3
Patellofemoral replacement (axial view).

RESULTS

The lack of long-term follow-up studies make sweeping statements unreasonable. Cartier's report featured an average follow-up of 4 years, and in Arciero's, the average follow-up was 5.3 years. Most patients developed their arthritis as a result of malalignment, very few as a result of trauma. It is, therefore, not possible to correlate results with etiology. Good to excellent results have varied from 72 percent to 92 percent depending on the interpretation. When results are good, they have the potential for providing remarkable function. Cartier and colleagues found that two-thirds of all patients had essentially full flexion, that 70 percent could climb stairs without hesitation, and that roughly half could perform deep knee bends.

COMPLICATIONS

Complications are divided into those pertaining to the patella and those relating to other knee structures.

Patellar complications are by and large related to technique, e.g., an excessively distal trochlear component (see Surgical Technique) or persistent subluxation/dislocation. Loosening and wear have *not* been problems in the short- and medium-term follow-up reports published to date.

Nonpatellar knee problems include degeneration of the other compartments (especially the medial compartment). Should it occur, placement of a TKR or addition of one or two femorotibial unicompartmental replacements becomes necessary. The propensity for such degeneration can often be detected on the preoperative clinical and radiologic evaluation.

SUMMARY

Compared to other arthroplasties, patellofemoral arthroplasty is a recent procedure. It is somewhat premature to be dogmatic with respect to its place in the orthopaedic armamentarium. It remains infrequently indicated due to the rare occurrence of isolated end-stage arthritis. The prevalence of patellar malalignment syndromes combined with the increasingly athletic tendencies of our population may change this. Moreover, when it is indeed indicated, very few alternatives exist and even fewer can match results of a successful patellofemoral arthroplasty.

Continued monitoring of patients and refinements of technique and indications remain the goals of surgeons interested in this procedure.

REFERENCES

1. Lewallen DG, Riegger CL, Myers ER, Hayes WC: Effects of retinacular release and tibial tubercle elevation in patellofemoral degenerative joint disease. *J Orthop Res* 8:856 1990.
1a. Ficat RP, Ficat C, Gedeon P, Toussaint JB: Spongialization: A new treatment for diseased patellae. *Clin Orthop* 144:74, 1979.
2. Duncan C, McKeever D: Patellar prosthesis. *J Bone Joint Surg* 37A:1074, 1955.
3. Aglietti P, Insall JN, Walker PS, Trent P: A new patella prosthesis. *Clin Orthop* 107:175, 1975.
4. Worrell RV: Prosthetic resurfacing of the patella. *Clin Orthop* 144:91, 1979.
5. Harrington K: Long-term results of the McKeever patellar resurfacing prosthesis used as a salvage procedure for severe chondromalacia patellae. *Clin Orthop* 279:201 1992.
6. Froimson MI, Jiang Y, Kelly MA, et al: Mismatch of material properties at the patellofemoral joint: Significance in the etiology of cartilage lesions. *Orthop Res Soc* 152, 1990.
7. Lubinus HH: Patella glide bearing total replacement. *Orthopedics* 2:119, 1979.
8. Blazina ME, Fox JM, Del Pizzo W, et al: Patellofemoral replacements. *Clin Orthop* 144:98, 1979.
9. Corpe RS, Engh GA: A quantitative assessment of degenerative changes acceptable in the unoperated compartments of knees undergoing unicompartmental replacement. *Orthopedics* 13:320, 1990.
10. Mansat CH, Bonnel F, Jaeger JH: *L'Appareil Extenseur du Genou.* Paris, Masson, 1985.
11. Cartier P, Sanouiller J-L, Grelsamer RP: Patellofemoral arthroplasty—2–12 year follow-up study. *J Arthroplasty* 5:49, 1990.
12. Arciero RA, Toomey HE: Patellofemoral arthroplasty: A three to nine year follow-up study. *Clin Orthop* 236:60, 1988.
13. Noyes FR, Wojtys EM, Marshall MT: The early diagnosis and treatment of developmental patella infera syndrome. *Clin Orthop* 265:241, 1991.

CHAPTER 21

Patellectomy

Marlene De Maio
David J. Drez, Jr.

INTRODUCTION

The role of patellectomy in the treatment of knee problems has been controversial in the orthopaedic literature. The popularity of patellectomy was greater when there was little understanding of its biomechanics. Today, with more information about the importance of the patella with respect to normal knee function, more emphasis is placed on its preservation. The patella is an important biomechanical link between the quadriceps mechanism and the patellar tendon; it increases the effective lever arm of the quadriceps for knee flexion and extension.[1,2] However, there are certain conditions in which the patella cannot be preserved or circumstances in which conservative therapy or operative management have failed and therefore patellectomy is indicated.[1–30] Such conditions include osteomyelitis, malignant tumors, or severely comminuted fractures (particularly if such fractures are open). Relative indications for which patellectomy is indicated include degenerative lesions secondary to trauma, osteoarthritis, previous infection, and avascular necrosis. A special indication for patellectomy occurs in the patient with a total knee replacement or a patellar replacement who sustains a comminuted patellar fracture with loosening of the component and disruption of the extensor mechanism.[31]

This chapter delineates the absolute and relative indications for patellectomy. An understanding of the biomechanics of the patellofemoral joint is essential to this discussion. Both the nonoperative and operative management of patients with lesions of the patellofemoral joint rely heavily on biomechanical principles.

HISTORICAL REVIEW OF PATELLECTOMY

The first known patellectomy was performed by Putz in 1860 for chronic dislocation of the patella.[32] Yet surgery on the patella was not common at this time. Patellar fractures were the first closed fractures to be treated operatively, often by open reduction and internal fixation.[10] But this was not reported until 1877, 17 years after the first patellectomy. Lister and Cameron performed the first known open reductions and wiring of closed patella fractures.[18,33] Patellectomy was rarely performed,[10] but the major indication was comminuted fractures.[1]

The next period was one of condemnation for patellectomy. This period encompassed the early twentieth century. One report in particular was responsible for this trend. In 1909, Heineck reviewed 1100 cases of surgically treated patellar fractures. Thirteen of these cases were treated by patellectomy (five for fractures, four for tuberculosis, three for osteomyelitis, and one for primary sarcoma).[34] He concluded that the removal of the patella resulted in functional impairment of the knee, loss of protection of the femoral condyles, unacceptable appearance, and loss of quadriceps strength. He asserted that patellectomy be reserved as a treatment of "last resort" for severely comminuted fractures. Interestingly, he felt that the patella seemed to be an unnecessary structure for gait. During the next two decades, little information was added to influence this trend.[10] However, Ludloff in 1925 suggested the application of patellectomy for chronic osteoarthritis.[10]

The 1930s and 1940s brought enthusiasm for patellectomy. This period also was responsible for the earliest scientific investigations regarding the functional and biomechanical importance of the patella. Several authors during this period reported on both the clinical and experimental results of patellectomy. These early reports showed relatively quick recovery, minimal loss of function, and minimal postoperative pain.[5,13,15,35–41] Some of these reports are worth discussing because they still have an impact on the literature of today.

Blodgett and Fairchild first reported a small series on patellectomy in 1936 with better results than Heineck.[38] However, no real series of the results of patellectomy showing favorable outcomes was published until 1937,[10] when Brooke published his results of patellectomy in 30 cases of patellar fractures.[37] He noted recovery in 2 to 3 weeks and almost complete functional recovery. Brooke believed that the patellectomized knee was more efficient in extension power and speed. Hey-Groves in the same year examined eight of Brooke's patients and supported Brooke's conclusions.[1,35] Not until 1945 did Haxton show that patellectomy actually caused a decrease in the extensor power of the knee.[11]

Earlier, Bruce and Walmsley in 1942 demonstrated that the patella was an integral part of the extensor mechanism.[42] It was not until the second half of this century that poor results following patellectomy for fracture were again published, about 50 years after Heineck cautioned its use.[16,21,43-45] In 1949, Scott published the results of 101 patellar fractures treated with patellectomy and only 5 percent considered the leg as good as the contralateral nonoperated side. In addition, 60 percent complained of giving way and 90 percent of continued pain. Currently, better results, some with long-term follow-up, are reported, with 50 percent to 92 percent good or excellent results, but patellectomy is recommended only for severely comminuted or open patellar fractures in which other treatment is not possible.[8,9,18,21,25,26,46,47]

However, additional early reports of patellectomy for fracture demonstrated good results and few complications.[33,45,46,48-50] Such good early results, most with short follow-up, led to the application of patellectomy in the ensuing decades for degenerative arthritis, chondromalacia patellae, recurrent dislocation, and malalignment. Successful results using patellectomy for osteoarthritis were reported by Haggart, Haliburton and Sullivan, Geckler and Queranta, and Boucher.[13,15,39,40] Good results in patients with isolated patellofemoral arthritis have been reported recently.[1,17,43] The results are best if the patellofemoral joint alone is affected.[15,17,18,43,51]

The reported success rates of patellectomy for degenerative arthritis are higher than those reported for other reasons. However, the success rates are variable. Thompson and colleagues, Stougard, Geckeler and colleagues, and Ackroyd and coworkers in relatively large studies with long-term follow-up achieved success rates of 53 percent to 90 percent.[15-17,52] The criteria used were pain, range of motion, ability to work, extensor lag, and need for reoperation.[15-17,52] Patellectomy for these patients has had better results in older patients in some studies but not in others. Boucher reported data on 76 patients who were 50 years or older and had good results.[40] Contrarily, a review by Kelly and Insall of 100 patellectomies done in patients with an average age of 49.3 years showed that 76 percent of the patients under 40 years of age achieved a good or excellent result. This compared to a good or excellent result in 70.5 percent in patients more than 40 years old.[1]

The use of patellectomy for patients with chondromalacia patellae has been advocated. Bentley described 24 such patients.[4] He achieved 83 percent good or excellent results. He recommends patellectomy for extensive involvement of 2 cm or more in diameter in the appropriate patient.[5] Other authors have also had good results using chondromalacia as an indication.[6,8,12,26,53-56] Other authors have cautioned against the use of patellectomy in these patients. Kelly and Insall "do not believe that patellectomy is indicated in the primary treatment of chondromalacia patellae. However, when other surgical procedures have failed to give the desired result, patellectomy may be indicated." This conclusion was based on a review of 100 patellectomies done at the Hospital for Special Surgery. The average age was 49.3 years and average follow-up was 5.1 years. Seventy-two percent of patients achieved a good or excellent result.[1]

Patellectomy for recurrent subluxation or dislocation and chronic or persistent dislocation has been suggested by several authors who have obtained good results.[7,14,29,41] McFarland concluded that patellectomy was the best procedure for recurrent dislocation.[41] Teal also advocated patellectomy for recurrent dislocation. Yet, McKeever felt that patellectomy had no place as a primary procedure for recurrent dislocation.[44] However, most authors today do not recommend patellectomy as a primary procedure.[1,6,10,57] Most authors currently recommend that the primary procedure be some type of realignment or lateral release.[1,57] As Fulkerson and Hungerford point out, the extensor apparatus can subluxate and dislocate after patellectomy.[57] This perhaps explains the poor results many investigators have obtained in patients with malalignment undergoing patellectomy.[58] Fulkerson and Hungerford currently recommend that patellectomy, in general, be avoided in patients with patellar instability with exceptions of severe arthrosis or if other surgical procedures cannot provide relief.[57]

The problems evaluating the role of patellectomy reflect the diverse patient population and heterogeneous indications for which it has been applied. There are limited numbers of long-term studies with good follow-up in homogeneous patient and treatment groups. Most early studies have inadequate patient numbers and years of follow-up to yield meaningful results. Few recent studies have large numbers, homogeneous diagnosis, and long follow-up. Yet, the literature still provides no consistent method of evaluation of the results, either clinically or radiographically. Furthermore, there is no consistent pattern of rehabilitation, even when similar operative procedures are used. Although a review of the literature is essential to a discussion of the role of patellectomy, the biomechanical considerations of the patellofemoral joint are more useful and informative to the clinician. Such an undertaking will help to decide when patellectomy is indicated and what goals may be accomplished by its application in the appropriate patients. This is particularly important in patients with degenerative lesions of the patella.

BIOMECHANICAL CONSIDERATIONS OF PATELLECTOMY

The role of the patella in normal knee mechanics was not evaluated until the 1940s. As mentioned above, in 1942 Bruce and Walmsley showed the patella to be an integral part of the extensor mechanism.[42] Other studies have shown that the patella increases the efficiency of the extensor mechanism and increases the mechanical advantage of the quadriceps. The patella is a sesamoid bone and as such increases the radius from the center of rotation of the knee by lengthening the lever arm of the extensor mechanism. The mathematical expression of knee extension power is the quadriceps force multiplied by the extensor moment arm.[11] Biomechanical studies on cadaver legs have been done to determine the quadriceps moment arm.[11,59] The moment arm is expressed in percent as compared to the intact knee (which is 100 percent by definition). The experimental studies have confirmed Maquet's calculations.[2,69] The quadriceps moment arm changes with flexion and extension. It is therefore variable throughout the range of motion. The moment arm is small in flexion but increases in extension. The patella accounts for 31 percent of the entire moment arm at full extension.[2] The patella's contribution to the moment arm is as little as 13 percent between 90 and 120 degrees of flexion.[2]

A patellectomy will decrease both the quadriceps force and the extensor moment arm, thereby decreasing the extension power. As the amount of knee flexion increases, the extensor mechanism sinks into the intercondylar region, resulting in relative quadriceps insufficiency.[60] This has been demonstrated in numerous clinical evaluations of patellectomized patients.[3,8,15,17,40,59–63,70] In addition, the patella increases the contact area between the patellar tendon and the femur, which distributes compressive stress over a wider area.[64,65] Refer to Chap. 1 for a more thorough review of normal patellar biomechanics.

Both partial and total patellectomy affect patellar biomechanics. Total patellectomy will be considered here. Without the patella, the effective radius of the extensor mechanism from the center of rotation of the knee is shortened as mentioned above. The quadriceps must therefore produce more force to maintain the same torque from 45 to zero degrees of extension.

(Recall the knee extension power equals the quadriceps force times the moment arm.) Kaufer in 1971 showed that to maintain this torque, 15 percent to 30 percent more quadriceps force is needed.[59] This additional necessary force may be beyond the capacity of some patients. This will cause a relative quadricep insufficiency. The quadriceps may have been weakened by preexisting atrophy, postoperative atrophy, or postoperative effects of patellectomy on the quadriceps. Atrophy will decrease the cross-sectional area of the muscle and will therefore result in a decrease in contractile force.[66,67,75]

Also, compressive stress generated by the quadriceps mechanism is concentrated over a much smaller area without the patella. The forces measured in the tibiofemoral joint after patellectomy have been found to be increased as much as 250 percent.[51] The peak torque generated by the tibia after patellectomy has been measured to be less.[68] This is due to the shortened moment arm but may also be due to the higher imparted forces on the tibiofemoral joint as described above.

After patellectomy the extensor mechanism must be repaired so that the link between the quadriceps tendon and the patellar ligament can be maintained. Biomechanical studies of the strength of repair and the effect on the function of the extensor mechanism are available. Transverse repairs are superior to longitudinal repairs.[3,59] However, despite the wide variety of specific repairs described, all types of transverse repairs are biomechanically similar.[3] Not surprisingly, all types of longitudinal repairs are also biomechanically similar. As Kaufer reminds us, restoration of the extensor mechanism by any type of repair does not fully restore the extensor power.[2,3] This is because the presence of the patella lengthens the moment arm, as described above. Even repairing the extensor mechanism does not address this consequence of patellectomy. In addition, patellectomy changes the contractile properties of the quadriceps muscle, the exact effect depending on the type of repair as described below. So, even with repair of the extensor mechanism, the moment arm of the quadriceps remains shortened and the contractile properties of the quadriceps are altered. The consequence of this is to decrease the extensor power.

Lengthening the moment arm of the extensor mechanism was eloquently described by Maquet and later by Kaufer.[2,3,59,69] Surgical lengthening of the moment arm has been described in a variety of procedures, including the Maquet procedure, the modified Maquet procedure,[69] the Blounth procedure, and the Fulkerson procedure.[57] These procedures either elevate the tibial tubercle or anteriorly displace the proximal tibia. Anterior displacement of the proximal tibia by osteotomy has the advantage in that it may be combined with varus or valgus osteotomy.[3] Maquet has demonstrated that anterior displacement of the patellar tendon can lengthen the quadriceps moment arm and therefore negate this effect of patellectomy.[69] In an experimental model, Bandi showed up to a 33 percent decrease in patellofemoral loading forces for 10 mm of anterior displacement.[57] Repairing the quadriceps tendon to the patellar ligament combined with elevation of the tibial tubercle of 1.5 cm results in complete correction of the quadriceps moment arm after patellectomy.[59] Ferguson and colleagues have shown in cadavers that anterior displacement of the tibial tubercle relieves contact stress and that the optimum amount of elevation is about one-half inch.[72]

Patellectomy also affects the quadriceps resting length. A decrease in a muscle's resting length will decrease the force (active tension and total tension) it may generate.[66,73] Shortened muscle fibers are also more susceptible to injury; they absorb less force before tearing.[73] Longitudinal closure of the extensor mechanism after patellectomy shortens the quadriceps resting length.[3] This may account for the reported strength deficits in the patellectomized knee despite adequate rehabilitation. Transverse closure of the defect in the extensor mechanism increases the resting fiber length of the quadriceps.[3] Although increasing the resting length of the muscle decreases the amount of active tension generated, the total tension is actually increased. This is because of the contribution of passive stretch, that is, preloading of the lengthened muscle. A muscle whose resting length is increased is preloaded and can therefore generate more total tension.[66,73] This has been documented in cadaver knees by Kaufer who showed that transverse repair requires 15 percent more quadriceps force to maintain the same torque while longitudinal repair requires 30 percent more quadriceps force.[59] Muscles in a lengthened position can absorb more force prior to tearing as compared to muscles in a shortened position.[73]

While various surgical procedures can negate some of the biomechanical effects of patellectomy, Kaufer cautions us that certain physiologic effects persist.[3] Transverse repair of the extensor mechanism can minimize loss of extensor power by maintaining the length of the quadriceps. Elevation of the tibial tubercle or anteriorization of the proximal tibial by osteotomy can increase the moment arm.[59] However, the amount of power that the quadriceps can generate remains decreased. This explains the extensor lag and 25 percent to 60 percent loss of extensor power

reported in postpatellectomy patients, regardless of procedure and rehabilitation.[3,8,15,17,40,59–63,70,74,75] Numerous investigations have documented the loss of strength after patellectomy evaluated by manual muscle testing, maximal weight-lifting measurements, isometric and isokinetic muscle testing, and strain gauges in clinical and cadaveric studies.[17,60,62,63,68,70] In general, extensor power loss should be expected and the degree of loss relates to the patient's functional result.[4,62] The loss of extensor power has been measured to be 25 percent to 60 percent as compared to the intact contralateral knee in clinical studies.[17,60,62,70,74] The peak torque generated by the quadriceps in patients after patellectomy was noted to be decreased by an average of 54 percent at the test speed of 30 degrees per second and by 49 percent at 180 degrees per second on the Cybex-II isokinetic dynamometer.[63] Additionally, torque values were lower throughout the range of motion except at or near full extension. In the same study, the peak torque generated by the ipsilateral hamstrings was normal at 30 degrees per second. Studies on cadaveric knees have yielded similar results.[68]

Knee motion after patellectomy has been studied; extensor lag and decreased flexion have been commonly documented.[15,17,18,59–63,76] Several explanations are given for this decrease in range in the postpatellectomy patient. First, a distortion in the path of the instant centers has been noted and it is strikingly so in the last 60 degrees of extension.[77] Second, extensor lag is a consequence of the shortened moment arm after patellectomy alone and the altered contractile properties of the quadriceps. (Recall that extensor power is decreased and this predisposes to extensor lag.[3]) Third, removal of the patella shortens the extensor mechanism and predisposes to a loss of flexion.[3] One study on cadaver knees after patellectomy documented a decrease in the excursion of the quadriceps of about 1.5 cm from zero to 90 degrees flexion.[68] This may be further accentuated by postoperative adhesions and influenced by any preexisting preoperative condition.[3] The average loss of motion has been measured at 18 degrees.[60]

Alterations in gait have been documented after patellectomy by high speed photography, by electrogoniometry, and by dynamic electromyography.[60,62] Hill and colleagues examined 12 patients who had undergone unilateral patellectomy. In the patient groups with 45 percent loss of extension power, walking velocity was 75.9 m/min. In comparison, the group with 60 percent loss of extension power had a walking velocity of 54.3 m/min. Single limb support time was increased in the group with less extension power. Eighty percent of the patients had early soleus firing before heel strike. Early soleus firing was hypothesized to decrease quadriceps demand at heel strike by placing the foot in more plantar flexion to decrease the knee flexion thrust at heel strike.[62] Decreased flexion and extension have been noted during normal gait, ascending and descending stairs, and active range of motion.[60] The greatest loss of flexion occurs during stance phase but the amount of loss is variable.[62] About 7 degrees on average (about 50 percent of the stance phase flexion) is lost.[60] The explanation for this also relates to the decreased moment arm after patellectomy. With knee flexion, the extensor mechanism sinks into the intercondylar notch, further reducing the extensor moment arm and causing a relative quadriceps insufficiency.[60]

Knee instability after patellectomy has also been investigated. Kaufer explains that the discussion of instability in the postpatellectomy patient encompasses both subjective and objective parameters.[3] The postpatellectomy patient will have the subjective feeling of instability due to extensor lag, decreased extensor power, and quadriceps weakness. This will manifest as giving way. Pain and apprehension will complicate this subjective feeling of instability.[3] Objective parameters that lead to pathologic laxity include preexisting conditions,[3] disturbed balance between extensors and flexors,[2,3,63] loss of the stabilizing effect of the patella,[60] and increased strain leading to increased ligamentous laxity.[2,60,61] The imbalance between the extensors and the flexors can be thought of as an imbalance between the agonists and antagonists.[2,3] This can lead to an increase in ligamentous strain.[2,3] This may lead to increased posterior tibial displacement.[1,2] Additionally, after patellectomy the course of the patellar tendon is no longer parallel to the posterior cruciate and therefore provides less resistance to anterior displacement of the distal femur.[78] Important preexisting conditions include abnormal primary restraints (cruciate ligament insufficiency), abnormal secondary restraints (meniscal or collateral ligament pathology), or certain systemic diseases (rheumatoid or other inflammatory arthritides and Ehlers-Danlos). Medial instability has also been noted in 25 percent of patients.[79] Sutton and colleagues found that 19 of 26 patients after patellectomy had clinical instability, but the breakdown (medial versus lateral, anterior versus posterior, and rotational) was not reported.[60]

INDICATIONS FOR PATELLECTOMY

The reported indications for patellectomy are numerous, yet they have not always been clearly stated in the literature. The published indications are listed in Table 21-1.[1-6,8-13,15-20,22-31,51,80,81,84] The indications for patellectomy in the patient with degenerative disease have been debated. Currently, it is best thought of as a procedure with limited indications. Numerous authors feel that the patella should be preserved whenever possible.[1-3,10,16,57] The relative lack of solid reproducible homogeneous clinical reports and gaps in experimental studies still makes it difficult to give absolute indications for patellectomy in the patient with degenerative disease. However, enough information suggests an approach to the patient with painful patellofemoral disease. In general, the goal is to relieve pain with minimal disturbance to the extensor mechanism.[2-5,10,12,15]

First, the etiology of the degenerative arthritis should be determined. A good history and examination of previous records and radiographs may provide the clinician with this information. Physical examination and appropriate diagnostic imaging will provide further information. Radiographs, bone scans, and magnetic resonance imaging (MRI) studies are all useful. (The evaluation of the patellofemoral joint is the subject of a previous section; the reader is referred there.) Specific diagnostic entities that will influence the outcome and treatment are sought. These include abnormalities of primary restraints (cruciate ligament insufficiency), abnormalities of secondary restraints (meniscal or collateral ligament pathology), disorders of cartilage (chondromalacia patellae, posttraumatic changes), disorders of bone (avascular necrosis, nonunion, osteochondritis dissecans, osteomyelitis), patellar maltracking (subluxation or dislocation), and systemic disease (inflammatory arthritis). If the patient has one of these disorders, treatment should first be directed toward solving this problem. Even if the patient does eventually require patellectomy, the effects of the above problems must be taken into account preoperatively.

The patient may have no apparent explanation for the degenerative lesions. For example, the patient may have primary osteoarthritis. In this case and in cases above, the extensor mechanism should be carefully evaluated for atrophy, imbalance with the hamstrings, and maltracking. Symptomatic therapy is prescribed, using a nonsteroidal drug in patients without contraindications to these medications. Aspirin given as a dose of 3 g/day for 6 weeks may be beneficial in patients with chondromalacia patellae.[6] Physical therapy is then prescribed to address any deficiencies or imbalance. Braces or orthotics may help control maltracking or valgus thrust, respectively.[57] Failure of this regimen may lead the clinician to consider operative interventions other than patel-

TABLE 21-1
Indications for Patellectomy Reported in the Literature

I. Trauma

  A. Acute fracture

    1. Comminuted

    2. Open

    3. Cannot reconstruct

  B. Sequela of trauma

    1. Intractable pain (in the absence of reflex sympathetic dystrophy)

    2. Symptomatic nonunion

    3. Osteomyelitis

    4. Severe patellofemoral osteoarthritis

    5. Persistent dislocation (irreducible)—rare

    6. Avascular necrosis—rare

    7. Traumatic chondromalacia patellae, Outerbridge grades III or IV

    8. Osteochondritis dissecans (juvenile and adult)

II. Nontraumatic Acquired Patellar Disorders

  A. Chondromalacia patellae

    1. Extensive involvement

      a. Outerbridge grades III or IV

      b. 2 cm or more

    2. Irreversible and advanced biomechanical or biochemical disorder (after Jackson)

  B. Tracking abnormalities associated with

    1. Patellar malposition

      a. Patella baja

      b. Patella alta

    2. Dislocation

      a. Recurrent

      b. Chronic

    3. Subluxation

      a. Recurrent

      b. Chronic

  C. Inflammatory arthritides—rheumatoid arthritis

  D. Osteoarthritis

  E. Infection

    1. Chronic bacterial osteomyelitis

    2. Tuberculosis

  F. Tumors—locally aggressive or malignant

    1. Aneurysmal bone cyst

    2. Chondroblastoma

    3. Giant cell tumor

    4. Osteoblastoma

    5. Malignant tumors—rare

  G. Hemophilic arthropathy

III. Total Knee Arthroplasty

  A. Primary excision

  B. Secondary excision

    1. Complication

      a. Rupture of patellar tendon

      b. Patellar fracture

      c. Component failure

      d. Infection (especially with adhesions)

IV. After Other Procedures Which Have Failed or Were Not Totally Successful (Persistent Pain)

  A. Fusion

  B. Resurfaced patella

    1. Metal or plastic

    2. Cemented or noncemented

  C. Soft tissue realignment

  D. Lengthening of the extensor moment arm

    1. Tibial tubercle elevation

    2. Anteriorization of the proximal tibia using an osteotomy

lectomy at this point. Such procedures depend on the patient's specific diagnosis. For example, maltracking might be treated by soft tissue realignment or lateral release. Degenerative lesions or nonunion without maltracking might be treated by a partial patellectomy.[6] Patelloplasty may also have a role.[6] These procedures have the advantage of preserving the moment arm of the extensor mechanism provided by the patella.

Other degenerative lesions may benefit from other procedures designed to alter the biomechanics of the patellofemoral joint. We feel that these procedures should be considered before patellectomy. In this manner, the patient retains the extensor mechanism and can be treated symptomatically. Patients with hypertrophic spurs may have these debrided. This may be combined with various osteotomies. The extensor moment arm may be lengthened by anteriorization of the tibial tubercle or proximal tibial osteotomy. The proximal tibial osteotomy has the advantage that it may be combined with a varus or valgus osteotomy.[3] These procedures also have the benefit of changing the area of contact of the degenerated patella on its femoral articulation. Studies of the patellar articulation on the unloaded[64] and loaded[82] patellofemoral joint have shown dramatic changes in the patellofemoral contact pattern with flexion and extension. As Dinham and French explained, the "worn patella can scour" the distal femur with movement.[51] It therefore follows that lengthening the moment arm will change some of the contact pattern, the amount of which will depend on the amount of lengthening. This has been demonstrated in studies on cadavers by Ferguson and colleagues.[72] Patellofemoral contact stress by anterior displacement of the tibial tubercle was achieved and the greatest relief of stress occurred at 90 degrees of flexion.[72] Depending on the osteotomy, or if debridement of the patella is done alone, the patient may be a candidate for postoperative continuous passive motion. This may promote cartilaginous repair.[67]

Should the patient not achieve success with any of the above procedures, the clinician should next determine the reason for failure. Although failure may be a consequence of the natural history of the disease process, that is, progressive osteoarthritis, other diagnoses may have influenced or caused the failure. For example, the patient may have developed a symptomatic loose body that is now causing effusion, locking, and pain. This can be treated and the consideration of patellectomy can be delayed. Should the patient have no other cause for failure, patellectomy can now be considered.

Before patellectomy, the patient should again be evaluated for quadriceps atrophy, extensor and flexor imbalance, extensor maltracking, and range of motion. Before patellectomy, these factors should be optimized by vigorous rehabilitation. Patients with symptomatic arthritis should be treated to "quiet down" their symptoms. In addition, contraindications to patellectomy must be ruled out. Patients with an uncertain diagnosis of patellofemoral pain are especially poor candidates. A subset of this category is the patient with reflex sympathetic dystrophy. Patients with minimal pathology of patellar cartilage as documented on arthroscopy, other surgery, or MRI are not candidates for patellectomy unless they have a severe, unresponsive maltracking disorder. Patellectomy should also be avoided in young patients; our impression is to limit patellectomy to patients over age 30 years. This is an arbitrary limit based on clinical impressions.

As Fulkerson and Hungerford point out, patellectomy "is rightfully considered the end of the line."[57] Kelly and Insall caution that alternatives for patellectomy can usually be found.[1] Partial patellectomy is sometimes an option. However, using the above guidelines (Table 21-2), we feel that patellectomy does have limited indications and can lead to a satisfactory outcome. In summary, Berkheiser's indications for patellectomy published in 1939 still provide one of the best descriptions of these surgical candidates.[85] His indications are listed below.

TABLE 21-2
Indications and Contraindications for Patellectomy: Guidelines

I. Absolute Indications
  A. Tumors
  B. Infections
  C. Salvage procedure
     1. Acute fracture—fixation not possible
        a. Open
        b. Severely comminuted
        c. Both
     2. Osteoarthritis
        a. Ankylosis of the patellofemoral joint
        b. Severe osteoarthritis of the patellofemoral joint
     3. As an alternative to patelloplasty
  D. Failure to achieve a successful result in a complaint patient after appropriate therapy
     1. Severe chondromalacia patellae in an older patient
     2. Inflammatory arthritis
     3. Severe patellofemoral pain after realignment

II. Relative Indications
  A. Failure to achieve a successful result with appropriate therapy in younger patient (<40 years old)—highly limited
  B. Acute fracture—fixation possible
     1. Severely comminuted
     2. Open
     3. Both
  C. Patient unable to comply with postoperative rehabilitation
  D. Patient elderly, sedentary, or bedridden

III. Contraindications
  A. Uncertain diagnosis of patellofemoral pain
  B. Noncompliant patient who had not had rehabilitation
  C. Failure to have undergone appropriate rehabilitation
  D. Young age (< 30 years old) and the absence of absolute indications
  E. Minimal cartilage pathology (in the absence of other pathology) diagnosed on
     1. Arthroscopy
     2. MRI
  F. Reflex sympathetic dystrophy

Berkheiser's Indications in Degenerative Lesions

- Degenerative lesions present for several years
- X-rays showing definite evidence of degenerative joint disease

- Recurrent symptoms after repeated conservative treatment
- Arthritis quiescent at the time of surgery
- Extension to within 20 degrees of normal
- Patient can stand and walk and cooperate with postoperative management

In general, the most recent clinical studies reviewing patellectomy for degenerative lesions have an overall success rate of 60 percent to 90 percent.[1,4,10,13,18,52,85] Patients with minimal radiographic changes at the tibiofemoral joint have been shown to have better results.[16] Age at the time of patellectomy has not been a consistent factor associated with outcome.[1,5,17,79]

SURGICAL TECHNIQUE

Various surgical techniques for excision of the patella and repair of the extensor mechanism have been reported. The goals of any procedure are to decrease or control the patient's symptoms with the least disruption of the extensor mechanism. If the patella is to be excised, the extensor mechanism can still be maintained. This can be accomplished by a strong repair, possibly with reinforcement, and by the selected use of procedures designed to minimize the biomechanical effects of patellectomy. These selected additional procedures have already been discussed in the biomechanics section of this chapter. They include elevation of the tibial tubercle and anteriorization of the proximal tibia via an osteotomy.

The basic procedure is probably best described by Boyd and Hawkins.[87] A midline vertical incision is used. The quadriceps tendon and the patellar ligament are identified and then incised in the direction of their fibers. Proximally, the extensor mechanism is incised in the midline. The trochlear surface is protected with a malleable retractor. The patella is then split in half lengthwise with an osteotome. The patella is excised by grasping it with a towel clip or bone clamp and first incising the extensor mechanism proximally to the patella's equator and then distally up to the equator. The extensor mechanism is repaired longitudinally by imbricating the vertical margins in a double row of interrupted sutures (Fig. 21-1). After the closure, the knee should achieve 90 degrees flexion without stressing the suture line.[57] The tracking of the extensor mechanism should also be evaluated prior to skin closure. A lateral retinacular release is rarely necessary.[57] The quadriceps tendon may be divided up to 10 cm proximally and

the patellar ligament may be divided to the tibial tubercle.[57]

Kaufer showed a greater reduction of extensor power with longitudinal closure than the transverse closure and stated that longitudinal repair does not restore the linking function of the patella.[2,59] Fulkerson and Hungerford explain that this may not be clinically significant.[57] In their discussion of Kaufer's results, they point out that Kaufer's closure was side-to-side, not imbricated, and that the transfer of quadriceps power may have been transferred to the tibia by the retinacula, rather than through a central tendon. This would decrease the extensor moment arm. In addition, they recognize two other important clinical points with longitudinal closure—better range of motion is possible and none of their patients developed an extensor lag.

Other types of extensor mechanism repair after patellectomy include transverse repair (as advocated by Kaufer)[2,3,59] and the Chari "double tourniquet" repair.[88] The extensor repair may be reinforced by an inverted v-plasty[89] or cruciate type.[77,90] The inverted v-plasty, cruciate repair (the "St. Andrews cross" method), or vastus medialis advancement are special types of transverse repairs and have no mechanical advantage over the simple transverse repair.[18,59,91]

Certain techniques may help prevent postoperative complications. The tube technique as described by Compere and colleagues has been reported to prevent excessive ossification of the quadriceps tendon with a good success rate.[92] Briefly, this technique involves a transverse incision through which the patella is exposed. First, a medial parapatellar capsular incision is made and then a lateral parapatellar incision. The patella is then enucleated. The medial border of quadriceps tendon is brought under the lateral border and sutured together to form a tube. The sutures lie deep to the repaired quadriceps tendon and superficial to the femoral sulcus. The vastus medialis is advanced to close the medial capsule. Ossification, when it occurs, will appear in the tube.

Prevention or delay of further osteoarthritis may be accomplished by procedures that increase the moment arm to optimize loading. Early motion and rehabilitation will help strengthen the quadriceps, promote range of motion, and prevent adhesions. It may promote cartilage healing.

POSTOPERATIVE REHABILITATION

The trend in postoperative management is for rapid mobilization and strengthening. Certainly, this must be individualized. However, the following general guidelines are useful. Initially, the patient has a compressive dressing and a knee immobilizer. The patient may perform quadriceps strengthening exercises immediately, including straight leg raises. The knee immobilizer is removed between days 5 and 7 postoperatively and gentle range of motion is begun. Both active extension and flexion can be performed. Fulkerson and Hungerford note that most patients achieve 90 degrees flexion by postoperative week 2.[57]

A knee immobilizer should be used for 6 weeks, although as little as 3 weeks has been reported with good results.[16,86] Weight bearing as tolerated is initially prescribed and full weight bearing can be obtained within the first 2 weeks. Continued range of motion and strengthening should be gradually increased. Maximum function usually occurs at 6 to 12 months after surgery, although some patients may note continued improvement up to 3 years.[21,43,93]

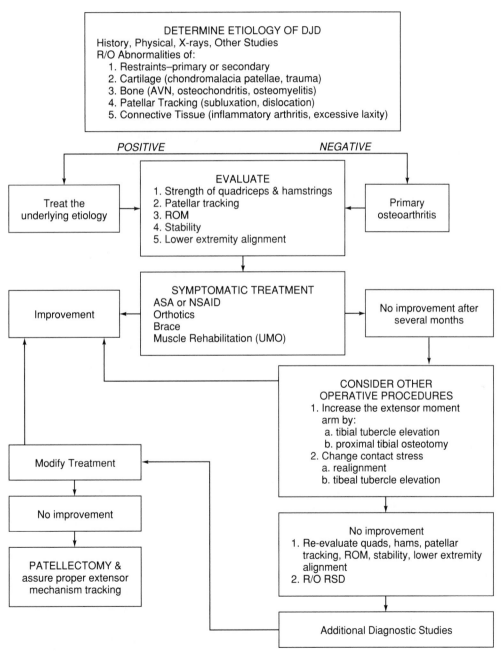

FIGURE 21-1
Patellectomy: Indications in Degenerative Disease.

TABLE 21-3
Complications of Patellectomy

I. Effects on the extensor mechanism	IV. Altered gait
A. Decreased extensor power (25–60%)	A. Walking
1. Decreased quadriceps contractile force and peak torque	1. Decreased stance phase flexion
2. Decreased moment arm	2. Decresed walking velocity
3. Imbalance between extensors (agonists) and flexor (antagonists)	3. Increased single limb support time
B. Intrinsic changes in the quadriceps	4. Early soleus firing before heel strike
1. Atrophy	B. Stairs
a. From preexisting atrophy	1. Decreased flexion
b. From inadequate postoperative rehabilitation	V. Degenerative changes
2. Shortened resting length	A. Tibiofemoral arthritis
a. From repair of the extensor mechanism after removal of the patella (loss of a biologic spacer)	B. Hypertrophic degenerative joint disease of the tibiofemoral joint
b. Longitudinal repair	C. Cartilage changes
C. Subluxation or dislocation of the remaining extensor mechanism	1. Chondromalacia patellae
II. Altered loading of the knee	2. Degenerative changes
A. Imbalance between the extensors (agonists) and flexors (antagonist)—increased strain on the ligaments	VI. Heterotopic ossification
B. Distorted paths of the instant centers	A. Of bony structures
C. Increased forces in the tibiofemoral joint	B. Of the patellar tendon
D. Decreased surface contact area for the extensor mechanism	1. Minimal
E. Increased laxity—posterior translation of the tibia	2. Excessive—decreases range of motion
III. Altered motion	VII. Other
A. Extensor lag	A. Pain
B. Decreased flexion	B. Boutonnière deformity
C. Decreased quadriceps excursion	C. Disruption of the extensor mechanism repair
	1. Infection
	2. Adequate repair
	3. Too rapid or vigorous rehabilitation
	D. Necrosis of the patellar tendon
	E. Adhesions
	F. Altered appearance

COMPLICATIONS

Besides the usual complications that accompany any surgery (infection, blood loss), certain complications are specific to patellectomy. The types of reported complications after patellectomy are listed in Table 21-3.[20,25,27,28,42,43,63,68,74,77,83,90,94,95] The biomechanical consequences of the procedure are discussed in the biomechanics section of this chapter. They are predictable and present to some degree in all postpatellectomy patients. The loss of extensor power is a significant consequence of patellectomy and is responsible for quadriceps weakness, altered gait, abnormal loading of the knee, and increased laxity. Some of these cannot be avoided and may be a cause

of postoperative pain. A decrease in both flexion and extension may be due to prolonged immobilization or the effects of the patellectomy alone.

Postoperative pain, while highly subjective, can be a complication of patellectomy. Several studies have documented pain to be the single most important factor in the functional outcome after patellectomy.[62] Pain may be responsible for decreased range of motion and altered patterns of gait. Hill and colleagues observed that persistence of pain in the poorest functional group was associated with prior meniscectomy, markedly decreased quadriceps power, abnormalities of gait, and arthritic changes on x-ray.[62] Persistent postoperative pain that is clinically significant (causing a change in activities of daily living, diminished range of motion, etc.) can be expected in about 20 percent to 45 percent of patients.[1,15,17,26]

A boutonniere deformity in which the femoral condyles buttonholed through a longitudinal defect in the extensor mechanism has been described.[94] The extensor mechanism repair may rupture[17] secondary to infection, inadequate repair, or too vigorous rehabilitation. Adhesions may develop and these can further limit range of motion.[3,17] Necrosis of the patellar tendon has also been described. The remaining extensor mechanism may dislocate or subluxate.[20,90]

Degenerative changes after patellectomy have been observed to progress more rapidly than the intact contralateral knee in clinical studies.[17,43,54,74] However, some authors dispute this finding.[15,16,18,21,23,25,26,83] One study with one of the largest follow-up periods reported (20 years) did not show any increased incidence of arthrosis.[26] However, experimental models in the rabbit have clearly documented synovial inflammation, proliferation of invasive pannus, destruction of articular cartilage, and limited spur formation.[95] This was also confirmed in the dog model by DePalma and colleagues.[97,98] Although these data cannot be directly applied clinically, they do lend credence to the dictum of patellectomy as a salvage procedure.

Heterotopic ossification has been documented in up to 50 percent to 66 percent of patients after patellectomy.[17,28,90,93] It may occur in the soft tissues or around patellar remnants. Stougard noted that 37 of 76 cases in 72 patients had visible bone formation at the site of the patella.[17] In one of his cases, the entire patella had regenerated.[17] Unless such ossification is extensive, the amount of calcification or ectopic bone formation does not affect function.[17,21,25,28,74,83] It may, however, be related to persistent postoperative pain.[93] Rupture of the extensor mechanism repair has been described in about 3 percent of cases.[28]

PROCEDURES AFTER PATELLECTOMY

Patellectomy does not exclude subsequent surgical procedures. Tibial tubercle elevation, proximal tibial osteotomy, fusion, total knee arthroplasty and arthroscopy can all be successfully performed in the postpatellectomy patient.[2,3,78,80,99–101] After patellectomy the joint capacity has been noted to be limited (about 40 cc as compared to 80 to 120 cc) as determined by saline injection.[101] This has clinical significance for arthroscopy and arthrography. Numerous authors have suggested that a posterior stabilized total knee arthroplasty system be used for those patients without patellae undergoing knee reconstruction.[1–3,60,78,80,99,100] It is thought that a posterior stabilized system will prevent posterior displacement of the tibia (and relative anterior displacement of the femur).[1–3,60,80,99,100]

SUMMARY

Patellectomy has been performed for numerous reasons with variable results. In the patient with degenerative lesions of the patella, patellectomy can be a successful alternative if all other therapeutic options have been exhausted.[1,6,10,26,59] Although it has been termed the procedure of "last resort,"[34] it may be the only option in the appropriate patient. Once the diagnosis has been confirmed, specific goals can be set. For the patient with documented degenerative patellofemoral disease who has failed a period of appropriate nonoperative management or other surgical procedures, patellectomy may be considered as a salvage procedure to alleviate pain. It does not prevent surgical intervention at a later date. However, it must be remembered that patellectomy always disrupts the extensor mechanism and can cause increased pathologic laxity and degenerative changes. For these reasons, patellectomy should be reserved for the "end of the line."[57]

REFERENCES

1. Kelly MA, Insall JN: Patellectomy. *Orthop Clin North Am* 17:289, 1986.
2. Kaufer H: Patellar biomechanics. *Clin Orthop* 144:51,1979.
3. Kaufer H.: Management of knee joint disorders, in *American Academy of Orthopaedic Surgeons Symposium of Reconstructive Surgery of the Knee.* St. Louis, Mosby, 1978, chap 12, pp 123–130.
4. Bentley G: Chondromalacia patellae. *J Bone Joint Surg* 52A:221, 1970.
5. Bentley G: Current concepts of etiology and treatment of chondromalacia patellae. *Clin Orthop* 189:209, 1984.
6. Chrisman OD, Snook GA: The role of patelloplasty and patellectomy in the arthritic knee. *Clin Orthop* 101:40, 1974.
7. Miller MD, Hausman M, Jokl P, Lindsey RW: Permanent post-traumatic patellar dislocation. *J Trauma* 28:1389, 1988.

8. Flinchum D: Patellectomy: When, why, and how. *South Med J* 59:897, 1966.

9. Marya SK, Bhan S, Dave PK: Comparative study of knee function after patellectomy and osteosynthesis with a tension band wire following patellar fractures. *Int Surg* 72:211, 1987.

10. Peeples RE, Margo MK: Function after patellectomy. *Clin Orthop* 132:180, 1978.

11. Haxton H: The function of the patella and the effects of its excision. *Surg Gynecol Obstet* 80:389, 1945.

12. Outerbridge RE, Dunlop JAY: The problem of chondromalacia patella. *Clin Orthop* 110:117, 1975.

13. Haliburton RA, Sullivan CR: The patella in degenerative joint diseases. A clinicopathologic study. *Arch Surg* 77:677, 1958.

14. Teal F: Treatment of dislocation of the patella. *Clin Orthop* 3:61, 1954.

15. Geckeler EO, Queranta AV: Patellectomy for degenerative arthritis of the knee—Late results. *J Bone Joint Surg* 44A:1109, 1962.

16. Ackroyd CE, Polyzoides AJ: Patellectomy for osteoarthritis. A study of 81 patients followed from two to 22 years. *J Bone Joint Surg* 60B:353, 1978.

17. Stougard J: Patellectomy. *Acta Orthop Scand* 41:110, 1970.

18. West FE: End results of patellectomy. *J Bone Joint Surg* 44A:1089, 1962.

19. Insall JN: Disorders of the patella, in *Surgery of the Knee,* edited by JN Insall. Churchill-Livingstone, 1984, pp. 191–260.

20. Hughston/Walsh/Puddu, personal communication.

21. Wilkinson J: Fracture of the patella treated by local excision. A long-term follow-up. *J Bone Joint Surg* 59B:352, 1977.

22. Bostman O, Kiviluoto O, Nirhamo J: Comminuted displaced fractures of the patella. *Injury* 13:196, 1981.

23. Khermosh O, Weissman SL: Total patellectomy in fractures of the patella. *Isr J Med Sci* 9:67, 1973.

24. Salerno DJ: Fractures of the patella: Closed and open repair. *J Am Osteopath Assoc* 74:538, 1975.

25. Mishra VS: Late results of patellectomy in fractured patella. *Acta Orthop Scand* 43:256, 1972.

26. Jakobsen J, Christensen KS, Rasmussen OS: Patellectomy—A 20 year follow-up. *Acta Orthop Scand* 56:430, 1985.

27. Jensen DB, Hansen LB: Patellectomy for chondromalacia. *Acta Orthop Scand* 60:17, 1989.

28. Chakraverty AC: Patellectomy for chondromalacia patellae. *J Royal Med Serv* 58:104, 1972.

29. Dandy DJ, Poirier H: Chondromalacia and the unstable patella. *Acta Orthop Scand* 46:695, 1975.

30. Gottschalk FA, Solomon L, Isaacson C, Schmaman A: Aneurysmal bone cysts of the patella secondary to chondroblastoma. *S Afr Med J* 67:105, 1985.

31. Rand JA: Knee and Leg: Reconstruction, in *Orthopaedic Knowledge Update 3*. Park Ridge, IL, American Academy of Orthopaedic Surgeons, 1990.

32. Cohn BNE: Total and partial patellectomy. An experimental study. *Surg Gynecol Obstet* 79:526, 1944.

33. Doobie RP, Ryerson S: The treatment of fractured patella by excision. *Am J Surg* 55:339, 1942.

34. Heineck AP: The modern operative treatment of fractures of the patella. *Surg Gynecol Obstet* 9:177, 1909.

35. Hey-Groves EW: A note on the extension apparatus of the knee joint. *Br J Surg* 24:747, 1937.

36. Watson-Jones R: *Fractures and Other Bone and Joint Injuries.* Baltimore, Williams & Wilkins, 1940.

37. Brooke R: The treatment of fractured patella by excision. A study of morphology and function. *Br J Surg* 24:733, 1937.

38. Blodgett WE, Fairchild RD: Fractures of the patella. Results of total and partial excisions of the patella for acute fracture. *JAMA* 106:2121, 1936.

39. Haggart GE: Surgical treatment of degenerative arthritis of the knee joint. *N Engl J Med* 236:971, 1947.

40. Boucher HH: Patellectomy in the geriatric patient. *Clin Orthop* 11:33, 1958.

41. McFarlan B: Excision of the patella for recurrent dislocation. *J Bone Joint Surg* 30B:158, 1948.

42. Bruce J, Walmsley R: Excision of patella. *J Bone Joint Surg* 24:311, 1942.

43. Burton VM, Thomas HM: Results of excision of the patella. *Surg Gynecol Obstet* 135:753, 1972.

44. McKeever DC: Recurrent dislocation of the patella. *Clin Orthop* 3:55, 1954.

45. Scott JC: Fractures of the patella. *J Bone Joint Surg* 31B:76, 1949.

46. Horowitz T, Lambert RG: Patellectomy in the military service. *Surg Gynecol Obstet* 82:423, 1946.

47. Sanderson MC: The fractured patella: A long term follow-up study. *Aust NZ J Surg* 45:49, 1975.

48. MacAusland WR: Total excision of the patella for fracture. *Am J Surg* 72:510, 1946.

49. O'Donoghue DH: The place of patellectomy in treatment of fractures of the patella. *South Surgeon* 15:640, 1949.

50. Schmier AA: Excision of the fractured patella. *Surg Gynecol Obstet* 81:370, 1945.

51. Dinham JM, French PR. Results of patellectomy for osteoarthritis. *Postgrad Med J* 48:590, 1972.

52. Thompson WJ, Schweigel JF: Patellectomy: A 21-year follow-up. *Can J Surg* 11:173, 1968.

53. Bronitsky J: Chondromalacia patella. *J Bone Joint Surg* 29:931, 1937.

54. Soto-Hall R: Traumatic degeneration on the articular cartilage of the patella. *J Bone Joint Surg* 27:426, 1945.

55. Gray C: Chondromalacia patellae. *Br Med J* 1:427, 1948.

56. DeNio AE, Hudson OC: An end result study of patellectomy. *Am J Surg* 94:62, 1957.

57. Fulkerson JP, Hungerford DS: *Disorders of the Patellofemoral Joint,* 2d ed. Baltimore, Williams & Wilkins, 1990.

58. Heywood AWB: Recurrent dislocation of the patella. *J Bone Joint Surg* 43B:507, 1961.

59. Kaufer H: Mechanical function of the patella. *J Bone Joint Surg* 53A:1551, 1971.

60. Sutton FS, Thompson CH, Lipke J, Kettelkamp DB: The effect of patellectomy of knee function. *J Bone Joint Surg* 58A:537, 1976.

61. Lewis MM, Fitzgerald PF, Jacobs B, Insall J: Patellectomy, an analysis of one hundred cases. *J Bone Joint Surg* 58A:736, 1976.

62. Hill JA, Mayness DR, Yocum LA, et al: Gait and functional analysis of patients following patellectomy. *Orthopedics* 6:724, 1983.

63. Watkins MP, Harris BA, Wender S, et al: Effect of patellectomy on the function of the quadriceps and hamstrings. *J Bone Joint Surg* 65A:390, 1983.

64. Wiberg G: Roentgenographic and anatomic studies on the patellofemoral joint. *Acta Orthop Scand* 12:319, 1940.

65. Goodfellow J, Hungerford DS, Zindel M: Patello-femoral joint mechanics and pathology. *J Bone Joint Surg* 58A:287, 1976.

66. Bechtol CO: Muscle physiology, in *American Academy of Orthopaedic Surgeons Instructional Course Lectures,* vol 5. JW Edwards, Ann Arbor, MI, 1948.

67. Jokl P, DeMaio M: Exercise and athletic conditioning, in *Orthopaedic Knowledge Update 3.* Park Ridge, IL, American Academy of Orthopaedic Surgeons, 1990.

68. Wendt PP, Johnson RP: A study of quadriceps excursion, torque, and the effect of patellectomy on cadaver knees. *J Bone Joint Surg* 67A:726, 1985.

69. Maquet PGJ: *Biomechanics of the Knee with Application to the Pathogenesis and Surgical Treatment of Osteoarthritis.* Berlin, Springer-Verlag, 1976.

70. O'Donoghue DH, Tompkins F, Hays MB: Strength of the quadriceps function after patellectomy. *West J Surg Obstet Gynecol* 60:159, 1952.

71. Ferguson AB: Elevation of the insertion of the patellar ligament for patellofemoral pain. *J Bone Joint Surg* 64A:766, 1982.

72. Ferguson AB, Brown TD, Fu FH, Rutkowski R: Relief of patellofemoral contact stress by anterior displacement of the tibial tubercle. *J Bone Joint Surg* 61A:159, 1979.

73. Garrett WE Jr, Jokl P, DeMaio M: Soft tissue trauma, in *Orthopaedic Knowledge Update 3.* Park Ridge, IL. American Academy of Orthopaedic Surgeons, 1990.

74. Einola S, Ado AJ, Kallio P: Patellectomy after fracture. *Acta Orthop Scand* 47:441, 1976.

75. Levack B, Flannigan JP, Hobbs S: Results of surgical treatment of patellar fractures. *J Bone Joint Surg* 67B:416, 1985.

76. DePalma AF, Flynn JJ: Joint changes following experimental partial and total patellectomy. *J Bone Joint Surg* 40A:395, 1958.

77. Steurer PA, Gradisar IA, Hoyt WA, Chu ML: Patellectomy: A clinical study and biomechanical evaluation. *Clin Orthop* 144:84, 1979.

78. Sledge CB, Ewald FC: Total knee arthroplasty experience at the Robert Breck Brigham Hospital. *Clin Orthop* 145:78, 1979.

79. Lind T: An evaluation of patellectomy for retropatellar pain. 78 patients followed from two to twelve years. *Acta Orthop Belg* 52:831, 1986.

80. Robinson SC, States JD: Epidemiology, treatment, and prevention of patellar fractures, in *American Academy of Orthopaedic Surgeons Symposium on Reconstructive Surgery of the Knee.* St. Louis, Mosby, 1978, chap 11, pp 111–120.

81. Scapinelli R: Blood supply of the human patella, its relation to ischemic necrosis after fracture. *J Bone Joint Surg* 49B:563, 1967.

82. Goodfellow J, Hungerford DS, Woods C: Patello-femoral joint mechanics and pathology. 2. Chondromalacia patellae. *J Bone Joint Surg* 58B:291, 1976.

83. Khong BT, Pillay VK: Patellectomy for fracture. A study of the results of 40 fractures. *Singapore Med J* 8:230, 1967.

84. Namey TC, Frogameni AD: Coexistent *Mycobacterium intracellulare* gonarthritis and patellar osteomyelitis in a patient with pulmonary sarcoidosis. A case report and literature review. *Orthopedics* 9:425, 1986.

85. Berkheiser EJ: Excision of the patella in arthritis of the knee joint. *JAMA* 113:2303, 1939.

86. Bickel WH, Johnson KA: Z-plasty patellectomy. *Surg Gynecol Obstet* June:985, 1971.

87. Boyd HB, Hawkins BL: Patellectomy—A simplified technique. *Surg Gynecol Obstet* 86:357, 1948.

88. Chari PR, Roy GK, Murty VS: Repair of the quadriceps apparatus following patellectomy in recent fractures of the patella: A new technique with results. *Aust NZ J Surg* 48:99, 1978.

89. Shorbe HB, Dobson CH: Patellectomy; repair of the extensor mechanism. *J Bone Joint Surg* 40A:1281, 1958.

90. Reiley RE, De Souza LJ: Patellectomy: An alternative technique. *Clin Orthop* 103:170, 1974.

91. Lewis RC, Scholz KC: Cruciate repair of the extensor mechanism following patellectomy. *J Bone Joint Surg* 48A:1221, 1966.

92. Compere CL, Hill JA, Lewinnek GE, et al: A new method of patellectomy for patellofemoral arthritis. *J Bone Joint Surg* 61A:714, 1979.

93. Duthie HL, Hutchinson JR: The results of partial and total excision of the patella. *J Bone Joint Surg* 40B:75, 1958.

94. Noble HB, Hajek MR: Boutonniere-type deformity of the knee following patellectomy and manipulations. *J Bone Joint Surg* 66A:137, 1984.

95. Garr EL, Moskowitz RW, Davis W: Degenerative changes following experimental patellectomy in the rabbit. *Clin Orthop* 92:296, 1973.

96. Crenshaw AM, Wilson FD: The surgical treatment of fractures of the patella. *South Med J* 47:716, 1954.

97. DePalma AF, Sawyer B, Hoffman JD: Reconsideration of lesions affecting the patellofemoral joint. *Clin Orthop* 18:63, 1960.

98. Worrell RV: A comparison of patellectomy with prosthetic replacement of the patella. *Clin Orthop* 111:284, 1975.

99. Bayne O, Cameron HU: Total knee arthroplasty following patellectomy. *Clin Orthop* 186:112, 1984.

100. Lennox DW, Hungerford DS, Krackow KA: Total knee arthroplasty following patellectomy. *Clin Orthop* 223:220, 1987.

101. O'Connor RL: Diagnostic procedures, in *American Academy of Orthopaedic Surgeons Symposium on Reconstructive Surgery of the Knee*. St. Louis, Mosby, 1978, chap 9, p 87.

CHAPTER 22

The Role of Arthroscopy in Patellofemoral Arthritis

Robert W. Jackson

INTRODUCTION

The patient who presents with anterior knee pain often provides a challenge in treatment. The treating physician must initially determine whether or not the cause of the anterior knee pain lies in the patellofemoral articulation or in another nonosseous source. All too often the term chondromalacia patellae is applied as a "catch-all" diagnosis to conditions that are not true chondromalacia. Most orthopaedic surgeons now reserve the term *chondromalacia* for situations with a proven breakdown of the articular cartilage of the patella, and patellofemoral arthritis for breakdown not only of the patella, but also the trochlea of the femur against which the patella articulates. It is also likely that chondromalacia patellae, despite its frequent onset in the younger age group, is the first manifestation of a degenerative process affecting the patellofemoral articulation. No evidence suggests that the breakdown of the articular cartilage of the patella is any different from the articular cartilage breakdown that occurs in joints elsewhere in the body. The only deviation from the more commonly seen osteoarthritic processes elsewhere is that degeneration in the patellofemoral joint occurs earlier, and symptoms are somewhat different over the first few years. Moreover, as people age and as the degenerative process progresses, pain usually diminishes, although crepitus and restricted range of motion might persist.

THE ETIOLOGY OF PATELLOFEMORAL ARTHRITIS

For practical purposes and to aid in the treatment of this condition, I believe that the process afflicting the patellofemoral joint that leads to degenerative changes can be attributed to one of three basic causes: direct trauma, instability, or malalignment.

Direct Trauma

Should the patellofemoral articulation be subjected to a direct blow of sufficient magnitude, the process of degeneration is set in motion. Direct trauma can split the surface of the articular cartilage, resulting in exposure of chondrocytes, the release of enzymes, and gradually the further destruction of the articular surface. This has been shown in experimental work by Gedeon, Repo, and others.[1,2] Direct trauma may occur from a fall on the flexed knee, a dashboard injury, or from any other cause. It can occur in a normally aligned and stable articulation. The clinical result of such direct trauma is a localized softening and breakdown of the articular cartilage, usually in the central area of the patella.

Instability

When the patellofemoral articulation is disjointed or dislocated due to trauma, the surface of the joint is not only affected by the trauma (see above), but also the soft tissues that guide and help to stabilize the patella in the trochlea of the femur are stretched, strained, or even ruptured. Recurrent instability is therefore a common problem and can lead to further breakdown of the articular cartilage. Even though the initial injury is relatively mild, if the soft tissue support mechanisms are not sufficient to stabilize the patella, the repetitive and cumulative action of the microtraumas produced by the subluxing patella can have deleterious effects. The most common reason for instability would be a dislocation due to trauma, but other reasons can also be identified, such as patella alta, with wobbling of the patella prior to its engagement in the trochlea of the femur on flexion movements.

Malalignment

If the extensor mechanism of the knee does not develop in a longitudinally aligned fashion during growth, and a rotational or angulatory component develops, there is a permanent tendency for the patella to sublux with each flexion-extension movement. This type of malalignment pathology can be detected by the presence of a high Q angle, genu valgus, tibial torsion, or femoral anteversion. Even later in life malalignment can occur due to partial epiphyseal arrests or fractures, which can cause angulatory deformity of the long axis of the leg. If the result of such malalignment is to cause repetitive lateral thrusts to the patella, the cumulative effect of the resulting microtraumas causes the breakdown of the articular surface, the release of enzymes, and further destruction of the cartilage. In this type of pathology, the most common finding is erosion of articular cartilage on the lateral facet, and fibrillation on the medial facet. The erosion is due to excessive lateral pressure, which has been recognized as a syndrome (ELPS) as described by Ficat.[4]

In the not too distant past, a fairly common problem following open medial meniscectomy was the development of chondromalacia on the medial facet of the patella. It is our belief that an open model meniscectomy often caused a collapse of the medial compartment, a tendency for the medial femoral condyle to sag backward into the deficient posterior horn region, thus creating a rotational angulation effect, increasing the Q angle and producing an acquired malalignment syndrome with the subsequent development of chondromalacia several months later. Hopefully, with arthroscopic treatment and preservation of a stable posterior rim, this complication will be minimized.

WHY IS CHONDROMALACIA PAINFUL?

Most of the pain is probably derived from the underlying trabecular bone of the patella. When the articular cartilage no longer has the ability to absorb the tremendous contact forces transmitted through the patellofemoral articulation, those forces must be transmitted to the underlying subchondral bone. The trabecular bone is therefore stressed, and microscopic fractures occur. A healing response is induced, and gradually the subchondral bone becomes thicker, as evidenced by increasing radiologic density. With the passage of time the subchondral trabecular bone becomes strong enough to withstand the forces to which it is being subjected. At this point the condition, which originally was known as chondromalacia, might be called degenerative arthritis, but it is no longer painful.

A second source of pain may be the soft tissues that are irritated by the debris fragments of articular cartilage and the enzymes that are released during the active phase of the degenerative process. Substance P and prostaglandin are two products known to have an effect in producing pain. The synovium is given the task of absorbing and digesting the microparticles of articular cartilage that are produced by the wear process and that are shed into the joint. A chronic synovitis is the common result, and this might also be an additional source of pain, if the synovial fronds are pinched by the articular surfaces.

DIAGNOSIS

The diagnosis of patellofemoral pathology is discussed elsewhere in this text. A careful history and physical examination must be performed. The radiologic evaluation must include a tangential view of the patellofemoral compartment.[3] It is our practice to take tangential x-rays of the patella with both knees in the same film, flexed to approximately 20 degrees to 30 degrees. As Ficat pointed out, this is the unstable position of the patellofemoral articulation and although not diagnostic, some valuable information can be obtained from tangential x-rays at this degree of flexion.[4] This view can indicate a tendency to lateral subluxation and tilting. Moreover, the width of the joint space can be more accurately measured when both patellae, at the same degree of flexion, are included on the same film.

Therefore, although normal x-rays do not rule out chondromalacia, the tangential view is important to augment the clinical information gained by history and physical examination. The newer diagnostic techniques of computed tomography scanning and magnetic resonance imaging may prove to be much more valuable than tangential x-rays in the ultimate assessment of patellofemoral problems.

The clinical diagnosis of chondromalacia is made on the basis of the three cornerstones of diagnosis (i.e., the history and the physical and radiologic examinations). However, the ultimate diagnosis requires arthroscopic visualization of the breakdown of articular surface. We suggest that clinically diagnosed chondromalacia (or degenerative arthritis) then be classified into one of the three etiologic categories—trauma induced, malalignment, or instability. If one can easily place the etiology of the problem into one of these categories, sound guidelines for future treatment can be developed.

MANAGEMENT OF CHONDROMALACIA

Conservative Treatment

The initial treatment of any disorder, except those that are life-threatening, should be conservative until one is absolutely sure that the symptoms are severe enough to warrant a more aggressive approach to treatment. The clinician should initially buy time with nonoperative measures of treatment, as the natural history of chondromalacia suggests that the individual has a good chance of becoming symptom free in time. Conservative treatment includes the relative restriction of activity, the use of analgesics, and the use of buttress pads to minimize lateral subluxation and to provide stability to the articulation. The use of physical therapy to strengthen the quadriceps mechanism (and in particular, the vastus medialis muscle) may enable a more uniform pull of the extensors and avoid a tendency for a lateral pull from the vastus lateralis. Therapy should concentrate on using isometric exercises or terminal short arc exercises. These exercises tend to minimize the contact forces between the patella and the trochlea of the femur that occur with restricted extension from the fully flexed position. It is not our policy to inject knees with steroid because there is reason to believe that the short-term beneficial effect on the inflammatory response is offset by the long-term detrimental effect of the steroid on articular cartilage.

If patients fail to respond to these conservative measures, they then become candidates for arthroscopy, which is still the gold standard in diagnosing chondromalacia patellae. Only by direct visualization can one truly determine that the articular cartilage has been disrupted, which by definition is the condition called chondromalacia. The extent of the degenerative process can also be determined at arthroscopy and as a bonus, an opportunity for relatively simple treatment is afforded.

Arthroscopic Classification

We have attempted to categorize or classify the severity of chondromalacia patellae, as seen arthroscopically, as one of three types. A fourth type has been identified, which is now included in our type I.[5,6]

1. *Type I chondromalacia* basically consists of a small area of fibrillation, usually in the central area of the patella. Type I can also include a "blister" type of lesion, which is a defect in the articular cartilage deep to the surface.[6] At a later stage the surface defect would become apparent.

2. *Type II chondromalacia* involves fairly widespread fibrillation or breakdown of articular cartilage, often of the crabmeat type of appearance. It is, however, still restricted to the patella itself.

3. *Type III chondromalacia* is basically a degenerative process in which the trochlea of the femur is involved, along with widespread degenerative change of the patella. This may also include those cases where exposed bone on the patella has resulted from excessive pressure. Exposure of bone is usually

seen on the lateral facet. Secondary changes may also be seen on the lateral femoral condyle.

Arthroscopic Treatment

In patients with degenerative changes who have been unresponsive to conservative measures and have a definitive diagnosis by arthroscopy, three possible arthroscopic treatments are available to the surgeon. One is lavage alone, the second is arthroscopic shaving of the degenerative area, and the third involves shaving and possible lateral release.[5,7,8]

Various methods of performing a lateral release are described elsewhere in this text. The primary purpose of any lateral release operation is to release the constricting lateral structures of the knee, thus allowing the patella to assume a more central and slightly different articulation with the trochlea of the femur. A lateral release allows the vastus medialis to exert a more positive action in pulling the patella toward the midline of its articulating path. Lateral release might therefore be considered for situations where a tight lateral compartment is evidenced on clinical and radiologic examination or in situations where malalignment is obvious either from developmental or acquired etiologies. Lateral release, plus or minus shaving, is therefore indicated when an element of malalignment can be determined. A secondary benefit from lateral release might be a degree of denervation of the painful patella.

Shaving is an extremely valuable treatment in the individual with chondromalacia due to direct trauma, with a normally aligned and stable extensor mechanism. An analogy often used to explain this to a patient is that of an apple that falls on the floor, and a few days later is seen to have a brown area of softening, secondary to the direct trauma and damage to its pulp. Removing the damaged area does not affect the rest of the apple. Similarly, the softened or deranged area of articular cartilage in the central area of the stable patella, can be removed surgically with a rotating suction shaver and the remaining articular cartilage functions extremely well. Shaving may also be used with lateral release to debride the patellofemoral articulation of the chondral fragments that would ultimately be shed into the joint. Theoretically, this minimizes the development of synovitis and the effects of the painful enzymes.

Lavage alone eliminates enzymes and washes out debris fragments, therefore minimizing the synovitis effect. It does little to correct the underlying problem of why the chondromalacia has occurred, and therefore lavage alone has little to offer by itself, in the treatment of chondromalacia.

RESULTS OF ARTHROSCOPIC TREATMENT

In a series of 319 patients with proven chondromalacia patellae, we were able to categorize the etiologic agent as direct trauma, instability, or malalignment in 50 percent. The other 50 percent were labelled idiopathic and mainly represented earlier cases in the series that were diagnosed before an etiologic delineation was established. A review of these patients at 1 year and at 5 years following arthroscopy was correlated with the degree and severity of pathology at the time of initial diagnosis.

Those patients treated with lavage alone showed an early remission but there was no long-term benefit. Symptoms had usually recurred by 1 year and were still present at 5 years.

Patients in the posttraumatic group, possessing normal alignment and stability, were treated by arthroscopic shaving and joint lavage. If the severity of the problem was relatively minimal, such as types I and II, the results at 1 year and at 5 years were equal. In such instances 76 percent to 82 percent of patients were in the good to excellent category. Those cases diagnosed with type III and therefore with more severe pathology at the time of treatment showed 42 percent satisfactory results at 1 year and a dramatic drop to 12 percent good results at 5 years.

In a group of patients with proven malalignment, the chosen treatment was shaving and a lateral release. The treatment was effective in the earlier stages (types I and II) of pathology. Good to excellent results were found in 85 percent to 90 percent in this category. However, although those patients at stage III showed a 70 percent good result at 1 year, only 15 percent were still good at 5 years. This would suggest that malalignment is best treated early, before the degenerative process becomes too extensive.

In those instances where true instability or dislocation had occurred, the results of shaving and lateral release were less beneficial. Lateral release produced good results in approximately 60 percent of cases at 1 year, but by 5 years the good to excellent results had fallen to 30 percent. Shaving alone gave no specific improvement.

The rationale of arthroscopic treatment was to remove the debris that causes synovitis by shaving, to eliminate the microparticles and the enzymes that could also create synovitis by the lavage process, and through a lateral release, improve the alignment of the articulation and theoretically decrease the wear on the patellofemoral articulation.

LATERAL RELEASE IN THE OLDER AGE GROUP

A series of 39 cases, involving patients 30 years of age and older, was reviewed 4 years following lateral release of the patella and again at 6 years.[7] These patients all presented with severe patellofemoral degenerative joint disease with malalignment and decreased joint space on tangential x-rays. A subcutaneous lateral release was performed according to the method described by Metcalf, with a foam rubber pad applied to the lateral aspect of the knee to minimize bleeding and to push the patella medially during the first 8 to 10 postoperative days.[9] Ambulation was immediate, and appropriate physical therapy was instituted after 1 week.

The results of the initial assessment at a mean of 4 years following surgery revealed 75 percent good to excellent results. However, when the same patients were reviewed at a mean of 6 years following surgery, only 56 percent of the knees were considered good or excellent results, and 12 knees (31 percent) had undergone further surgery.

We concluded that although the results are not ideal, lateral release has the advantage of being a low morbidity procedure, easily performed as outpatient surgery; it does not hinder further procedures being carried out at a later date, if necessary.

TREATMENT AFTER FAILED ARTHROSCOPIC SURGERY

Should the symptoms continue after arthroscopic treatment, the surgeon should look toward some form of open operative treatment. For the knees that show extensor malalignment one might consider the medial transposition of the patellar tendon (Elmslie-Trillat) or elevation of the tibial tuberosity (Maquet procedure).[10,11] Both of these procedures can produce good results. My personal preference is toward the Elmslie-Trillat, which changes the alignment and (presumably) the longitudinal compression forces, without producing an elevation of the tibial tuberosity. The Maquet procedure creates several problems with inability to kneel, difficulty in closing the skin over the elevated bump, fracture of the tuberosity, and others. The complication rate reported with Maquet procedures has been fairly high, whereas the complication rate with the Elmslie-Trillat is relatively low.

If such procedures also fail to improve the situation, I believe that a patellectomy is the final treatment of choice. Our results with "purse-string" patellectomies have been extremely gratifying.[12] The patella is removed through an enucleation process and the defect is closed with a purse-string suture so that all of the slack in the extensor mechanism, produced by removal of the patella, is taken up in a uniform way. The end result is one in which an excellent range of motion can be obtained with good function and much less pain. The major drawback to a patellectomy is the observed decrease in power, once the fulcrum of the patella has been removed.

Other surgical procedures must be considered experimental. Patellar resurfacing and patellar osteotomy may provide alternative answers in the future. Arthroscopic abrasion and drilling of the patella has purposely not been advocated because this has not been a successful treatment method in my hands, and to my knowledge, no good scientific evidence indicates that this is any better than debridement alone.

SUMMARY

Our basic concept is that chondromalacia patellae is merely the first stage of degenerative arthritis of the patellofemoral articulation. The reasons for the development of chondromalacia patellae (and ultimately degenerative arthritis) are grouped in one of three categories—direct trauma, malalignment, and instability. Such grouping provides rational indications for further treatment. Chondromalacia due to malalignment can effectively be treated by shaving and lateral release at the time of arthroscopy. Those cases due to direct trauma can best be treated by shaving alone. Instability must be treated by stabilizing the patella through therapy or surgery. Should the arthroscopic procedure fail to produce adequate results, surgical realignment procedures might be contemplated and if these also fail to improve the results then a patellectomy, with a purse-string type of closure, is the treatment of choice for the final procedure.

REFERENCES

1. Gedeon P: Les contusions du cartilage articulaire. Thesis, University of Toulouse, France, 1977.

2. Repo RV, Finlay JB: Survival of articular cartilage after controlled impact. *J Bone Joint Surg* 59A:1068, 1977.

3. Laurin CA, Dussault R, Levesque HP: The tangential x-ray investigation of the patellofemoral joint: X-ray technique, diagnostic criteria and their interpretation. *Clin Orthop* 144:16, 1979.

4. Ficat P, Hungerford DS: *Disorders of the Patellofemoral Joint.* Baltimore, Williams & Wilkins, 1977, pp 63–110.

5. Ogilvie-Harris DJ, Jackson RW: The arthroscopic treatment of chondromalacia patellae. *J Bone Joint Surg* 66B:291, 1976.

6. Goodfellow J, Hungerford DS, Woods C: Patellofemoral joint mechanics and pathology. *J Bone Joint Surg* 58B:291, 1976.

7. Jackson RW, Kunkel S, Taylor G: Lateral retinacular release for patellofemoral pain in the older patient. *Arthroscopy* 7:283, 1991.

8. Merchant CA, Mercer RL: Lateral release of the patella. *Clin Orthop* 40:103, 1974.

9. Metcalf RW: *Operative Arthroscopy of the Knee,* vol. 30. Instructional Course Lectures. Chicago, American Academy of Orthopaedic Surgery, 1981, p 357.

10. Trillat A, Dejour H, Conette A: Diagnostic et traitement des subluxations recidivantes de la rotule. *Rev Chir Orthop* 50:813, 1964.

11. Maquet PGJ: *Biomechanics of the Knee.* Berlin, Springer, 1976.

12. Blatter G, Jackson RW, Bayne O: Patellectomy as a salvage procedure, in *Surgery and Arthroscopy of the Knee: 2d Congress of the European Society,* edited by W. Muller and W. Hackenbruch. Berlin-Heidelberg, Springer-Verlag, 1988, pp 476–485.

SECTION VIII
Rehabilitation

CHAPTER 23

Rehabilitation of the Knee Extensor Mechanism

Letha Y. Griffin

INTRODUCTION

Rehabilitation of the extensor mechanism received increased attention during the 1980s. Several excellent articles emphasized the advantage of properly managed nonoperative care in the treatment of subluxation and dislocation of the patella.[1,2] Those involved in reconstructing the anterior cruciate ligament found patella pain to be a common complication.[3] They investigated ways to more effectively rehabilitate the extensor mechanism to avoid postoperative patella pain. At about the same time, Cooper, DeLee, and Ramamurthy[4]; Schutzer and Gossling[5]; and others stressed the role of physical therapy in treating reflex sympathetic dystrophy of the knee, an entity that consistently involves the patellofemoral mechanism.

Moreover, as our population increased its interest in athletics and fitness activities throughout the 1970s and 1980s, increased numbers of patients with overuse injuries of the patellofemoral joint were seen.[6] These patients, aware of conditioning principles, sought exercise protocols to decrease their symptoms and improve the function of their knees. The exercise boom also brought with it a greater availability of exercise equipment, both for use in fitness clubs and for home purchase.

During this same time, a change occurred in the prevailing attitude that limitations in physical performance were inevitable if one had a congenital variant (e.g., patella subluxation) or an acute injury (e.g., patella tendon rupture). Patients demanded a chance to return to an active life-style.

THE REHABILITATION PROGRAM: AN OVERVIEW

Goals of a Rehabilitation Program

The goals of a rehabilitation program are to decrease inflammation, to restore range of motion, and to regain muscular strength, endurance, power, and flexibility while maintaining the patient's overall fitness (i.e., cardiovascular endurance).[7] In the final stage of rehabilitation, attention must be given to regaining proprioceptive awareness, as well as agility and functional skills, including sport-specific skills in the athlete.[8]

Rehabilitation Goals
Decrease inflammation
Restore range of motion
Regain muscular strength
   endurance
   power
   flexibility
Maintain or improve cardiovascular fitness
Develop proprioceptive awareness
   agility
Perfect functional skills, including sport-specific
   skills

To meet these goals, rehabilitation programs must be individualized.[9] One must consider the patient's age, the prior level of muscular and cardiovascular fitness, the familiarity with exercise equipment, and the degree of motivation.

An understanding of the psychology of rehabilitation is extremely important because maximum mo-

279

tivation is needed to achieve desired results. The physician and therapist must win the patient's confidence and be sensitive to the patient's emotions, but they must be firm in their approach to gain the patient's commitment to the rehabilitation effort.

They must help the patient to overcome the denial, anger, and depression that frequently accompany an injury or disease.[10] Moreover, they must motivate the patient even during periods of discouragement, which often occur when rehabilitation goals are more slowly achieved than expected. They must make the patient realize that the injury is the patient's and not theirs. Although it is their role to instruct the patient in proper rehabilitation techniques and to aid in the performance of same, it is the patient who must faithfully adhere to the rehabilitation protocol if he or she is to recover.[11]

Phases of a Rehabilitation Program

It is helpful to divide any rehabilitation program into various phases, with the goals and the techniques used to achieve these goals defined for each phase.[12] The total number of phases into which a program is divided or the exact points of division between these phases is not critical. What is critical is to realize that the rehabilitation effort is a progression of activities, which must be divided into some logical scheme of goal-oriented steps to allow the physician, the therapist, and the patient to more easily assess the patient's progress.

Although at first such a scheme seems far too complex for the adolescent with a common problem such as Osgood-Schlatter disease, one finds that it is really not. The patient with a less severe problem will merely be able to move more rapidly through the phases.

An example of a rehabilitation progression follows. The scheme is a general one and applicable to the rehabilitation of most joints. It can be easily adapted to construct exercise protocols for the patellofemoral mechanism.

Phase I: Immediate postinjury or postoperative period (first 24–48 h)
  Goals: •To decrease inflammation and pain
  •To attempt to maintain muscle tone

Phase II: Early rehabilitation (1–2 weeks)
  Goals: •Continue to decrease inflammation and pain
  •Slowly restore range of motion

•Maintain muscle tone
•Maintain cardiovascular endurance if possible

Phase III: Intermediate phase
  Goals: •Continue to decrease inflammation and pain if needed
  •Restore final degrees of motion
  •Emphasize increasing strength and flexibility
  •As strength increases, work toward developing muscular endurance and power
  •Begin aerobic (functional) skills such as biking, swimming, walking for muscular endurance, as well as overall cardiovascular endurance
  •Begin emphasizing techniques that enhance proprioceptive awareness

Phase IV: Advanced rehabilitation
  Goals: •Should have very little residual pain or swelling
  •Should have full range of motion
  •Emphasize maximizing muscular performance, strength, endurance, power, and flexibility
  •Further develop proprioceptive awareness and agility
  •Further advance performance of functional skills (run, jump, cut, half squat), and in athletes add sport-specific drills
  •Continue activities to maintain cardiovascular fitness

The rehabilitation principles used to develop muscular strength, power, endurance, and flexibility, as well as to gain return of proprioceptive awareness and agility are similar to those used in training and conditioning programs.

An understanding of certain terms is critical in a discussion of such principles. *Strength* refers to the maximal force that can be generated by a muscle during a single maximal contraction. *Endurance* is the ability to perform repetitive muscular contractions against a resistance, and *power* is the strength developed by the muscle over time, that is, strength times speed.[13]

Typically, for activities of daily living it is more critical to develop muscular endurance than maximal muscular strength or power. For successful return to sports participation, all are needed.

A *motor unit* consists of a motor nerve and the group of muscle fibers it innervates. Each motor unit has type I and type II muscle fibers within it. Type I are slow twitch fibers. They take longer to generate a force, but are more resistant to fatigue. Their energy metabolic pathways are primarily aerobic. Type I fibers are lost rapidly with immobilization and are thought not to be preserved by isometric contractions.[14] Type II fibers, or fast twitch fibers, produce quick, forceful contractions over a short period of time, but they fatigue rapidly.[15] There are three types of type II fibers: type IIa, type IIab, and type IIb. Type IIa have some endurance, as well as power capacities. Type IIb are primarily glycolytic or anaerobic, and hence, are power generators only.[13] Type IIab are somewhat in between.

The percentage of each muscle fiber type in a particular muscle varies from individual to individual and is largely genetically determined. Training may be able to maximize on the development of one muscle fiber type over another, however.[16] Type II fibers are critical to short bursts of activity, such as kicking a can, but type I fibers would be needed to continuously kick that can for two to three miles. In reality, both type I and type II fibers function in everyday activities to complement each other. Skills must be incorporated into a rehabilitation program that will develop both types.

Overload Principle of Building Muscular Strength

A progressive gradual increase in effort is used in rehabilitation, as well as in training and conditioning.

Atrophy is the decrease in size of the muscle fibers resulting from disuse, whereas *hypertrophy* is the increase in muscle fiber size (i.e., its diameter). Strength is a function of both the number and the diameter of muscle fibers within a given muscle fiber,[13] as well as the efficiency of the neuromuscular system. The number of muscle fibers is genetically determined, but training can maximize on the diameter of fibers and on the neuromuscular efficiency of the system, and hence, improve strength.

In addition, strength depends on such mechanical factors as the distance from the joint at which the tendon is attached, or the angle of application of force,[13] both of which are genetically determined anatomic factors that cannot be influenced through rehabilitation.

Muscle length also influences muscle strength. In general, a muscle is capable of generating its maximal force when it is in the midrange of motion. If it is stretched beyond its normal length, it may be incapable of generating a muscular force. Hence, the interrelationship of resting tone between antagonists and agonists is critical and must be addressed during rehabilitation; that is, the rehabilitation effort may concentrate initially on the injured joint, but must be broadened to include return to normal function of the entire extremity and indeed, the body as a whole.[17]

The exercises used to build strength in training and rehabilitation programs are similar. Both use the principle of requiring a progressive, gradual increase in effort—the overload principle.[18] Overload can be implemented by increasing resistance, increasing repetitions or sets, or increasing the duration of the exercise.

Types of Exercises Used to Build Strength

Isometric
    muscle length remains constant with contraction
Isotonic
    muscle length changes with contraction
Isokinetic
    speed of motion is set and resistance is
    accommodating.

Three types of exercises can be used to build strength: isometric, isotonic, and isokinetic.[19] An *isometric exercise* involves a muscle contraction in which the length of the muscle remains constant while tension develops toward maximal force against an immovable resistance. The disadvantage to this exercise is that strength gains are specific only to the joint angle at which the training is performed.[20]

Isotonic exercise involves a muscle contraction in which the force is generated when the muscle is changing length. Equipment used for isotonic exercise includes free weights, bar bells, dumb bells, and machine equipment such as Nautilus.

There are two types of isotonic contractions: a *concentric contraction* in which the muscle shortens when generating force and an *eccentric contraction* in which the muscle lengthens when generating force.[21] A person sitting on a weight bench with his knee and ankle flexed to 90 degrees and a 5-lb weight on his ankle must concentrically contract his quadriceps to extend his knee. The quadriceps performs eccentrically, that is, contracts as it lengthens, as the weight is lowered and the knee returns to the 90 degree flexed position. Eccentric contractions generate greater force than do concentric contractions and have been reported to be associated with a greater risk of injury.[22] However, when rehabilitating athletes performing jumping or kicking sports, many feel it is essential to rehabilitate the quadriceps both concentrally and eccentrically.

The obvious difficulty with isotonic exercise is that a constant weight is used. Yet, it is known that the amount of force needed to move a weight through a range of motion changes according to joint angle, and hence, in isotonic exercises, loads encountered by exercising muscle vary throughout the range of motion.[9] Nautilus equipment tends to decrease this inequity somewhat by building a cam into the pulley system.

Isokinetic exercise is one in which the speed of motion is set and resistance accommodates to move the force applied. Theoretically, maximal resistance is provided throughout the range.[23] This equipment works on either a hydraulic, pneumonic, or mechanical pressure system. When isokinetic equipment is used, speed (not resistance) is set by the therapist. Hence, an exuberant patient can potentially generate higher forces than desired during the early stage of rehabilitation. Therefore, these devices are generally reserved for more advanced rehabilitation phases.

Stretching techniques include ballistic, static, and proprioceptive neuromuscular facilitation.[10] Ballistic stretching, or stretching through repetitive bouncing motion, is infrequently used because it may cause tearing of the muscle fibers. Static stretching involves a slow gentle stretch of the muscle to a point of discomfort and holding this point for a count of 10 to 12. The patient relaxes the muscle for a count of 3 to 5, and then repeats the stretch.

Stretching Techniques
Ballistic
Static
Proprioceptive neuromuscular facilitation (PNF)

There are several variations of proprioceptive neuromuscular facilitation stretching techniques, but all involve alternating contraction and relaxation of both agonist and antagonist muscles.[24] This technique can be used for the patient who finds it difficult to relax into a slow static stretch. The therapist acts as the patient's partner for this stretching technique. For example, when stretching the quadriceps muscle, the therapist first slowly stretches the muscle to the point where the patient feels slight discomfort, and holds this point for a count of 10 to 12. The patient then contracts his quadriceps against the therapist's resistance for another 10 to 12 count, after which the therapist repeats the passive quadriceps stretch.

During the first phase of rehabilitation, pain can be decreased with medications, ice, or electrical stimulation. Frequently, muscle tone can be maintained by isometric exercises or by muscle stimulation units, as demonstrated by Eriksson and Haggmark,[25] as well as Gould and colleagues.[26]

In phase II, range of motion can be initiated by gentle active or passive means. Heat, ultrasound, and electrical stimulation may be used before initiating range of motion exercises. Isometric exercises are used to maintain tone until there is sufficient range of motion to allow for beginning isotonic exercise. For rehabilitation following lower extremity injuries, cardiovascular endurance can be maintained by techniques such as one leg biking (put the injured extremity on a chair and bike with the well leg only), walking with a water vest in water, or using leg buoys and swimming with arms only. Begin stretching muscle groups in the injured extremity. Start with a gentle, slow relaxation stretch.

In phase III, when muscle strength in the injured extremity is increasing, muscular endurance as well as cardiovascular endurance can be developed through interval training, circuit training, continuous sustained training, or a combination of these techniques. *Interval training* involves alternating periods of relatively intense work (heart rate approximately 85 percent of maximum) with low intensity work periods for recovery (heart rate at 35 percent to 40 percent maximum).[27] A *circuit training* program involves moving through a series of stations incorporating flexibility exercises, calisthenics, brief aerobic exercise periods, and strength training.[13] A recovery period is present between each station. Generally a circuit consists of 8 to 12 stations repeated three times for one set.

Techniques to Develop Muscular and Cardiovascular Endurance
Interval training
Circuit training
Continuous sustained training

In phases III and IV, proprioceptive and agility skills are begun and can consist of running patterns with fast changes in direction, side-to-side hopping, or rapid stepping motions up and down using step stools (e.g., step aerobics), as well as partner skills in which one partner runs or cuts to catch a ball thrown by another.

REHABILITATION OF THE EXTENSOR MECHANISM

Because of the unique biomechanical properties of the patellofemoral joint, created in part by the patella being a sesamoid bone housed in the quadriceps and patella tendon mechanism, special consideration needs to be given in adapting general rehabilitation programs to injuries of this joint.

From the work of Hungerford and others, one learns that at no point in time does the entire retropatellar hyaline cartilage articulate with the hyaline cartilage of the femoral condyle. Contact between the hyaline cartilage surfaces of this joint begins between 10 degrees and 20 degrees flexion. The first contact is between the inferior margin of the patella, but as flexion increases, the contact area moves proximally on the patella.[29,30]

These points of patellofemoral contact can be altered by changing the contribution to contraction made by each of the four heads of the quadriceps.[31] The degree to which forces on the patellofemoral joint can be altered by changing the vector of contraction force produced by these four heads has not been thoroughly documented. However, research has shown that the radiographic position of the patella in the femoral groove on a skyline view depends not only on the degrees of knee flexion, but also on the degree of quadriceps contraction at the time the film is taken[32,33] (Fig. 23-1). Moreover, clinically it is known that if one emphasizes vastus medialis obliquus development in patients with patella alignment problems, a great majority will be symptomatically improved. This is true not only in those patients with multiple patella dislocations or subluxations, but

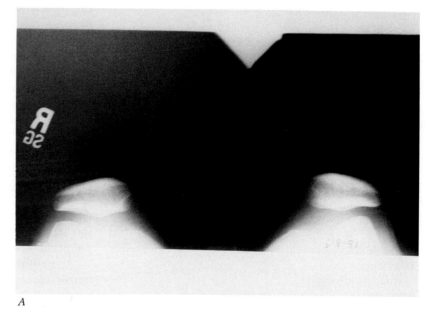

A

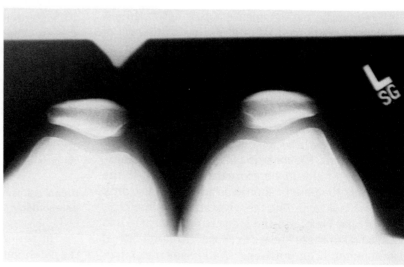

FIGURE 23-1
Same patient with two skyline views. *A.* Complete relaxation of quadriceps; *B.* Slight quadriceps contraction. Note influence of degree of quadriceps contraction on the position of the patella in the femoral groove.

B

also in patients with the lateral patella compression syndrome.[34]

The vastus medialis obliquus fibers contract maximally in terminal extension.[35] Hence, most rehabilitation programs for patellofemoral malalignment problems apply straight leg raises, short arc extensions (30 degrees to 0 degrees) and quadriceps setting exercises.[36]

However, in some patients symptoms seem to worsen with quadriceps sets or straight leg raises; that is, merely maximizing patellofemoral force even in the absence of patellofemoral articular contact seems to result in pain. In these patients, rapid full range of motion exercises may be tried. These exercises can also be used to complement the short arc extensions, quadriceps setting exercises, and straight leg raises in patients who can perform these exercises without difficulty.

A bike with the seat elevated (to minimize knee flexion on the up stroke),[21] the tension low to moderate, and the speed rapid or a stair stepper machine with rapid setting, minimal elevation of the foot, and low to moderate tension can be used for this purpose. The bike and stair steppers have the advantage of exercising multiple muscle groups, as well as maintaining cardiovascular fitness while altering mechanics of the patellofemoral joint.

Endurance Exercises
Bike
Swim
Walk
Jogging
Stair stepper
Rowing (stationary)
Water walking

Frequently, patients can use rowing machines, but only if the forced flexion portion of the arc of motion does not aggravate symptoms. Swimming has been used as a cross-training technique in runners with acute symptoms of patellofemoral stress syndrome who cannot return immediately to their sport. However, swimming does not seem to maximally develop the vastus medialis obliquus or even lower extremity strength because it is primarily an upper extremity sport. Kickboards can be used to force maximal effort of the lower extremity muscles. While swimming, the patient should be advised to use only the crawl kick, avoiding the whip kick, the frog kick, breaststroke kick, and the sidestroke (scissor) kick, because all of these kicks can cause increased lateral patellofemoral compression.[37] Walking or running in chest deep water or walking or running in deeper water with a water vest may be a good transitional exercise to augment weight routines in running athletes or in patients who need to return to jobs requiring such walking skills.

Rehabilitate the entire extremity, not just the injured part.
Include aerobic and anaerobic exercise in the rehabilitation protocol.

When using a free weight program for extensor mechanism rehabilitation, one must remember to rehabilitate the entire extremity, not just target exercises for the patellofemoral joint.[38] Exercises should be incorporated into the protocol that strengthen the hip adductors and abductors, as well as the hip flexors and extensors, the hamstrings, and muscles of the lower legs.[17] Even if using primarily an aerobic exercise routine for rehabilitation of the patellofemoral joint, it may be advisable to include at least some anaerobic exercises for all these muscle groups because type I and type II fibers need to be balanced.

Some investigators feel short arc extensions and quadriceps isometrics exercises for patellofemoral tracking should be done from 90 degrees to 40 degrees knee flexion.[39] They argue that even though contraction of the vastus medialis obliquus is maximal during terminal extension, so is contraction of the vastus lateralis maximal. Currently this is not the most widely used exercise scheme, but this controversy emphasizes the need for greater research in the biomechanics and the pathophysiology of pain of the patellofemoral joint.

Flexibility exercises are started very early in extensor mechanism rehabilitation programs because many feel it is the combination of the tight lateral retinaculum and vastus lateralis fibers, as well as the lack of adequate strength of the vastus medialis obliquus that leads to altered tracking, and hence, to increased patellofemoral compression forces.[17,40] In addition, tight hamstrings have been shown to increase patellofemoral forces.[1] As previously noted, a tight or overly powerful agonist can prevent its antagonist from achieving an ideal resting length, and hence, put it at a mechanical disadvantage. Balancing of forces both in strengthening and flexibility exercises is essential during a rehabilitation program.[38]

Balance strength and flexibility of agonist and antagonist.

In patients with essentially normal anatomy of the patellofemoral joint who sustain an acute dislocation, some recommend immediate repair of the medial retinaculum.[41] Others have written that if there are no osteochondral fractures, aspiration of the hemarthrosis and initial immobilization in extension with a lateral pad to closely approximate the medial retinaculum to the patella are advised.[42] During this stage of immobilization, which may last up to 2 to 3 weeks, isometric strengthening of the quadriceps and hip adductors, as well as other muscles of the lower extremity, can be started. Muscle-stimulating units can also be used to maintain tone in the quadriceps. Even in the patient who still has significant pain in the medial quadriceps following a dislocation, hip adductor exercises can generally be done by having the patient lie on the affected side with the foot dorsiflexed to 90 degrees and the knee in extension. The patient raises the heel of the affected lower extremity 4 to 6 inches off the bed or floor (Fig. 23-2). Another exercise that can be used following an acute dislocation with immobilization, as well as in other patients with patellofemoral alignment problems, to simultaneously strengthen both the vastus medialis obliquus and the hip adductors is to have the patient sit with

both hips flexed and both knees extended. In this position, the patient should try to push the metatarsophalangeal joints of the right and left great toes together (Fig. 23-3). This will cause an isometric contraction of the hip adductors and vastus medialis obliquus.[43] Such a contraction should be held for a count of 10; three sets of ten repetitions should be done several times throughout the day. Alternately, a ball of about 8 to 10 inches in diameter can be placed between the thighs just above the knee, and the patient instructed to squeeze the ball with both thighs, tightening the hip adductors as well as the vastus medialis (Fig. 23-4). If there is no history of low back pain or lumbar disc disease, the patient can,

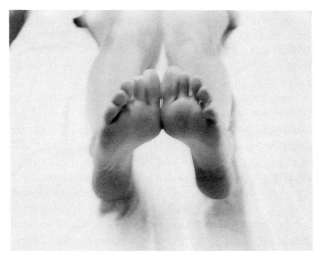

FIGURE 23-3
Exercise to strengthen vastus medialis and hip adductors. Sitting with knees extended and feet dorsiflexed, push MTP joints of great toes together.

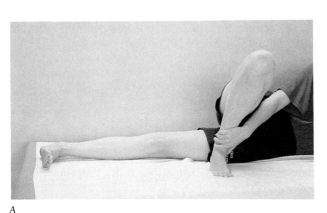

A

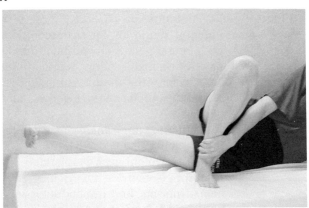

B
FIGURE 23-2
Hip adduction exercise. *A.* Lie on affected side with the foot dorsiflexed 90 degrees and the knee in extension. *B.* Raise the heel of the affected lower extremity 4 to 6 inches off the bed or floor.

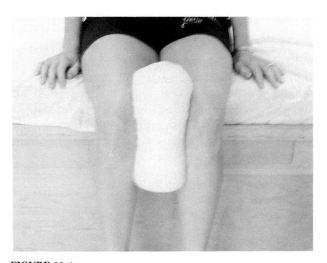

FIGURE 23-4
Strengthen hip adductors and vastus medialis by squeezing ball or similar object placed between thighs.

while squeezing the ball, attempt to lift the heels off the floor. This exercise has the potential for aggravating underlying sciatica and, therefore, should be used with caution.

Similarly, in cases of patella fractures or following surgery on the patellofemoral joint, isometric exercises emphasizing the vastus medialis obliquus should be started early, as soon as the acute inflammation has subsided. Use of a neuromuscular stimulator may help maintain tone if a period of immobilization is required. Also, in patients in whom immobilization results in tightening of the parapatellar retinacular structures, mobilization of these structures using manual massage, ultrasound, and other modalities should be started early in the initial stages of rehabilitation. When healing will permit, range of motion exercises should be started. Braces that can limit motion to protect the injury yet allow some motion in an attempt to diminish scar formation and permit early isotonic exercises are helpful in these patients.

Chronic patella tendinitis is often frustrating to treat. Some believe successful rehabilitation must incorporate not only concentric but also eccentric strengthening exercises to allow the muscles to adapt to achieving tension while lengthening, the type of activity typically implicated in causing the injury.[22] For example, the patient can jump off a block, lower a weight gradually from 0 degrees to 90 degrees knee flexion, or practice kicking a ball slowly at first, and then increasing both the speed and force of the kick. Ultrasound, phonophoresis, electrical stimulation, or iontophoresis at the target point of pain may also be tried to decrease inflammation.

Warm up tissue before exercise.
Ice injured area following exercise.

During all phases of any rehabilitation, the general rules for warming up before exercise and icing following exercise to decrease inflammation should be followed. Use of oral anti-inflammatories, although most helpful during the initial phases of rehabilitation, may also be used during any stage of rehabilitation if the patient overexerts with resultant inflammation and pain.

Key to Treating Patient with Patellofemoral Compression Syndrome
Alter patella tracking by muscle strengthening program, braces or tape, or orthotics

To help alter patella tracking, braces and orthotics are frequently recommended to complement the muscle strengthening programs.[44–46]

Patients with patellofemoral problems should also consider modifying some of their daily activities that can cause increased patellofemoral forces. For example, they should be encouraged to avoid the flexed knee position.[31,47] They should not sit Indian style or with the affected leg tucked under their buttocks. They should be encouraged to sit on the aisles of theaters to be able to periodically straighten their knee and to buy cars with cruise control that allows them to occasionally flex and extend the knee while driving. Also, in some cases of chronic patellofemoral pain, elevating the seat of the car with a pillow or blanket or using bench seats instead of bucket seats to decrease the extent of knee flexion while driving may be helpful. There are cases of patients becoming symptomatic from patellofemoral pain in the left leg when they have changed from driving an automatic to a manual gear shift, particularly if they drive in heavy traffic where they must use the clutch frequently. Moreover, when acutely symptomatic, taking elevators rather than walking down stairs should be encouraged.

When appropriate, nutritional counseling should be recommended, as certainly patellofemoral forces are greater when quadriceps contraction has to balance a greater amount of body weight.

INJURY-SPECIFIC REHABILITATION PROGRAMS

Acute Traumatic Dislocation of the Patella (nonoperative case)

Phase I: 24 to 48 hours
- Immobilization in knee immobilizer with lateral pad. Ace wrapped to hold patella against medial retinaculum; ice, electric stimulation unit, or other modalities to decrease swelling and pain
- Anti-inflammatory/analgesic, e.g., ibuprofen, naproxen if needed
- Crutches, weight bear as tolerated
- Attempt isometric quadriceps sets, hamstring sets, and hip abductor sets; hold each for count of 10; do 3 sets of 10 each
- May use neuromuscular stimulation unit to help retard atrophy, as well as decrease pain and swelling

Phase II: 1 to 3 weeks
- May change to patella-stabilizing brace under knee immobilizer
- Take immobilizer off 3 times a day for range of motion 0 degrees to 30 degrees
- Continue ice, transcutaneous electrical stimulation (TENS) or neuromuscular stimulation unit to reduce atrophy and/or pain control
- Perform quadriceps setting in full extension
- Increase to full weight bearing
- Continue isometric exercises as well as isotonic exercises in 0 degrees to 20 degrees
- Can start short arc extensions 30 degrees to 0 degrees using a rolled towel under the knee
- Continue isometrics for hamstrings
- Begin isotonic hip abduction and adduction exercises
- Progress to 3- to 5-lb weights and do 3 sets of 10 repetitions for each muscle group
- Do range of motion and strengthening for ankle (dorsi and plantar flexors, as well as invertors and everters)
- Do cross leg biking for cardiovascular fitness and cross-training effort
- Passive and active assisted knee flexion exercises to 90 degrees

Phase III: 3 to 6 weeks
- Use patella-stabilizing brace only when swelling and tenderness along medial retinaculum are resolved
- Do full range of motion exercises
- Do stretching exercises for hamstrings, quadriceps, hip abduction, hip adduction, flexion, and extension
- Advance isotonic quadriceps exercises (from 45 degrees to 0 degrees); progress to 3-lb weight; as can do 3 sets of 10 easily, advance by 2 lb up to 10 to 15 lb, depending on patient body weight and prior level of exercise
- Continue isotonic exercises for all other muscles of lower extremity
- Stair stepper with short steps, walking, or biking with elevated seat for cardiovascular fitness when patient has 95 degrees to 100 degrees of knee flexion passively and actively; begin fast step-

ping side to side and up and down a small step (4–6 inches)

Phase IV: 6 weeks
- Achieve full range of motion
- Achieve strength equal to noninjured side by advancing isotonic exercises
- Work for muscular endurance and power by alternating long, slow workouts with short bursts of activity for each muscle group
- Continue cardiovascular fitness by biking, walking, or stair stepper
- May attempt to jog and increase running over next 4 to 6 weeks if desired
- Add skills such as cut, squat
- Start jumping at 8 to 12 weeks, depending on advancement of other parameters
- Develop proprioceptive skills in weeks 8 through 10
- Try step aerobics, functional sports skills, etc.
- Can return to full activity (anticipate 8–12 weeks) if range of motion equal to opposite side; no swelling, no pain; strength 95 percent to 100 percent of opposite extremity; can hop, skip, squat and jump without difficulty

Osgood-Schlatter Disease

Phase I: 1 to 5 days
- If acutely symptomatic with limp, immobilize until acute symptoms decrease
- Oral anti-inflammatories if needed to reduce inflammation and pain
- Ice
- Crutches if needed

Phase II: Out of immobilization
- Infrapatellar strap or protective brace with inferior horseshoe pad may be used
- Try TENS or high voltage electrical stimulation to decrease inflammation if desired (may use in phase I also)
- Continue to use ice or oral anti-inflammatories to decrease inflammation
- Do straight leg raises
- Perform resisted plantar flexion of ankle with tubing

- Begin short arc extension exercises, progressing to 1- to 2-lb weight, and advancing by 2-lb increments
- Begin isotonic exercises for hip flexors, extensors, abductors, and adductors and for muscles of the lower leg
- Achieve full range of motion
- Walk in chest high water, use water vest, or swim to maintain cardiovascular fitness, or bike if biking does not cause pain
- Stretching exercises for hip and knee muscles

Phase III: Continue to brace and use ice if needed
- Continue range of motion exercises
- Strengthening exercises for hip and knee flexors, extensors, abductors, adductors, doing 3 sets of 10 repetitions of each starting with 3- to 5-lb weights and increasing by 2 lb when exercise is done easily for the 3 sets
- Start isometric exercises 0 degrees to 90 degrees and include eccentric exercises for quadriceps; e.g., lift 5 lb from 90 degrees to 0 degrees knee flexion, then slowly lower weight from 0 degrees to 90 degrees (i.e., eccentric quadriceps activity) as tolerated

Phase IV: Add jumping, hopping, stepping
- Jump off 8-inch step then jump back up, first slowly and then more rapidly
- Sport-specific skills where appropriate

Patellofemoral Stress Syndrome

Phase I: 1 to 2 days
- Knee immobilizer if acutely symptomatic
- Ice and oral anti-inflammatories to decrease inflammation and pain
- TENS unit if needed for pain control
- Begin quadriceps sets, straight leg raises when pain permits

- Hip adductor/abduction, flexion, and extension exercises

Phase II: Out of immobilizer
- Infrapatellar strap or patella-stabilizing brace
- Continue ice, especially following exercise periods
- Continue TENS and oral anti-inflammatories if needed
- Straight leg raises, quadriceps sets, short arc extensions
- Flexibility exercises for quadriceps, hamstrings, iliotibial band, gastrocnemius, soleus
- Start to bike with seat elevated, swim (crawl only), use stair stepper (small steps done rapidly)
- Advance isotonic exercises for hip flexors, extensors, abductors, adductors, as well as muscles of the lower leg and foot, increasing weight as tolerated, doing 3 sets of 10 and increasing weight by 2 lb

Phase III: Use brace if needed
- Continue quadriceps isotonics from 30 degrees to 0 degrees, increasing weight as tolerated to a maximum of 20 lb to 30 lb
- Advance hamstring strengthening exercises
- Continue biking, swimming, stair stepper, or walking for cardiovascular and muscle endurance; increase duration, then speed
- Continue flexibility exercises

Phase IV: Add slow return to running if desired; increase distance, then speed
- Warm up well
- Ice following workout
- Continue to aerobically cross train
- Start to jump, cut, half squats, kick, and other sport-specific skills if applicable
- Wear brace or tape for sport participation if desired

REFERENCES

1. Henry J: Conservative treatment of patellofemoral subluxation. *Clin Sports Med* 8:261, 1979.
2. Henry J, Crosland J: Conservative treatment of patellofemoral subluxation. *Am J Sports Med* 7:12, 1979.

3. Sachs R, Daniel D, Stone M, Garfein R: Patellofemoral problems after anterior cruciate ligament reconstruction. *Am J Sports Med* 17:760, 1989.

4. Cooper D, DeLee J, Ramamurthy S: Reflex sympathetic dystrophy of the knee. Treatment using continuous epidural anesthesia. *J Bone Joint Surg* 71A:365, 1989.

5. Schutzer D, Gossling H: The treatment of reflex sympathetic dystrophy syndrome. *J Bone Joint Surg* 66A:625, 1984.

6. Schmidt D, Henry J: Stress injuries of the adolescent extensor mechanism. *Clin Sports Med* 8:343, 1989.

7. Knight K: Total injury rehabilitation. *Phys Sportsmed* 7:111, 1979.

8. Roy S, Irvin R: *Sports Medicine.* Englewood Cliffs, NJ, Prentice-Hall, 1983.

9. Steadman J, Forster R, Silferskiold J: Rehabilitation of the knee. *Clin Sports Med* 8:605, 1989.

10. American Academy of Orthopaedic Surgeons. *Athletic Training and Sports Medicine,* 2d ed. Park Ridge, IL, American Academy of Orthopaedic Surgeons, 1991.

11. Kulund D: *The Injured Athlete,* 2d ed. Philadelphia, Lippincott, 1988.

12. Knight K: Guidelines for rehabilitation of sports injuries. *Clin Sports Med* 4:405, 1985.

13. Prentice W: *Rehabilitation Techniques in Sports Medicine.* St. Louis, Times/Mirror Mosby, 1990, pp 34–61.

14. Eriksson E: Sport injuries of the knee ligaments: Their diagnosis, treatment, rehabilitation, and prevention. *Med Science Sports* 8:133, 1976.

15. Lamb D: *Physiology of Exercise,* 2d ed. New York, Macmillan, 1984, pp 19–37.

16. Gollnick P, Saltin B: Skeletal muscle physiology, in *Scientific Foundations of Sports Medicine,* edited by C. Teitz. Toronto, Decker, 1989.

17. Beckman M, Craig R, Lehman R: Rehabilitation of patellofemoral dysfunction in the athlete. *Clin Sports Med* 8:841, 1989.

18. Arnheim D: *Modern Principles of Athletic Training,* 6th ed. St. Louis, Times/Mirror Mosby, 1985.

19. Torg J, Vegso J, Torg E: *Rehabilitation of Athletic Injuries.* Chicago, Year Book Medical Publishers, 1987, pp 1–8.

20. Gould J, Davies G (eds): *Orthopaedic and Sports Physical Therapy.* St. Louis, Mosby, 1985, pp 181–198.

21. Brunet M, Stewart G: Patellofemoral rehabilitation. *Clin Sports Med* 8:319, 1989.

22. Stanish W, Rubinovich R, Currwin S: Eccentric exercise in chronic tendonitis. *Clin Orthop* 208:65, 1986.

23. Hislop H, Perrine J: The isokinetic concept of exercise. *Phys Ther* 47:114, 1967.

24. Prentice W, Kooima E: The use of proprioceptive neuromuscular facilitation techniques in the rehabilitation of sport-related injury. *Athletic Training* 21:26, 1986.

25. Eriksson E, Haggmark T: Comparison of isometric muscle training and electrical stimulation supplementing isometric muscle training in the recovery after major knee ligament surgery. A preliminary report. *Am J Sports Med* 7:169, 1979.

26. Gould N, Donnermeyer D, Pope M, Ashikaga T: Transcutaneous muscle stimulation as a method to retard disuse atrophy. *Clin Orthop* 164:215, 1982.

27. Mellion M, Walsh W, Shelton G (eds): *The Team Physician's Handbook.* Philadelphia, Hanley and Belfus, 1990, pp 27–33.

28. Malek M, Mangine R: Patellofemoral pain syndromes: A comprehensive and conservative approach. *J Orthop Sports Phys Ther* 2:108, 1981.

29. Hungerford D, Barry M: Biomechanics of the patellofemoral joint. *Clin Orthop* 144:9, 1979.

30. Huberti H, Hayes W: Patellofemoral contact pressures: The influence of Q-angle and tendofemoral contact. *J Bone Joint Surg* 66A:715, 1984.

31. Percy E, Strother R: Patalgia. *Phys Sportsmed* 13:43, 1985.

32. Kettelkamp D: Management of patellar malalignment. *J Bone Joint Surg* 63A:1344, 1981.

33. Merchant A, Mercer R: Roentgenographic analysis of patellofemoral congruence. J Bone Joint Surg 56A:1391, 1974.

34. Yates C, Giana W: Patellofemoral pain in children. *Clin Orthop* 255:36, 1990.

35. Muller W: *The Knee.* Berlin, Springer-Verlag, 1983.

36. Hunter-Griffin L: The patellofemoral stress syndrome in women. *Your Patient and Fitness* 4:9, 1990.

37. Stulberg S, Shulman K, Stuart S, Culp P: Breastroker's knee: Pathology, etiology, and treatment. *Am J Sports Med* 8:164, 1980.

38. Stanitski C: Rehabilitation following knee injury. *Clin Sports Med* 4:495, 1985.

39. Irrgang J: The patello-femoral joint: Strategies for rehabilitation. *Sports Medicine Update* 2:4, 1990.

40. Fulkerson J: Awareness of the retinaculum in evaluating patellofemoral pain. *Am J Sports Med* 10:147, 1982.

41. Jackson J, Waugh W: *Surgery of the Knee Joint.* Philadelphia, Lippincott, 1984.

42. Hughston J, Walsh W, Puddu G: *Patellar Subluxation and Dislocation*. Philadelphia, Saunders, 1984.

43. Hanten W, Schulthies S: Exercise effect on electromyographic activity of the vastus medialis oblique and vastus lateralis muscles. *Phys Ther* 70:561, 1990.

44. Lysholm J, Nordin M, Ekstrand J, Gillquist J: The effect of a patella brace on performance in a knee extension strength test in patients with patellar pain. *Am J Sports Med* 12:110, 1984.

45. Palumbo P: Dynamic patellar brace: A new orthosis in the management of patellofemoral disorders. *Am J Sports Med* 9:45, 1981.

46. James S, Bates B, Osterling L: Injuries to runners. Am J Sports Med 6:40, 1978.

47. Bentley G, Dowd G: Current concepts of etiology and treatment of chondromalacia patellae. *Clin Orthop* 189:209, 1984.

CHAPTER 24

Patellofemoral Rehabilitation

Todd J. Molnar

INTRODUCTION

The treatment of patellofemoral pain and dysfunction can be the most challenging as well as frustrating situation encountered by physicians and therapists alike. Although surgery may become necessary, this option should only be considered when all possible conservative methods have been exhausted.[1-3] The term "conservative," however, should not be confused with passive or nonaggressive treatment.[4] This chapter discusses the many options available in the nonsurgical treatment of anterior knee pain.

As our knowledge of patellofemoral anatomy, pathophysiology, and biomechanics has expanded, so too have the techniques for rehabilitating this complex joint. We must stray away from the old trap of calling all anterior knee pain "chondromalacia patellae," and then prescribing a standardized "cookbook" type rehabilitation program.[5-7] Chondromalacia patella should be used only as a pathologic description of softening and fissuring of the undersurface of the patella when directly seen during arthroscopy or implied by magnetic resonance imaging (MRI) scan. It should not be used as a clinical diagnosis.[8,9] In fact, the correlation of patellofemoral pain and the degree of chondromalacia patella is poor. Instead, emphasis should be placed on the precise pathophysiologic and pathomechanical dysfunction that occurs throughout the patellofemoral joint.[10-12] A successful rehabilitation program must start with an accurate diagnosis followed by an individually tailored program.

BASIC PRINCIPLES OF REHABILITATION

To develop a successful rehabilitation program for patellofemoral pain, one must first understand all the therapeutic exercises available and then determine which will be the most appropriate for the given condition. Basmajian defines *therapeutic exercises* as any motion of the body or its parts used to improve functional ability to relieve symptoms.[13,14] These may take the form of passive or active exercises. To achieve and gain strength, however, one must perform an *active resisted exercise,* either statically or dynamically. Static strength may be developed through *isometric contractions* where tension is increased in a muscle without any change in its length.

Dynamic strength may be achieved through *isokinetic* or *isotonic contractions. Isotonic strengthening* refers to a constant tension in the muscle with a concomitant change in muscle length. When this occurs during muscle shortening, it is considered a *concentric contraction* and during lengthening an *eccentric contraction.* Both types of contractions occur throughout typical activities of daily living as well as sports and may need to be addressed during rehabilitation. First described in the late 1940s, the DeLorme principle, using *progressive resistance exercise* (PRE), remains the standard method of isotonic strengthening.[15-17] Emphasis on endurance is achieved by low resistance and a high number of repetitions, whereas emphasis on strength uses heavy resistance and a lower number of repetitions. Much debate still occurs over eccentric training techniques. Eccentric contractions place high loads and greater tension on muscle fibers and tendons. In fact, electron microscopy has shown myofibril damage after eccentric loading versus concentric loading.[18] The problem of eccentric loading cannot be ignored, however, because many of life's activities involve eccentric contractions. Any decelerating action of the leg, such as descending stairs (a hallmark of patellofemoral pain), will require eccentric quadriceps contraction. However, clinical studies of patellofemoral pain patients demonstrates significant weakness in eccentric strength compared to concentric.[19] Following eccentric training significant symptomatic improvement occurred.

The other form of dynamic strengthening is isokinetic, whereby the speed of motion is kept constant and the force applied can be varied. Use of specialized equipment from various manufacturers can achieve this effect for both strength testing and training. Isokinetic techniques can play a role in the more advanced stages of patellofemoral rehabilitation.

The principle of specificity of training must be kept in mind in designing a rehabilitation program. It is well established that there is not complete crossover of training effect when going from one strengthening type to another.[20,21] For example, if isometric training techniques are used, optimal performance will be achieved isometrically not isotonically and vice versa. Therefore, patients must be trained according to the type of activity they will be performing.

BIOMECHANICAL CONSIDERATIONS

In considering rehabilitation programs for patello-femoral dysfunction, one must focus not only on the knee but on all of its surrounding and supporting structures.[22] Malalignment of any portion of the lower extremity should be assessed and dealt with accordingly. Findings highly associated with patellofemoral dysfunction include femoral anteversion, increase genu valgus or varus, increased Q angle, excessive tibial torsion, foot pronation/supination,[23] and pes planus/cavus deformities. In a study on the three-dimensional tracking pattern of the human patella, Van Kampen and Huiskes showed complex and consistent motion patterns that are greatly influenced by internal and external rotation of the tibia.[24] Often custom foot orthotics can be prescribed to correct or lessen the malalignment and have a significant effect on patellofemoral symptoms.[25-27] Patellofemoral tracking is thought by many to play a large role in the etiology of patellofemoral symptoms.[8,9,28-31] Physical examination may give some clues by observation of patellar position relative to the femur and tibia. Extreme out-pointing or in-pointing of the patella from femoral malalignment may have dramatic effects on patellar position in the femoral groove. Conventional radiography gives additional information regarding patellofemoral relationships.[32-34] However, it is fraught with its own shortcomings. These include distortion and an inability to access the joint at knee angles less than 25 degrees.[28] In addition, measurement of congruence angle, sulcus angle, and other objective measures becomes difficult and unreliable in the presence of condylar dysplasia, a finding often seen in patients with patellar subluxation or malalignment. Computed tomography (CT) has given us additional information on the patellofemoral relationships but has limited clinical usefulness.[35-37]

Recent advances in MRI technology have allowed excellent visualization of the patellofemoral joint and surrounding soft tissues.[38-40] This has been particularly helpful at joint angles of 0 degrees to 30 degrees where most maltracking appears to occur.[36,37,41] Shellock and coworkers have used kinematic MRI to evaluate patellar tracking abnormalities.[39,40] They describe a spectrum of maltracking in clinically symptomatic patients that range from lateral to medial subluxation. These include lateral subluxation, excessive lateral pressure, medial subluxation, lateral to medial subluxation, and dislocation. This has become extremely useful information in designing rehabilitation programs. The old theories that all patellae maltrack only in a lateral direction may no longer hold true.

Medial subluxation was first described by Hughston as a complication of lateral release procedures,[42] but is now well documented to occur in the absence of any surgical intervention.[39,40] Special modifications must therefore be made in the approach to the rehabilitation of patellofemoral dysfunction.

All patients with anterior knee pain must not be considered equal. Following detailed history, meticulous physical examination, radiography, and possibly MRI evaluations, a precise diagnosis is made and *only then* can the most appropriate rehabilitation program be created.

THERAPEUTIC EXERCISES

The primary goal in the rehabilitation of patellofemoral dysfunction is to decrease symptoms, improve strength and endurance, and return the individual to maximal functional potential.[43] The emphasis must be on an *active* exercise program that safely increases quadriceps strength and corrects, or at least optimizes, the patellofemoral tracking mechanism.[44,45] The key principle to be followed is the avoidance of pain during the actual exercises. The "no pain—no gain" philosophy fails miserably when applied to patellofemoral rehabilitation. In fact, through a reflex inhibition, the force of the quadriceps contraction is reduced in the presence of pain.[46-48] Thus, sound mechanical principles must be followed to minimize patellofemoral pressures while maximizing quadriceps strengthening. Biomechanical analysis has shown that patellofemoral contact forces are lowest in extension from 0 degrees to 30 degrees.[49,50] Thus, leg extension exercises at 90 degrees are avoided and replaced by quadriceps sets, straight leg raising (SLR) (Fig. 24-1) and short arc quadriceps (SAQ) extensions (Fig. 24-2).[51,52] Hip abductors and adductors are also strengthened using ankle weights (Fig. 24-3) or appropriate gym equipment (Fig. 24-4). However, many patients do not do well with these traditional *open kinetic chain* exercises. They may have exacerbation of their patellofemoral symptoms as well as poor carryover into functional daily activities. Research conducted in a *closed kinetic chain* with the subject's foot in contact with the ground shows distinctly different biomechanics of tibial rotation and subtalar motion.[48,53] In addition, less patellofemoral contact stresses have been demonstrated from 30 degrees to 60 degrees knee flexion in a closed kinetic chain versus an open kinetic chain.[54] Although patellofemoral joint reaction forces increase with knee flexion, so does surface contact areas which in turn will actually decrease the force per square inch since the force

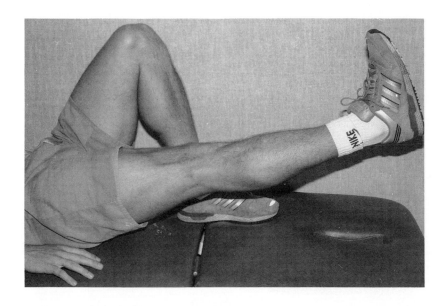

FIGURE 24-1
Straight leg raising exercise for quadriceps strengthening.

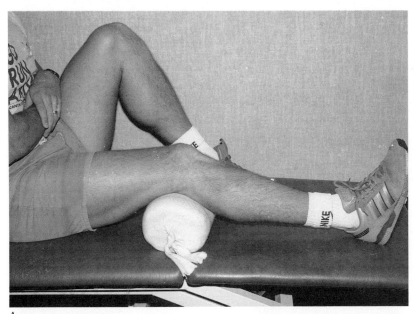

A

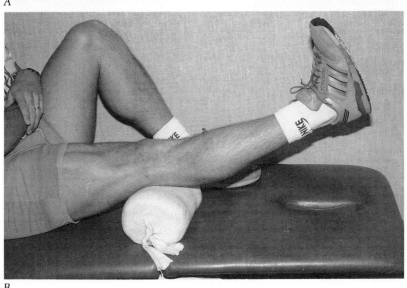

B

FIGURE 24-2
Short arc quadricep exercises are performed starting at 30 degrees flexion (*A*) to full extension (*B*).

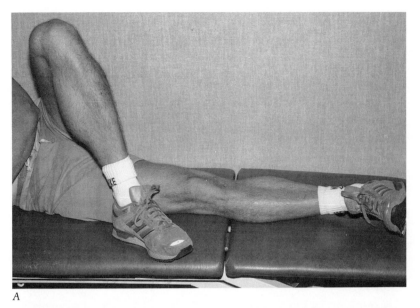

A

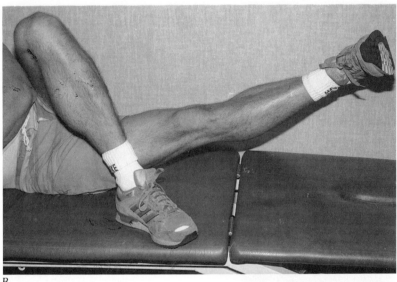

B

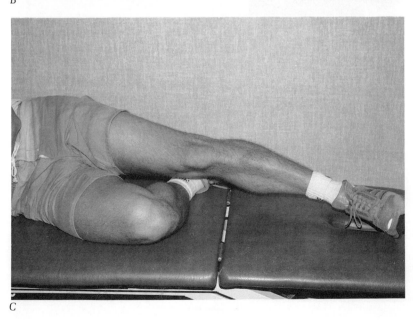

C

FIGURE 24-3
Hip abductor (*A* and *B*) and adductor (*C* and
D) exercises. Resistance may be increased by
adding ankle weights.

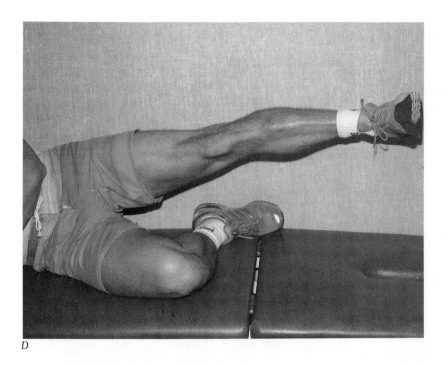

FIGURE 24-3 *D*

D

is distributed over a greater surface area. It follows that quadriceps strengthening exercises should include closed kinetic chain activities. These are generally used in the most advanced stages of quadriceps femoris muscle rehabilitation. Closed kinetic chain exercises include step downs (Fig. 24-5*A*), lunges (Fig. 24-5*B*), partial squats (Fig. 24-5*C*), and leg presses. Additional endurance training can be achieved on Stairmaster-type equipment (Fig. 24-6). Precautions should be taken to minimize patellofemoral forces on such equipment by using short steps,

thereby limiting the amount of knee flexion. Stationary cycling (Fig. 24-7) is useful for warm-up for an exercise program as well as conditioning. Care should be taken to keep pedal resistance low and seat position appropriate to avoid unnecessary patellofemoral stresses.

Aqua therapy can also be considered as part of the rehabilitation program.[55] Therapeutic exercises when performed in the limited gravity environment of the pool produce much less stress on the patellofemoral tissues. Exercises include walking against

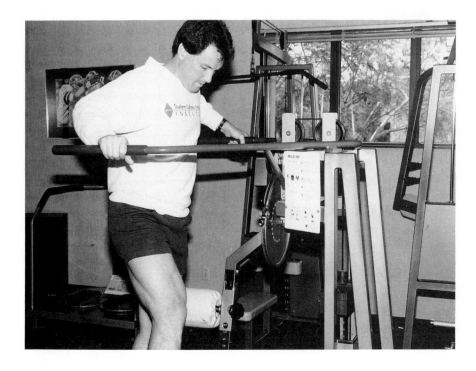

FIGURE 24-4
Standing four-way hip machine pictured here strengthening the hip adductors.

295

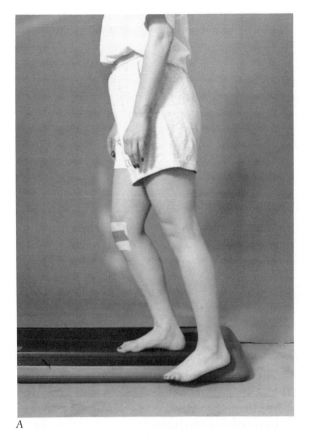

A

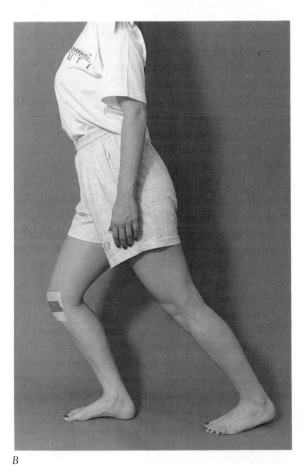

B

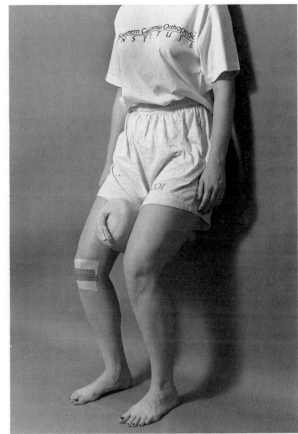

C

FIGURE 24-5
Closed kinetic chain exercise for advanced stages of quadriceps strengthening include step downs (*A*), lunges (*B*), and partial squats (*C*).

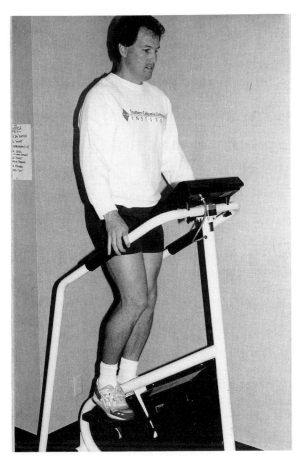

FIGURE 24-6
Stairmaster-type step machine for closed kinetic chain functional strengthening and conditioning.

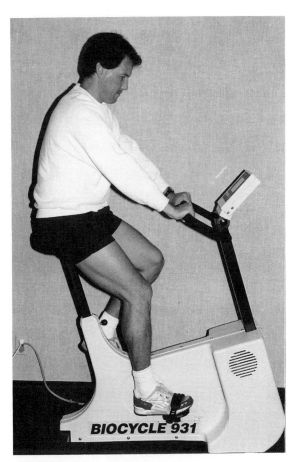

FIGURE 24-7
Stationary bicycle can be helpful for patellofemoral rehabilitation in selected patients. Pedal resistance should be kept low.

water resistance at various depths, freestyle swimming, and kick board use with and without swim fins (Fig. 24-8*A*). More advanced training progresses toward running in place in deep water with flotation vests or use of underwater treadmill and other resistive equipment that have recently become available (Fig. 24-8*B* and *C*). Use of such equipment is best done under the supervision of an experienced pool therapist. The drawback of aqua therapy is its limited availability. Few physical therapy centers are equipped with a pool. Patients can be instructed on proper exercises in a home pool if available or at their local gym if so equipped.

In monitoring any patient going through a course of rehabilitation for patellofemoral pain, one must not underestimate the patient's level of frustration and need for reassurance. It is helpful to reevaluate these patients in the office every 6 weeks to reassess their symptoms and extensor mechanism function and encourage their continuation in the exercise program. The extra time spent educating the patient, including the parents of adolescents, is helpful in relieving the fears, anxieties, and frustration so often present. This will usually result in better compliance

with the total rehabilitation program. The physician must quell the temptation to perform invasive procedures even in the face of the patient's desperate pleas to "do something." Nothing may be more disheartening in orthopaedics than having to face the patient whose patellofemoral pain has been made worse by surgery. The indications for surgery are beyond the scope of this chapter. Suffice it to state that operating on the patellofemoral joint should remain a last ditch effort and only considered when the appropriate rehabilitation efforts have all been tried and failed.

SPECIAL TECHNIQUES

Even after following all of the above recommendations for therapeutic exercises, many patients continue to be symptomatic. In fact, many may be unable to tolerate even the simplest and apparently least stressful of exercises. Jenny McConnell, a physical therapist from Australia, has developed a treatment program using taping and exercise techniques that boast a 96 percent success rate.[56] The taping is based on an assessment of patellar position and maltrack-

297

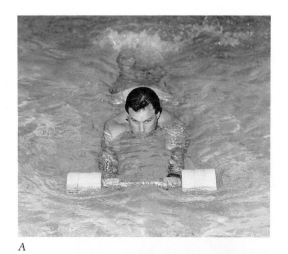

A

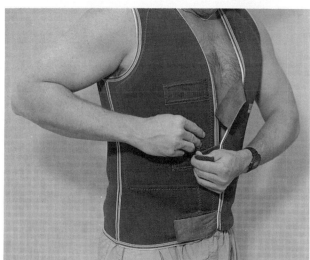

B

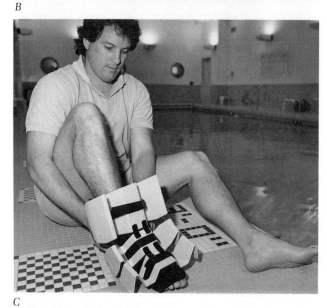

C

FIGURE 24-8

Aqua therapy is an excellent medium to rehabilitative patellofem-oral disorders. *A*. Use of kickboard with swim fins for additional resistance. Flotation vests (*B*) are useful for deep water exercises such as running in place. Hydrotone equipment (*C*) allows for much greater resistance for higher level strengthening programs.

ing. Three abnormal patellar orientations are exam-ined: glide component, tilt component, and rotation component. The critical test is performed in a sitting position with the patient's legs dangling free. Isomet-ric quadriceps contractions are performed at knee flexion angles of 0, 30, 60, 90, 120 degrees while the femur is externally rotated (Fig. 24-9). Pain reproduc-tion is noted for each angle tested. The patient's leg is then brought to full extension resting on the exam-iner's knee to allow for complete quadriceps relax-ation. The patella is then passively glided medially (see Fig. 24-9C). While the examiner maintains this position, the patient again performs isometric con-tractions at the positions previously noted to be pain-ful. Pain should be dramatically reduced if its origin is lateral patellofemoral maltracking. The patella would then be taped from its lateral border medially (Fig. 24-10A). When excessive lateral tilt is encoun-tered, taping is done from midpoint of the patella to the medial knee (Fig. 24-10B). Abnormal rotation components are taped toward a neutral position (Fig. 24-10C). If the taping has been applied appropriately, correcting each abnormal patellar component, the pa-tient should then be able to begin the exercise pro-gram and activities in a pain-free state. Emphasis is placed on training the vastus medialis obliquus (VMO) in weight-bearing positions using closed ki-netic chain techniques. Specific attention is placed on foot supination and pronation, which is incorpo-rated into the exercises (Fig. 24-11). Patients progress to eccentric training by performing step downs (see Fig. 24-5A). The tape is readjusted as necessary to ensure that pain does not increase. Training may be advanced to sports-specific activities as indicated. McConnell taping techniques appear to work favor-ably in patients with lateral malalignment syn-dromes. However, a subset of patients with patello-femoral pain seems to respond poorly. Using medial patellar glide taping may aggravate their symptoms. These patients have tenderness over their medial reti-naculum and medial patellar facet. Further evalua-tion using kinematic MRI studies may reveal *medial* subluxation (Fig. 24-12A). We have found success in these patients by reversing the standard McConnell taping protocol. The patella is taped with a *lateral* glide technique (Fig. 24-13) and the patient is pain free and able to exercise. The key to success is the individual assessment and treatment of each painful patellofemoral joint.

In addition to taping, other therapeutic modali-ties have joined the physical therapist's armamentar-ium to battle patellofemoral problems. Electromyo-graphic (EMG) biofeedback has become increasingly popular in patellofemoral rehabilitation programs. Studies have shown patients can selectively train the VMO using EMG biofeedback.[57,58] This may be com-

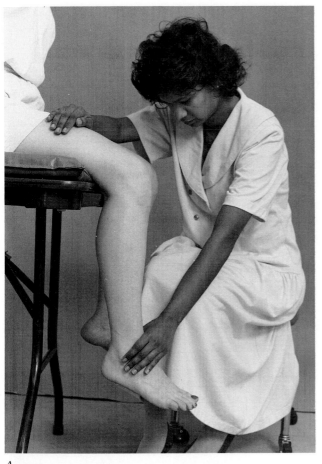

A

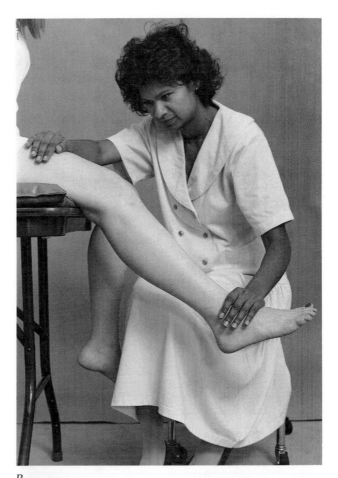

B

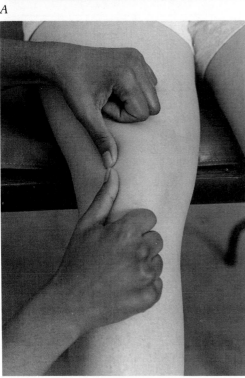

C

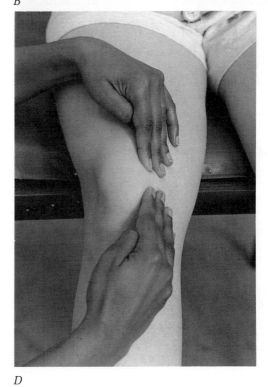

D

FIGURE 24-9
Early evaluation for McConnell taping includes assessment of pain, reproduction at joint angles of 0, 30, 60, 90, and 120 degrees during isometric quadriceps contraction (*A* and *B*). The patella is then passively glided medially by examiner (*C* and *D*) as patient performs isometric quadriceps contraction.

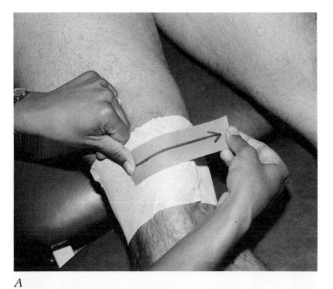

A

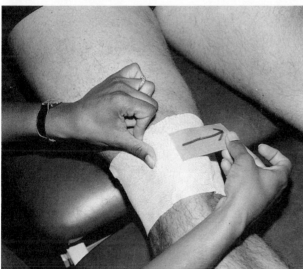

B

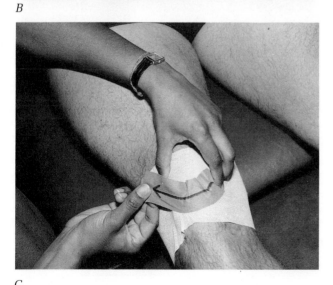

C

FIGURE 24-10
Components of McConnell taping include (*A*) medial glide to correct for lateral tracking, (*B*) medial tilt to correct for lateral patellar tilt, and (*C*) rotation to tape toward a neutral position.

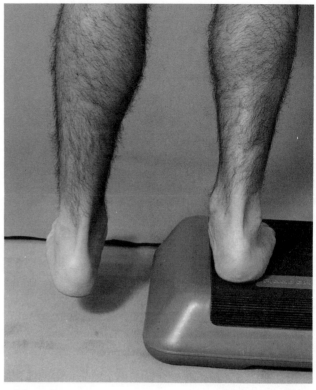

FIGURE 24-11
Patients with excessive foot pronation require additional assistance by therapist to maintain a neutral foot during exercises. Orthotics may be necessary for optimal correction.

bined with the McConnell taping program to help patients reeducate the quadriceps mechanism.

BRACING FOR PATELLOFEMORAL PAIN

Use of knee braces for the treatment of patellofemoral problems remains a controversial issue. Opinion varies greatly regarding which braces to use as well as when and how to use them.[59] The variations of brace design are countless, raging from simple straps to elastic or neoprene sleeves to more complicated buttresses and pads that attempt to influence patellar alignment (Fig. 24-14). Many theories have been proposed to explain how knee braces may improve symptoms. The warming effect to soft tissues and joints may offer some relief. Some advocate sensory feedback as a factor, whereas others claim bracing may improve alignment and patellofemoral tracking. Very few studies are available that scientifically assess the benefits of bracing. Lysholm and colleagues used isokinetic testing with and without an elastic knee brace and claimed 88 percent improved performance with the brace.[60] Palumbo designed a brace that applies medial displacing forces to the lateral border of the patella.[61] He reports 93 percent of 62 patients had reduced patellar symptoms. Other at-

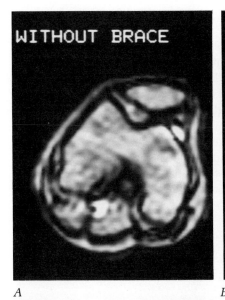

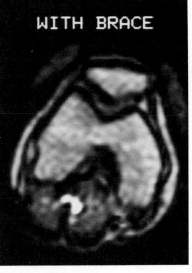

FIGURE 24-12
Kinematic MRI study demonstrates *medial* patellar subluxation (*A*). Same patient with a laterally displacing patellar brace demonstrates adequate correction (*B*).

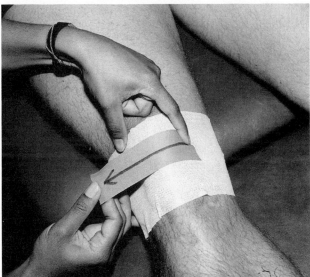

FIGURE 24-13
Lateral glide technique for patients with medial subluxation.

tempts at studying brace efficacy used radiography and cineradiography and were unable to document any significant mechanical advantage to bracing.[62] Kinematic MRI may be a more useful method for assessing patellofemoral bracing. Figure 24-12*A* and *B* shows a patient with significant medial maltracking that is markedly improved by a soon-to-be released brace by Bauerfeind Inc. (Fig. 24-15). It is obvious that additional scientifically valid studies are needed to substantiate patellofemoral bracing. When braces are used, they should be considered only as an adjunct to the full treatment plan. Patients must be encouraged to focus less on the brace and more on their active participation in the rehabilitation process.

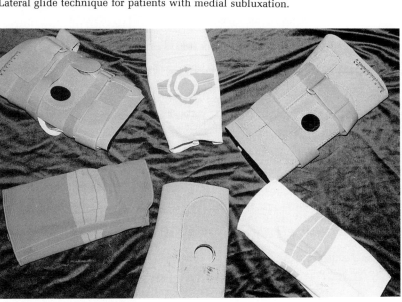

FIGURE 24-14
A multitude of braces is available, claiming to help reduce patellofemoral pain.

301

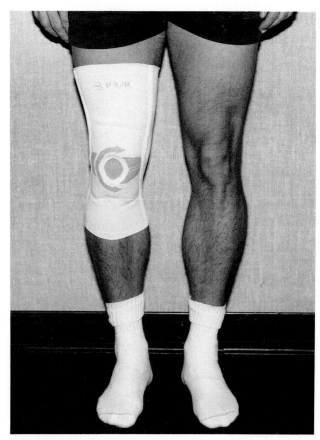

FIGURE 24-15
Experimental brace by Bauerfeind Inc. that attempts to improve patellar tracking by placing a directional force on the patella, as denoted by arrows.

SUMMARY

Patellofemoral dysfunction should not be considered a simple or straightforward problem; nor should it be treated as such. This chapter has emphasized the importance of making an accurate diagnosis followed by a specific treatment program. Patients must be followed closely with frequent reassurances by both physician and therapist. The temptation to operate must be controlled. Surgical intervention should be reserved for only those patients in whom an appropriate and extensive source of rehabilitation has failed.

REFERENCES

1. Fisher RL: Conservative treatment of patellofemoral pain. *Orthop Clin North Am* 17:269, 1986.
2. Gruber M: The conservative treatment of chondromalacia patellae. *Orthop Clin North Am* 10:105, 1979.
3. Heckmann TP: Conservative versus postsurgical patellar rehabilitation. *Physical Therapy of the Knee.* pp 127–143; 19.
4. Malek M, Mangine R: Patellofemoral pain syndromes: A comprehensive and conservative approach. *J Orthop Sports Phys Ther* 2:108, 1981.
5. Insall J: "Chondromalacia patellae": Patellar malalignment syndrome. *Orthop Clin North Am* 10:117, 1979.
6. Outerbridge RE: Further studies on the etiology of chondromalacia patellae. *J Bone Joint Surg* 46B: 179, 1964.
7. Outerbridge RE: The aetiology of chondromalacia patellae. *J Bone Joint Surg* 43B:752, 1961.
8. Merchant AC: Classification of patellofemoral disorders. *Arthroscopy* 4:235, 1988.
9. Radin EL: Anterior knee pain: The need for a specific diagnosis, stop calling it chondromalacia! *Orthop Rev* 14:128, 1985.
10. Goodfellow J, Hungerford DS, Woods C: Patello-femoral joint mechanics and pathology. 2. Chondromalacia patellae. *J Bone Joint Surg* 58B:291, 1976.
11. Goodfellow J, Hungerford DS, Zindel M: Patello-femoral joint mechanics and pathology. 1. Functional anatomy of the patello-femoral joint. *J Bone Joint Surg* 58B:287, 1976.
12. Kummel BM: The diagnosis of patellofemoral derangements. *Primary Care* 7:199, 1980.
13. Basmajian JV: *Therapeutic Exercise;* 4th ed. Baltimore, Williams & Wilkins, 1984.
14. Basmajian JV, DeLuca CJ: *Muscles Alive: Their Functions Revealed by Electromyography.* Baltimore, Williams & Wilkins, 1985.
15. DeLorme TL: Heavy resistance exercises. *Arch Phys Med* 27:607, 1946.
16. DeLorme TL: Restoration of muscle power by heavy-resistance exercises. *J Bone Joint Surg* 27:645, 1945.

17. DeLorme TL, Watkins AL: Techniques of progressive resistive exercises. *Arch Phys Med* 29:263, 1948.

18. Pavone E, Moffat M: Isometric torque of the quadriceps femoris after concentric, eccentric and isometric training. *Arch Phys Med Rehab* 66:168, 1985.

19. Bennett JG, Stauber WT: Evaluation and treatment of anterior knee pain using eccentric exercise. *Med Sci Sports Exerc* 18:526, 1986.

20. DeLateur B, Lehmann JF, Stonebridge J, et al: Isotonic versus isometric exercise: A double-shift-transfer-of-timing study. *Arch Phys Med Rehab* 53:212, 1972.

21. DeLateur B, Lehmann JF, Warren CG, et al: Comparison of effectiveness of isokinetic and isotonic exercise in quadriceps strengthening. *Arch Phys Med Rehab* 53:60, 1972.

22. Fulkerson JP: Awareness of the retinaculum in evaluating patellofemoral pain. *Am J Sports Med* 10:147, 1982.

23. Tiberio D: The effect of excessive subtalar joint pronation on patellofemoral mechanics: A theoretical model. *J Orthop Sports Phys Ther* 9:160, 1987.

24. Van Kampen A, Huiskes R: The three-dimensional tracking pattern of the human patella. *J Orthop Res* 8:372, 1990.

25. Buchbinder R, Naporo N, Bizzo E: The relationship of abnormal pronation to chondromalacia patellae in distance runners. *J Am Podiatr Med Assoc* 69:159, 1979.

26. Cox JS: Patellofemoral problems in runners. *Clin Sports Med* 4:709, 1985.

27. Wallace L: Foot Pronation and Knee Pain, in *Introduction to Sports Medicine,* edited by L. Wallace. Cleveland, Case Western Reserve University, pp 101–122, 1976.

28. Ficat RP, Hungerford DS: *Disorders of the Patellofemoral Joint.* Baltimore, Williams & Wilkins, 1977.

29. LeVeau BF, Rogers C: Selective training of the vastus medialis muscle using EMG biofeedback. *Phys Ther* 60:1410.

30. Reider B, Marshall J, Ring B: Patellar tracking. *Clin Orthop* 157:143, 1981.

31. Wiberg G: Roentgenographic and anatomic studies on the femoropatellar joint, with special reference to chondromalacia patellae. *Acta Orthop Scand* 12:319, 1941.

32. Insall J, Falvo KA, Wise DW: Patellar pain and incongruences. II. Clinical application. *Clin Orthop* 176:225, 1983.

33. Merchant AC, Mercer RL, Jacobsen RH, Cool CR: Roentgenographic analysis of patellofemoral congruence. *J Bone Joint Surg* [Am] 56:1391, 1974.

34. Newberg AH, Seligson D: The patellofemoral joint: 30°, 60°, and 90° views. *Radiology* 137:57, 1980.

35. Brunet ME, Stewart GW: Patellofemoral rehabilitation. *Clin Sports Med* 8:319, 1989.

36. Delgado-Martins H: A study of the position of the patella using computerized tomography. *J Bone Joint Surg* 61B:443, 1979.

37. Martinez S, Korobkin M, Fondren FB, et al: Diagnosis of patellofemoral malalignment by computed tomography. *J Comput Assist Tomogr* 7:1050, 1983.

38. Shellock FG, Mink JH, Deutsch A, Fox JM: Kinematic magnetic resonance imaging for evaluation of patellar tracking. *Physician and Sportsmed* 17:99, 1989.

39. Shellock FG, Mink JH, Deutsch AL, Fox JM: Patellar tracking abnormalities: Clinical experience with kinematic MR imaging in 130 patients. *Radiology* 172:799, 1989.

40. Shellock FG, Mink JH, Fox JM: Patellofemoral joint: Kinematic MR imaging to access tracking abnormalities. *Radiology* 168:551, 1988.

41. Laurin CA, Dussault R, Levesque HP: The tangential x-ray investigation of the patellofemoral joint: X-ray technique, diagnostic criteria and their interpretation. *Clin Orthop* 144:16, 1979.

42. Hughston JC, Deese M: Medial subluxation of the patella as a complication of lateral release. *Am J Sports Med* 16:383, 1988.

43. Beckman M, Craig R, Lehman RC: Rehabilitation of patellofemoral dysfunction in the athlete. *Clin Sports Med* 8:841, 1989.

44. Radin EL: A rational approach to the treatment of patellofemoral pain. *Clin Orthop* 144:107, 1979.

45. Steadman JR: Non-operative measures for patellofemoral problems. *Am J Sports Med* 7:374, 1979.

46. Antich TJ, Brewster CE: Modification of quadriceps femoris muscle exercises during knee rehabilitation. *Phys Ther* 66:1246, 1986.

47. DeAnrade J, Grant C, Dixon A: Joint distension and reflex inhibition in the knee. *J Bone Joint Surg* 47A:313, 1955.

48. Stokes M, Young A: Investigations of quadriceps inhibition: Implication for clinical practice. *Physiotherapy* 7:425, 1984.

49. Hungerford DS, Barry M: Biomechanics of the patellofemoral joint. *Clin Orthop* 144:9, 1979.

50. Huberti H, Hayes W: Patellofemoral contact pressures. *J Bone Joint Surg* 66A:715, 1984.

51. Montgomery JB, Steadman JR: Rehabilitation of the injured knee. *Clin Sports Med* 4:333, 1985.

52. Pevsner DN, Johnson JRG, Blazina M: The patellofemoral joint and its implications in the rehabilitation of the knee. *Phys Ther* 59:869, 1979.

53. Olerud C, Berg P: The variation of the Q angle with different positions of the foot. *Clin Orthop* 191:162, 1984.

54. Hungerford DS, Lennox DW: Rehabilitation of the knee in disorders of the patellofemoral joint: Relevant biomechanics. *Orthop Clin North Am* 14:397, 1983.

55. Huey L, Knudson RR: *The Waterpower Workout.* New York, New American Library, 1986.

56. McConnell J: The management of chondromalacia patellae: A long term solution. *Aust J Physiother* 33:215, 1986.

57. Lieb FJ, Perry J: Quadriceps function. An anatomical and mechanical study using amputated limbs. *J Bone Joint Surg* 50A:1535, 1968.

58. Wise HH, Feibert IA, Kates JL: EMG biofeedback as treatment for patellofemoral pain syndrome. *J Orthop Sports Phys Ther* 6:95, 1984.

59. Podesta L, Sherman MF: Knee bracing. *Orthop Clin North Am* 19:737, 1988.

60. Lysholm J, Nordin M, Ekstrand J, Gillquist J: The effect of a patella brace on performance in a knee extension strength test in patients with patellar pain. *Am J Sports Med* 2:110, 1977.

61. Palumbo PM: Dynamic patellar brace: A new orthosis in the management of patellofemoral disorders. *Am J Sports Med* 9:45, 1981.

62. Chenf J, Paulos L: Bracing for patellar instability. *Clin Sports Med* 9:813, 1990.

SECTION IX
Surgical Technique

CHAPTER 25

A Technique for Arthroscopic Surgery of the Patellofemoral Joint

J. Whit Ewing

The patient is placed supine on the operating table. General or regional anesthesia is used. A tourniquet is placed on the proximal thigh but not inflated unless necessary during the procedure. A padded low profile leg holding device is used. This device is placed over the tourniquet. Placing the leg holder in this fashion aids in controlling external rotation of the leg and allows more room for instrumentation during proximal approaches to the patellofemoral joint (Fig. 25-1).

After routine prepping and draping, the portals are outlined with a marking pencil. Proximal portals are placed approximately three finger breadths above the superior pole of the patella, along the patellofemoral joint line. These portals are marked out using a marking pencil with the knee in full extension (Figs. 25-2 through 25-4). The inflow portal is made superomedially (Fig. 25-5). Routine diagnostic arthroscopy is carried out to evaluate the menisci as well as the articulation of the femoral-tibial joint. Following this portion of the procedure, the leg is brought into full extension and the foot is placed on a sterile, draped, padded surgical stand (Fig. 25-6). The inflow cannula is now transferred to the anteroinferolateral portal, which is located at the level of the inferior pole of the patella, immediately adjacent to the lateral border of the infrapatellar tendon (Fig. 25-7). The superolateral portal is now used for placement of the camera-equipped arthroscope (Figs. 25-7 and 25-8). A 70 degree fore-oblique lens is best suited for visualization of the patellofemoral joint from this portal.

A proximal medial portal is now created for

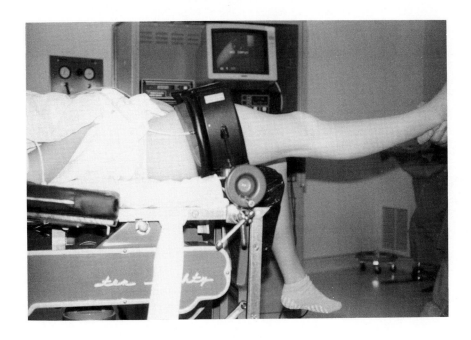

FIGURE 25-1
Patient positioned on the operating table with the tourniquet and the leg holder in proper position.

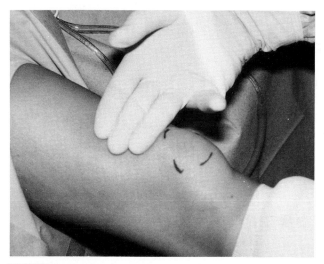

FIGURE 25-2
Measuring the proper positioning for proximal portals. Three finger breadths above the superior pole of the patella with the knee fully extended.

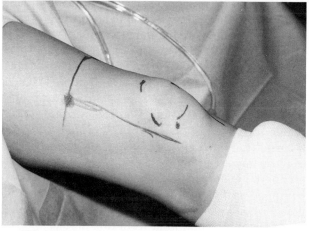

FIGURE 25-3
Lateral view of the leg with the portals outlined in relation to the patella.

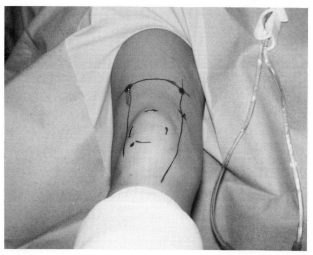

FIGURE 25-4
Anterior view of the knee illustrating the proximal medial and lateral portals as well as the anterior inferolateral portal.

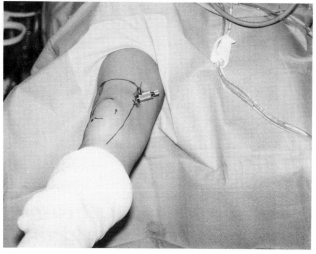

FIGURE 25-5
Placement of the superomedial inflow portal.

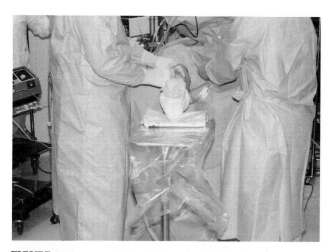

FIGURE 25-6
View from below the patient illustrating the placement of the patient's foot on a padded surgical stand to maintain the knee in full extension during the surgical procedure.

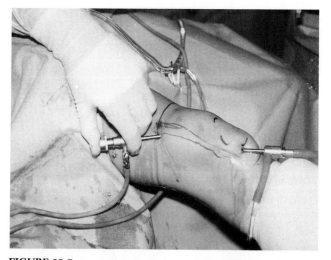

FIGURE 25-7
This figure shows the inflow cannula having been moved to the inferoanterolateral portal. The arthroscope cannula is shown in the superolateral portal.

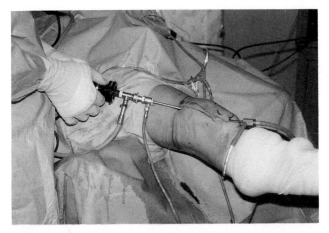

FIGURE 25-8
The surgical assistant holds the arthroscope camera assembly in position to give the surgeon a good visual field of view.

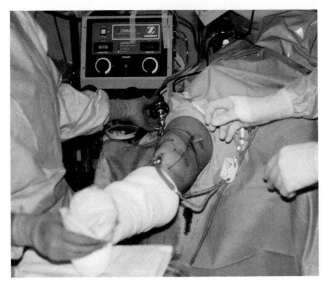

FIGURE 25-9
The surgeon uses an 18 gauge spinal needle to select the optimum medial portal position.

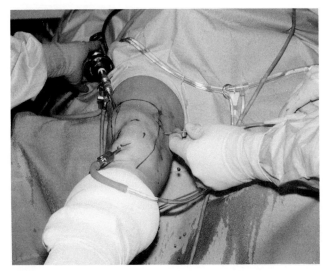

FIGURE 25-10
Insertion of a cutting electrode for lateral retinacular release.

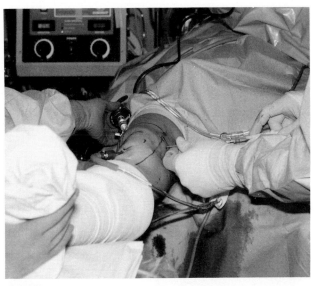

FIGURE 25-11
The lateral release is begun.

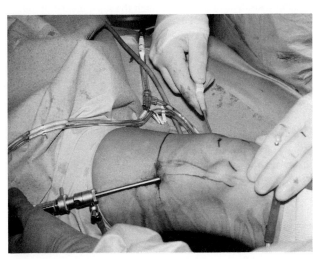

FIGURE 25-12
Bimanual surgical technique is important both in the lateral release and the patellar debridement.

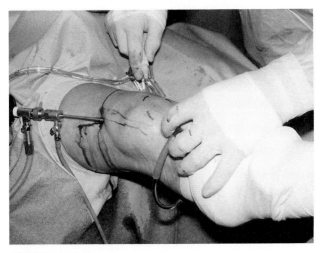

FIGURE 25-13
The surgeon moves the inflow cannula to mark the distal extent of the release.

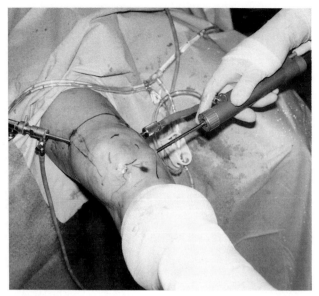

FIGURE 25-14
Patellar debridement is done through the same medial portal.

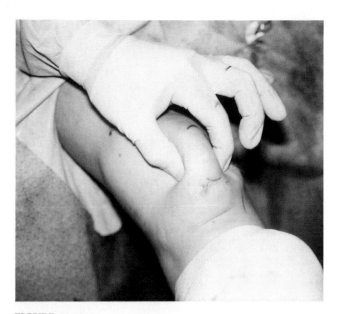

FIGURE 25-15
The patellar "tip" test. The patella is able to be tipped to 90 degrees in the trochlea following release.

surgical instrumentation. This portal is somewhat empirical. Occasionally, the proximal medial portal originally used for inflow is appropriate. At other times, the medial portal is located in a different position, being selected by probing with an 18 gauge spinal needle until the optimum position is found (Fig. 25-9). After creation of the operative portal, surgical instruments are inserted to perform the desired techniques (Figs. 25-10 through 25-14). The surgeon's assistant holds the arthroscope, permitting the surgeon to use bimanual techniques. At the conclusion of the lateral release procedure, the patella tip test is performed to ensure adequacy of the release (Fig. 25-15). A routine soft tissue dressing completes the procedure.

CHAPTER 26

Lateral Retinacular Release

Richard D. Ferkel

INTRODUCTION

The lateral retinacular release is not a new procedure. It has been used in patellofemoral joint surgery since Roux's article first appeared in the French literature in 1888.[1] Pollard[2] and Goldthwait[3] both used the lateral release as a component of treatment for recurrent dislocating patella. In the past, lateral retinacular release was used as a part of various patellofemoral reconstructive procedures, including proximal realignment, fascial transfers, quadriceps plasty, distal realignment, and patellectomy.

Isolated lateral retinacular release is a relatively recent procedure, which was first described in 1970 by Willner, who reported on the technique in which he removed a strip of the lateral capsule approximately 0.6 by 6 inches long.[4] In 1974, Merchant and Mercer reported preliminary results from an isolated lateral release done through a lateral skin incision, leaving the synovium intact.[5] Since that time, both open and arthroscopic lateral retinacular procedures have been performed with increasing frequency.[6–8]

Harwin and Stern presented a series in which a blind subcutaneous lateral release (SLR) was performed through an anterolateral arthroscopic portal by extending that portal approximately 1.5 cm.[9] Arthroscopic lateral release was reported by McGinty and McCarthy in 1981. The release was done blindly with scissors to the equator of the patella, with the completion of the proximal release being done with arthroscopic visualization. They had two significant hemarthroses.[10] In 1982, Metcalf reported SLR on 903 knees using a blind release with scissors with completion of the proximal portion of the release under arthroscopic control. Ninety-two percent of the patients reported significant subjective improvement at an average 48 month follow-up, but 20 percent developed significant permanent quadriceps weakness postoperatively. Nine patients had difficulty with postoperative hemarthrosis.[28] In 1981, an electrosurgical instrument to perform arthroscopic SLR was developed at the Southern California Orthopedic Institute (SCOI). It was felt that by directly coagulating the bleeding vessels during the release, the high rate of hemarthrosis (10 to 33 percent) could be significantly diminished.[11]

Grana and colleagues reported their results of SLR in 43 patients, with an average postoperative follow-up of 30 months. In this series, there were 90 percent satisfactory results, but all patients developed a postoperative hemarthrosis, which with one exception subsided within 4 to 6 weeks.[12] Henry and coworkers described a three-year study with 100 patients undergoing SLR. Good results were obtained in 88 percent, but a 13 percent complication rate was documented. This included 9 patients with severe hemarthrosis; 4 developed reflex sympathetic dystrophy.[13] Sherman and colleagues presented the results from SCOI on 39 patients and 45 knees with recurrent patellar subluxation using electrosurgical lateral release. Seventy-five percent of the patients were improved, and there were no postoperative hemarthroses.[22]

SURGICAL ANATOMY

The general anatomy of the patellofemoral joint has been discussed in Section I, but certain critical aspects should be reinforced to understand the procedure of lateral retinacular release. The lateral peripatellar retinaculum is comprised of two major layers, the superficial oblique retinaculum and the deep transverse retinaculum. The superficial oblique retinacular fibers originate from the iliotibial tract, interdigitating with the longitudinal fibers from the vastus lateralis and patellar tendon (Fig. 26-1*A*). The deep transverse retinaculum runs from the deep portion of the fascia lata and inserts on the lateral patella. It is comprised of three major components. The deep transverse layer of retinacular fibers runs through the deep portion of the iliotibial band and has a dense fibrous attachment to the lateral patella. At the inferior border of the deep transverse retinaculum, the patellotibial ligament stems from the inferior aspect of the patella distally to the anterior corner of the ligament, the lateral meniscus, and the anterior margin of the tibia. An expansion of the deep transverse retinaculum, the epicondylopatellar ligament, also known as the lateral patellofemoral ligament, runs from the lateral intermuscular septum and lateral epicondyle to the lateral patella, and was originally described by Kaplan[14] (Fig. 26-1*B*).

With knee flexion, these lateral retinacular bands are drawn posteriorly along with the iliotibial band, causing the patella to be displaced laterally. This lateral displacement force is counteracted by the medial stabilizers. However, when the medial stabilizers have been stretched, the static lateral stabilizers will create lateral tilt and displacement of the patella, which may lead to subluxation, excessive tilt, dislocation, or excessive lateral pressure syndrome (ELPS). There is a critical balance between the medial and lateral static stabilizers in maintaining normal alignment of the extensor mechanism within the trochlea, but there is a stronger lateral retinacular support laterally than medially. Although the structures previously discussed are primarily passive stabilizers, both the medial and lateral retinaculum are partially affected by active stabilizers, especially the lateral retinaculum, which originates in the iliotibial tract and provides both active and passive stabilization of the patella.

The primary complication with lateral retinacular release is hemarthrosis. This can be avoided by understanding the normal vascular anatomy of the patellofemoral joint. Superiorly in the patellofemoral joint, the lateral superior genicular artery passes through the insertion of the lateral intermuscular septum and gives a branch to the superolateral aspect of the patella. This branch anastomoses anteriorly and through the quadriceps insertion with branches of the supreme genicular and medial superior genicular arteries approaching the superior medial aspect of the patella. Inferiorly, the medial inferior genicular artery encircles the patella and sends anastomosing branches both superiorly, paralleling the medial border of the patella, and laterally, behind the patellar tendon, to anastomose with the lateral inferior genicular artery[15] (Fig. 26-2).

INDICATIONS

The indications for lateral retinacular release have evolved over the last 20 years. Originally, it was recommended for all symptomatic patients with patellar subluxation and dislocation and later advocated for treatment of all patellofemoral pain. More recently, the initial enthusiasm has been diminished by reports that indicate failure of the lateral release to relieve pain and instability, and the fact that some results deteriorate with time. McGinty and McCarthy followed 39 patients for an average of 17 months after SLR. Initially, the patients were 82 percent good and excellent, but a repeat follow-up of the same patients at 40 months postoperatively revealed significant de-

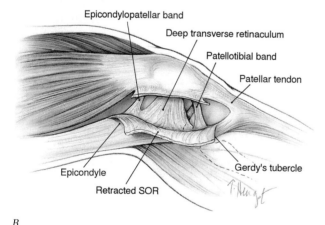

B

FIGURE 26-1
A. Extensor mechanism demonstrating the superior oblique retinaculum interdigitating with the longitudinal fibers from the vastus lateralis and patellar tendon. *B.* Deep transverse retinaculum with the epicondylopatellar band and patellotibial band. Note that the superior oblique retinaculum has been retracted to demonstrate the deep structures.

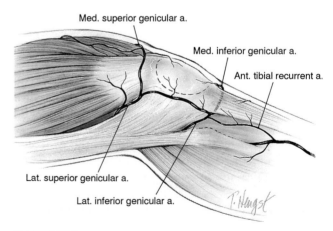

FIGURE 26-2
Arterial blood supply to the patellofemoral joint.

terioration with a satisfactory result in only 69 percent. In 1987, results from SCOI for patellar instability treated by SLR were reported. Twenty-five percent were rated as poor, and these were primarily patellar dislocators.[22]

It is now clear that very specific indications for lateral retinacular release are needed to ensure reproducible satisfactory results. This procedure does little more than release a tight lateral restraint. Therefore, preoperatively the physical examination must confirm the presence of an excessively tight lateral restraint to predict a successful outcome. The physical findings associated with a successful outcome after lateral retinacular release include: (1) normal lateral glide (≤two quadrants); (2) normal tubercle-sulcus angle; (3) medial patellar glide one to two quadrants; (4) passive patellar tilt negative or neutral (see Chap. 4). The lateral pull test should be superior or superolateral, with a ratio of no more than 1:1, although this is not critical.[16]

The indications for lateral retinacular release include: (1) patellofemoral pain with patellar subluxation, with no articular lesion or grade I to II chondromalacia; (2) patellofemoral pain with patellar tilt with no articular lesion or grade I to II chondromalacia; (3) patellofemoral pain with patellar tilt and subluxation, with no articular lesion or grade I to II chondromalacia. This includes the patients with ELPS. It is still controversial whether lateral release should be performed on patients with chronic patellofemoral pain but no malalignment and no articular lesion. In general, these patients should continue nonoperative care and lateral release should be avoided.

CONTRAINDICATIONS

Lateral retinacular release is contraindicated and can make the patient worse under the following circumstances: (1) deficient medial restraint; (2) patella alta; (3) small hypermobile patella; (4) severe malalignment; (5) physical examination with a positive patellar tilt, three quadrant or greater medial and lateral patellar glide, and abnormal tubercle-sulcus angle (90 degree Q angle) test.

TECHNIQUE

Lateral retinacular release can be performed via open or closed techniques. The open technique includes either an incision, excision, or Z-plasty. The closed techniques include percutaneous, arthroscopic incision, and arthroscopic electrosurgical release.

The arthroscopic lateral release can be done by either scissors with or without electrosurgery, knife, or totally by electrosurgery. Although each technique has advantages and disadvantages, the electrosurgical technique appears to have more advantages and fewer disadvantages than other techniques. Because of this, arthroscopic SLR via electrosurgery will be discussed in this chapter. However, to use electrosurgery correctly and safely, its principles and practices must be understood.

Principles of Electrosurgery

A detailed discussion of the use of electrosurgery in arthroscopy is beyond the focus of this chapter. However, the reader is referred to detailed references for such information.[17-19] A brief description of the principles will be presented to facilitate an understanding of the surgical technique to be performed. The use of heat to obtain coagulation dates back to the fourth century B.C. with Hippocrates' use of a hot poker. William Gilbert was called the "father of electrotherapy" for his work with magnetism and electricity during the sixteenth century. Electrosurgery itself was developed in the 1890s by d'Arsonval when he passed 1 ampere of 500-kHz current through two human volunteers, causing a 100-watt lightbulb to light. Subsequent research showed that a current of <10,000 Hz delivered to a patient produced muscular contractions, whereas a current greater than this caused no muscular stimulation but could produce an electrosurgical effect on local tissue. Harvey Cushing, a neurosurgeon, and William T. Bovie, a physicist, working in conjunction, developed the first "spark-gap" generator in 1926. However, acceptance of electrosurgical techniques was initially slow until the development of nonexplosive anesthetic agents in the 1950s and 1960s, and solid state electrosurgical generators in the 1970s. Aritomi and associates developed the first arthroscopic electrosurgical instrument called the rectoscope in 1973. In 1981, an electrosurgical system specifically for arthroscopic knee surgery was developed at SCOI.[11]

The effect of electrosurgery is based on the flow of current, which is defined as the flow of electrons in living tissue. This consists of the transfer of charged ions between or within cells. Two types of currents are available, direct and alternating. Direct current implies flow of electricity in one direction only; alternating current changes direction in regular cycles. High frequency alternating current that oscillates above 10,000 Hz can be passed through cellular material without causing neuromuscular activation. The electrosurgical tip itself does not produce heat, but instead carries and projects a current that cuts or cauterizes depending on its waveform and frequency and resistance of the tissues through which the current is passed. Resistance of the various cells to the flow of electricity causes their heat-related mechanical destruction.

LOOP PRINCIPLE

The term *loop principle* was coined to illustrate how electrosurgery works in the human body. This loop consists of the generator source, conductive cable, active electrode, patient, return or dispersive electrode, and return cable to the generator (Fig. 26-3). As long as this loop is intact, the patient and surgeon are safe. However, if the loop is broken, a hazard can be created for the patient or surgeon or both. As the surgeon initiates the electrosurgery device, a high current density is generated at the electrode tip. This produces the effects of cutting or coagulation. Heat is produced by the resistance to current flow as electrical energy is absorbed and converted to thermal energy. The higher resistance of current density, the greater the local heating. As the current diffuses through the body, over a larger surface area, a low current density is achieved, which then exits at the dispersive electrode pad.

TISSUE RESPONSE

Tissue response is defined as the speed and depth of cutting or degree of coagulation and depends on several factors, including: (1) power generated at the active electrode tip; (2) waveform with the electric

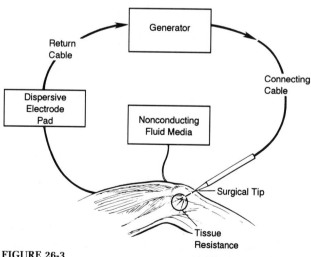

FIGURE 26-3
Applied loop principle. Note high current density at the active electrode (surgical tip) and the low current density at the dispersive electrode pad.

current; (3) duration of exposure to the current; (4) depth of electrode penetration; and (5) cooling due to blood circulation. Other factors that determine the response the tissue will have when exposed to electrosurgery include the type of tissue and its environment, the age of the patient, and whether the tissue involved is diseased.

ELECTROSURGICAL ACCESSORIES

Today's solid state generators have replaced all other types because they are safer, have both cut and coagulation control, and operate in the frequency of 0.5 to 5 MHz. With the advent of electrosurgery for intra-articular procedures, the concept of "impedance matching" became an important consideration. Since the resistance in the knee joint is approximately 750 to 1200 Ω, generators for electrosurgery must work most efficiently in this range. Today these generators are the isolated or floating type, which means that the generator has an isolated output that is not referenced to the ground. If the loop is interrupted, the entire system becomes inoperative, thereby protecting both the patient and the physician. This was not the case in the older "aggressive" generators. The active electrode is composed of the handheld unit, with a coagulation/cut switch with one of various tip designs. The electrode is connected to the generator by well-insulated conductive cable or wire. It is critical that, with the abundance of fluid present in arthroscopy, the handheld unit and all its wiring be fluid resistant. The active electrode imparts its thermal effect on the tissue by "throwing a wave" of energy from its tip. The majority of the metal tip is insulated to prevent inadvertent cutting or cauterizing tissue, and to allow the current to be concentrated at the small exposed tip. This permits the use of lower current settings to effect cutting and coagulation.

Today, an inherent "capacitative couple" type of passive electrode is used in electrosurgery. It contains no gel and has its circuitry connected to the generator, so that if the skin contact is lost, the current flow is immediately stopped. It is important that the adherent pad be placed in an area that is well profused and free of bony prominences.

ELECTROSURGICAL FLUIDS

If electrosurgery is to be used, a nonconductive fluid must be used. Normal saline and Ringer's lactate, because they have free ions in solution, are conductive and their use in electrosurgery is contraindicated. The reason for this is that these electrolyte solutions may conduct current to other parts of the body and reduce the efficiency of the local electrical

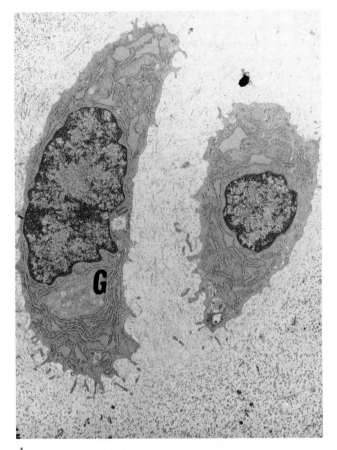

A

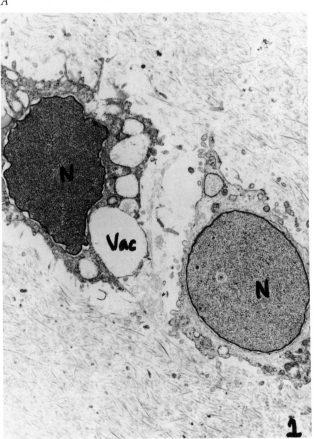

B

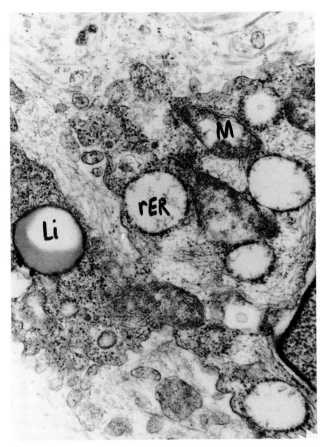

C

FIGURE 26-4

Electron microscopy of articular cartilage. *A*. Normal cartilage electron micrograph of two chondrocytes near the articular surface. These cells have intact cytoplasmic membranes, dilated and nondilated rough endoplasmic reticulum (*rER*), and a well-developed Golgi complex. *B*. Sterile water electron micrograph. Pictured are two chondrocytes whose nuclei (*N*) are swollen with the loss of a distinct chromatic pattern and the cytoplasm contains numerous vacuoles (*Vac*). *C*. Higher magnification shows a loss of membrane integrity, swollen and empty rough endoplasmic reticulum (*rER*), damaged mitochondria (*M*) and lipid droplets (*Li*). Reprinted with permission from Reference 17.

action. In the past, sterile water (*p*H 7) has been used in electrosurgery; however, recent studies have demonstrated that even short-term use of sterile water causes dramatic changes in the synovial surface cells and the superficial chondrocytes[20] (Fig. 26-4*A–C*). Although the use of sterile water has been advocated, this fluid is highly unphysiologic, as it does not support proteoglycan synthesis and it is extremely hypoosmolar (around zero). With sterile water, the intraarticular surface (articular cartilage and synovium) absorbs large amounts of water causing swelling, nuclear disruption, and in some cases, destruction. Glycine (1.5 percent) has also been used for electrosurgery, but has potential problems because it is hypoosmolar (approximately 200 mOsm/L compared to synovial fluid, which is around 300, and *p*H, which is approximately 7.2). However, this has been the fluid most commonly used until recently. The two best solutions for electrosurgery appear to be HEPES Buffer 0.3 *M*, and glycerol.[21] Both solutions allow proteoglycan synthesis to continue at a rate at least consistent with that provided by normal saline, particularly if the procedure does not extend beyond 2 h. Marshall, Snyder, and colleagues also found that a glycerol solution was a satisfactory irrigant for arthroscopy and have developed a fluid termed Synovisol, which has been extensively tested on laboratory animals with excellent results, and presently is close to being released for general use in the United States[20] (Fig. 26-5*A* and *B*).

Subcutaneous Lateral Release Technique

The advantages of electrosurgery include improved visualization during operation, less postoperative pain allowing rehabilitation, no tourniquet, possibly decreased infection, and reduced hospital costs by avoiding hemarthrosis.

ARTHROSCOPIC TECHNIQUE

The patient is placed in the supine position and satisfactory general, epidural, or spinal anesthesia is used. In some cases, a selective sensory epidural has been used, although this is usually only done when more extensive procedures such as medial reefing and distal realignment are anticipated. The reader is referred to elsewhere in the book for this discussion (see Chap. 27). Local anesthesia is generally not used for electrosurgical procedures because it includes a base of sodium chloride, which has a high electrolyte content and thus conducts energy through the tissue. A pneumatic tourniquet is placed on the upper thigh but is not inflated. The procedure is done without a leg holder to allow for evaluation of the patellofemoral relationships through a complete arc of movement while avoiding tethering and compressive forces on the quadriceps musculature.

INSTRUMENTATION

The instruments used in arthroscopy and SLR are listed in Table 26-1 and are shown in Figure 26-6. A variety of electrosurgical tips are available. The author's preference is the 90 degree coated tip because it concentrates the energy in a smaller area, thus allowing a lower power setting. The coating also

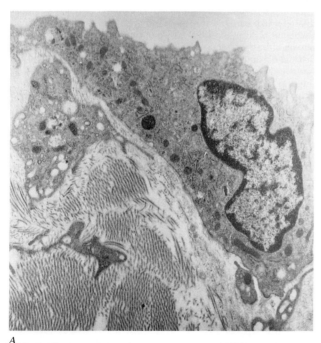

A

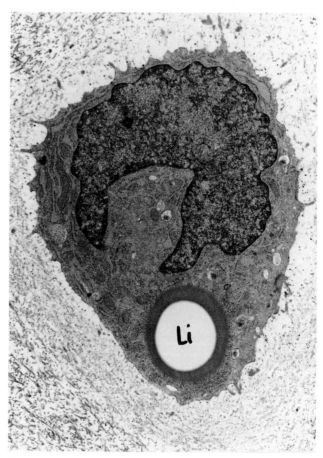

B

FIGURE 26-5
Effect of Synovisol. *A.* Synovisol effect on synovial lining cell. Lining cell has normal morphology and cytoplasmic integrity. *B.* Synovisol effect on cartilage. A normal chondrocyte with lipid (*Li*) accumulation. Reprinted with permission from Reference 17.

TABLE 26-1
Instruments for Subcutaneous Electrosurgery

1. Motorized intra-articular shaver
2. 30° 4-mm arthroscope with high flow cannula
3. Light-weight chip videocamera
4. 18-gauge spinal needle
5. Nonconductive inflow cannula
6. Nonconductive large bore cannula for electrosurgery instrument
7. Active electrode
8. Dispersive electrode
9. Arthroscopic probe

protects against articular cartilage scuffing and inadvertent burns (Fig. 26-7).

PROCEDURE

Standard preparation and draping are performed, and a large inflow cannula (4 mm diameter) is inserted via the superomedial portal. Diagnostic arthroscopy is performed through a standard anterolateral portal using high flow irrigation with gravity inflow and

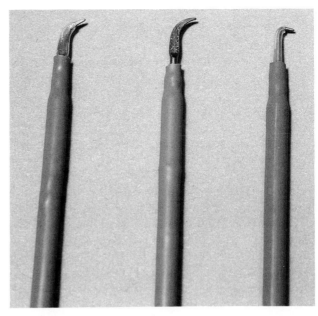

FIGURE 26-7
Electrosurgical tips. The one on the left was developed for electrosurgery, the middle for subacromial decompression, the right for meniscal surgery. Any of these tips, however, can be used for any of the functions, depending on surgeon preference.

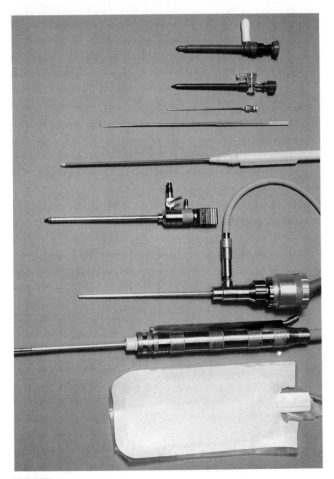

FIGURE 26-6
Instruments for electrosurgery. These include arthroscope, shaver, nonconductive cannulae, and electrosurgery dispersive pad and tip.

suction through the arthroscope for rapid irrigation of the joint. Complete arthroscopic evaluation is performed, with special attention to patellofemoral articulation, lateral facet compression, and areas of chondromalacia. The anteromedial portal is used for instrumentation. Frequently, patellar debridement will be necessary as part of the procedure. It is important that this is done prior to lateral release. If this is done afterward, occasionally there is a problem with excessive extravasation of fluid through the retinacular defect caused by the lateral release.

Patellar debridement is most easily accomplished by switching the arthroscope to the anteromedial portal and using the motorized shaver through the anterolateral portal. Once this has been accomplished, the arthroscope is inserted through the superomedial portal and a nonconductive inflow cannula is placed in the inferior medial portal for the arthroscopic fluid. The conductive fluid is turned off, and glycine or glycerol is turned on to be used throughout the electrosurgical procedure. A nonconductive cannula is then inserted through the anterolateral portal, and the electrosurgery instrument is inserted through this portal to initiate the procedure (Fig. 26-8). The patellofemoral articulation is now evaluated through the superomedial portal and the amount of patellar tilt and chondromalacia is again assessed. Further debridement of the patella can be effected while visualizing through this portal, and if needed, the shaver can be switched with the arthroscope to facilitate complete debridement.

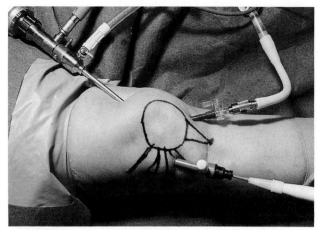

FIGURE 26-8
Typical setup for subcutaneous lateral release using electrosurgery on a right knee. Note the arthroscope visualizes the patellar tracking from the superomedial portal and the lateral release is performed from the inferior lateral portal.

Subcutaneous lateral release using electrosurgery is performed with the isolated generator set at 10 watts for cutting and 10 watts for coagulation (a digital readout generator for confirmation is recommended). The operating surgeon must personally verify the settings on the generator visually before initiating electrosurgery.

It is important to "throw the wave" before the electrode to facilitate efficient use of the electrosurgery device. Technically, electrosurgery is activation of the energy source prior to touching the tissue, allowing the surgeon to affect a cutting mode approximately 1 mm from the tip of the electrode without actually touching the tissue directly. The result is a much sharper and finer cutting line with diminished chance of tissue carbonization. The power setting should be limited to the lowest setting that still effectively produces energy. A spinal needle can be inserted at the superior pole of the patella for orientation. The release is performed from proximal to distal, maintaining a straight line as the cutting is performed. The release should be performed approximately 5 mm from the palpated lateral border of the patella and is carried normally from the superior border of the patella to the bottom of the inferior lateral portal (Fig. 26-9). In some cases, the release may need to be carried to the beginning of the vastus lateralis muscle, but extensive resection of this muscle should never be done, even if patellar centralization is not achieved. In addition, overrelease must be avoided.

Sequentially, the synovium, and the lateral peripatellar retinaculum, both the deep and superficial portions, are released (Fig. 26-10). Further cutting into the fat should be avoided, particularly in skinny patients, because this can lead to either partial or full thickness thermal burns. Extreme caution must be

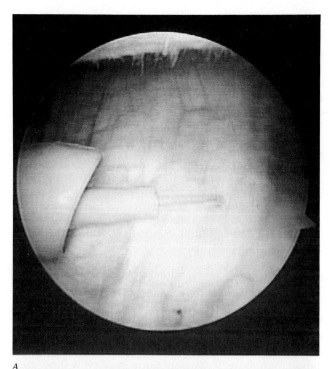

A

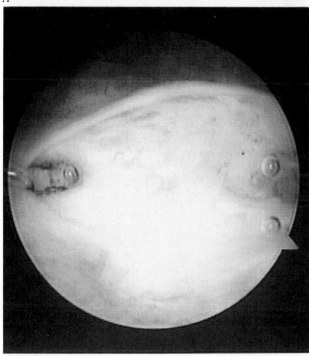

B

FIGURE 26-9
Subcutaneous lateral release using electrosurgery. *A.* The release is started at the superior pole of the patella. *B.* The superficial oblique retinaculum is released.

exercised throughout the procedure, but particularly at the inferior anterolateral portal, to avoid thermonecrosis.

The tourniquet is not inflated during the procedure unless hemostasis cannot be secured rapidly. Normally, bleeders are coagulated as encountered,

316

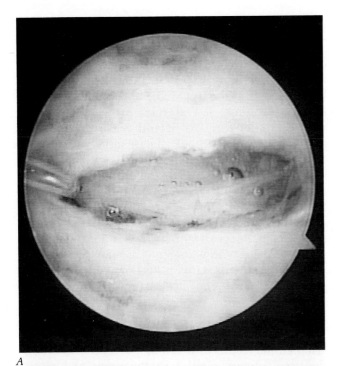

A

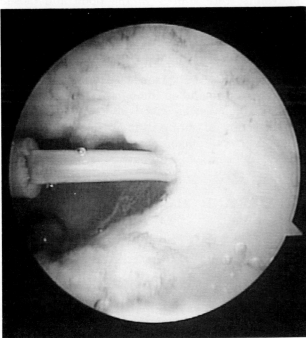

B

FIGURE 26-10
Release of the superficial oblique retinaculum and deep transverse retinaculum. *A*. Release of superficial oblique retinaculum, coagulating bleeders as encountered. *B*. Release of the deep transverse retinaculum, epicondylopatellar band, and patellotibial band.

but if the visual field becomes obliterated by blood, the tourniquet may be temporarily inflated and the knee irrigated clear. Once the area of bleeding is identified and coagulated, the tourniquet is slowly deflated until it is completely released and coagulation has been achieved (Fig. 26-11). At the end of the

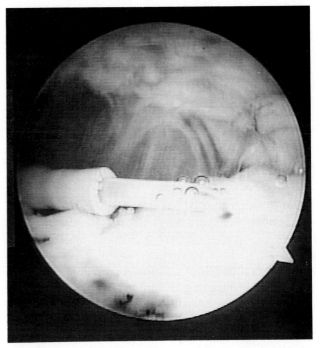

FIGURE 26-11
Coagulation of bleeding vessels using electrosurgery. Note the branch of the lateral superior genicular artery that is preserved during the lateral retinacular release.

release, the passive patellar tilt test is performed with an intraoperative tilt of 60 degrees to 90 degrees the usual goal (Fig. 26-12). This will result in an optimal postoperative tilt of approximately 30 degrees to 45 degrees. The release site is then again carefully checked for bleeders and the patellofemoral articulation is evaluated with flexion and extension. The knee is then irrigated free of the glycine or glycerol, with either normal saline or lactated Ringer's.

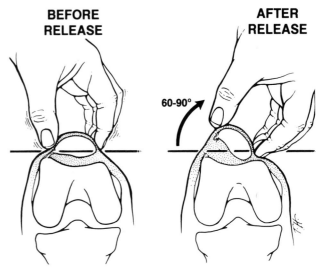

FIGURE 26-12
Turn up test. At the end of the release, passive patellar tilt is done to achieve a goal of 60 degrees to 90 degrees tilt.

TABLE 26-2
Tips to Avoid Complications

1. Use nonconductive fluid
2. Use impedance matched isolated generator
3. Use capacitive couple dispersive electrode
4. Have electrosurgery instrument insulated except at the tip
5. Avoid extensive sectioning of the vastus lateralis
6. Use low settings on the generator to avoid thermal burns
7. Use the superomedial portal for arthroscopic visualization

Surgical incisions are closed with adhesive tape, and a sterile padding is applied over the incisions and held in place with an elastic support stocking previously measured for the patient. No drains are inserted nor are sutures normally used. The patient is usually discharged home approximately 1 to 2 hours after the procedure.

Tips to avoid complications in electrosurgery are summarized in Table 26-2.

POSTOPERATIVE MANAGEMENT

In the postoperative period, the patient is encouraged to begin an isometric exercise program with active flexion of the knee. Electromuscle stimulator electrodes also may be applied to further facilitate rehabilitation of the quadriceps. The compressive stocking is maintained for 1 week, and then a patellar brace may be applied if knee swelling is minimal. One of the advantages of electrosurgery is to minimize swelling or hemarthrosis and allow the rehabilitation to begin immediately. The elastic stocking may be removed 48 hours postoperatively for showering, and then afterward reapplied. The patient is usually seen in the office 1 week following surgery. At this time, the majority of patients have regained an arc of 95 degrees to 100 degrees of flexion with the incidence of hemarthrosis being <3 percent. Rehabilitation is then continued with formal therapy beginning at 1 week postoperatively with the principles that have been discussed in the rehabilitation section.

RESULTS

Results have been published from SCOI, which reviewed a group of 39 patients and 45 knees for patellar instability. Seventy-five percent of the patients were improved, but 25 percent were graded poor postoperatively. Dislocators had a more frequent rate of poor results. The complication rate was 4.4 percent, but there were no postoperative hemarthroses.[22] In another study done at SCOI, 100 consecutive cases of electrosurgical lateral releases were compared with a similar series of lateral releases performed arthroscopically without electrosurgery. The two groups were otherwise comparable with respect to sex, age, and activity level. The hospital stay was reduced from 1.9 day average to 100 percent outpatient basis with electrosurgery. In addition, the incidence of hemarthrosis was reduced from 12 percent to 3 percent. Range of motion 1 week postoperatively was >90 degrees in 90 percent of the electrosurgery patients, compared with only 34 percent of the other group. Moreover, the electrosurgically treated patients had a significant increase in their ability to return to their preoperative level of activity.[23]

Aglietti reviewed the literature in 1989 and grouped the results as listed in Table 26-3. Although the results were similar in the open and closed groups, different methods of evaluation were used, and the activity level and hemarthrosis rates were not discussed for the various studies. Bray reported a 46 percent satisfactory result in workers' compensation cases after SLR.[24] Fulkerson used preoperative and postoperative computed tomography scans to show that lateral release can effectively correct lateral tilt, but correction of subluxation was less consistent. Grade IV chondromalacia and facet collapse presented a poor prognostic sign.[25]

PITFALLS AND COMPLICATIONS

Failure of the electrosurgical instrument to work may be the result of: (1) incorrect fluid medium with a

TABLE 26-3
*Results of Lateral Release**

Symptom	No. of Studies	Total No. Knees	Range of Follow-up (yr)	Range of Satisfactory Results (%)
Pain (open)	5	383	0.5–3.0	60–82
Pain (closed)	7	235	1.0–5.0	66–90
Instability (closed)	5	148	1.0–6.0	44–86
Pain and Instability (closed)	3	182	1.0–1.4	85–87
Pain and Instability (open)	5	408	1.4–3.4	65–88

*Modified from Aglietti[30]

Method of release in parentheses

nonconductive fluid not being used; (2) passive electrode becoming loose, or its connection to the generator failing; or (3) loosening of the connection of the surgical tip to the electrosurgery pencil. In addition, sometimes the electrode may be difficult to maneuver, and the anterolateral portal capsular incision may need to be enlarged or slight flexion of the knee may be needed to improve access of the electrosurgery knife to the area of the release.

Subcutaneous lateral release is not without complications. A variety of problems have been reported after this procedure, including rupture of the quadriceps tendon, reflex sympathetic dystrophy, deep vein thrombosis and pulmonary embolism, fascial herniation, medial subluxation of the patella, hemarthrosis, recurrent lateral patellar compression syndrome, patella baja or infrapatellar contracture syndrome, thermal burns, and persistent pain.

Hemarthrosis

Hemarthrosis is the most commonly cited complication after SLR, other than a poor result (Fig. 26-13). Although hemarthrosis is usually not associated with a long-term poor outcome, the knee usually requires aspiration if it is painfully distended, or if the hemarthrosis persists. In the rare instance, the hemarthrosis may lead to arthrofibrosis and loss of motion. Occa-

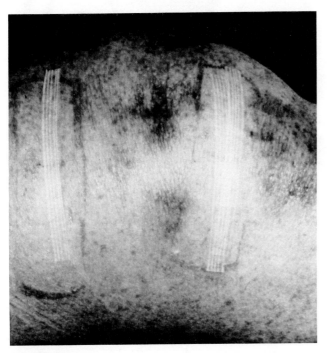

FIGURE 26-13
Postoperative hemarthrosis after lateral retinacular release done using a knife.

sionally, a severe hemarthrosis may require operative drainage because aspiration will usually be inhibited by clotted blood. Subsequently, this can lead to patellar entrapment syndrome, reflex sympathetic dystrophy, or significant loss of knee motion.

Since the advent of electrosurgery for SLR, the incidence of this complication has diminished.[28,29] Small reviewed data on 446 lateral retinacular release patients and found 32 complications, for an incidence of 7.2 percent. A higher complication rate was noted with the use of the tourniquet and with the use of a postoperative suction drain for 24 h or longer. He did not find the use of electrosurgery to be associated with a lower incidence of hemarthrosis. However, this was not a controlled study at a single center, but rather a compilation of multicenters with 21 arthroscopic surgeons involved. Our experience has continued to demonstrate a very low incidence of postoperative hemarthrosis since the advent of its use over 11 years ago.

Insufficient Release

It is important both before and after SLR to observe patellar tracking from the superomedial portal, to see if the patella centralizes at 30 degrees of flexion. Usually, the release must extend above the superior pole of the patella 1 to 2 cm, and if the patella still tracks laterally, one may have to extend it further slightly into the vastus lateralis to weaken its overpull. In addition, if lateral tethering persists, further release may be necessary to avoid recurrence of the lateral patella compression syndrome.

Overrelease

Overrelease of the vastus lateralis may lead to permanent quadriceps insufficiency and is a very serious complication of SLR. The patient may present with complaints of giving way, vague anterior knee pain, and persistent weakness, and most will feel their operative knee is worse than it was before surgery. Examination may demonstrate passive patellar tilt between 80 degrees and 135 degrees, and a defect in the vastus lateralis, extending 5 to 10 cm proximal to the patella or curving around the superior pole of the patella, may be palpated. This may also lead to medial subluxation and reoperation to repair the vastus lateralis tendon.

Medial Patellar Subluxation

This complication occurs if an excessive lateral release has been performed or if a lateral release has been performed on a patient with preoperative subtle medial subluxation that has not been appreciated. In addition, patients with patellar hypermobility have a higher chance of developing medialization after a lateral release. The diagnosis can usually be made by a history of the type of patellar pain, as well as watching the patella track and the persistent quadriceps weakness. In these patients, the patellar tilt mobility is significantly increased, and the patellofemoral Merchant x-ray may confirm medial subluxation or tilting. At SCOI over the last several years, we have used kinematic magnetic resonance imaging (MRI) of the patellofemoral joint, preoperatively to assess patients with patellar subluxation, medial and/or lateral. We have also used it to evaluate patients with persistent symptoms after lateral release (Fig. 26-14). Shellock and colleagues recently published results on a group of 40 patients with persistent symptoms after lateral retinacular release. It was found that 63 percent of the patients had medial subluxation of the patella on the operative side, and 43 percent had the same on the unoperated side.[26] Therefore, it is critical to evaluate the patients preoperatively before consid-

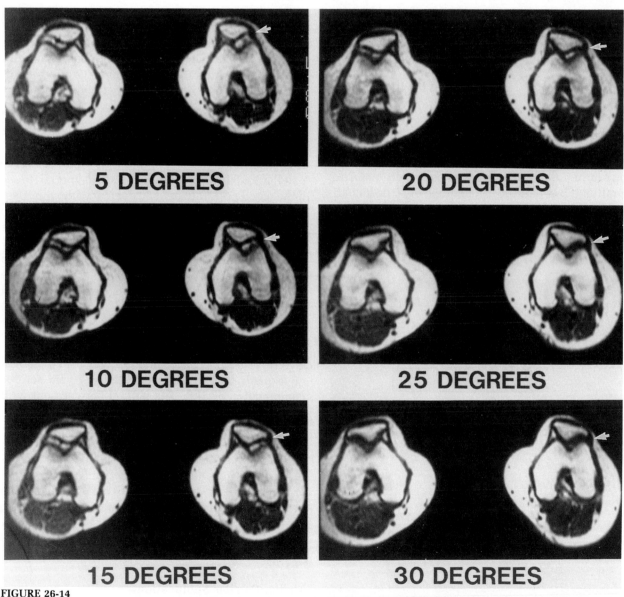

FIGURE 26-14
Kinematic MRI of the patellofemoral joint. Note both knees have medial patellar subluxation, but only the knee on the right is status post lateral retinacular release. The arrows demonstrate thickened retinaculum where the previous release has been performed. *Courtesy of Frank Shellock, PhD; Tower MRI Imaging.*

ering SLR. Hughston and others have documented the need for reoperation for medial patellar subluxation.[27]

Patella Baja

Patella baja may also occur after SLR (Fig. 26-15). The etiology is not clear, but it may be due to scar and adhesion formation termed the patellar entrapment syndrome. With this problem, scar tissue and adhesions form between the patellar tendon and the anterior tibia, effectively shortening the patellar tendon. The problem can be either caused or worsened by inappropriate or inadequate postoperative rehabilitation. Another etiology may be a release too far medially so that the cut wanders into the vastus medialis and rectus femoris. This may lead to patellar rotation and displacement distally, with a contraction of the patellar tendon.

Patients will complain of pain, weakness, and loss of motion. Physical examination will show a distal position of the patella, particularly at 90 degrees flexion. A lateral radiograph of the knee may also be helpful in making this diagnosis. If the situation is severe enough, further surgery may be necessary in the form of an open procedure, to do lysis of adhesions, release of the patella and infrapatellar

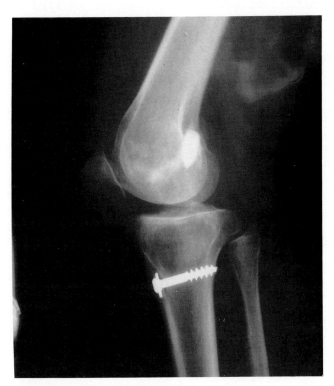

FIGURE 26-15
Patella baja in a patient who has undergone anterior cruciate ligament reconstruction and subcutaneous lateral release.

tendon, and occasionally even transposing the tibial tubercle proximally.

Reflex Sympathetic Dystrophy (RSD)

Development of RSD can occur after any surgical procedure. Several studies of SLR have demonstrated cases of this. Typically, there is a diffuse dysesthetic sensation and aching around the knee and a cold intolerance with changes in color and temperature of the knee. Physical therapy is important to try to relieve this problem, but sympathetic blocks may also be necessary.

Thermal Injury

Thermal injury to the skin is an avoidable complication that should never occur. All electrosurgical equipment should have preventive maintenance and periodic inspections. The operating room personnel must be familiar with the equipment to be able to confirm that it is properly functioning at all times.

Flammable anesthetic agents should never be used with electrosurgical instruments, and electrocardiography (ECG) electrodes should be placed as far from the operating site as possible, and never between the active and passive electrodes. Nonconductive towel clips should be used at all times in any patient undergoing electrosurgery. After the procedure, the circulating nurse must check the patient at the passive electrode placement site, the ECG electrode sites, and other areas where conductive material came in contact with the skin to make sure there is no evidence of skin burns.

Power settings on the generator should be kept as low as possible to reduce the risk of burning the skin at the passive electrode or at the active electrode surgical tip. This is particularly important when performing a lateral release where only a fine layer of subcutaneous fat separates the electrosurgical instrument from the skin. In addition, the use of a nonconductive cannula through the anterolateral portal will also diminish the risk of burning the skin at this site (Fig. 26-16).

Indiscriminate Use

Lateral release is not a panacea for all patella problems. In the past, it has been recommended for any type of patella pain and even severe patellofemoral dislocation. With the advent of numerous studies to document poor results, the indications are now much stricter.[28,29]

If arthroscopic findings do not correlate with the preoperative symptoms, the release should not be

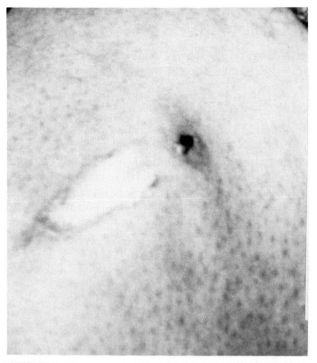

FIGURE 26-16
Full thickness skin burn from incorrect use of electrosurgery for a subcutaneous lateral release.

done. A preoperative kinematic MRI is helpful to make sure that the patient's patella is subluxing laterally and is not going out medially instead. A release should never be done just because at arthroscopy the patella looks like it is subluxating, but the patient has no clinical signs of this occurring.

SUMMARY

Arthroscopic lateral release is an effective procedure in the properly selected patient and can treat both patellar pain and instability in the appropriate cases. Short-term results appear to be comparable between the open and closed techniques, although the complication rate appears to be slightly less in the arthroscopic procedures. The results after SLR are highly dependent on rehabilitation and correct preoperative diagnosis. Lateral retinacular release is not a simple procedure and should not be treated as such. It has potentially serious complications that are difficult to treat once the procedure has occurred. And finally, one should not use lateral release as a panacea for all anterior knee pain. Indiscriminate use will lead to poor results and complications.

REFERENCES

1. Roux C: Luxation habituelle de la rotule: Traitemente operatoire. *Rev Chir* 8:682, 1888.
2. Pollard B: Old dislocation of the patella by intra-articular operation. *Lancet* i:17, 1891.
3. Goldthwait JE: Dislocation of the patella. *Trans Am Orthop Assoc* 8:237, 1895.
4. Willner P: Recurrent dislocation of the patella. *Clin Orthop* 69:213, 1970.
5. Merchant AC, Mercer ND: Lateral release of the patella, a preliminary report. *Clin Orthop* 103:40, 1974.
6. Betz R, Magill J, Lonergan R: The percutaneous lateral retinacular release. *Am J Sports Med* 15:477, 1987.
7. Ceder L, Larson: Z plasty lateral retinacular release for the treatment of patellar compression syndrome. *Clin Orthop* 144:110, 1979.
8. Fulkerson JP, Schutzer SF: The failure of conservative treatment for patello-femoral malalignment: Lateral release or realignment. *Orthop Clin North Am* 17:283, 1986.
9. Harwin SF, Stern RE: Subcutaneous lateral retinacular release for chondromalacia of the patella. A preliminary report. *Clin Orthop* 156:207, 210, 1981.
10. McGinty JB, McCarthy JC: Endoscopic lateral retinacular release: A preliminary report. *Clin Orthop* 158:120, 1981.
11. Miller GK, Dickason JM, Fox JM, et al: The use of electrosurgery for arthroscopic subcutaneous lateral release. *Orthopedics* 5:301, 1982.
12. Grana WA, Hinkley B, Hollingsworth S: Arthroscopic evaluation and treatment of patellar malalignment. *Clin Orthop* 186:122, 1984.
13. Henry JH, Goletz TH, Williamson B: Lateral release in patello-femoral subluxation. *Am J Sports Med* 14:121, 1986.
14. Kaplan E: Some aspects of functional anatomy of the human knee joint. *Clin Orthop* 23:18, 1962.
15. Shim SS, Leung G: Blood supply of the knee joint. A microangiographic study in children and adults. *Clin Orthop* 298:119, 1986.
16. Kolowich PA, Paulos LE, Rosenberg TD, et al: Lateral release of the patella: Indications and contraindications. *Am J Sports Med* 18:359, 1990.
17. Fox JM, Ferkel RD: Use of electrosurgery in arthroscopic surgery, in *Arthroscopic Surgery,* edited by JS Parisien. New York, McGraw-Hill, 1988, pp 315–324.
18. Fox JM, Ferkel RD, Del Pizzo W, et al: Electrosurgery in orthopedics: Part 1—Principles. *Contemp Orthop* 8:37, 1984.

19. Fox JM, Ferkel RD, Del Pizzo W, et al: Electrosurgery in orthopedics: Part II—Applications to arthroscopy. *Contemp Orthop* 8:37, 1984.

20. Marshall GJ, Kirchen ME, Sweeney JR, Snyder SJ: Synovisol as an irrigant for electrosurgery of joints. *Arthroscopy* 4:187, 1988.

21. Reagan B, Zarins B, Mankin HJ: Low conductivity irrigating solutions for arthroscopy. *Arthroscopy* 7:105, 1991.

22. Sherman OH, Fox JM, Sperling H, et al: Patellar instability: Treatment by arthroscopic electrosurgical lateral release. *Arthroscopy,* 3:152, 1987.

23. Gallick GS, Brna JA, Fox JM: Electrosurgery in operative arthroscopy. *Clin Sports Med* 6:607, 1987.

24. Bray RC, Roth JH, Jacobsen RP: Arthroscopic lateral release for anterior knee pain: A study comparing patients who are claiming worker's compensation with those who are not. *Arthroscopy* 3:237, 1987.

25. Fulkerson JP, Schutzer SF, Ramsby GR, et al: Computerized tomography of the patellofemoral joint before and after lateral release or realignment. *Arthroscopy* 3:19, 1987.

26. Shellock FG, Mink JH, Deutsch A, et al: Evaluation of patients with persistent symptoms after lateral retinacular release by kinematic magnetic resonance imaging of the patellofemoral joint. *Arthroscopy* 6:226, 1990.

27. Hughston JC, Deese M: Medial subluxation of the patella as a complication of lateral release. *Am J Sports Med* 16:383, 1988.

28. Metcalf RW: An arthroscopic method for lateral release of subluxating or dislocating patella. *Clin Orthop* 167:9, 1982.

29. Small NC: An analysis of complications in lateral retinacular release procedures. *Arthroscopy* 5:282, 1989.

30. Aglietti P, Pisaneschi A, Bussi R, et al: Arthroscopic lateral release for patellar pain or instability. *Arthroscopy* 5:176, 1989.

CHAPTER 27

Tibial Tubercle Transfer Technique

Marc J. Friedman

INTRODUCTION

Tibial tubercle osteotomy is performed for three basic pathologic conditions: patellofemoral instability, patellofemoral arthritis, and infrapatellar contracture syndrome.

PATELLOFEMORAL INSTABILITY

Variables to consider in evaluating surgical treatment for patellofemoral instability include:

1. Medial glide in one, two, or three quadrants and patellar tilt (Fig. 27-1)[1] give an accurate indication as to how "tight" the lateral retinaculum is and lead one to consider starting out with a lateral retinacular release, as discussed by Dr. Ferkel (see Chap. 26).

2. Lateral glide in one, two, or three quadrants gives an indication as to the degree of laxity of the medial retinacular structures in a passive situation (Fig. 27-2).[1] In most instances, if there is three quadrant glide, the author recommends definitely performing a proximal realignment since the "degree" of medialization of the tibial tubercle would, in most cases, have to be excessive to control the disposition toward the lateral instability.

3. The Q angle at 90 degrees should be approximately 0 (Fig. 27-3).[1] If this is dramatically increased, and the lateral glide is only one quadrant, then consider "starting" with medialization of the tibial tubercle and carefully assessing patellar tracking at the time of surgery, reserving reefing of the medial retinaculum as a backup procedure.

4. Computed tomography scans or dynamic magnetic resonance imaging is used preoperatively, and as Fulkerson has demonstrated, one can classify a patellofemoral instability related to the posterior femoral condyle as either: lateral shift, lateral tilt, or lateral shift and tilt (Fig. 27-4).[2] He states that in his hands, a lateral shift can be handled with an "isolated" lateral release, whereas either a tilt or shift

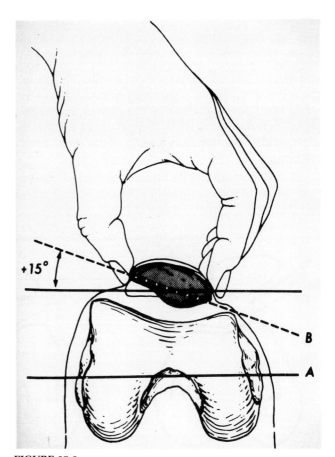

FIGURE 27-2
When the patella is everted and crosses a line parallel to the transcondylar axis, it is felt to be "positive." If it is less than this line, it is termed "negative."

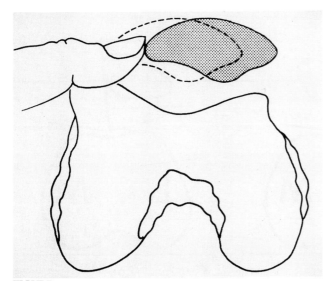

FIGURE 27-1
Demonstrates one quadrant *medial* "glide."

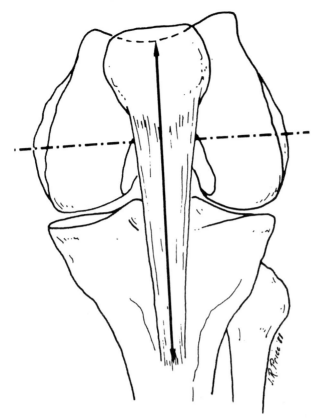

FIGURE 27-3
Q-angle is measured in flexion; it is generally zero degrees.

patella alta, hyperlax tissues and a "flat" trochlear groove, it is unreasonable to expect any degree of proximal or distal realignment without some form of "static" procedure being added to prevent patellar instability. We have used both the semitendinosus and medial third of the patellar tendon as "static" supports in this condition.

Technique—Semitendinosus

In most cases, arthroscopic evaluation is carried out from above (see selective epidural technique). Lateral release is carried out. The medial retinaculum is incised 1 cm from the border of the patella, synovium not being violated, coming three finger breadths up into the quadriceps tendon itself and a no. 1 Maxon suture in a mattress fashion is used to bring the medial structures on the surface of the patella (Fig. 27-5). Prior to tying, with the arthroscope in the superomedial portal, we attempt to "centralize" the patella at approximately 35 degrees to 40 degrees flexion in the trochlear groove. Various combinations of "reefing" are used to achieve this position (Fig. 27-6).

A 3-inch vertical incision is made two finger breadths medial to the tibial tubercle. The semitendinosus tendon is isolated with a right angle clamp, and a Concept blunt-tipped closed end tendon stripper is then inserted from below, and the tendon taken as high as possible. It is then delivered into the wound, with sutures of no. 1 Ticron placed in the end, and delivered subcutaneously. The fascia above the tibia is then incised, and the tendon is placed below the sartorius gracilis tendons up to the patella at approximately 8 o'clock (left knee). A guidewire is then drilled from this point obliquely to the 2 o'clock position; a 6-mm cannulated reamer is then used once the guidewire position has been checked. The tendon

and tilt requires a distal transfer of the tibial tubercle.[3] We agree with this as a general principle; however, we feel that careful evaluation from the superomedial portal arthroscopically is indicated to determine whether this also requires reefing of the medial retinaculum.

5. Degree of patella alta and general ligamentous laxity. In some adolescent patients with marked

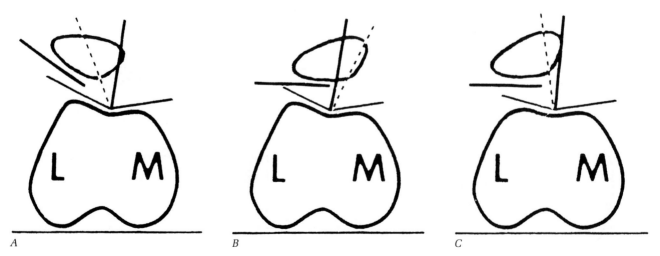

A   *B*   *C*

FIGURE 27-4
A. Lateral shift without tilt. *B.* Tilt without shift. *C.* Lateral tilt *and* lateral shift.

326

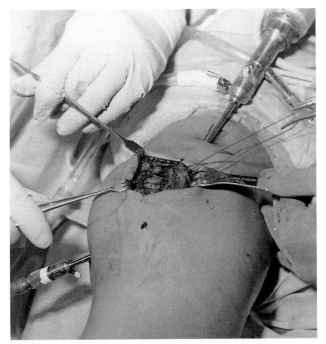

FIGURE 27-5
The medial retinaculum is incised leaving the synovium intact to allow arthroscopic visualization after reefing the medial retinaculum.

is then passed with a tendon passer brought in overlapping fashion on top of the patellar tendon where the loose fascia is incised so that the tendon goes below the bursa on the patella back down to be tied onto itself with no. 1 Ticron. It is extremely important to flex the knee through a full range of motion before tying the tendon, so that the patella is not "captured" in an inferior medial position. Our goal is to have

some tension at approximately 50 degrees flexion and very little tension at 20 degrees to 30 degrees flexion. Multiple interrupted no. 1 Ticron sutures are then used to sew this tendon onto itself.

The patient is placed in a range of motion from 0 degrees to 30 degrees and a knee immobilizer. Weight bearing is as tolerated. The knee is flexed from 0 degrees to 30 degrees for the first month, and then progresses through a full range of motion as tolerated from this point on.

Medial Patellar Tendon Transfer

Slocum has described taking the medial third of the patellar tendon coming medially and sewing or stapling this under the pes tendon in a similar fashion, performing a check rein against lateral subluxation. We have accomplished this in a number of ways. Mitek sutures can be placed in the medial tibia, brought up and then sewn through the transferred medial patellar tendon in whipstitch fashion. We have also taken the medial third of the tibial tubercle with its tendon and placed a 4-O cancellous screw in the medial tibia. The postoperative course is entirely similar to the semitendinosus procedure.

In estimating the degree of patellar medialization, we have found the technique of *selective* epidural anesthesia extremely helpful. "Selective" epidural anesthesia of 1% xylocaine and 0.25% marcaine with epinephrine with 2 cc sublimaze is given (sublimaze potentiates blockade of the dorsal horn cells). This produces total sensory block with maintenance of motor function. Normal epidural anesthesia uses 2% xylocaine with epinephrine (or ½% marcaine with epinephrine).

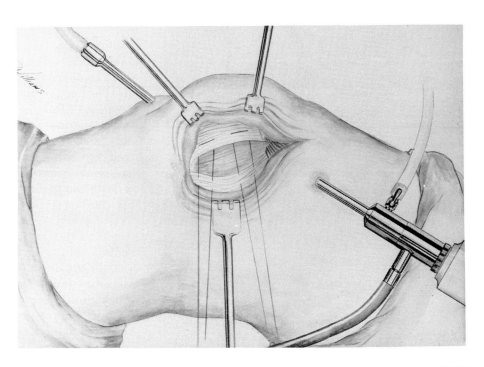

FIGURE 27-6
Mattress sutures of vicryl are used to "medialize" the patella.

In our experience, patients best suited to this procedure are those in whom (on active quadriceps extension) audible click or subluxation can be appreciated. In these cases, after selective epidural, the patient is then able to actively extend the knee and produce the same click and subluxation. Our procedure is to analyze carefully the various factors that could produce the patellar instability, perform an arthroscopic evaluation if indicated, and then leave the arthroscope in the superomedial portal.

The superomedial portal is made 3 to 4 cm above the superomedial portion of the patella (Fig. 27-7), angling into the joint so that this is in the central trochlear groove. With the arthroscope in the superomedial portal, patellar tracking is observed with the patient "actively" extending and flexing the knee. In some cases, it appears that the lateral retinaculum is unduly tight and a lateral retinacular release is performed under arthroscopic control, and patellar tracking is again observed with active extension. If after a lateral release tracking is still "lateral," then consideration for a medial plication with a 2- to 3- inch incision over the medial retinaculum is made, leaving the synovium intact. This goes 2 inches above the superior pole of the patella, down to the inferior pole. If the synovium is left intact, then arthroscopic examination is still possible. The medial retinaculum is then reefed with no 1. Maxon sutures and tracking

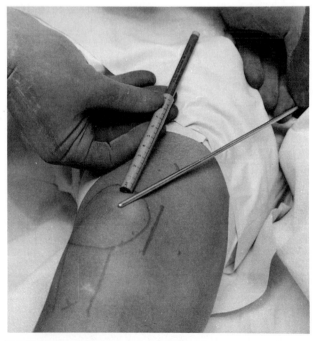

FIGURE 27-7
The superomedial portal is placed 3 to 4 cm above the superomedial portion of the patella so as to allow more "central" visualization of patellofemoral tracking.

is evaluated as noted previously. We strive to have the patella "centralized" by 35 degrees to 40 degrees flexion. In cases that have significant Q angles, the tibial tubercle is generally osteotomized, left attached distally and then with finger pressure on the tibial tubercle, tracking is observed arthroscopically and the lateral border of the medial displaced tibial tubercle is fixed with a smooth K wire and tracking again observed. In this way, the localization can be very precise and after adequate tracking is ensured, the tibial tubercle is generally fixed with a large flat-headed 6.5 cancellous screw.

Postoperatively, range of motion starts immediately from 0 degrees to 60 degrees. Hemovacs are generally not used. Weight bearing is as tolerated regardless of whether or not the tibial tubercle has been moved or medial retinacular plication has been performed.

Our first case is illustrative of the advantage of this particular technique. The patient was referred for a chronic dislocating left patella. She was 32 years old and, as a child, had three attempts (two proximal and one distal) at realigning her right patella. Her left patella continued to dislocate; however, after the experience with her right knee, she declined to have anything done until this became very symptomatic. An orthopaedic surgeon outside our office "medialized" the tibial tubercle, which stopped the dislocations; however, it produced active and dramatic *medial* subluxation of her patella. She was taken to the operating room and given selective epidural anesthesia and the tibial tubercle was osteotomized, left attached and brought back slightly laterally, and active extension still left the patient with medial subluxation. The tibial tubercle was then brought back almost to its original position and then the patient easily subluxed and could dislocate her patella laterally. The medial retinaculum was exposed and reefed in various combinations until it could be seen that with appropriate tightening of the medial retinaculum, the patella tracked quite nicely. The patient was treated in a range of motion machine as mentioned and has done quite well, with ideal patellar tracking on the left and no patellar instability symptoms. What this case has dramatized was that if one were to simply go by an increased Q angle and "medialized" the patella in this patient, one is left with significant medial subluxation of the patella. In this particular case, the tibial tubercle was placed almost within its precise anatomic location and reefing of the medial retinaculum was required.

It is important to note that we still perform arthroscopic subcutaneous lateral release under standard general anesthesia without the selective epidural technique. We feel that unless the patient manifests significant patellar instability findings on active quadriceps extension, the real advantage of the procedure is minimal. We therefore have only done 21 cases in the past 3 years. Of those 21, 8 had medialization of the tibial tubercle (4 without repeat lateral release, 4 with repeat lateral release), and 13 had combinations of proximal realignment.

In cases without significant chondromalacia or arthralgia pain, we have found the Trillat osteotomy technically easy with minimal morbidity. A 3-cm incision is made lateral to the tibial tubercle. Full thickness flaps are developed, visualizing both medial and lateral borders of the tibial tubercle. Extreme care is taken on the medial side to avoid the anterior tibial recurrent artery. An oscillating saw is used starting on the lateral aspect of the tibial tubercle, at an approximate 30 degree angle to the anterior cortex, and passed from lateral to medial under direct visualization. The subcondylar anterior region of the tibia is carefully visualized to complete the cut proximally. This is then "green sticked," allowing mobilization of the tibial tubercle with it still being attached to the anterior tibia. Digital pressure is then placed against the lateral border of the osteotomized tibial tubercle, "medializing" it and stabilizing this with a 5/32-inch Steinmann pin at its lateral border (e.g., *not* through the transferred tubercle). Arthroscopic patellofemoral tracking is observed from above, and when the patella centralizes by 40 degrees, the tibial tubercle is drilled, tapped, and fixed with a 6.5 flat-head Richards cancellous screw, catching the posterior cortex. Intraoperative x-rays are taken to check the length of the screw. This type of fixation allows full weight bearing with range of motion as tolerated. If this type of screw is not available, we use a 6.5 A-O cancellous screw with a metal washer. It is important to "bevel" the cortex of the transferred tubercle to allow adequate seating of the screw to prevent anterior skin irritation. We do not feel that staples give secure enough fixation to allow full range of motion and weight bearing as tolerated.

Further tracking is observed, and if additional medial reefing proximally is required, this is carried out. All our tubercle osteotomy patients are placed in range of motion (0 degrees to 45 degrees), knee immobilizer for ambulation, and weight bearing as tolerated for 6 weeks.

PATELLOFEMORAL ARTHRITIS

If significant chondromalacia or patellofemoral arthrosis is present in addition to patellofemoral insta-

bility, "anteriorization" is carried out in one of two ways:

1. *Fulkerson osteotomy*—An oblique lateral incision is made posterior to the iliotibial band, coming distally and anteriorly past the distal tibial tubercle. Flaps are developed visualizing the medial tibial tubercle subcondylar patellar tendon region and the entire lateral subcondylar region of the tibia. This exposure is similar to that during which a proximal tibial osteotomy is performed. Guidewires are then drilled from medial to lateral at an approximate 60 degree angle, starting anteriorly, coming posteriorly, laterally. A curved Homan retractor is placed across the posterior tibia. This is done under direct visualization to protect the neurovascular structures posterolaterally. A saw cutting block is then applied to the pins, and an oscillating saw used to cut the tibia (Fig. 27-8). The distal tibia is "green sticked" and the tubercle is brought medial and anterior (Fig. 27-9) and evaluated from above arthroscopically, as in pa-

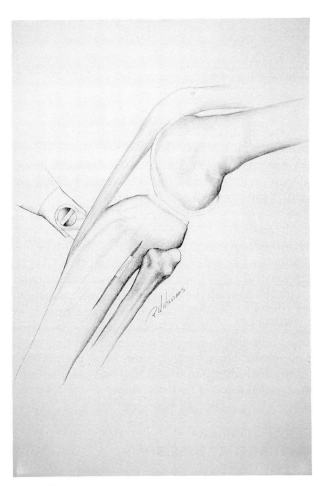

FIGURE 27-8
Oblique cut angle posteriorly for Fulkerson osteotomy.

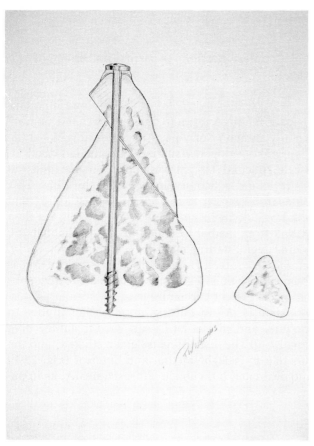

FIGURE 27-9
Anterior medialization of the tibial tubercle after Fulkerson osteotomy fixed with a 6.5 flat head AO cancellous screw.

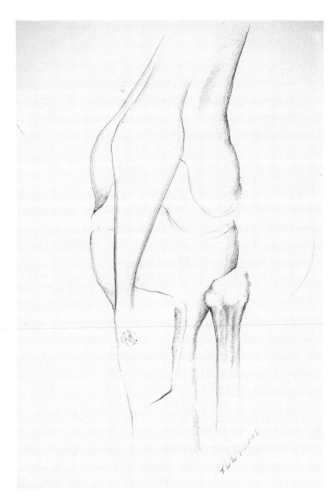

FIGURE 27-10
The completed Fulkerson osteotomy.

tellofemoral instability. The tubercle is stabilized similarly with 6.5 A-O flat-head cancellous screws and washers (Fig. 27-10). At times, two are used. Range of motion and immediate weight bearing are begun, protecting with an immobilizer.

2. *Trillat osteotomy*—may be performed as in patellofemoral instability, and a localized bone graft harvested from below the tibial tubercle with an oscillating saw and flexible osteotomes[4,5] (Fig. 27-11). This cortical cancellous bone block is then rotated and placed beneath the tibial tubercle and again fixed with the 6.5 A-O flat-head cancellous screw. It is important when using the bone graft to have this sloped and also to move it proximally so that there is no excess bone overlying the bone graft. Other authors, including Bandi[6] and Maquet,[7] use iliac crest bone graft instead of the local bone.[8–11]

INFRAPATELLAR CONTRACTURE SYNDROME

In cases of severe infrapatellar contracture syndrome,[12] an open lateral release is performed first.

The entire fat pad and subchondral region of the patellar tendon is then excised. Often, the medial incision is also used. Patellar mobility is then assessed. Lateral x-rays are taken to see if there has been any change in the height of the patella. In most cases, the inferior pole is almost down to the level of the joint line (see x-rays; Fig. 27-12).

In most cases, the *proximal* advancement of the tibial tubercle must also be performed. This is accomplished in two ways:

1. *Previously performed Trillat osteotomy*—is taken and proximally placed on the anterior surface of the tibia and fixed with a small K wire. X-rays are repeated to assess the *precise amount* of proximal movement. As a general rule, with the knee flexed 90 degrees, the inferior pole of the patella should be approximately one to two finger breadths above the joint line. The tubercle is then fixed, again with a bicortical 6.5 A-O flat-head screw. Range of motion is 0 degrees to 30 degrees in a range of motion machine; weight bearing is as tolerated and fixed with a knee immobilizer.

330

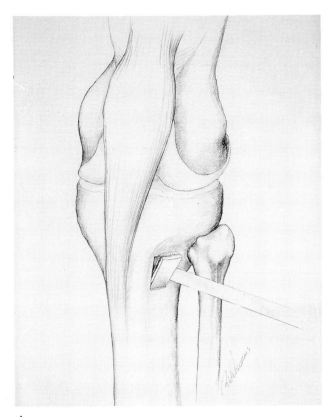 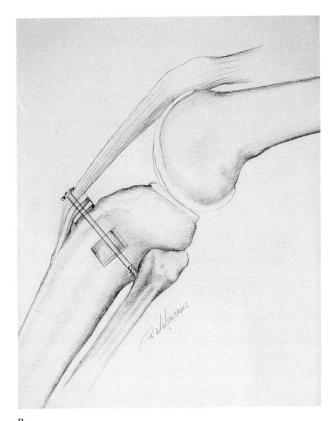

A   *B*

FIGURE 27-11
A. Maquet tibial tubercle osteotomy with localized cortical cancellous bone graft taken from below Gerdy's tubercle. *B*. Lateral view of bone graft and screw in place with Maquet tibial tubercle elevation.

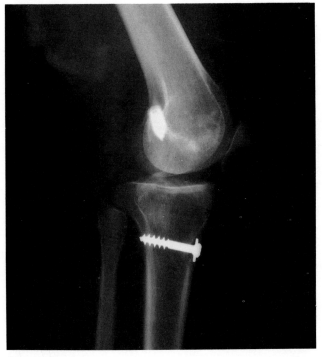 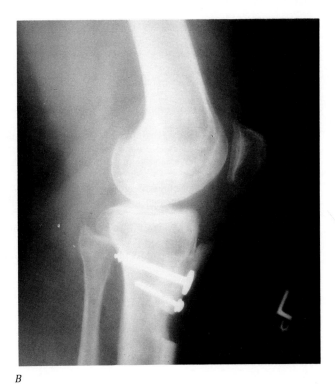

A   *B*

FIGURE 27-12
A. Infrapatellar contracture syndrome post-ACL reconstruction (note the inferior position of the patella relative to the joint line). *B*. Post-osteotomy of the tibial tubercle *proximally* (note increased patella height above the joint line).

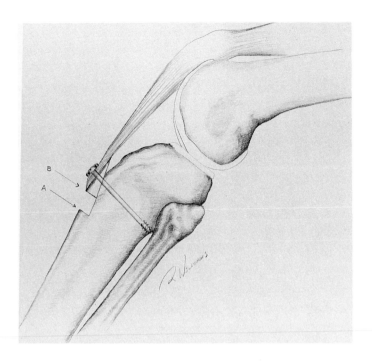

FIGURE 27-13
DeLee osteotomy. An oblique osteotomy is made such that with proximal advancement of the tibial tubercle, this is moved both proximally and anteriorly.

2. *DeLee osteotomy*—Since patellofemoral arthralgia often accompanies infrapatellar contracture syndrome, anterior advancement can be helpful. Straight osteotomes are used to start an osteotomy below the patellar tendon and obliqued at a 45 degree angle posteriorly (Fig. 27-13). The tubercle is then advanced proximally and anteriorly and fixed with a 6.5 A-O screw.

REFERENCES

1. Kolowich P, Paulos L, Rosenberg T, Farnsworth S: Lateral release of the patella: Indications and contraindications. *Am J Sports Med* 18:359, 1990.
2. Shutzer S, Ramsby G, Fulkerson J: Computed tomographic classification of patellofemoral pain patients. *Orthop Clin North Am* 17:235, 1986.
3. Fulkerson J: Anteromedialization of the tibial tuberosity for patellofemoral malalignment. *Clin Orthop* 177:176, 1983.
4. Ferguson AB: Elevation of the insertion of the patellar ligament for patellofemoral pain. *J Bone Joint Surg* 64A:760, 1982.
5. Ferguson AB, Brown TD, Fu FH, Rutkowski R: Relief of patellofemoral contact stress by anterior displacement of the tibial tubercle. *J Bone Joint Surg* 61A:159, 1979.
6. Bandi W: Chondromalacia patellae und femoro-patellare arthrose. *Helv Chir Acta* (suppl 1):3, 1972.
7. Maquet P: Advancement of the tibial tuberosity. *Clin Orthop* 115:225, 1976.
8. Radin EL: Anterior tibial tubercle elevation in the young adult. *Orthop Clin North Am* 17:297, 1986.
9. Hadjipavlou A, Helmy H, Dubravcik P, et al: Maquet osteotomy for chondromalacia patellae: Avoid the pitfalls. *Can J Surg* 25:342, 1982.
10. Cameron HU, Huffer B, Cameron GM: Anteromedial displacement of the tibial tubercle for patellofemoral arthralgia. *Can J Surg* 29:456, 1986.
11. Lund F, Nilsson BE: Anterior displacement of the tibial tuberosity in chondromalacia patellae. *Acta Orthop Scand* 51:679, 1980.
12. Paulos L, Rosenberg T, Drawbert J, et al: Infrapatellar contracture syndrome: An unrecognized cause of knee stiffness with patellar entrapment and patella infera. *Am J Sports Med* 15:331, 1987.

CHAPTER 28

Tibial Tubercle Elevation

Kenneth M. Singer
Mary Isham
Thomas Helpenstell

The surgical technique advocated by Maquet consisted of a 2.5 cm elevation of the tibial tubercle based on a 10- to 13-cm long pedicle of tibial crest using a longitudinal anteromedial incision and autogenous iliac crest bone.

Modifications have been described and the technique that is described has been that used by the senior author.

The procedure may also be combined with chondroplasty of the patellofemoral joint, realignment of the extensor mechanism, or occasionally with valgus osteotomy. The initial portion of the procedure should include arthroscopy and arthroscopic debridement when appropriate.

SKIN INCISION

The skin incision should be long and gradually sloping. If there are old scars, we suggest using the scars and elongating them, making the skin flaps deep and avoiding tension on the skin. If the patient has no other incisions, we prefer a long parapatellar incision, either coming down the lateral aspect of the tibia staying just lateral to the tibial crest or, as Radin describes, crossing over well below the tibial tubercle. It cannot be overemphasized that the skin flaps must be deep and there must not be tension on the skin flaps.

RETINACULAR RELEASE

It is important to do both medial and lateral retinacular releases. Remember, this is a decompressive surgical procedure and it is necessary to do a fairly extensive lateral retinacular release and a medial release up to the border or perhaps the midportion of the patella. One should not release the vastus medialis fibers. At the completion of the procedure, flexion and extension of the knee should not produce undue patellofemoral pressure.

OSTEOTOMY

The osteotomy should be long and tapered. Our recommendation is that the length of the osteotomy be a minimum of 6 cm long. Radin's shingle is much longer, and he first predrills it and then elevates it. Our preference is to use a saw and osteotomes, leaving it attached distally so that it will elevate forward without detaching at its distal end. It will be necessary to divide some of the periosteum, and since the shingle will communicate with the anterior compartment, it is important that the anterior compartment be adequately decompressed. Compartment syndromes have been reported as a complication of this procedure.

If the osteotomy is short, the cosmetic deformity will be greater and the patella will be lowered. If one imagines the radius of the circle starting at the distal tip of the osteotomy and extending to the distal pole of the patella, it becomes apparent that the shorter this length, the greater the lowering of the patella as the tubercle is elevated.

The amount of elevation advocated is varied in the literature as noted above. Based on our review of the literature, we would advocate a 1.5- to 2.0-cm elevation. The previous discussion outlines the various experimental evidence for patellofemoral pressure changes with varying amounts of tubercle elevation.

BONE GRAFT

It is strongly recommended that the osteotomy be grafted. Occasionally, the graft site can be taken from the proximal tibia and at other times it is necessary to take it from the iliac crest. With a long osteotomy, a double thickness piece of iliac crest can be obtained, turned sideways, and placed just beneath the osteotomized tongue, holding it anteriorly.

Another method is to take a square block of bone from the proximal tibia to use as the major portion of the bone graft with additional cancellous bone from the proximal tibia packed in along the graft. It is not necessary to fill the entire defect, but there must be good bone contact at the superior aspect of the osteotomy. We have had no experience with allograft bone.

The bone graft should be contoured so that it fits snugly with good contact between the tongue and the proximal tibia. It should also be placed high, because if the bone graft is more distal than the tendon–bone junction, a stress riser will be created at the superior aspect of the graft and fracture may occur.

INTERNAL FIXATION

Unless the elevated tubercle is very stable with the bone graft in place, internal fixation is advised. The authors' preference is to use a bicortical screw without compression. The flat head of the screw will make it less likely that the screw will have to be removed later, but removing it is not a problem. The thickness of the osteotomy is such that countersinking the screw is not advisable, and therefore it is preferable to avoid the large-headed screws in this instance.

WOUND CLOSURE

Suction drainage for 24 to 48 h is strongly recommended. The wound should be closed loosely, but with a sufficiently secure closure to allow motion early after the procedure.

POSTOPERATIVE CARE

A postoperative knee splint is applied, preferably with the knee in slight flexion initially. As soon as the patient has developed quadriceps control, we allow removal of the brace several times a day to institute early range of motion. Partial weight bearing is allowed immediately and this can progress to full weight bearing as tolerated. It has been our practice to protect the patient on crutches for a minimum of 6 weeks, even when full weight bearing, and to continue use of a protective splint until there is good evidence of union of the osteotomy. The initial dressing should be well padded so that there is no pressure over the tibial tubercle area, and the initial dressing should be changed on the day following surgery to be certain that no skin problems have developed.

CHAPTER 29

Arthroscopic Evaluation of the Patellofemoral Articulation

Lanny L. Johnson

Arthroscopy provides an important means of assessment of the patient with a patellofemoral problem.[1] The arthroscopic inspection of the patellofemoral joint is a diagnostic adjunct to other previously performed methods of evaluation but should not initiate the investigation, substitute for the clinical assessment, nor be the sole determinate concerning treatment decision-making.

Arthroscopy provides a unique and unparalleled opportunity to inspect the patellofemoral articular surfaces, palpate by probing, and evaluate patellar position (medial/lateral and proximal/distal). An additional value is visualization of the dynamics of patellar tracking in the surgical environment, both active and passive. The juxtapositional structures of synovium and plica can be assessed. The remainder of the comprehensive arthroscopy provides evaluation and discovery in the other compartments, including posterior medial and lateral.

Arthroscopy provides an accurate means of intraoperative evaluation of the repositioning of the patella.

There are no accurate and reproducible measures of patellar position, so the surgeon is advised to perform patellar arthroscopy on all patients so that "normal" in the arthroscopic environment can be appreciated. A correlation with physical findings, including manual manipulation of the patella, will school the surgeon concerning subtle abnormalities (Fig. 29-1).

This chapter can only give guidelines of assessment as a benchmark for each surgeon to establish an individual experience. Therefore, each surgeon is encouraged to view patellar status from both positions as a routine in all knee arthroscopy cases.

HISTORICAL BACKGROUND

The patellofemoral joint was one of the first areas for application of arthroscopic techniques.[1-3] This area of the knee was easily visualized with the knee extended and the large size of the suprapatellar pouch. The patella was chosen for the first arthroscopic debridement procedures performed by motorized instrumentation.[1]

Arthroscopic lateral release was one of the first surgeries popularized.[2-4] Plica resection became a common surgical procedure in the 1970s with series numbering in the hundreds.[5,6]

Each of these surgical procedures has been redefined from the surgical indications, the method, and the frequency. Arthroscopic debridement procedures are rarely primary procedures but are performed as adjuncts during correction of other problems. The arthroscopic lateral release is infrequently performed as an isolated procedure and is usually combined with medial imbrication procedures (open and arthroscopic). The plica is now recognized as a normal structure that rarely produces symptoms. The main indication for plica resection now is a fenestrated plica or an enlarged one that erodes on the medial femoral condyle. Isolated plicectomy is an infrequent operation.

While these three procedures were being reshaped, there was no less interest in the patellofemoral problems, which are common presenting complaints in most orthopaedic surgeons' office

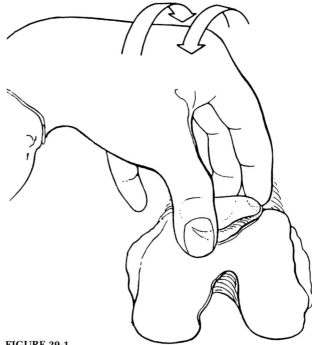

FIGURE 29-1
External manipulation of patella enhances viewing or stabilizes it for surgery. [From Johnson LL: *Arthroscopic Surgery, Principles and Practice*, 3rd ed. St. Louis, Mosby, 1986. Used with permission. (See Ref. 1.)]

335

practices. Anterior knee pain constituted 10 percent of my new office patients in one 2-year span (1986 to 1987). Of this group, it should be also added that only one in ten came to surgery if there was no preoperative evidence of maltracking. Of those without malalignment who underwent arthroscopy, only one (1 percent) of the original group had arthroscopically identified abnormality. This convinced me that patients with anterior knee pain rarely have arthroscopically identifiable problems.

INDICATIONS FOR ARTHROSCOPY

Anterior knee pain alone or patellar crepitus, without physically identifiable malalignment on examination or by imaging technique, rarely comes to arthroscopy in my practice.

The main indications for patellofemoral arthroscopy in my practice are those related to malposition of the patella. They include **dislocation**—acute, chronic, developmental: **subluxation**—traumatic and dynamic; and **lateral patellar position**—developmental and degenerative. The most frequent indication is **failure of previous surgery** on the patellofemoral joint (Table 29-1).

ARTHROSCOPIC TECHNIQUE

Two routine approaches are used for patellofemoral viewing. One is the routine anterior inferior portal. The other is the superior (medial) portal. Occasionally the anterior medial portal is used for another perspective.

Routine Inferior Portal

The routine arthroscopic approach provides access to most areas of the knee joint.[1] It is possible to visual-

ize the patellofemoral joint from inferior and lateral portal (Fig. 29-2*A–C*). The customary 30 degree inclined arthroscope is rotated to view both under the patella and the trochlear surface. Penetration provides view of the suprapatellar bursa including viewing for suprapatellar plica, if present. The dynamics of patellar tracking can be inspected through a limited range of motion from the inferior position. The easiest view of the patellofemoral joint is with the knee in extension. The patella sits in a lateral and proximal position to the femur (see Fig. 29-2*A*). In the past this was interpreted as an abnormal position, giving rise to many unnecessary lateral releases. As the knee is taken to flexion, the patella moves lateral and distal to center in the trochlea. The patella has not closed the medial opening at 20 degrees flexion (Fig. 29-3). At 45 degrees flexion, the patella has moved medial so it is centered and closes the medial gap (Fig. 29-4). Often before this degree of flexion, the inferior viewing portal is compromised by compression of the anterior tissues. This is precisely why the auxiliary superior portal is indicated for patellofemoral arthroscopic assessment.

The patellofemoral joint may be palpated with an inflow cannula if it was placed in the suprapatellar pouch (Fig. 29-5*A* and *B*). A probe may also be used (Fig. 29-6*A* and *B*).

Advantages: The advantages of this portal are limited to the initial assessment of the patellofemoral joint. It provides the best view of the suprapatellar plica with the knee in extension. The distal trochlea area is viewed when the inspection is combined with passive knee flexion. The flexion moves the fat pad away from the trochlea.

Disadvantages: The disadvantage is the incomplete view of the patella and dynamics of tracking.

Superior Medial Portal

In my routine arthroscopic technique of the knee, I use a separate superior inflow cannula from the medial side connected to gravity flow from a suspended fluid reservoir.

This method provides a means of applying suction to the arthroscope to cleanse the joint, while bringing hidden loose bodies into sight for removal. Loose bodies often accompany patellar problems. The medial portal goes through the wider tissue of the vastus medialis, which eliminates leakage. I prefer the medial approach over the lateral, which has a thicker, tough but thin lateral fascia. The medial portal provides a view of the entire patellofemoral joint while allowing opposite side viewing if a surgical lateral release would be performed. Simultaneous

TABLE 29-1

Arthroscopic Indications

Dislocation

Acute
Chronic
Developmental

Subluxation

Traumatic
Dynamic

Lateral Patellar Position

Developmental
Degenerative

Failed Previous Surgery

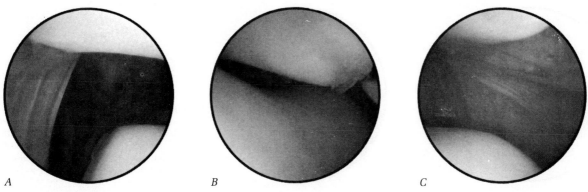

A   B   C

FIGURE 29-2
Normal patellar extension viewed from below. *A.* Lateral. *B.* Central. *C.* Medial. (From Ref. 1, with permission.)

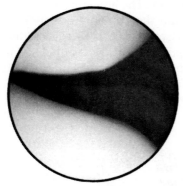

FIGURE 29-3
Normal patellofemoral joint at 20 degrees flexion; viewed from below. (From Ref. 1, with permission.)

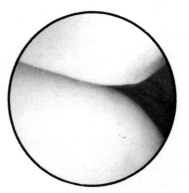

FIGURE 29-4
Normal patellofemoral joint at 45 degrees flexion; viewed from below. (From Ref. 1, with permission.)

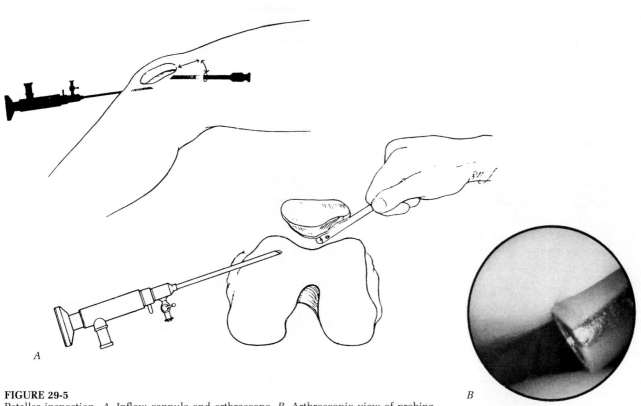

A

B

FIGURE 29-5
Patellar inspection. *A.* Inflow cannula and arthroscope. *B.* Arthroscopic view of probing. (From Ref. 1, with permission.)

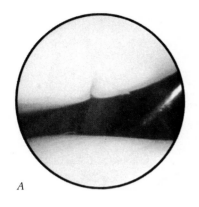

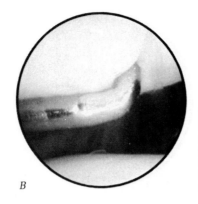

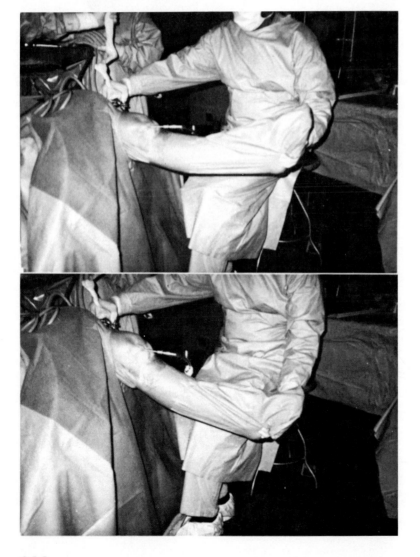

A

B

FIGURE 29-6
Probing of patella. *A.* Small crack or defect in articular cartilage in patient with subluxation at time of lateral release. *B.* Probe palpation of small defects in articular cartilage. Patellar shaving was not performed. (From Ref. 1, with permission.)

viewing and cutting from the lateral side is technically clumsy.

The arthroscope is interchanged with the inflow adapter with use of switching sticks.[1] This takes only a moment. The surgeon moves to the medial side of the extremity to be positioned behind the arthroscope and provide for free knee flexion and extension.

I perform the initial superior inspection with a 30 degree inclined scope, but if any surgery is to be

performed, the 90 degree anthroscope provides ease of orientation of patellofemoral joint.

Advantages: The advantages of the superior medial portal are the panoramic view of the joint for diagnostic assessment of the surfaces, the plica, membranous ligament, but especially tracking. Surgical debridement, lateral release, and medial imbrication are all performed from this one position.

Disadvantages: The disadvantages are minimal,

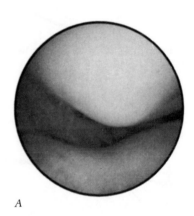

A

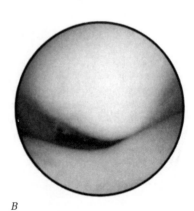

B

FIGURE 29-7 *A* and *B*

including some difficulty in seeing the distal femoral trochlea.

Combined Arthroscopic Inspection with Manipulation of the Knee

Additional information can be gained from combining arthroscopic inspection with manipulation of the knee. The knee can be taken through a range of motion while viewing from superior. Under local anesthesia the patient may actively perform flexion and extension while the surgeon views the patellar position to assess the dynamic restraints (Fig. 29-7A–D).

Patellar position also can be evaluated with viewing combined with external manipulation of the patella from side to side and proximal and distal to assess the static restraints (see Fig. 29-1).

Normal Arthroscopic Findings: The normal arthroscopic findings include a firm smooth white articular surface of both the patella and femoral trochlea.

The tip of the fat pad is fimbriated and protrudes between the distal patella and femur (see Fig. 29-7). The patella is positioned lateral and superior to the femur with knee in extension. (See description of evaluation of tracking later in this chapter.)

The suprapatellar plica is a normal anatomic structure. It is usually arch shaped. It may be present on the lateral, medial, or both walls of the suprapatellar pouch. It may be nearly complete with a small

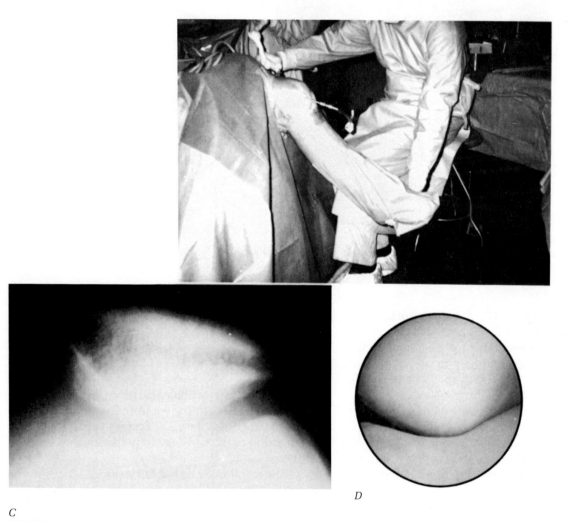

C

D

FIGURE 29-7

Normal patellar tracking—superior view of right knee. *A.* 0 degrees. No contact. Lateral position. *B.* 20 degrees. Lateral contact. Lateral position. *C.* 45 degrees. Central contact. Central position. *D.* Normal 45-degree Merchant axial view correlates with 45-degree athroscopic position. (View reversed for correlation.) Normal patellar tracking—superior view of right knee. (From Ref. 1, with permission.)

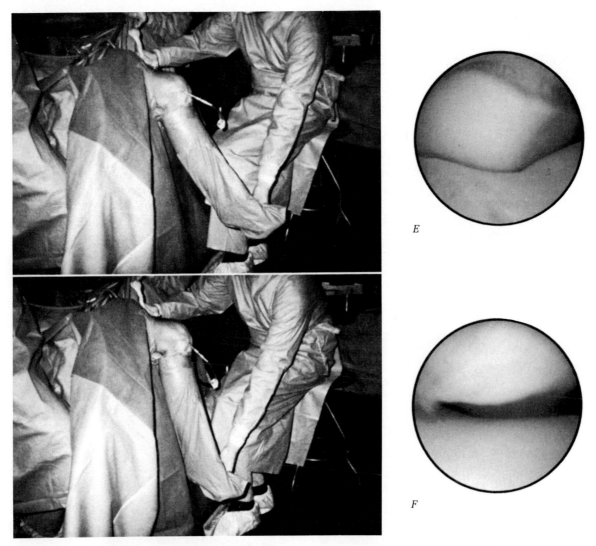

FIGURE 29-7 (continued)
E. 60 degrees. Central contact. Distal position. *F.* 90 degrees. Central contact. Disappears distally.

fenestration (see Fig. 29-17). On a rare occasion it forms an imperforate wall with no visible opening. This plica should be evaluated from below with first distention and then decompression of the joint, so that the dynamics of movement toward the patellofemoral joint can be assessed.

The medial plica is a normal anatomic structure. It is usually single, but may show double or triple folds in parallel. It extends anterior to the medial femoral condyle and is continuous with the alar ligament that attaches superior in the intercondylar notch.

Dynamic evaluation is necessary to inspect the plica with flexion and extension to see its relationship to the medial femoral condyle. In the decompressed joint, it normally glides over the medial femoral condyle.

PATHOLOGIC FINDINGS IN THE PATELLOFEMORAL AREA

Articular cartilage

The most common articular cartilage lesion is a bacon strip material hanging down from the superior aspect of the patella (Fig. 29-8). The first sign of degeneration is softening of the cartilage to palpation (see Fig. 29-5*B*).

This is followed by bubbling (Fig. 29-9). Fissures develop (Fig. 29-10). Fragmentation has been described as having the appearance of crabmeat (Fig. 29-11). Complete loss of articular cartilage results in a sclerotic lesion on bone (Fig. 29-12). This is often accompanied by osteophytes on patella or lateral femoral condyle.

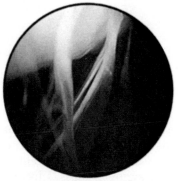

FIGURE 29-8
Bacon strip changes seen superiorly. (From Ref. 1.)

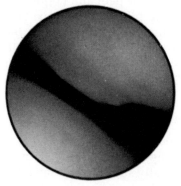

FIGURE 29-9
"Bubble" defect. (From Ref. 1, with permission.)

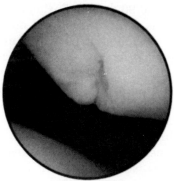

FIGURE 29-10
Fissuring. (From Ref. 1, with permission.)

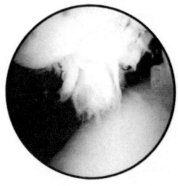

FIGURE 29-11
Fragmentation. (From Ref. 1, with permission.)

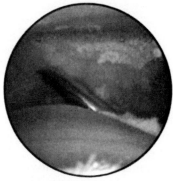

FIGURE 29-12
Exposed bone patellofemoral joint. (From Ref. 1.)

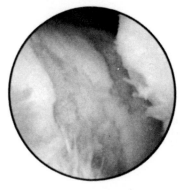

FIGURE 29-13
Degeneration partial thickness patella and femur. (From Ref. 1.)

The trochlear lesions go through the same staging as the patella, but are usually central in location. The configuration is frequently loss of tissue central with overhanging edges of adjacent articular cartilage (Fig. 29-13). The lateral trochlea can be denuded of cartilage with chronic lateral patellar position (see Fig. 29-12). Loose bodies may be in any compartment, including posterior. With dislocation, they are often attached to the lateral femur or in a lateral gutter (Fig. 29-14).

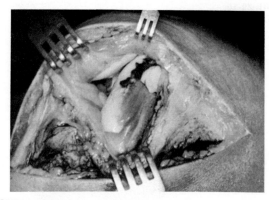

FIGURE 29-14
Lateral view showing avulsed portion of patella healed down to synovial overgrowth in lateral femoral condyle 1 week following injury. (From Ref. 1, with permission.)

Synovium

The most common finding is a villous synovitis. Small cartilaginous loose bodies may be engulfed in the synovium. The synovium may be scarred from previous surgery, showing fibrous bands that span the joint in either the suprapatellar pouch or the medial or lateral gutters (Fig. 29-15).

A localized mass of proliferative synovium may produce symptoms in this area. The cause may be trauma, reactive synovitis, or even localized pigmented villi nodular (Fig. 29-16).

Plica

The plicae are rarely pathologic. A large suprapatellar plica may be palpable by physical examination (Fig. 29-17A and B). A rare sensitive patient may identify its presence as a synovial mass. I have seen a large plica fold down between the patella and femur with joint decompression, providing a mechanism for the symptom of patellar pain and crepitus.

The medial plica (shelf) may be fenestrated, causing popping with flexion and extension while mimicking a torn meniscus[6] (Fig. 29-18A–D). It is rarely thickened due to direct trauma. On rare occasions it will erode on the medial femoral condyle.

Malalignment

The patellar position is assessed in the resting position from the superior medial portal. In extension the patella is normally superior and lateral to the femur (see Fig. 29-2A). In degenerative arthritis it rests more central, even with the knee extended (Fig. 29-19). In patella alta the knee cap is superior and is still visualized even at 90 degrees flexion (Fig. 29-20). In patella baja it is distal and almost out of view at only 45 degrees flexion (Fig. 29-21). In most cases of previous alignment surgery the patella is not normal, but positioned medial and distal, even in the resting extended position. The patella may rest medial as a postoperative complication of lateral release (Fig. 29-22). This occurs when patella alta also exists with a shallow trochlea.

External manual pressure will move the patella in all directions (see Fig. 29-1). It is less movable following previous surgery and in patella baja. It may be dislocatable lateral in pathologic conditions. Me-

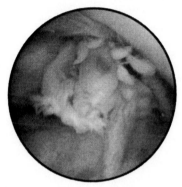

FIGURE 29-15
Postarthrotomy adhesions. (From Ref. 1.)

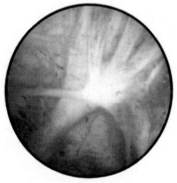

FIGURE 29-16
Localized nodular synovitis. (From Ref. 1.)

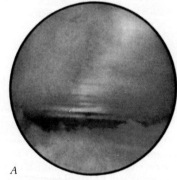

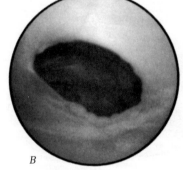

A   *B*

FIGURE 29-17
Suprapatellar plica. *A*. Large plica with small opening at lateral base. *B*. Large plica with central opening. (From Ref. 1, with permission.)

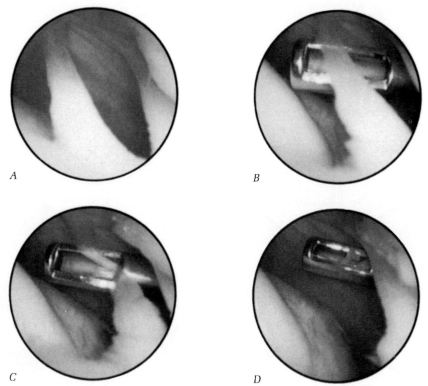

FIGURE 29-18
Fenestrated medial plica. *A.* Separation in body of plica. *B.* Resection. *C.* Motorized instrument removes only separated tissue. *D.* Intact margin preserved.

dial subluxation or even dislocation is possible after extensive lateral release.

PATELLAR TRACKING

Local Anesthesia Dynamic Assessment

The study of patellofemoral tracking under dynamic conditions may be performed under local anesthesia. A study was performed by Kevin Sprague, Leonard Pickering, and myself. It was presented as a scientific exhibit at the annual meeting of the American Academy of Orthopaedic Surgeons in 1984.[7]

We observed the patellofemoral tracking in 11 volunteers by arthroscopy under local infiltrative anesthesia. There was no intraarticular injection of anesthetic agent. The joint was distended with an intermittent bolus of normal saline solution. Viewing was from both inferior and superior portals.

The knee was first taken through a passive range of motion with patellar position recorded at various degrees of flexion. The patient was then asked to perform flexion and extension. This was intentionally a slow maneuver. A second range was performed with stopping at various degrees of flexion to determine more accurately the patellar position.

A second test was performed by asking the patients to contract their quadriceps against resistance at both extended and 10 degree flexion starting position. This was an isometric contracture at two different starting positions.

RESULTS

The patellar positioning under passive motion was the same as if the patient were anesthetized (see below). The presence or absence of tourniquet inflation did not alter the observations of patellar tracking.

The major difference was observed during active motion. During active flexion, the patella centered into the femoral trochlea when the patient flexed the knee only 20 degrees. This is compared to centering at 45 degrees by passive motion of the knee in either the local or general anesthetized patient.

A secondary observation showed a difference in the result of quadriceps contraction depending on the starting position. At 0 degrees (extended position), the patella moved superior and lateral. When the knee was flexed to 10 degrees and quadriceps contraction was performed against resistance, the patella centered into the trochlea.

CLINICAL SIGNIFICANCE

The nonoperative treatment of patellofemoral problems often includes isometric exercises. In the past they have been prescribed with the starting point

343

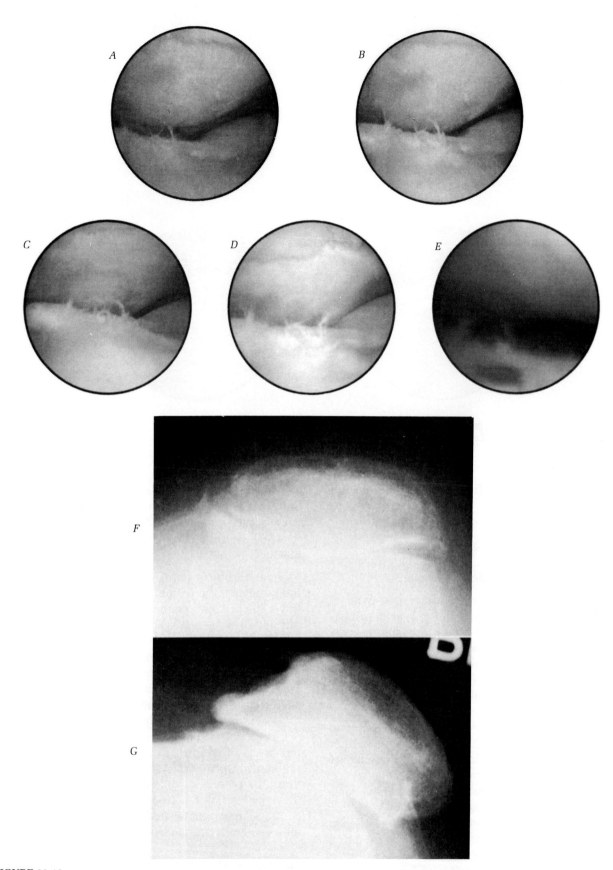

FIGURE 29-19
Patellar tracking in knee with severe degeneration. *A.* 0 degrees. No contact. Centered. *B.* 20 degrees. Minimum contact, Centered. *C.* 45 degrees. Contact. Centered. *D.* 60 degrees. Contact. Compressed. *E.* 90 degrees. Patella not visible. *F.* Merchant x-ray film at 45 degrees. *G.* Lateral x-ray film. (From Ref. 1, with permission.)

344

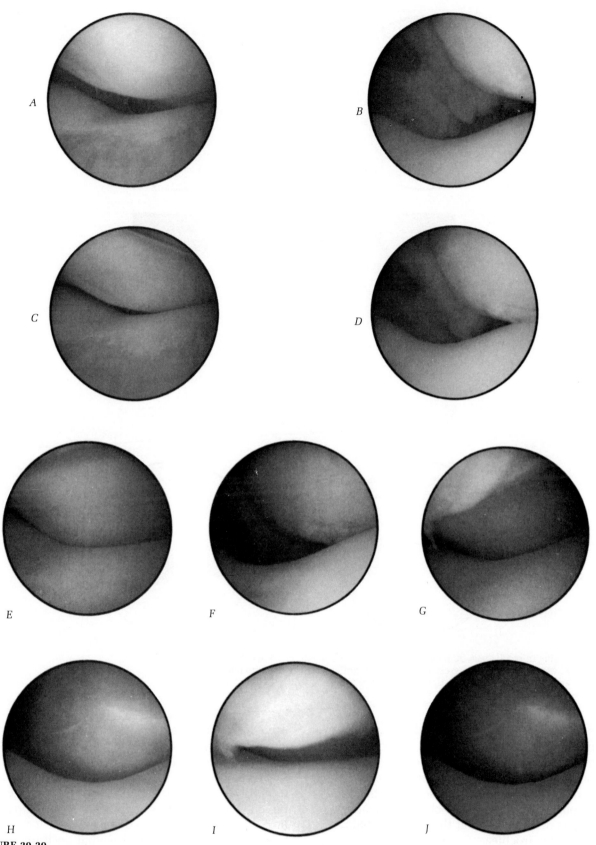

FIGURE 29-20

Comparison of normal knees and knee with subluxed patella alta at various degrees of flexion. *A*. Normal at 0 degrees. *B*. Patella alta at 0 degrees. *C*. Normal at 20 degrees. *D*. Patella alta at 20 degrees. *E*. Normal at 45 degrees. *F*. Patella alta at 45 degrees. *G*. Normal at 60 degrees. *H*. Patella alta at 60 degrees. *I*. Normal at 90 degrees. *J*. Patella alta at 90 degrees. (From Ref. 1, with permission.)

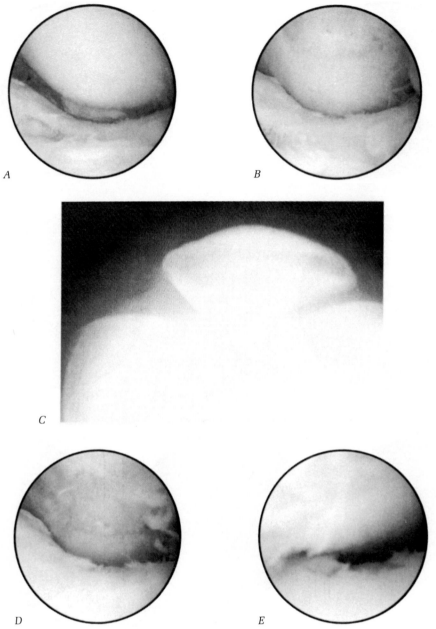

FIGURE 29-21
Patellar tracking in patella baja. *A*. 0 degrees. No contact. Centered. *B*. 20 degrees. Contact. Centered. *C*. Merchant x-ray 45 degrees for correlation. Notice compression into notch. *D*. 45 degrees. Contact. Distal. *E*. 60 degrees. Contact. Out of sight.

the extended knee. This has two disadvantages over isometrics being performed with the knee slightly flexed. In extension the patella moves superior and lateral, which is counterproductive for treatment of subluxation or dislocation. In addition, the slightly flexed position produces a mechanical advantage for the vastus medialis, so that the patella dynamically centers in the trochlea.

This test showed the "normal" active motion produces patellar tracking that centers the patella at 20 degrees flexion. This is compared to centering with passive motion at 45 degrees. Therefore, inter-

pretations of patellar tracking under general anesthesia must consider this difference during diagnostic arthroscopy. Also, this same fact must be considered during surgical correction of patellar tracking so as to not overcorrect the patella. If the surgery corrects the patella so it centers at 45 degrees during passive motion, the postoperative dynamic quadriceps function may produce abnormal medial position.

General Anesthesia Passive Assessment

The arthroscopic observation of patellar tracking was reported by William Dunbar. At the same time, Patrick Hergenroeder and I reviewed 201 of my private patients during routine arthroscopy.[1]

There were 201 patients undergoing knee joint arthroscopy between March 8 and July 27, 1982. The average age of the 118 men and 73 women was 40 years (range, 13–84 years). The right knee was involved 98 times and the left knee 103 times. The diagnosis varied with only a few patients having primary patellofemoral problems. Those with known patellar tracking problems were not included in the assessment of normal tracking, but served as a representation of abnormalities.

In this study, the Merchant axial patellar view on plain film radiography served as a benchmark of clinical patellar position. Since the patella is centered at this position in normal patients, the 45 degree position was considered the benchmark for arthroscopic position determination. It was observed that when this group of patients had a normal Merchant view, there were no signs or symptoms of patellofemoral abnormality in 86 percent.

The arthroscopy was performed under general anesthesia with pneumatic tourniquet applied high on the thigh. The thigh was held in a mechanical body part securing device. Therefore, the knee motion was independent of hip motion.

Diagnostic arthroscopy was performed from the routine anterior inferior portal. The patellofemoral joint was observed from this portal as well as the superior medial portal. Distention was provided by gravity flow from fluid reservoir of two 3-L bags of sterile normal saline. The inflow cannula inside diameter was 4.2 mm.

All the examinations were performed with recording on television ¾ inch U-matic tape and preserved for subsequent review. At the time of arthroscopic inspection, a master tape was constructed by electronic switching. This provided a continuous tape of each case's patellofemoral tracking, one after the other. The master tape included the patient's name, the Merchant view x-ray at 45 degrees, and the segment of the patellofemoral tracking from both above and below. This method eliminated the subsequent need to pull hundreds of cases for review. This method provided a continuum of study without interruption in the series of observations.

PILOT STUDIES

Three pilot studies were performed to direct this investigation. An intraoperative goniometer was used to measure the exact positions of flexion at 0, 20, 45, 60, and 90 degrees. It was abandoned because

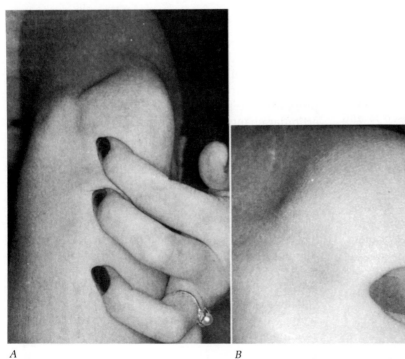

A   *B*

FIGURE 29-22

Complication of lateral release with postoperative medial dislocation. *A.* Patient shows mechanism of medial dislocation after lateral release. *B.* Close-up view of complication shown in *A.* (From Ref. 1, with permission.)

attempts at measurement were inexact due to technical difficulties of placing the goniometer along the draping and guessing the position of the femur or tibia in the sterile environment. Approximations of motion were used at various positions.

Various positions of Merchant view were taken. The 45 degree position correlated best with the arthroscopic observations of centering under general anesthesia. This position was chosen as the benchmark for this study.

The possibility of discrepancy between the patellar position on 45 degree Merchant x-ray in the non-distended and distended state was considered a possible variable. To evaluate this potential discrepancy, patients were taken to x-ray immediately prior to arthroscopy for Merchant view in both the undistended and maximally distended state. There was no difference between these two conditions. It is possible the patients were actively contracting their quadriceps muscle in response to the distention, thereby producing centering in the distended state. This correlation at 45 degrees supported our use of this position for correlation of x-ray and arthroscopic findings. The variable of anesthesia produced potential discrepancy.

VARIABLES

There were other variables in this study. The patients were under general anesthesia. They were in the supine position, unlike the normal daily activity of sitting or standing. The tourniquet could restrict the quadriceps muscle. In addition, the thigh was held in a mechanical holding device that made the knee motion independent of hip flexion, the normal activity. The joint was distended. The arthroscope and cannulas penetrated the joint. The exact position of knee flexion was not possible to record.

CONSTANTS

Each variable listed above is also the constant for any future arthroscopy. The routine arthroscopic environment would be the same as the test environment.

PATELLOFEMORAL TRACKING

In this environment, in extension, the normal patella rests superior and lateral to the femur (see Fig. 29-7A). There is a slight lateral tilt and lateral offset. The entire patellar surface can be seen. The patella is mobile to passive external force (see Fig. 29-1).

At 20 degrees flexion the lateral patella engages the lateral femoral condyle (see Fig. 29-7B). The patella is still lateral. There is no medial patellar contact

with the femur. The patella is still movable in all directions.

At 45 degrees flexion the patella centers in the femoral notch (see Fig. 29-7 C and D). This correlates with the Merchant view at this same position (see Fig. 29-7C). The medial patellar surface makes contact with the femur. Only half the patellar surface is visualized from above. The patella is stable from side to side or proximal to distal passive motion.

At 60 degrees flexion, the patellofemoral engagement becomes more secure (see Fig. 29-7E). Only the superior patellar surface is visualized from above. There is little motion possible by external force.

At 90 degrees flexion, the patellar surface disappears from view (see Fig. 29-7F). The central position is maintained. The patella is mechanically secure in the notch.

Pathologic Tracking

Experience gained by viewing many normal patients provides a benchmark for determination of abnormalities.

The arthroscopic assessment provides a means of viewing articular surfaces in contact areas. The viewing of tracking at various positions is coupled with external manual manipulation to evaluate coexisting capsular tightening.

PATELLAR SUBLUXATION

Patellar subluxation is a clinical diagnosis. Confirmation is possible at arthroscopy (see Fig. 29-23). The patella is usually in alta position. The capsular tissue permits considerable mobility by external manual pressure. The patellar surface may or may not have articular changes. The tracking shows failure to center at 45 degree flexion position. At 90 degrees the assessment of alta is confirmed, in that the patellar surface is visible similar to the 60 degree position of normals.

PATELLAR DISLOCATION

This diagnosis is confirmed at arthroscopy by ease of manual reproduction of the dislocation (see Fig. 29-22). The articular surface will be uninjured if the capsular tissues are congenitally loose. The articular cartilage is commonly damaged in the traumatic case when capsular tissues are inherently tight, thereby causing a compressive force.

DEGENERATIVE ARTHRITIS

The arthroscopic view of patellar position in severe degenerative arthritis is a premature centering of the patella (see Fig. 29-19). The patella is centered even in the extended position. Often this is accentuated by slight knee flexion contracture.

PATELLA BAJA

Patella baja is determined by clinical and x-ray findings. It is confirmed by arthroscopic viewing of tracking and patellar position (see Fig. 29-21). The

patellar position in baja is distal, so that at zero degree extension, the patella is centered. It looks like a comparable view in normal at 45 degrees flexion.

PATELLA ALTA

This condition is established by clinical and x-ray determination. Arthroscopy confirms the diagnosis (see Fig. 29-20). The patella is markedly superior and

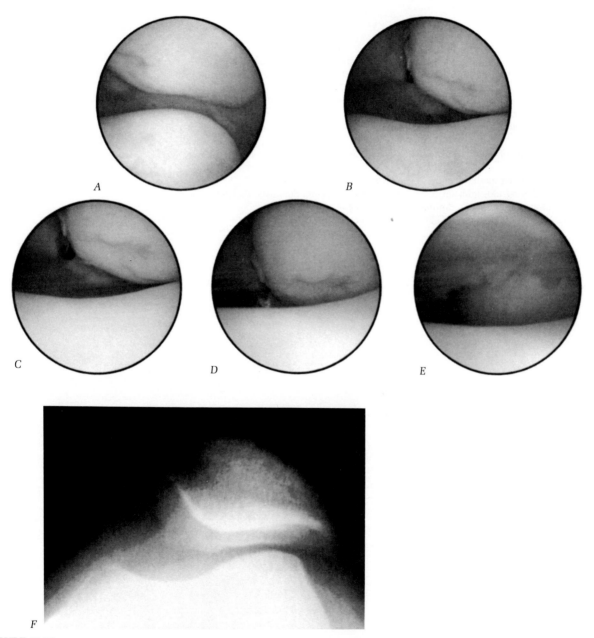

FIGURE 29-23
Patellar tracking. Patellar subluxation viewed from superior. Patient had previous arthroscopic debridement of medial facet. *A.* 0 degrees. No contact. Lateral. *B.* 20 degrees. No contact. Lateral; medial offset. *C.* 45 degrees. Contact. Lateral. *D.* 60 degrees. Contact. Medial offset. *E.* 90 degrees. Contact. Medial offset. *F.* Merchant x-ray view at 45 degrees. (Reversed for correlation).

lateral in extension. The patella is delayed in the normal centering phenomena. It often takes near 90 degrees flexion to center the patella. Because of this delay in centering, the patella is mobile to external manipulation.

sist in making the correct diagnosis and proper treatment program. This information assists the surgeon during surgical correction of the patellar position. The restoration of anatomic position should reproduce normal function.

CLINICAL SIGNIFICANCE

The addition of this arthroscopic knowledge to the armamentarium of the orthopaedic surgeon will as-

REFERENCES

1. Johnson LL: *Arthroscopic Surgery, Principles and Practice.* St. Louis, Mosby, 1986.
2. Sherman OH, Fox JM, Sperling H, et al: Patellar instability: Treatment by arthroscopic lateral release. *Arthroscopy* 3:152, 1987.
3. Metcalf RW: An arthroscopic method for lateral release of the subluxation or dislocating patella. *Clin Orthop* 9:167, 1982.
4. McGinty JB, McCarthy JC: Endoscopic lateral retinacular release: A preliminary report *Clin Orthop* 158:120, 1981.
5. Patel D: Arthroscopy of the plica—synovial folds and their significance. *Am J Sports Med* 6:217, 1978.
6. Barber FA: Fenestrated medial patella plica. *Arthroscopy* 3:253, 1978.
7. Sprague KJ, Pickering LM, Johnson LL: Patellofemoral Tracking, Scientific Exhibit. American Academy of Orthopaedic Surgeons, Annual Meeting, 1984.
8. Dunbar W: Arthroscopic patellar tracking (personal communication).

SECTION X
Case Presentations

The following are illustrative cases of eight commonly encountered problems of the patellofemoral joint to serve as a highlight and supplementation to the appropriate chapter.

We have presented each case to a discussor. They have been asked to review the information presented as if received from a colleague looking for additional opinions and recommendations.

CASE #1

History

A 17-year-old female high school basketball player who, when performing a layup, fell and collapsed with severe pain in the knee. According to her coach, the patella was noted to be sitting laterally. As the knee was slowing extended, the patella spontaneously reduced.

The patient presented to the orthopaedic surgeon 3 days after injury with an acute hemarthrosis.

Physical Exam

The patient presents with an acutely painful knee. There is a large hemarthrosis. Range of motion is from 10 degrees extension to 60 degrees flexion with pain. Lachman's test is negative. There is no varus or valgus laxity. There is marked tenderness along the medial facet of the patella and over the lateral femoral condylar area.

Examination of the opposite extremity demonstrates no stigmata of hyperlaxity or extensor mechanism dysfunction. There is range of motion from 0 degrees extension to 140 degrees flexion. Patella appears to be tracking well within the femoral groove.

X-Rays

The standing AP views are essentially within the limits of normal. The lateral view suggests a possible osteochondral fracture within the joint of the right knee. The patellar view, performed at 30 degrees of flexion, demonstrates bilateral patellar tilt with the right knee showing subluxation and, again, a suggested osteochondral fracture in the patellofemoral space (Fig. 1).

Surgical Findings

The patient was taken to surgery, at which time arthroscopic evaluation of the joint was performed. A large hemarthrosis was evacuated. An osteochondral fracture of the medial facet of the patella was noted, along with a contusion type lesion on the rim of the lateral femoral condyle compatible with dislocation and spontaneous reduction (Figs. 2 and 3). (For additional information, please review video supplement, Case History #1.)

CASE DISCUSSION

Richard Caspari, MD

I certainly concur with your decision to arthroscope this young lady, a decision which I think is borne out by the fact that you did remove some bone fragment from the joint. She would appear to have no overriding predisposition to patellar instability, other than that she is female and participates in sports. I think that this is a traumatic dislocation. Arthroscopy, in my opinion, is appropriate in order to define the pathology precisely, so that a good management program can be outlined and loose bodies can be removed, as was done in this case. At this point, I would not recommend lateral release or any reconstructive procedure, after a one time dislocation. However, I would rehabilitate her vigorously after the medial retinaculum has healed and return her to sports with a patella brace. If she has further episodes of patellar subluxation, or dislocation, then I would recommend a reconstructive procedure. In these circumstances, I have not found that isolated lateral release has been efficacious in my hands.

Peter A. Indelicato, MD and Chip Christian, MD

If the patient presented with (1) no evidence of an anterior cruciate ligament tear, and (2) no evidence of hyperlaxity or anatomic predisposition to patellar dislocation on the contralateral side, I would recommend that the patient have plain film radiography to assess the patella for intra-articular fragments. I usually recommend standard four-view knee series (AP, lateral, tunnel and patellofemoral views). If I am concerned that an osteochondral fracture off the

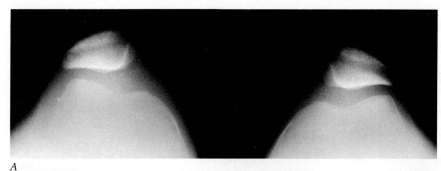

A

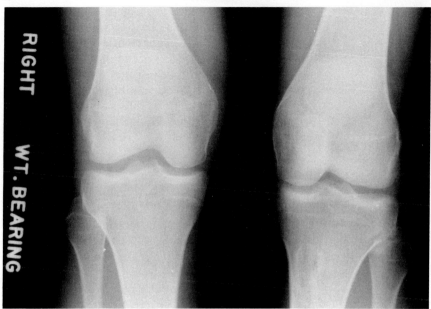

B

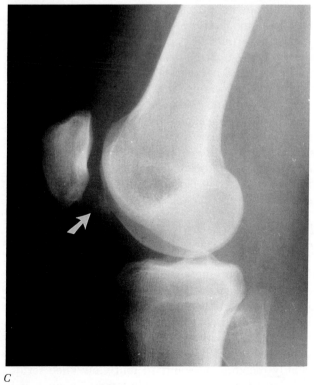

C

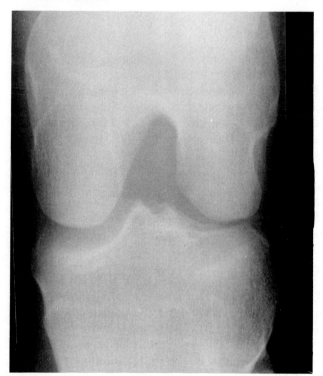

D

FIGURE CP-1
A. The Patellofemoral view shows a bilateral patellar tilt with increased subluxation on the right. *B*. AP view. *C*. On the lateral view, an osteochondral fragment is noted on the inferior patella. *D*. Tunnel view.

patella might not be well visualized on these views, I usually add oblique views. If these films are negative, then I assume no evidence of an osteochondral fracture. Certainly I could miss a purely cartilaginous lesion, but I have not found this to be a problem clinically. The AP and lateral views presented on the videotape do not demonstrate to me any evidence of an osteochondral fracture. With this in mind, I would treat the patient as follows: The patient should be placed in a knee immobilizer for several days until comfortable. I have usually found this varies anywhere from 1 to 2 weeks at the most. I then take the patient out of the knee immobilizer and begin range of motion therapy as tolerated. I believe that the benefits of early motion far outweigh the possible benefits of increased scarring along the medial retinaculum with prolonged immobilization. Once full motion has been reestablished, I generally begin active resistive quadriceps strengthening exercises, all within the limits of pain. This usually consists initially of straight leg raising and terminal extension-type exercises to which resistance can be added as time progresses. I inform patients such as this with acute first time traumatic dislocations that our usual course is one of conservative nonoperative care. They are, of course, at increased risk for future dislocations, but in the patient with no anatomic predispositions, I feel it is best to proceed with nonoperative care.

I must add at this point that if we do see any evidence of an osteochondral fracture within the joint, we would proceed to arthroscopy. We would not, however, recommend a medial repair at that time but would go on to the early motion and early strengthening physical therapy protocol as outlined above. I have been quite satisfied with the results of my treatment plan as outlined above for first-time traumatic patellar dislocators without anatomic predisposition.

If, however, the patient presented with a questionably positive Lachman, I would in all likelihood obtain an MRI of the knee to rule out significant cruciate ligament damage rather than proceed with an arthroscopy. At this point I would be able to assess both the patellofemoral articulation and the cruciates and menisci and feel that this nonoperative approach is preferable to proceeding with an arthroscopy. We have been quite satisfied with the results of our MRI scans at the University of Florida. If on the MRI scan an osteochondral fracture was noted that was not evident on the plain films as mentioned above, I would probably proceed with an arthroscopy at that point to further delineate the nature of the injury.

In most cases, I have just gone ahead and removed the osteochondral fractures of the patella, rather than trying to reduce and fix them. The only other point that I would like to bring up is that of what to do if conservative treatment fails. In this particular young woman, as I have outlined above, hopefully we would be able to get by with conservative treatment without a recurrent patellar dislocator

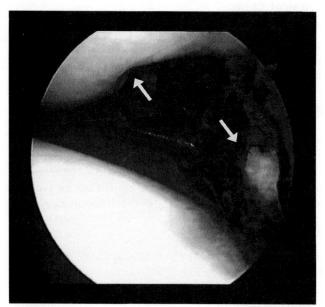

FIGURE CP-2 Viewed from the arthroscopic inferolateral portal, an osteochondral fracture of the medial facet can be seen.

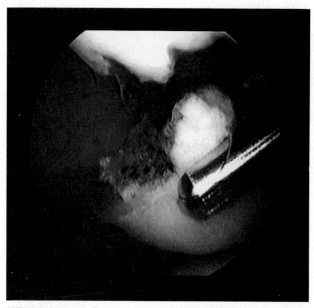

FIGURE CP-3 Arthroscopic view of removal of the osteochondral fracture.

or subluxator resulting. If she did have problems with recurrent subluxations or dislocations, I would probably proceed with a proximal realignment including a lateral release and medial reefing. In another possible scenario, if the patient had evidence of an anatomic predisposition, such as an increased Q-angle, I might consider a distal realignment as well, but this of course would be highly individualized.

In summary, for the case as outlined as you present it to me today, if conservative treatment failed, I would proceed only with a proximal realignment. I must emphasize again in closing that it is my sincere belief that immobilization for long periods of time (4 to 6 weeks in a cast) should be condemned for this type of problem. I would much rather have a mobile knee that has a problem with patellar dislocation or subluxation than a stiff knee with a stable patella. I feel that it is much easier to alleviate the problem of subluxation and dislocation as compared to one of arthrofibrosis. I believe that these types of patients, as with anterior cruciate ligament surgery, are at risk for developing arthrofibrotic problems if one injury, surgery, is superimposed on a prior injury such as the acute dislocation. I would caution all those who intervene surgically early that motion therapy should be instituted as soon as possible to attempt to alleviate these types of problems.

Editorial Comment

It has been our experience also that MRI has been helpful in the diagnosis of acute patellofemoral dislocation. MRI often will demonstrate the chondral fracture sometimes not visualized on routine radiography and also the contusion to the lateral femoral condylar surface and disruption of the medial patellar retinaculum. However, this is obviously an expensive diagnostic maneuver which, with cost restrictions, may become more and more limited in its availability.

In patients with acute patellar dislocation, hemarthrosis, and no stigmata of hyperlaxity, it has been our experience that, approximately 75 percent of the time, a chondral fracture occurs with a loose body present within the joint. This fracture is secondary to the compressive shear forces involved with the dislocation in this "normal" anatomy. Therefore, we recommend the frequent use of arthroscopic evaluation of the joint, evacuation of the hemarthrosis, and removal of the frequently found loose bodies. It has also been our experience over the last several years that with a limited medial arthrotomy incision (approximately 1 to 2 inches) the retinacular attachment to the patella can be explored and repaired with

arthroscopic visualization of the reduction of the patellofemoral joint. A range of motion brace is applied from 0 to 40 degrees flexion. The patient is allowed immediate weight bearing, and range of motion is encouraged and rapidly progressed. The procedure has been performed on an outpatient basis. Long-term advantages for this approach remain to be decided. The initial benefits from evacuation of the hemarthrosis, removal of loose bodies not visualized on radiography, and retinacular repair have been rewarding at this time. (For additional information on this condition and its treatment, please see Chapter 7 on acute patella dislocation.)

CASE #2

History

The patient is a 21-year-old female nurse at the treating physician's hospital. In high school basketball, she had an episode of dislocation of her patella, which reduced spontaneously with an associated hemarthrosis. It was treated by an orthopaedic surgeon with an immobilization splint for a three-week period and then physical therapy. Since that time she has had recurrent episodes of lateral patellar dislocation. She enjoys recreational sports such as tennis and skiing. She "works out" at her local health club approximately twice a week in an aerobic dance program and also exercises with isokinetic-type equipment.

Physical Exam

She is a normal weight female, 5′5″ in height. Range of motion of both knee joints is from 5 degrees hyperextension to 140 degrees flexion. There is no ligamentous laxity. When the patient stands, there is a genu valgus position of both knees, approximately five degrees. Q angle is approximately 20 degrees. With lateral digital pressure on the patella there is apprehension and lateral luxation of both patellae. Both patellae can be transferred approximately one-half the width of the patella surface within the femoral groove. There is a minimal lateral tilt to the patella and mild tightness of the lateral retinaculum.

X-Rays

Radiography demonstrates bilateral patellar tilt with lateral luxation (see Fig. 4).

Surgical Findings

Arthroscopy was performed. With superolateral view, lateral luxation of the patella is noted with

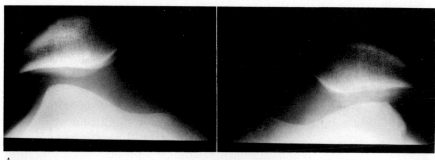

A

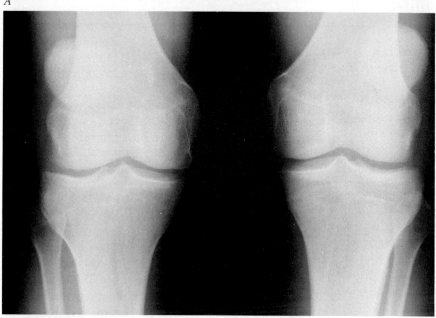

B

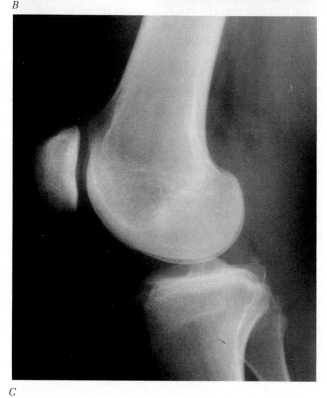

C

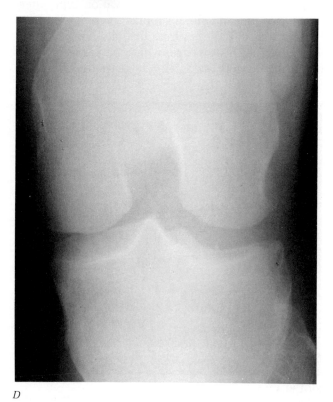

D

FIGURE CP-4
A. The patellofemoral view demonstrates bilateral patellar subluxation with patellar tilt and flattened femoral grooves. *B.* AP view. *C.* Lateral view. *D.* Tunnel view.

overhang across the lateral femoral condyle. The patella does not reduce until approximately 60 degrees of flexion (Fig. 5).

CASE DISCUSSION:

James Andrews, MD and Judson Ott, MD

We would initially treat this patient with a 6- to 12-month structured rehabilitation program with emphasis on dynamic patellar stabilization. The primary stabilizer to lateral patellar subluxation is the vastus medialis oblique, which resists the excessive valgus vector force commonly seen with patellofemoral malalignment. The VMO has recently been shown to be most active during knee extension at 50 degrees flexion for males and 70 degrees flexion for females. Based on these findings, patients are placed on a knee extension exercise program, with range of motion from 40 degrees to 90 degrees. This also represents an area of low compressive force and maximal patellofemoral joint contact. In addition, quad set straight leg raises and hip adductor exercises are performed, as well as stretching exercises of the hamstrings, gastrocs, and soleus. A patient may also benefit from a dynamic patellar stabilization type knee brace used to limit lateral subluxation episodes during sporting activities or from flexible shoe orthotics with a medial heel wedge, which may improve the biomechanics and artificially decrease the Q angle.

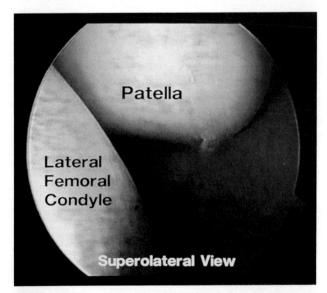

FIGURE CP-5
Arthroscopic superlateral view: note lateral subluxation of the patella with overhang across the lateral femoral condyle.

If the patient returns with persistent symptoms despite a minimum of 6 to 12 months of a compliant rehabilitation program, we would then involve the patient in an intensive, supervised program for an additional 8 to 12 weeks. If significant symptoms persist, surgical options would finally be explored. When discussing surgical options, strict attention must be paid to the individual's anatomy, the radiographic appearance, and the presence or absence of articular cartilage changes in the patellofemoral joint. This patient demonstrates both lateral subluxation and tilt, demonstrated by a tight lateral retinaculum and an abnormal Q angle.

Initially ligamentous examination would be undertaken under anesthesia, followed by arthroscopic evaluation. This is done in order to rule out associated meniscal pathology and to evaluate tracking and the presence or absence and location of any patellofemoral articular cartilage changes. A decision as to a minimal lateral release versus a full proximal and distal reconstruction would then be made. Following arthroscopic evaluation, if an open realignment would be indicated, the leg would be exsanguinated, and a tourniquet inflated. In this skeletally mature patient we would combine a distal tibial tubercle transfer with a proximal realignment consisting of a lateral release and VMO advancement. It is important to emphasize that the lateral release be performed no higher than the superior pole of the patella and that the release is performed close to the patellar border and not through the vastus lateralis. The lateral patellomeniscal ligament should be included in the lateral release. A lateral release alone or combined with a VMO advancement only in this patient, however, would lead to inconsistent results.

Postoperative protocol following a proximal and distal realignment is progressive and cautiously aggressive. Immediate postoperative motion is allowed from 0 degrees to 60 degrees for 2 weeks. Motion is progressed to 0 degrees to 95 degrees by week 4, and 0 degrees to 125 degrees by week 6. Weight bearing as tolerated is allowed immediately postoperatively, and crutches are discarded by week 3. In addition to the standard quad sets and straight leg raises, electrical stimulation is utilized to facilitate and augment the quadriceps contraction. The bicycle is encouraged by week 5; leg extensions from 40 degress to 90 degrees and leg presses from 0 degrees to 60 degrees by week 8; and return to functional sports is gradually initiated at 6 months. In essence, our approach is to try a conservative program, and we would be disappointed if any surgery would be necessary in this patient.

Frank R. Noyes, MD and John J. Larkin, MD

The AP view x-ray is unremarkable, showing no evidence of osteoarthrosis involving the tibiofemoral joint, either medially or laterally. The joint space is well preserved with no evidence of narrowing and no evidence of subchondral sclerosis. There is no evidence of bony abnormality as documented by an AP view.

An additional axial view, which is assumed to be a Merchant view, reveals lateral subluxation of what is assumed to be the left patella. Review of these films reveals a shallow femoral sulcus with a sulcus angle of approximately 165 degrees (compared to a maximum normal of 138 degrees +/− 6 degrees as per Merchant, *et al*, JBJS 1974). Comparison with the contralateral right Merchant view reveals a sulcus angle of 151 degrees. The congruence angle involving the left patella (involved) is markedly abnormal with a congruence greater than the 16 degrees maximum Merchant states as abnormal (JBJS 1974).

This young woman presents with a history consistent with recurrent lateral patellar subluxation. There is one episode of documented patellar dislocation based upon the presenting history. The physical examination is pertinent for no evidence of hyperlaxity of the other joints. The patellar tilt, which is measured in the supine position, is apparently minimal in nature, thus it is assumed to be approximately +10 degrees, which is normal in a female. Of note also is a medial and lateral patellar glide of approximately two quadrants or 50 percent of the width of the patella. This is assumed to be performed with the knee at 30 degree flexion. In general, a lateral patellar glide of one quadrant or 25 percent of its width suggests a competent medial restraint. A lateral patellar glide greater than three quadrants or 75 percent of the patella's width is consistent with evidence of incompetent medial restraints. This patient demonstrates a lateral patellar glide of two quadrants. These findings, when examined arthroscopically, often correspond to a three-quadrant or greater lateral subluxation. In addition, there is evidence of a positive apprehension sign (Fairbank's) on attempted lateral subluxation. The apprehension test simulates a subluxation episode and results in a positive response from a patient with lateral patellar instability.

The physical examination does not include an initial visual examination of both lower extremities. Visual examination of both lower extremities should document evidence of excessive femoral anteversion or excessive tibial torsion, which can give the appearance of a "squinting patella" or "grasshopper eye" patella as described by Hughston. Foot position should also be documented. Excessive forefoot pronation can lead to medial knee strain with a relative increase in the dynamic Q angle. It is important also to document in the sitting position, with the knees flexed at 90 degrees, the presence of patella position and rule out possible patella alta or baja. Routine radiographs should include a lateral view taken at 30 degrees flexion to allow calculation of the patellar tendon length to diagonal length of the patella (upper limit of normal 1.2, Ficat and Hungerford).

Review of the radiographs is consistent with a lateral patellar subluxation, revealing a shallow femoral sulcus with an abnormally high sulcus angle. The congruence angle is markedly abnormal, showing marked lateral subluxation of the patella as documented by both Merchant's and Aglietti's and Cerrulli's criteria. On review of the radiographs, no evidence of patellar tilt is seen, although radiographically the patellar tilt angle (the lateral patellar facet angle relative to the posterior femoral condylar line) cannot be measured based on the radiographs presented. However, based on the clinical examination and the radiographs presented with the Merchant axial views, the patient exhibits no evidence of patellar tilt.

In conclusion, the initial assessment of this patient reveals lateral subluxation with chronic instability of the left patella secondary to a dysplastic femoral sulcus. The initial conservative recommendation would consist of a quadriceps strengthening program with emphasis on the VMO, which is the primary stabilizer for patella centralization in the femoral sulcus. VMO strengthening is maximum at terminal extension. Thus, initial physical therapy begins with an isometric program at 0 degrees extension, which is supplemented by electrical stimulation, isolating the VMO using 40 Hz. Straight leg raises at 0 degrees extension are added to the protocol with 3 sets of 10 repetitions adding ankle weights in 1- to 2-pound increments. The realistic goal is approximately 3 sets of 10 straight leg raises with a total of 10 pounds of ankle weights. It is important to include a flexibility and stretching program specifically concentrating on the hamstring musculature. Presence of either tight hamstrings or tight gastrocnemius musculature has been well documented to increase patellofemoral contact forces.

Once straight leg raises are tolerated without associated pain or swelling, progressive short arc closed chain 0 to 30 degree squats are added to the program. Closed-chain kinetic exercises, specifically for the patellofemoral joint, prevent abnormal patel-lofemoral contact stresses (based upon the work of Hungerford) in a protected arc of 0 degrees to 30 degrees. Additional exercises included in the proto-col are standing wall slides or minisquats, which emphasize primarily concentric strengthening.

Bicycling is then instituted for increased endur-ance. It is recommended that this be controlled with the use of a stationary bicycle. Cycling is not added unless straight leg raise and short arc closed chain kinetics are pain free and not associated with swell-ing. The initial cycling program begins with no resist-ance with an initial 10 minutes of cycling, which is increased by 5-minute increments twice a week.

It is important during cycling that the height of the seat be maximized to minimize knee flexion. A good rule of thumb is to have the seat no lower than the patient's greater trochanter when standing beside the bicycle. Once cycling is tolerated with no pain or swelling for a 30-minute interval, a progressive resistance program may be instituted. Resistance in low gear is increased with the overall goal of toler-ance for a 30-minute interval.

During the intitial phase of rehabilitation, non-steroidal anti-inflammatory drugs may be of benefit to decrease pain and swelling. Generally, an initial trial period of 10 days to 2 weeks is recommended. In addition, post-exercise icing is routinely used to minimize inflammation.

Once cycling is tolerated with resistance for a 30-minute interval, a progressive weight program using closed-chain short arc squats is begun. Weight is added until an equivalent of approximately 25 per-cent of body weight is tolerated with short arc squats using closed chain kinetics. The program is then ad-vanced to straight-on running.

In this patient, because of the degree of dysplasia involving the femoral sulcus and associated high Q angle, initial therapy and strengthening should be performed with the use of a knee sleeve using a lateral patella support bar. If the patient responds to conser-vative measures, then participation in recreational sports along with her aerobics program should be supplemented with the use of a knee sleeve.

Overall goals of conservative treatment are full range of motion without pain along with a minimum symmetrical strength of 80 percent as documented by Cybex or Biodex testing. Once straight-on running is tolerated, sport-specific exercises are then added. The presence of either persistent pain or swelling (or both) is a contraindication to advancement of the program or return to athletics.

The second portion of this case presentation in-volves the same patient who now presents 6 months after failure of a conservative treatment protocol. An arthroscopic evaluation is performed revealing lat-eral subluxation of the patella with failure of the patella to centralize between 40 degrees and 50 de-grees. Of note on the arthroscopic examination is patellar tilt in the range of 0 degrees to 30 degrees flexion. There is no evidence of articular damage or chondrosis as seen arthroscopically.

ASSESSMENT

The presence of recurrent episodes of instability de-spite completion of a conservative treatment protocol now presents the patient with two alternatives. If the episodes of instability are associated only with participation in athletics, behavioral and activity modification is an alternative. If, however, the epi-sodes are associated with activities of daily living, then activity modification alone is not a viable alter-native. In this patient with failure of a conservative, 6-month physical therapy treatment program and the desire to continue her present life-style, surgical in-tervention now appears indicated. Three alternatives exist as to patellar realignment procedures that are offered in the literature. These consist of:

1. Isolated lateral retinacular release performed either open or arthroscopically
2. A proximal VMO advancement and imbrication
3. Both proximal VMO advancement and distal re-alignment that includes medialization of the tib-ial tubercle

In this patient, the initial surgical approach would be for arthroscopic evaluation, which is cru-cial in a patient with a history of recurrent lateral patellar subluxation. Arthroscopic examination should document the absence or presence of patello-femoral articular chondrosis. This is specifically im-portant with regard to realignment procedures and with overall prognosis in terms of pain relief.

Following arthroscopic examination in this pa-tient, there was no evidence of patellofemoral articu-lar degeneration or chondrosis involving either me-dial or lateral facets. The arthroscopic examination revealed evidence of true lateral subluxation with failure to centralize by 40 degrees flexion. In addition, lateral tilt was seen in the initial range of 0 degrees to 30 degrees.

Initial surgical recommendations would be for an arthroscopic lateral release with patellar tracking documented arthroscopically. Failure of the patella to centralize by 40 degrees flexion when viewed arthroscopically along with the history of recurrent lateral subluxation is an indication to proceed to lateral retinacular release whether openly or arthroscopically. The release should be completed up to, but not including, the vastus lateralis attachment. Release of the vastus lateralis itself will not only result in a strength loss but also may cause overcorrection with medialization of the patella. Patellar subluxation medially will often be the final result.

It should be noted that patellar tracking under arthroscopic examination is somewhat biased because the quadriceps is not active during routine arthroscopic evaluation. Two options exist to simulate quadriceps contraction. These include stimulation of the femoral nerve with a nerve stimulator during lateral release or quadriceps stimulation with the use of a muscle stimulator. A third option in patients in whom the lateral release is being performed arthroscopically is for the procedure to be performed under local anesthesia. This allows the patient to actively flex and extend the knee following the procedure so that patellar tracking can be observed dynamically arthroscopically. Based on the clinical examination of this patient and her subsequent arthroscopic evaluation with failure to centralize by 40 degrees flexion and evidence of patellar tilt in the range of 0 degrees to 30 degrees, it is doubtful that a lateral retinacular release alone would be sufficient to prevent lateral subluxation of the patella. The decision now involves whether to proceed with distal tibial tubercle medialization or to attempt a proximal soft tissue correction. If the lateral patellar glide had been on 25 percent of the patella width, giving evidence of competent medial restraints, then one could proceed distally to a distal tibial tubercle medialization if the Q angle is greater than 20 degrees. However, in this patient with evidence of 50 percent of lateral patellar subluxation, the use of a proximal VMO advancement may avoid a more extensive distal realignment procedure.

RECOMMENDATION

Failure of the lateral retinacular release to centralize the patella and the presence of two quadrants of lateral patellar glide support the use of a vastus medialis imbrication (advancement) as an excellent alternative for proceeding distally. The VMO is advanced through a limited 3-inch proximal midline incision. This allows a limited dissection with an excellent advancement of the VMO both distally and laterally. Care must be taken not to overtighten the medial restraints. Once the VMO is advanced, the knee is placed throughout full range of motion. Lateral patellar glide must not be restricted less than one quadrant

or 25 percent of the patella width. In addition, medial tilt is not acceptable once the medial restraints have been tightened. This is best assessed arthroscopically. If centralization is not achieved without undo medial advancement, then a distal realignment is indicated. With the patella now centralized within the femoral sulcus, the true Q angle can be measured, for the first time, since the patella was previously laterally subluxated. A Q angle greater than 20 degrees would be an indication to proceed with distal realignment. The preferred method of distal realignment is the Cox modification of the Elmslie-Trillat. The tibial tubercle is medialized to neutral with the knee flexed at 90 degrees. Patella centralization is then documented. Care must be taken to ensure that the tibial tubercle height is not elevated or depressed in the medialization. The use of elevation and medialization as described by Fulkerson is best reserved for patients with evidence of patella chondrosis or arthritis.

Fixation distally is provided by one or two cortical bone screws incorporating the posterior tibial cortex. The patient is placed in a bulky compressive dressing with a knee extension splint. Partial weight bearing with use of crutches is used for the initial 3 weeks with the advancement to full weight bearing in the knee splint during the subsequent 3- to 6-week period. Passive flexion exercises four times a day are performed under the guidance of a physical therapist. A goal of 90 degrees passive flexion should be reached by approximately 4 weeks. Once radiographs document satisfactory healing of the tibial tubercle medialization, full weight bearing without protection may be advanced based on quadriceps strength. The usual course for radiographic healing is 6 weeks.

To summarize, initial surgical approach in this patient would be for an arthroscopic lateral retinacular release. Based on her clinical examination and subsequent arthroscopic findings, the success of a lateral retinacular release alone in this patient would be doubtful. Failure of the lateral release to ensure centralization of the patella within the femoral sulcus as documented arthroscopically would then be an indication to proceed to a VMO imbrication/advancement. If centralization fails to occur without excessive tightening of the medial restraints, then a distal realignment tibial tubercle medialization would be indicated.

Roger Larson, MD

Radiographs were obtained and reviewed. The AP view shows lateral displacement of the involved patella. Axial views reveal marked lateral displacement of the involved patella laterally. There is a lateral overhang of the patella of greater than 1 cm compared to no lateral overhang on the opposite knee. There does not appear to be appreciable tilt of the patella.

Recurrent lateral subluxation of the patella with previous history of patellar dislocation—the problem that the patient relates is one of apprehension and instability, with pain complaints not being a major factor. There is radiographic evidence of lateral patellar displacement.

Diagnosis was thoroughly discussed with the patient. In addition, a discussion of patellofemoral biomechanics was carried out. The importance of quadriceps rehabilitation, especially of the VMO, was discussed with the patient and the importance of flexibility, particularly of the hamstrings and the gastrocnemius-soleus complex was discussed. She understands the concepts well and has been on previous rehabilitation programs but is willing to again participate in rehabilitation with an attempt to further optimize the regimen. I have also suggested that she obtain a patellar stabilizing brace, which will most importantly consist of a lateral buttress for the patella. She is encouraged to wear this when participating in sports or other activities that she has found to produce subluxation events. I have told her that due to her frequent bouts of subluxation and her abnormal radiographic findings that surgical intervention may be needed in the future, but I have also stressed that this is not absolutely the case: she may respond adequately to therapy and braces. If she does not respond satisfactorily to therapy, it will still be advantageous to obtain maximal rehabilitation of the quadriceps prior to operative intervention.

Note for second visit 6 months after initial evaluation: The patient presents today and relates that she has had no appreciable improvement in her symptoms. She continues to have episodes of patellar subluxation. She feels that she is unwilling to compromise her goal of an active life-style and would like to consider operative intervention if I feel that this might help her situation.

The plan will be to take this patient to the operating room for extensor realignment. In my experience in cases of recurrent subluxation it is usually necessary to perform a tibial transfer in addition to a lateral retinacular release. This will be preceded by an arthroscopic inspection of the knee joint to treat any associated pathology and to consider debriding any cartilaginous lesions of the patellofemoral joint. It will also be important to inspect the retropatellar surface to be sure that there is not a lesion that may come under more force following a tibial tubercle transfer. Assuming that there are no cartilage lesions

that would prohibit it, I would proceed to do a limited open lateral retinacular release under arthroscopic control. This would involve a small transverse incision at the superior lateral border of the patella. Through that incision, a scissor will be placed to perform a retinacular release under direct arthroscopic viewing. The release will be carried proximally only enough to allow patellar tilt of 70 degrees. Special care will be taken to be sure the inferolateral retinaculum is completely released. Following this, a transverse incision will be made at the tibial tubercle. The tubercle will be osteotomized and shifted medially according to the technique of Trillat. The goal will be to decrease the Q angle to approximately 10 degrees; however, this almost always represents a medialization of approximately 1 cm. The tibial tubercle will be fixed by two bicortical screws.

Postoperatively, the patient will be immobilized for approximately 5 days with a compressive dressing. This is to lessen the chance of hemarthrosis. Following that, the patient will be in a removable immobilizer, which she will wear while ambulating with crutches and weight bearing as tolerated. She will start quadriceps isometric exercises and straight leg raising. She will remove the brace several times a day to work on obtaining a full passive range of motion. She will be seen approximately three times a week in physical therapy to help her in obtaining the passive range of motion. At physical therapy, modalities such as electrical stimulation will be used as necessary to ensure that she is making good quadricep contractions. She will be started on patellar mobilization maneuvers. If tibial tubercle fixation is felt to be secure, she can start low resistance stationary bicycling as soon as motion permits, using her other extremity as the primary motor. It is anticipated that she would be able to come off crutches approximately 6 to 8 weeks postoperatively.

Editorial Comment

The three discussors emphasize the importance of trying a conservative program of strengthening and conditioning, trying to rehabilitate the vastus medialis musculature, and using appropriate bracing. Also, such things as femoral anteversion, pronation of the forefoot, and other generalized malalignment need to be recognized at the clinical examination. These patients can benefit from shoe orthoses to improve their gait function and mobility. In those patients who, after extensive trial of conservative treatment, have continued instability problems, surgical intervention becomes a viable additional alternative (please see Chaps. 4, 23, and 24).

As for the type of surgical intervention for this particular patient with tightness of the vastus lateralis, the common denominator of all the discussors is a lateral release, whether performed arthroscopically or open. This must not proceed beyond the superior pole of the patella due to the risk of weakening the vastus lateralis musculature and losing control of patellofemoral tracking (please refer to Chaps. 9 and 26).

The incompetence of the medial restraints is indicated by the ability to displace the patella laterally more than 50 percent of its width. Two of the discussors emphasize the aspects of tibial tubercle transfer prior to proximal medial tightening. It has been our experience that this procedure is performed in a sequential manner. First is the lateral release: The arthroscope is maintained superolateral to follow the tracking of the patellofemoral joint. If the reduction is not achieved (we would not expect it to be in this patient with incompetence of the medial restraints), then a medial incision 1 to 2 inches in length is made and advancement of the medial retinaculum and the vastus medialis with sequential sutures are done. Each suture is clamped to observe the reduction of the patellofemoral joint from the superolateral portal before tying the sutures. If the reduction is not maintained through the arc of movement, then a medial tibial tubercle transfer with compression screw fixation is done.

The decision-making process can be enhanced using a selective sensory epidural-type anesthesia. This allows the patient to have motor control to actively flex and extend the knee without pain. However, not all patients are comfortable with this approach, because they do have some sensation and are obviously aware of the operating room environment. Most patients, though, are quite enthusiastic about this anesthetic approach (see Chaps. 8 and 27).

CASE #3

History

A 57-year-old woman in good general health. She is a commercial real estate sales representative. For general conditioning, the patient walks approximately 4 miles per day, three times per week, and plays doubles tennis once a week with her friends. Over the last 2 years, she has had chronic low grade pain along the anterior aspect of her patella. This has become more and more progressive. The patient has tried anti-inflammatory medication and developed gastrointestinal complaints. She has tried a physical therapy program emphasizing quadriceps strengthening without any benefit.

Her activity level has progressively diminished. She is no longer able to participate in tennis and has had to stop her walking program over the last 6 months because of the increasing pain. She is frustrated with her inactivity.

Physical Exam

There is bilateral retropatellar crepitation of a marked severity, both palpable and audible. The patient volunteers that she has noted "grinding" in both her knees since adolescence, with progression over the last 10 years.

Range of motion is from 0 degrees extension to 130 degrees flexion bilaterally. There is no ligamentous laxity. A minimal effusion is present within both knee joints. The patient demonstrates marked tenderness over the lateral facet of the left patella.

X-Rays

Radiographs demonstrate lateral luxation, lateral tilt of the patella, lateral facet compression bilaterally, and marked narrowing of the patellofemoral joint (see Figure 6).

Surgical Findings

Arthroscopic surgery superolateral view demonstrates marked erosion of the articular surfaces of the lateral facet of the patella and lateral femoral condyle, with narrowing of the space between the lateral facet of the patella and its femoral articulation (Fig. 7).

CASE DISCUSSION

Richard Laskin, MD

This 57-year-old woman has degenerative changes involving at least two compartments of her left knee. She has marked joint space narrowing in the retropatellar space and milder narrowing in the medial tibial femoral joint space. Her patella is subluxed laterally from the trochlear groove. Her femoral-tibial axis measures approximately 0 degrees, thereby placing her in about 4 degrees to 5 degrees of functional varus. Her symptoms have proved recalcitrant to the usual nonoperative therapy and she presently has had to limit her sporting and walking activities.

I feel that the treatment offered to her must be targeted to three particular problems: her lateral patellar subluxation, her marked patellofemoral arthritis, and the medial tibio-femoral degenerative changes. I do not feel that a further arthroscopic procedure would be of value. Furthermore, in view of her medial compartment disease I do not feel that

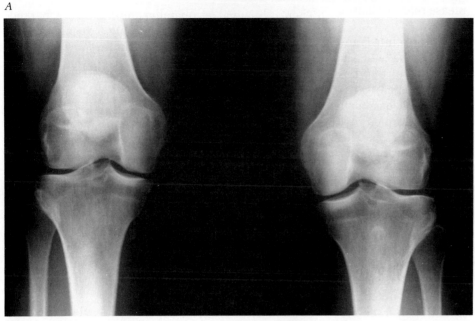

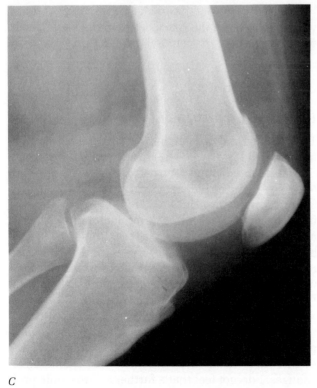

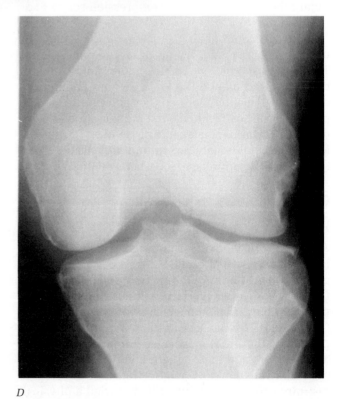

FIGURE CP-6
A. The patellofemoral view demonstrates bilateral patellar subluxation with patellar tilt and flattened femoral grooves. *B.* AP view. *C.* Lateral view. *D.* Tunnel view.

A

B

C

D

a procedure to decrease the patellofemoral contact stresses (i.e., a Maquet osteotomy) would be effective. A high tibial osteotomy combined with a Maquet-type oesteotomy would address both her medial compartment and patellofemoral problems; however, in my experience this combined type of operation (and indeed high tibial valgus osteotomies by themselves) are not well tolerated by women, especially as related to cosmesis. Arthrodesis is to be mentioned only for completeness; however, I do not feel that it is a reasonable suggestion in a patient of this age with bilateral disease.

This leaves the only surgical alternative to be a total knee replacement. My current thinking is to perform the arthroplasty cement-free in patients of this age if the underlying bone is of sufficient quality to allow stable fixation of the individual implants. Her knee has neither ligamentous laxity nor a flexion contracture, so I feel we could probably use an implant that retained the posterior cruciate ligament. Her patella is subluxed laterally so that the appropriate soft tissue balancing of the quadriceps expansion would be paramount at surgery. This might include a lateral retinacular release (preserving the lateral superior genicular artery) and/or a medial capsular imbrication.

The patient would have to be well aware, however, of the potential of long-term loosening in a woman of her age as well as the usual potential complications of infection, phlebitis, anesthetic reaction, etc. In view of this she should not consider returning to jogging, tennis or racquet sports after the knee arthroplasty since the impact loading that would occur could be expected to increase the potential for component loosening. For an athletic patient such as she, I would recommend golf, swimming, and walking as suitable exercises after a knee replacement. Even with these reasonable limitations on her activities after surgery there is the potential that she will require revision as the years progress. The two most common causes at this time for long-term revision in a young patient such as she are tibial component loosening and polyethylene wear and debris formation.

The final recommendation for total knee arthroplasty would have to be based on the patient's decision that her pain has significantly diminished her own personal ability to participate in most of the activities of daily living and could not be made from radiographs alone.

James A. Rand, MD

The options for management of this patient would include continued nonoperative management, arthroscopic debridement with lateral release, patellectomy, or total knee arthroplasty. Additional information that would be helpful in deciding on the appropriate treatment modality would include the presence or absence of rest or night pain, extent of impairment of function of walking ability, the need for ambulatory aids, and the adequacy of her participation in a quadriceps strengthening program. Additional important considerations would be her overall medical health and projected life expectancy. Although the patient has tried some limited nonoperative management, she has not exhausted this modality. The use of an ambulatory aid such as a cane, activity modification to avoid stairs and bent-knee activities under load, weight reduction if she is overweight, and a change of her recreational conditioning to swimming or walking in the swimming pool would be helpful.

If the patient fails these nonoperative measures, then a consideration for arthroscopy of the knee with debridement of the patellofemoral joint and a lateral retinacular release could be performed. This would provide the opportunity to visualize the tibiofemoral joint and determine the extent of arthrosis in this articulation, as this will influence the subsequent management. The patient may receive some temporary benefit from the lavage and lateral release, although this is less predictable than in the patient with only chondromalacia without advanced arthrosis. The results of arthroscopic debridement for advanced patellofemoral arthritis are probably no more than 20 percent successful.

If there were no evidence of tibiofemoral disease and the trochlear surface of the femur was only mini-

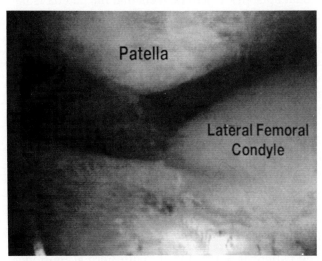

FIGURE CP-7
Superolateral view at arthroscopy demonstrates marked erosion of articular surfaces of lateral facet and lateral femoral condyle.

mally involved and the patient had intractable pain, then patelletomy could be considered. Unfortunately, patellectomy will decrease the quadriceps lever arm, necessitating an increased quadriceps force for knee function. That effect of this increased force will be an increased tibiofemoral reaction force which can accelerate preexisting arthrosis in this articulation. Therefore, before considering a patellectomy, the extent of arthrosis in the tibiofemoral joint needs to be defined, and arthroscopy would provide the most information referable to this articulation. The patient needs to be cautioned that patellectomy may not relieve all of her pain, and she may have some residual discomfort from the extensor mechanism articulating on the trochlear surface of the femur. She also needs to be advised that if patellectomy were performed this would complicate subsequent management by total knee arthroplasty if needed in the future and provide a less satisfactory functioning knee.

Total knee arthroplasty is a reasonable management for the elderly patient with advanced osteoarthritis in the patellofemoral joint. In general, this approach would be applied to the patient who is in the late 60s or older age group or the physiologically equivalent age group. This would provide excellent relief of the patellofemoral pain without concerns about subsequent degeneration in the tibiofemoral joint. However, at age 57, the patient is younger than most patients who would be selected for total knee arthroplasty for this diagnosis. Total knee arthroplasty would only be considered if this patient failed less aggressive surgical as well as conservative management and only if she had evidence of significant tibiofemoral disease at the time of arthroscopic evaluation.

Patellofemoral arthroplasty is not a particularly good choice for this patient because it provides all the limitations of a total knee arthroplasty without all of the advantages. Salvage of the failed patellofemoral surfacing can be difficult due to the loss of bone stock.

Maquet osteotomy is not a good choice for a patient in this age group due to the frequent soft tissue complications and the fact that this will potentially make subsequent knee arthroplasty more difficult.

Therefore, I believe the best choice for this patient is initially continued nonoperative management at the present time. If the symptoms progress, then arthroscopic evaluation with debridement and lateral release should be performed. This will allow evaluation of the tibiofemoral joint and the ability to subsequently plan for additional surgery, if necessary. Hopefully, the patient will be able to manage with the nonoperative measures until she is older and

becomes a more suitable candidate for knee arthroplasty.

Editorial Comment

Lateral facet compression and lateral luxation with the severe articular surface loss is an extremely frustrating situation for the patient and for the treating orthopaedic surgeon. This latter statement is supported by both prominent discussors.

This patient has a high risk for proceeding to total joint replacement. It is our opinion that if that can be delayed or avoided, it is to the patient's advantage. The patient needs to understand that all of the procedures available to her are "salvage" procedures. The choices for this patient are arthroscopic debridement, lavage of the joint, intraarticular shaving, and lateral release to try to decompress the lateral patellar compressive forces. Approximately 65 to 70 percent of the patients do benefit from this procedure over a minimum of 2 to 3 years. About 35 percent obtain no significant benefit and do proceed to more aggressive surgical procedures. (Please refer to Chaps. 18 through 22 in the section on Degenerative Lesions.)

CASE #4

History

The patient is a 38-year-old male accountant who participates in recreational sports such as skiing, golf, and racquetball. His chief complaint is an aching pain over the anterior aspect of both knee joints for the last 10 years, increasing in discomfort with all of his sporting activities over the last year. He has occasional episodes where he feels that his patella is becoming displaced.

Fifteen years previously while wrestling in college, he suffered a lateral dislocation of his patella with hemarthrosis. This reduced spontaneously and was treated with immobilization for a six week period of time and a strengthening and rehabilitation program.

The patient has been previously treated by another orthopaedic surgeon prior to presenting to your office, with a rehabilitation program three times per week, emphasizing strengthening of the quadriceps musculature. He has also been tried in various patellar knee supports without benefit.

Physical Exam

The patient is 5'10", 165 lb, with normal muscular development. Range of motion of the uninvolved knee is from 0 degrees to 140 degrees flexion; the involved knee is 0 degrees to 130 degrees flexion. There is no evidence of ligamentous laxity. There is marked tenderness over the lateral facet of the patella and the patella can be displaced approximately one-third of its width within the femoral groove laterally. There is noted to be a mild patellar tilt.

X-Rays

Radiographs demonstrate lateral displacement of the patella with tilt and narrowing of the lateral facet space (Fig. 8).

Surgical Findings

Articular surface wear changes of the patella and lateral femoral condyle are noted from the superolat-

eral view. Lateral tracking of the patella with lateral overhang is noted (Fig. 9).

CASE DISCUSSION

Champ Baker, MD

ASSESSMENT

Recurrent lateral subluxation of the patella.

RECOMMENDATIONS

This patient has had multiple years of complaints referable to his patella. In particular, he has feelings of subluxation in addition to his discomfort. After having a patellar dislocation several years ago, he

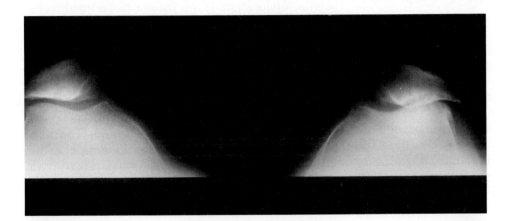

A

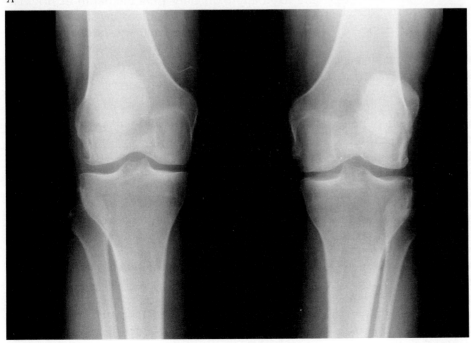

B

FIGURE CP-8
A. Patellofemoral view, demonstrating bilateral subluxation, left greater than right, and marked narrowing of the patellofemoral joint with sclerosis. *B.* AP view.

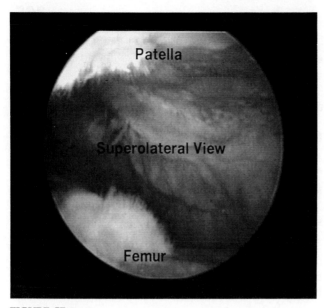

FIGURE CP-9
Superolateral view demonstrating articular surface wear changes and lateral tracking of the patella.

began a modified exercise program and began wearing a patellar knee support without benefit. The patient is presently 38-years-old and is active in recreational sports, including racquetball and golf. It is my feeling that, if the patient's symptoms have increased to or remain at a point where he wants to have them corrected, he is a surgical candidate at this time.

Options for surgery would include arthroscopic lateral release only, open lateral release, or lateral release combined with medial advancement of the vastus medialis obliquus (VMO). The patient's radiographs show a lateral patellar tilt but do not show a patella alta; therefore, he would not require a distal tibial tubercle transfer.

It is my impression that the patient's symptoms of subluxation coupled with the arthroscopic visualization of the malacic changes of the lateral patella indicate that he is continuing to have subluxation episodes with contact between the lateral aspect of the patella and the femoral condyle. In this patient, I believe that a pure lateral release, whether arthroscopic or open, would not completely alleviate these symptoms and that a medial reefing combined with a lateral release is indicated.

My surgical intervention would involve a lateral parapatellar incision and a medial arthrotomy with identification and removal of any medial synovial bands that could be causing retinacular symptoms. An open lateral release would then be performed with care taken not to completely detach the vastus lateralis, but to merely decompress the lateral joint by lengthening the lateral retinaculum. The VMO is advanced and attached to the medial edge of the patella, taking care to attach it no lower than the proxi-

mal third of the patella. The advancement is usually secured with nonabsorbable sutures in a pants-over-vest manner. The ligatures are then placed and the leg is flexed and extended with pressure on the patella to ensure that lateral subluxation has been controlled.

The postoperative regimen would include immobilization of the knee for approximately 2 weeks. During that time, however, the straight leg immobilizer would be removed while the patient worked on passive flexion exercises. He will be allowed partial weight bearing on crutches. After 2 weeks, he will begin wearing a protective patellar stabilization brace and start more active rehabilitation. I would anticipate limited activities for this patient for 6 weeks and a return to full activities at a minimum of 3 months.

Bertram Zarins, MD

The patient has recurrent lateral patellar subluxation and has had a past history of a single episode of lateral patellar dislocation. If the patient has a quadriceps angle of 20 degrees or more (not noted in physical examination) and if he has apprehension on lateral pressure on the patella, I would recommend proximal and distal patellar realignment. The proximal realignment would consist of: (1) Z lengthening of the lateral retinaculum and capsule as described by Slocum, leaving the synovium intact (not a lateral release), and (2) medial retinacular and capsular reefing. The distal realignment would be an Elmslie-Trillat type medial transfer of the tibial tuberosity. I would perform a 6- or 8-cm long osteotomy of the tibial tuberosity, leaving the periosteum intact distally. The tibial tuberosity would be angled medially and fixed approximately 1 cm medial to its original position using an A-O cancellous lag screw. I would use a knee immobilizer for 6 weeks but remove it several times daily for passive range of motion exercises.

John B. McGinty, MD

In summary, we have a 38-year-old man with chronic lateral subluxation of the patella with a moderate degree of secondary chondromalacia. This situation is producing pain, which is aggravated by athletics and is becoming increasingly bothersome. He has morphologic change and degeneration of his articular cartilage in the form of chondromalacia, documented arthroscopically. He has no real degenerative arthritis of his patellofemoral joint.

Assuming that this individual has not responded to a good conservative program, he is a candidate for operative intervention. However, before considering operative intervention, I would be certain that he had at least 6 months of short arc quadriceps exercises on a regular basis with no response.

366

This is an individual on whom I would first consider a lateral retinacular release. This could be done arthroscopically without a tourniquet and controlling the bleeding with electrocautery. He should then be put on an intensive rehabilitation program postoperatively with isometric quadriceps exercises, progressing to short arc quadriceps exercises and on to a program of bicycling and swimming. I think that this may improve his symptomatology so he can participate in athletics as he desires.

If this program were unsuccessful after 6 to 12 months, I would consider a Maquet tibial tubercle elevation. I think this knee, with chronic subluxation and chondromalacia, is an ideal candidate for a Maquet osteotomy. In our experience, the patients who do best with a Maquet are those who have not yet gone on to radiologic changes but show morphologic changes of chondromalacia arthroscopically, even as advanced as Grade III.

However, I suspect that his response to a lateral retinacular release and a good rehabilitation program would be sufficient to obviate any need for further surgery.

Editorial Comment

Once again, there is obviously no universal approach to this difficult problem. It has been the editor's experience in those patients who appear to have an adequate medial restraint (i.e., lateral subluxation of the patella within the femoral groove less than one-third the width of the patella), that there is no advantage to medial arthrotomy and reefing. Without a markedly increased Q angle and lateral displacement of the patellar tendon insertion, we have noted approximately 70 percent of the patients benefitted from a limited lateral release (see Chap. 26).

If this is not successful and the patient continues to have functional disability, we have performed a transfer of the tibial tubercle medially with associated elevation with internal fixation. This is an oblique osteotomy, allowing the tibial tubercle to be transferred medially approximately 1 cm and elevated depending on the angle of the osteotomy, up to approximately 1 cm (please refer to Chaps. 19 and 28).

CASE #5

History

The patient is a 27-year-old woman with a "previous history of recurrent subluxation of her patellofemoral joint." According to the patient, this was treated initially with a conservative strengthening program and physical therapy for 4 months. Subsequently, because of continued pain and disability, the orthopaedic surgeon performed a lateral release without benefit. She continues to have pain and "instability."

The patient is a former bicyclist, skier and tennis player. She has had to stop all of her recreational activities because of increasing pain and discomfort with all bent knee activities. She is also noting increased pain and discomfort with climbing and descending stairs and continues to have feelings of instability.

Physical Exam

The lateral retinaculum is widely separated with retraction of the vastus lateralis. There is marked thigh atrophy with associated visible atrophy of the vastus medialis. Range of motion is from 0 degrees extension to 130 degrees flexion as opposed to 3 degrees recurvatum to 140 degrees flexion on the opposite side. There is no ligamentous laxity. Q angle is 10 degrees bilaterally.

X-Rays

Radiography demonstrates the patella to be questionably medially situated (see Fig. 10).

FIGURE CP-10
AP view.

A special MRI study was performed with ultrafast technique to evaluate patellofemoral joint motion. It demonstrates the patella to track medially bilaterally, with a greater extent on the operated side (Fig. 11). (For additional view of the MRI study, please refer to the video supplement.)

Inspection of the knee following the patient walking on a treadmill demonstrates both patellae to be pointing inward, "squinting patellae," with pronation in gait and apparent femoral anteversion (Fig. 12). (Please refer to video supplement.)

CASE DISCUSSION

H. Royer Collins, MD

First of all, this is an extremely difficult problem. As you watch this young lady walk, she has a miserable malalignment as described by Stan James. There is a considerable amount of hip anteversion, which is noted by the internal rotation of the femur and the squinting patellae. It appears from this short segment which we saw, with her walking, that she is a little worse on the right side than on the left. As I reviewed the tape, I looked to see if there was a great deal of atrophy of the vastus lateralis, and if there was any evidence that the lateral release extended up into the vastus lateralis with some loss of vastus lateralis function, but was unable to really determine any difference between the right knee, which is her operated knee, and the other one. She also has the external rotation deformity of the tibia, and in walking, she

exhibits more of a Q angle than she does in the static phase, which only measures 10 degrees.

We have approached these patients by first seeing if we might be able to build up the thigh musculature to try to balance the patella, having our therapist use a technique of taping the patella to allow it to track more normally, so that they can undergo terminal extension exercises and isometric exercises, to be able to develop the thigh musculature without causing increased patellofemoral pain. We also include stretching of the hamstrings and the quadriceps mechanism during this period. Although she has been on a controlled program in the past, I think this is still worthwhile to attempt with just some of these variations as mentioned. If this is not successful, we have often resutured the vastus lateralis release, attempting, arthroscopically, to rebalance the extensor mechanism and the tracking of the patella. Sometimes it has been necessary to even do something on the medial side, arthroscopically, to achieve balancing of the extensor mechanism, allowing a more normal synchronous motion.

If this type of surgery were to fail and symptoms persisted to the point that something more were required, we have done further studies to determine the amount of femoral anteversion and the relationship of the hip to the knee and to the lower extremity. In two instances, we have done distal osteotomy of the femur and a proximal osteotomy of the tibia, the "floating knee operation" to correct the alignment of the entire extremity, so that the extensor mechanism can ride as smoothly as it should. Admittedly, this is a big operation and one not to be undertaken lightly. In both of these instances, the patient was very sat-

FIGURE CP-11
MRI study shows patella tracking medially bilaterally and to a greater extent on the operated side.

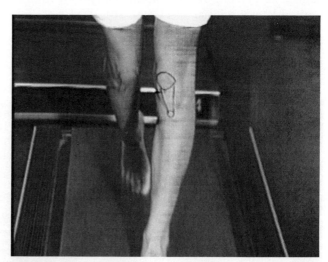

FIGURE CP-12
This photo of the patient on a treadmill shows "squinting patellae," with pronation in gait and femoral anteversion.

isfied with the result following the surgery, but this is admittedly a drastic technique to help solve this problem.

Robert Larson, MD

IMPRESSION/RECOMMENDATION

The patient has patellofemoral abnormality of tracking as demonstrated on her kinetic MRI as well as her arthroscopic evaluation. I feel the problem is primarily related to the femoral torsion causing the sulcus to point medially and causing the patella to take this track with selective tension, thereby causing a pain syndrome as well as a feeling of instability. The lateral retinacular release has obviously contributed to this feeling of instability. It is difficult to make some recommendations without further evidence of her physical examination, such as how her patella lines up with the feet externally rotated and how much hip rotation is noted with the knees flexed 90 degrees.

On the basis of the present information it would appear that if she stood with her patella pointing straight ahead, there would be rather marked external tibial rotation present. If this were the case and she had adequate hip rotation, then a high tibial osteotomy done between the tibial tubercle and the joint line would be an appropriate procedure. This should be done carefully to realign her tibial tubercle with the sulcus to provide a more normal tracking mechanism for the extensor apparatus.

Treatment following the surgical procedure includes immobilization until healing has occurred, followed by an extensive rehabilitation program to redevelop the vastus medialis and quadriceps strength.

Editorial Comment

This patient with anteversion of the femur and the patella tracking along the medial facet of the femoral groove can easily be confused with lateral luxation as she does have marked pain and symptoms and is unresponsive to a conservative program. It has been our experience that the lack of response in therapy is secondary to strengthening of the vastus medialis, which further enhances the aspect of the medial tracking.

Prior to any surgical intervention, we have had success with alteration of the physical therapy exercise program by emphasizing strengthening of the vastus lateralis and de-emphasizing the vastus medialis. Also shoe orthoses, working on gait patterns, and lateral taping of the patella have helped.

Vastus lateralis release needs to be conscientiously avoided. If there is any question by the treating physician regarding the possible medial tracking of the patella, an MRI study of the patellofemoral motion can be extremely beneficial. It is important to separate medial tracking from a medial tilt secondary to tightness of the lateral retinaculum.

If, unfortunately, these patients have undergone previous lateral retinacular release, then secondary surgery may become necessary. On five occasions we have performed medial retinacular release under arthroscopic control. In these five cases, four have benefited.

Another choice is formal arthrotomy with repair of the lateral retinaculum and repositioning of the patella with either high tibial osteotomy and/or tibial tubercle repositioning and elevation.

Regardless of the chosen treatment program, a heightened awareness of this entity needs to be maintained so that the inadvertent diagnosis of lateral luxation and subsequent lateral release may be avoided. (Please refer to Chaps. 9 and 24.)

CASE #6

History

The patient is a 10-year-old girl who 4 years previously had undergone open lateral release and medial side reefing of the left patella for recurrent patellar dislocations. She had been suffering recurrent lateral dislocation of the left patella since age 5. With the initial surgical procedure, she seemed to do well for a year. The episodes of dislocation have recurred and increased rapidly over the past 3 years, with frank dislocation now occurring three to four times per month.

The patient has had a previous dislocation of the right patella on one occasion.

Physical Exam

She has a guarded gait. The patient does not achieve complete extension of the left knee joint, stopping at approximately 10 degrees because she is afraid that the patella will "dislocate." The patient is able to flex to 120 degrees. She is extremely apprehensive to any examination. An audible and palpable pop is noted with the intial degrees of flexion. With the knee in complete extension, the patella can be seen seated laterally.

There is noted to be generalized ligamentous laxity with hyperextension of the thumb and recurvatum of both elbows. Range of motion of the opposite extremity is hyperextension of 10 degrees and flexion, heel to buttocks. The patient has been evaluated for connective tissue disorders and all studies have been negative, including biopsies.

X-Rays

Radiography demonstrates the lack of formation of the femoral groove, corresponding dysplasia of the patella, and lateral position (Fig. 13).

Surgical Findings

At surgery, the gross lateral position of the patella is noted. In complete extension under anesthesia, the patella is sitting laterally and reduces spontaneously with progressive flexion. The patella digitally can be held laterally. Visible stretching of the skin scars are so noted. Repeat lateral release does not center the patella. With medial reefing, it still remains uncentered (Fig. 14).

CASE DISCUSSION

Neil Green, MD

This 10-year-old girl with a recurrent dislocation of her patella presents a significant problem. She has marked hyperlaxity of her joints and has had recurrent dislocations of her left patella beginning at age 3. Because of the long history of recurrent patellar

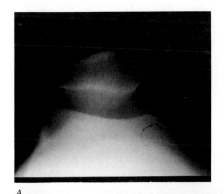
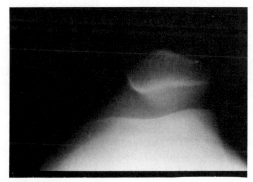

A

FIGURE CP-13
A. Patellofemoral view, demonstrating bilateral subluxation, left greater than right, with patellar tilt. *B.* AP view showing open physeal plates and patella alta. *C.* Lateral view demonstrating patella alta.

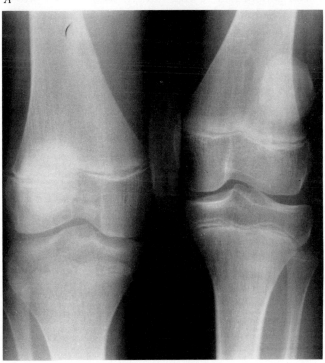

B

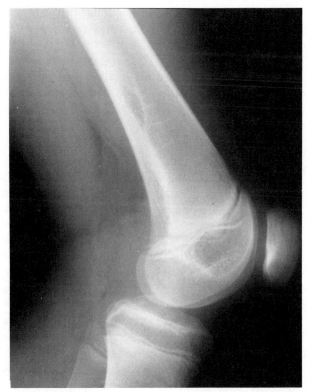

C

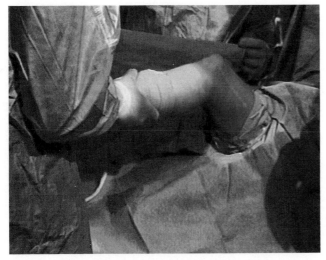

A

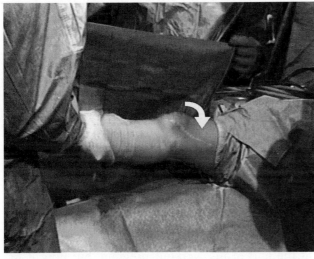

B

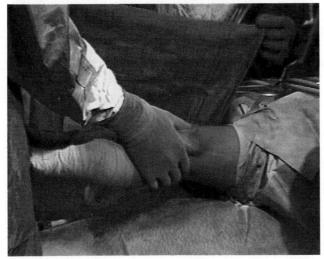

C

FIGURE CP-14
A. Patella in a grossly lateral position. B. Complete extension under anesthesia. C. The patella held laterally by hand. Repeat lateral release and medial reefing did not manage to center it.

dislocations, the femoral groove will probably not be normally developed. In addition, she has already undergone a previous lateral release and medial side reefing 4 years ago with subsequent recurrence of the dislocations.

She is, however, disabled because of the recurrent patellar dislocations and therefore stabilization of her patella is imperative. Her patella tracks laterally towards the end of knee extension and actually subluxates. The patella is high riding and laterally situated on the AP radiograph.

The treatment, therefore, would require repeat release of the lateral retinaculum and this should go well up into the attachment of the vastus lateralis. The medial side should be tightened again, and the pull of the quadriceps mechanism must be altered. She is skeletally immature and, therefore, transfer of the tibial tubercle is not possible. There are two alternatives to transfer of the tubercle itself. The first is transfer of the lateral half of the patellar tendon as in the Roux-Goldthwaite. The lateral half of the patellar ligament is sharply detached from its attachment on the tibial tubercle without injuring the tibial tubercle apophysis. It is passed medially underneath the medial half of the patellar tendon and then sutured to the periosteum on the medial side. The vector pull of the quadriceps mechanism has been altered to a more medial direction.

An alternative to this is the use of the semitendinosus tendon as a tenodesis. This works very well to help keep the patella from tracking laterally. The semitendinosus is detached at about its musculotendinous junction and pulled distally. The cut end of the semitendinosus is then passed through a drill hole in the patella and pulled back onto itself and sutured. It is sutured with enough tension to allow the patella to track normally in the femoral groove.

The last thing that I cannot determine completely from the radiographs is the femoral tibial angle. If the patient has a significant amount of genu valgum, then one should consider stapling the medial side of the distal femur to allow for correction of the valgus deformity. Correction of genu valgum, if it is present, will help to prevent recurrence of the patellar dislocation.

Steven Schopler, MD

Nonoperative treatment will not succeed in a child with this type of patellar instability. While bracing and exercise may be attempted to reassure the relucant family that all nonoperative means have been explored, surgery is required to fix this.

First, it is important to distinguish a patella which dislocates in extension from one which dislocates in flexion. A patella dislocating laterally in

371

flexion is accompanied by a contracted quadriceps mechanism and a restricting lateral retinaculum, both of which must be dealt with by lengthening or releasing the restraining soft tissues. In contradistinction, this patient whose dislocation is occurring in extension, has hypermobility, not restriction, of the patella. Neither shortening of the quadriceps nor a contracted lateral retinaculum are present, and thus, a lateral releasing procedure or proximal realignment will be ineffective in stabilizing the patella.

Radiographically, the standing AP radiograph demonstrates patella alta, genu valgum, and lateral patellar subluxation. An axial view of the patellofemoral joint will show a hypoplastic trochlear groove and lateral tracking of the patella in flexion. Dislocation of the patellofemoral joint in full extension would be seen on a kinematic study using MRI or CT.

This case demonstrates that lateral dislocation of the patella in extension is a manifestation of rotatory malalignment of the extensor mechanism around the mechanical axis of the extended limb. Additionally, patella alta contributes to this patient's instability, which can be clinically demonstrated by blocking the proximal migration of the patella in full knee extension with the examiner's finger. This maintains the patella within the trochlear groove, eliminating the dislocation.

To treat the dislocating patella, it must be restrained from assuming its unstable position in extension. This can be accomplished by reducing the patella alta and restricting its lateral mobility. In skeletally immature patients, advancement and medial displacement of the tibial tubercle is not acceptable, and, therefore, soft tissue realignment distally is the preferred surgical treatment. We have found an arthroscopically guided distal realignment to be superior in our hands. This consists of an arthroscopic examination of the patellofemoral joint with documentation of patellar tracking, followed by distal semitendinosus tenodesis to the patella through a transverse drill hole in the inferior pole. Where necessary, this is augmented with a Slocum or Roux-Goldthwaite transfer of half of the patellar tendon to further restrain the patella distally, but possible damage to the apophysis of the tibial tubercle is a risk with the addition of this transfer.

Usually, the tenodesis is adequate and afterward patellar tracking improves arthroscopically and clinically. A limited medial retinacular shortening procedure may also be added when distal realignment is insufficient, but, with medial reefing, care must be taken to avoid overcorrection.

Postoperatively, continuous passive motion equipment and patient-controlled analgesia are helpful to comfortably restore motion during the hospitalization, along with physical therapy to regain knee flexion and maintain ankle range of motion. The patient is discharged from the hospital in a restricted-motion knee brace, limiting motion to patient tolerance. Isometric quadriceps exercises are instituted immediately postperatively, and active knee extension is resumed 2 to 4 weeks postoperatively. Aqua therapy is useful in restoring flexion and for progressive resistance quadricep and hamstring rehabilitation.

Editorial Comment

This is an extremely disabling phenomenon of congenitally dislocating patella. With soft tissue procedures, there is a high probability of progressive stretching. Tenodesis, whether through transferring a portion of the patellar tendon or, in our experience, utilizing the semitendinosus tendon, had afforded satisfactory benefit.

CASE #7

History

The patient is a 24-year-old male competitive volleyball player of Olympic capabilities. He was scheduled to try out for the Olympic team, but for the past 2 years has been troubled by progressive anterior knee pain. Originally this anterior knee pain occurred at the end of his workout program, but now it has progressed to the point that he has pain with climbing and descending stairs in his daily life and any type of jumping maneuver. The patient has had to discontinue his participation in volleyball workouts. Not only is this extremely frustrating from a participant point of view, but it is also frustrating from a financial point of view as the patient with his Olympic potential had already signed endorsement contracts dependent upon his participating with the Olympic team.

The patient has had an extensive trial in strengthening and conditioning programs, quadriceps strengthening, anti-inflammatory medication including nonsteroidals, and various types of knee supports including compressive wraps across the patellar tendon. His physical therapy has also included ultrasound, phonophoresis, ionophoresis, heat prior to participation, and icing after participation.

X-Rays

Routine radiographs are normal. MRI scans demonstrate marked increased activity within the patellar tendon compatible with patellar tendinitis (Fig. 15).

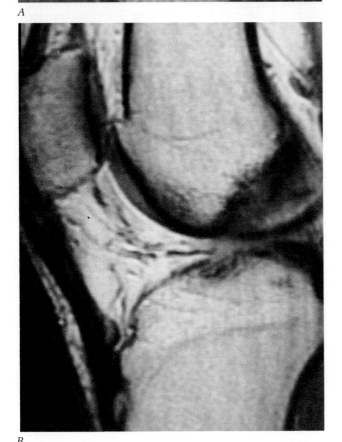

A

B

FIGURE CP-15
MR scans demonstrating the increased activity in the patellar tendon seen in tendinitis.

Stephen Lombardo, MD

After the prescribed course of evaluation, management, and therapy in this 24-year-old Olympic-caliber volleyball player with a diagnosis of patellar tendinitis, I would attempt to establish whether (1) an adequate period of low or no impact activities has taken place, to see if this condition would improve; (2) if it hadn't I would be sure that the physical therapy program included electrical muscle stimulation of the quad and hamstring muscles and a course of phonophoresis (maximum 9 treatments); (3) if he continued to need to participate and was not able to rest the extremity because of the upcoming Olympic trials, then I would consider one or two cortisone injections in the area of presumed tenderness of the tendon spaced 2 weeks apart. I would inform him that this had the potential to weaken the tendon in addition to pre-disposing it to rupture. In some cases I've seen significant improvement when this "last ditch effort" was utilized. I personally have never had anyone sustain a rupture from an injection I gave, but on the other hand I have seen people and patients who have sustained ruptures with a history of cortisone injections. It's most important to realize that this approach is reserved for individuals who are at the highest competitive levels or who may be candidates for scholarships and otherwise would not receive them if they did not compete. Additionally, those rare cases in which people had chronic knee pain from patellar tendinitis, that did rupture and went on to repair, in my limited experience, all returned to the same competitive sport at essentially the same competitive level. This includes both collegiate and professional athletes. This is a very limited number of patients, five or under, and in no way should it be conveyed that this form of management is recommended or acceptable for most people.

In summary, with the exception of the elite athlete, no recommendations other than a well-defined therapy program for anterior knee pain and patellar tendinitis would be made beyond what is outlined in our usual physical therapy management protocol.

Frank M. Ivey, MD

I will assume that the patient is seeing me for the first time. He has symptoms of an end stage (Blazina 3) patellar tendinitis (jumper's knee) which can, if left untreated, progress to catastrophic patellar tendon rupture. In the patient's history I would like to ascertain the specific exercises involving his quadriceps and hamstring muscles and whether he had been involved with eccentric quadriceps strengthening exercises. Physical examination would be focused on

373

the extensor mechanism to determine if any subtle malalignment was present but should encompass all areas of knee pathology, including ligamentous stability, meniscal function, and overall limb alignment. The most specific test I have found to confirm my diagnosis of patellar tendinitis is the tilt test performed by pushing distally on the patella and then palpating the inferior pole of the patella with the opposite examining index finger. The patient specifically relates this as the pain they experience during stair climbing or jumping activities.

My first reaction to this patient's clinical problem would be to be sure that he had been given a full comprehensive conservative treatment program including moderation of activities, a therapeutic dose of an anti-inflammatory medication, ice massage, flexibility exercises of the quadriceps and hamstrings plus eccentric quadriceps exercises prior to resuming training activities. If the patient has gone through a comprehensive, well-supervised nonoperative program, and is at the stage where he presents today with MRI evidence both on T1- and T2-weighted signals of hemorrhage and edema within the patellar tendon at the distal pole of the patella, then surgical treatment is indicated. After examination of the knee under anesthesia and diagnostic arthroscopy to rule out any intra-articular pathology, a lateral longitudinal peripatellar incision is made to explore the proximal aspect of the patellar tendon. This incision preserves sensation to the anterior aspect of the knee and is cosmetically acceptable. The peritenon is incised and longitudinal incisions are made within the proximal tendon substance looking for areas of tendon degeneration, which are excised. The distal pole of the patella is exposed and numerous drill holes are made in this area to stimulate a vascular healing response.

Postoperative full weight bearing is allowed with a 4-point crutch gait. Isometric exercises in full extension are begun the day after surgery. Gravity-assisted flexion is encouraged. Eccentric quadriceps contraction using the weight of the leg only is started after 2 weeks. Isotonic exercises are started after 4 weeks and gradual resumption of activity after 3 months.

Concern for the patient's Olympic and/or professional career is reasonable but should not take precedence over proper management of this condition as outlined.

K. Donald Shelbourne, MD

Generally, patellar tendinitis in a young competitive athlete is something that should be avoided and kept under control rather than treated only once it be-

comes severe. When cases progress from stage I and II to stage III, generally, a period of rest and rehabilitation can get the athlete back to the stage I level. For in-season athletes, stage III patellar tendinitis is difficult to treat without restricting playing time. The rehabilitation program should be designed to first get the tendon pain under control with appropriate relative rest and activity modification and avoiding the forces that are causing the pain, such as jumping in volleyball. Unfortunately, if the athlete is in-season it is difficult to balance the amount of time out of sports with the need for continued participation and attempting to treat the symptoms as they occur. In our clinic, rehabilitation almost always uniformly works to take care of the problem when it is seen in the acute phase and not the chronic recurrent phase. Rehabilitation should not be prescribed to develop quadriceps muscle strength but more to involve strengthening the patellar tendon. We have had extensive experience in treating patellar tendon strength programs from harvesting autogenous patellar tendon grafts for ACL reconstructions. The closed kinetic chain rehabilitation program which involves biking, Stairmaster, leg press, etc., and then gradually returning to running activities keeping the pain under control has worked uniformly well in almost all cases.

The case presented is somewhat of a problem in that the athlete is a year-round athlete who does not have time to take time off, and therefore is going to be more difficult to treat. It was not stated when the Olympic tryouts are and how much time he has between presentation and the actual need to be 100 percent for the tryouts. It appears that this is a chronic problem which has not gotten better with nonoperative treatment to this point and the MRI scan does appear to show an area of focal degenerative changes in the patellar tendon which would be indicative of a chronic partial tear. We do not have progressive MRI scans to show if this is a healing lesion or progression lesion and therefore do not have an indication if this is getting better with time or worse. If this is an acute finding then conservative treatment is initially warranted to see if this focal area of degenerative change can heal. If this is a chronic problem, which has not gotten better with appropriate conservative treatment and appropriate relative rest and the athlete feels that in his present condition he cannot participate in the sport at the level he would like, and he has sufficient time (i.e., 6 months or so prior to his need to be 100 percent) then surgical consideration would be warranted. Surgery, if deemed necessary and appropriate, should consist of excising the area of degenerative tendon. We normally would excise this as we would a patellar tendon graft, taking off the distal portion of the patellar bone itself as well as the attached patellar tendon region that shows the change. As is the case in harvesting a patellar tendon graft for ACL surgery, this almost always uniformly works well but takes approximately 6 months of rehabilitation afterward to obtain a final good result.

In summary, I feel that if the athlete is disabled to the point that he cannot participate in his sport at the level he would like to and can definitely not make the Olympic tryouts with the present pain that he has and the treating physician, therapist, and athlete all feel that appropriate conservative treatment at this point has not helped and further treatment would not be beneficial, then surgical considerations should be given, understanding the limitations of surgery as far as time to return to full activities. Again, in our hands this problem rarely gets to this point. When it does, in the acute phase, treatment is designed to return the patient's tendinitis back to the stage I level and keep it in this level with activity modification and further treatment. Since from this history, I am not sure how the past rehabilitation correlates with our rehabilitation program, I am not sure if continued conservative treatment would suffice. Also, I am not sure of the time from presentation until participation in Olympic tryouts. If surgery were necessary, is there an appropriate time for this? Rarely does the tendinitis get bad enough that the athlete cannot participate but frequently it is bad enough that he cannot participate at the level of consistency that he would like. Again, I think because of the difficult position the athlete, physician, and therapist are in at this point, this case should emphasize the importance of avoiding a chronic patellar tendinitis rather than attempting to treat it once it develops.

Editorial Comment

The frequency of patients presenting to the sports medicine physician with chronic patellar tendinitis or "jumper's knee" appears to be markedly decreased compared to the early 1970s when this entity gained prominence. The reason for this is probably mutifactoral (i.e., a change in conditioning programs, surfaces, footwear, physician and athletic trainer awareness). However, the physician still encounters high level competitive athletes with unresponsive patellar tendinitis. It is our feeling that this patient fits this category. The aspect of steroid injections can be discussed with the patient, as there are pros and cons to this treatment.

Regarding the surgical exposure, our procedure is very similar to Dr. Ivey's suggestion. However, we have had success using a procedure under local anesthesia. Significant chondromalacia of the patella does occur with patellar tendinitis. Arthroscopic evaluation of the intra-articular aspects of the joint, and intra-articular shaving of the patella may be done. Following this, exploration of the patellar tendon under local anesthesia, looking for a localized nidus (inflammatory tissue) within the patellar tendon is done. The patient can help to confirm this area with the surgeon progressively "pinching" various areas of the patellar tendon with small forceps. It is surprising how many patients can specifically localize the area of nidus we have surgically excised and, if necessary, resected small bone spurs at the inferior pole of the patella.

We then proceed with the rehabilitation program similar to those outlined by the discussors. We indicate to our patients that we have approximately a 70 percent satisfactory result. The end-stage procedure of surgical intervention with complete detachment of the patellar tendon and resection of the inferior pole of the patella has been an ultimate salvage procedure with a limited probability, in our opinion, of return to high level competitive participation.

CASE #8

History

The patient is a 27-year-old woman who denies previous knee problems or difficulties until injured at work. She bumped the anterior aspect of her knee on a desk. She was evaluated by an orthopaedic surgeon who noted marked pain and discomfort in attempting to examine the patient. His initial evaluation demonstrated a range of motion from −5 degrees extension to 90 degrees flexion with no ligamentous laxity and a questionable effusion present. Radiographs were interpreted as being normal. A subsequent MRI study was apparently also within the limits of normal. The patient had been tried on a physical therapy program but continued to complain of marked pain and discomfort. She was unable to return to her usual occupation as a secretary. The orthopaedic surgeon performed an exploratory arthroscopic evaluation, finding no significant pathology. Since that time, the patient has remained in a physical therapy program and has remained on disability because of increasing pain and discomfort. She notes increased pain and discomfort with any type of bent knee activities and reports being unable to walk more than 15 to 20 minutes.

Physical Exam

There is an antalgic gait. The knee is held in slight flexion, never achieving complete extension in ambulation. There is noted to be increased warmth with palpation across the anterior aspect of the knee joint, thickening of the soft tissue, but no palpable effusion. There is no ligamentous laxity. Range of motion is from 5 degrees extension to 60 degrees flexion. There is tenderness of a diffuse nature over the medial and lateral joint line area and increased sensitivity over the peripatellar tissue.

X-Rays

There is diffuse osteopenia (Fig. 16). A bone scan demonstrates increased uptake, primarily involving the patellofemoral joint area. (Fig. 17)

CASE DISCUSSION

Alexander Kalenak, MD

ASSESSMENT

My impression is that this represents a reflex sympathetic dystrophy of the knee joint. The historical data of minor trauma followed by unrelenting pain is typical. Negative arthroscopy, osteoporosis indicated by radiography, and increased activity on radioactive isotope further substantiate a diagnosis of reflex sympathetic dystrophy.

PLAN

She was counseled extensively with regard to the diagnosis, management, and prognosis. She was en-

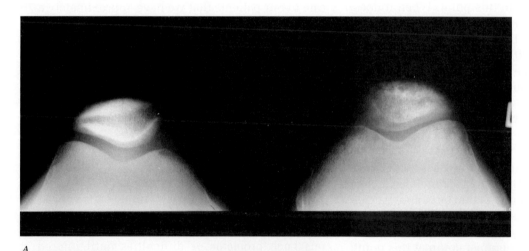

A

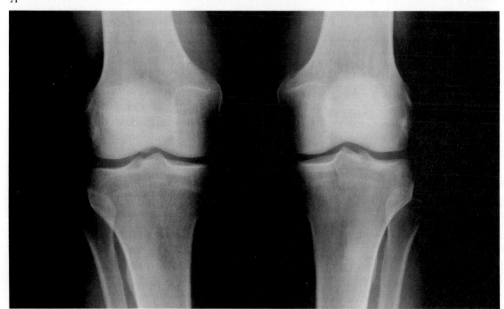

B   **FIGURE CP-16**

couraged to continue with physical therapy and to understand that the problem will most likely resolve. But with persistence of symptoms over a year or two, it will be less likely that the symptoms will completely resolve. I stressed the importance of a physical therapy regimen to maintain her present range of

motion and to work at restoring complete range of motion. Anti-inflammatory medication must be continued on a daily basis. I suggested an immediate consultation with our Pain Management Service to prescribe a sympathetic lumbar block or a series of sympathetic lumbar blocks. Epidural blocks may also be warranted to effect relief of pain and permit the patient to work on her range of motion. She may need to be in the hospital in order to receive these sympathetic lumbar blocks. At that time, she will need the help of a skilled and dedicated physical therapist or physical medicine rehabilitation specialist who will guide her and encourage her through her range of motion activities. She is to use whatever modalities and exercise equipment she can utilize to work on her range of motion effectively.

Finally, she was reassured again this was a treatable problem, but it will require dedication and firm resolve on her part to effectively alleviate her symptoms.

Mark Pitman, MD

DIAGNOSIS

It is my impression that this young lady is suffering from reflex dystrophy (RSD). Her symptoms, signs and course are typical. She developed severe anterior knee pain immediately after relatively mild trauma. Her pain was increased by physical therapy. Arthroscopy was performed as is frequently the case and was entirely normal. Arthroscopy did not relieve the pain

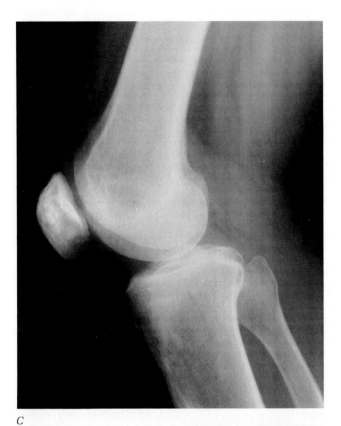

C

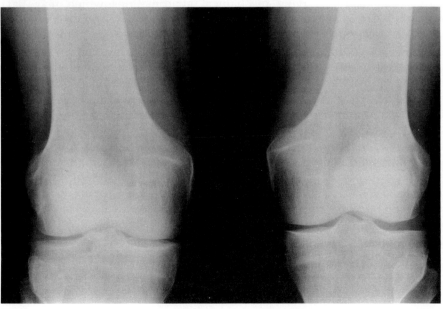

D

FIGURE CP-16
A. Patellofemoral view, demonstrating bilateral marked osteoporosis of the patella and femoral groove. *B.* AP view; osteoporosis present. *C.* Lateral view; again, diffuse osteoporosis in the femur and patella. *D.* Patellar view.

and she continued with a progressive course of increasing pain and increasing disability.

Increased sensitivity about the anterior knee joint to light touch, such as the wearing of heavy jeans, washing or shaving her leg, is also a very frequent finding in RSD.

THERAPY

The patient was told that the most effective and efficient diagnostic and therapeutic test is a course of paravertebral lumbar sympathetic blocks. Certainly, if these blocks relieve the pain, the diagnosis is confirmed. It was recommended that she be hospitalized for a period of 5 days. During this time, daily lumbar paravertebral blocks will be performed and the effects evaluated. Skin temperatures will be measured. There should be a rise of at least 1°C in the affected limb to confirm that sympathetic activity has actually been blocked. Immediately after the block she will be placed on physical therapy. Our physical therapists are skilled in treating these patients. Basically, therapy consists of active encouragement and gently assisted active range of motion. If pain is relieved and the patient realizes that she is able to move her leg without increasing her knee pain, then I think we are on the way.

An alternative means of blockade would be that suggested by DeLee wherein a paravertebral lumbar sympathetic block is first performed for diagnosis, and, if the pain is relieved, this is followed by continuous epidural analgesia during which time physical therapy is continued. Hopefully, as she improves during that week she can be placed in more active exercises utilizing closed chain activity such as the treadmill, the bicycle, and mini-squats.

The patient was told that I do not feel we should temporize with medication at this time but should proceed directly to the blocks. It is 6 months since her injury and this is still the period in which Schwartzberg feels the primary pathology is within the sympathetic ganglion and can be helped by sympathetic blocks. Later as it proceeds to the substantia gelatinosa of the spinal cord, it is a more central disease, a greater problem, and often not helped by sympathetic blockades.

She is also told that sympathetic blockades may work for a variable period of time. Her relief may be permanent or it may last for a few months or a few days. It is not uncommon that as symptoms recur after a period of time, occasionally repeat courses of sympathetic blocks are needed. We have found that some patients return once a year or so and require another course of blocks. Our patients to date have not required surgical sympathectomy.

There is a possibility that a neuroma of the infrapatellar branch of the saphenous nerve occurs from direct trauma or possibly from damage in the making of an arthroscopic portal. I am not able to ascertain this at this time. However, if sympathetic blockade removes most of her reflex dystrophic pain, then sometimes the area of pain localizes to a smaller area and an underlying neuroma can be perceived.

She was also told that it is rare that the knee returns completely to normal even after successful treatment. She can expect to have occasional discomfort and if this occurs it can, as mentioned above, be treated with further blocks or with oral or occasionally intravenous regional blockades. We have also had some success in relieving mild, intermittent residual discomfort with the use of topical Capsaicin 0.025% cream, which works as a topical analgesic probably by the depletion of substance P in the peripheral sensory neurons. Substance P is thought to be a neuropeptide principle transmitter of pain impulses and its depletion is at times effective in relief of mild residual symptoms.

Editorial Comment

The patient has the symptomatology and physical findings compatible with reflex sympathetic dystrophy. It is extremely important to eliminate any underlying mechanical abnormalities which may have been missed, therefore one must review the previous MRI studies to make sure they are within the limits of normal. If the previous arthroscopy was videotaped, it is our recommendation to review that, also.

Surgical intervention should be avoided. These patients are extremely sensitive to any type of manipulation and further trauma. It is very important to treat this aggressively, with appropriate physical therapy modalities and other associated modalities. (Refer to Chapter 17 on feflex sympathetic dystrophy or "Sudecks atrophy" by Gary Poehling, MD.)

The patient and "third parties" need to understand the prolonged recovery involved. Appropriate consultations, vascular specialist, neurologists, and even psychological counseling are to be considered.

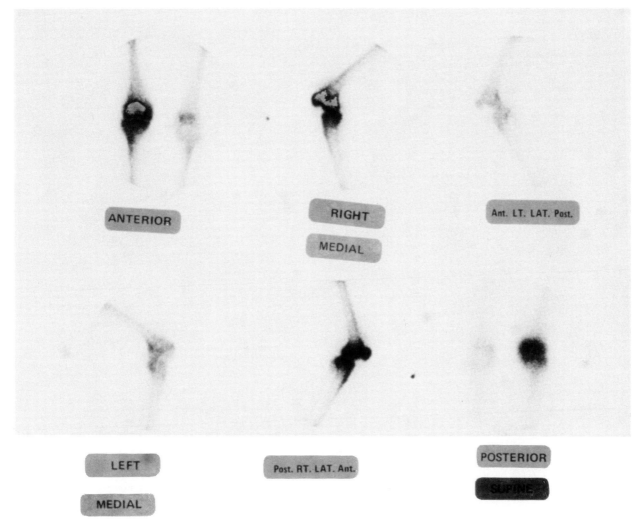

ANTERIOR

RIGHT

MEDIAL

Ant. LT. LAT. Post.

LEFT

MEDIAL

Post. RT. LAT. Ant.

POSTERIOR

SUPINE

FIGURE CP-17
Increased uptake shown on bone scan.

INDEX